ABNORMAL PSYCHOLOGY

A South African perspective

T Austin • C Bezuidenhout • K Botha • E Du Plessis • L Du Plessis • E Jordaan
M Lake • M Moletsane • J Nel • B Pillay • G Ure • C Visser • B Von Krosigk • A Vorster

Edited by Alban Burke

OXFORD
UNIVERSITY PRESS
SOUTHERN AFRICA

OXFORD
UNIVERSITY PRESS

Oxford University Press is a department of the University of Oxford.
It furthers the University's objective of excellence in research, scholarship,
and education by publishing worldwide. Oxford is a registered trade mark of
Oxford University Press in the UK and in certain other countries

Published in South Africa by
Oxford University Press Southern Africa (Pty) Limited

Vasco Boulevard, Goodwood, N1 City, Cape Town, South Africa, 7460
P O Box 12119, N1 City, Cape Town, South Africa, 7463

First published 2009
Second edition published in 2012

Abnormal Psychology: A South African perspective 2e Revised

ISBN 978 0 19 599837 5

Typeset in Minion Pro 10 pt on 12.5 pt
Printed on 70 gsm woodfree paper

Acknowledgements
Publishing manager: Alida Terblanche
Publisher: Marisa Montemarano
Project manager: Sarah Floor
Editor: Viv O'Neill
Designer: Louise Topping
Cover designer: Louise Topping
Cover image: Inspirestock
Typesetter: The Purple Turtle
Printed and bound by ABC Press, Cape Town

123581

CONTENTS

CHAPTER 7: NEUROCOGNITIVE DISORDERS 240

Basil Pillay

CHAPTER 8: DISSOCIATIVE AND SOMATIC SYMPTOM AND RELATED DISORDERS 266

Larise du Plessis & Conrad Visser

FOREWORD

It suffices to openly state that each generation and society has its unique needs and aspirations. This textbook reflects the nature and depth of psychopathology today. The critical scientific, technical and transcultural knowledge shared by the authors attests to its uniqueness and demonstrates a revolution in the way psychopathology is understood and dealt with. This book is written in an accessible register without losing the scientist-practitioner model.

The authors have gone beyond their borders in searching for knowledge on their particular subject expertise. This book is centrally important for our context; it incorporates a vast amount of information (e.g. introduction to neuro-anatomy, general medical conditions, ethics and South African legislation, as well as highlighting cultural issues). It also enables a global exchange of ideas, opinions and knowledge. Respect for diversity and its celebration throughout this book is gratifying.

Having taught the subject of psychopathology for more than 15 years at undergraduate and postgraduate levels I have found the book to be useful even in my clinical practice as a quick reference book.

Congratulations to the authors for producing such a sterling book. I highly recommend this book to all those who have the interests of mental health care users at heart.

Professor Humphrey Siphiwe Bafanabenkosi Ngcobo
President
Psychological Society of South Africa (PsySSA)

PREFACE

The authors would like to thank the users of the first edition for their valuable feedback. We tried, as far as possible to address all the comments. Based on the feedback there have been substantial changes to the book. These include, inter alia, a new chapter on Mental Wellness. The thinking behind this inclusion was that we felt it would contribute to a more balanced view of Abnormal Behaviour. Another substantial change is that etiological models are now discussed in a separate chapter as opposed to only a section in Chapter 1 of the previous edition. We deliberated about the timing of the second edition, especially because of the advent of DSM-5, however we felt that we should proceed as there will always be more foreseen changes to the classification systems. What we have done, though, is to include, as far as possible, the proposed changes from DSM-IV to DSM-5.

As was the case with the first edition, this book is the product of collaboration between practitioners and experienced academics from various universities. The aims of the second edition, which are in line with those of the previous edition, are as follows:

- A diverse undergraduate student population will use the book: To meet this aim, we keep the book as simple as possible, without compromising important facts and terminology. To assist students, we provide a glossary of important terminologies and concepts, case studies, and helpful hints. In addition, at the end of each chapter, we supply multiple-choice questions and essay questions to help students prepare for assessments and assess how well they have understood the content.
- The content will be relevant to South Africa: To this end, we include as much South African research as possible and present a South African, cross-cultural view on the various pathologies. We also present the South African code of conduct, the legislation regarding mental health care, and aspects of the South African Constitution as these are relevant to our readership.
- The book will be inclusive: We include diagnostic criteria from both the American Psychiatric Association's *Diagnostic and Statistical Manual of Mental Disorders* (DSM) and the World Health Organisation's *International Classification of Diseases* (ICD). We adopted this dual approach because there is a slight anomaly between what is typically taught and what is needed in practice. The textbooks from which students typically learn include only DSM criteria, whilst in practice the ICD system is used for medical aid claims. We present both classification systems, as each adds to our understanding of disorders. Throughout the book, we compare these two classification systems, pointing out similarities and differences between them. This should enable students to move between the two systems in both research and practice.

A few cautionary notes:

- Firstly, many academics and practitioners subscribe to a particular paradigm or theory, and might expect this book to share their enthusiasm for their specific choice. Some might be tempted to criticise the book for not providing sufficient information on a particular approach. We emphasise that this book is an introductory text for undergraduate students, and the aim is to introduce as wide a variety of theories as possible. The book cannot, therefore, be expected to reflect the details of every theory and approach.

- Secondly, various constraints have prevented us from covering all disorders. A survey was done to establish the disorders considered in the undergraduate curricula at the different universities, and we include only disorders that appear in these curricula.
- Finally, owing to space constraints, we cannot provide every detail of the disorders. We rely on lecturers to provide students with further information, and on students to read beyond the content of this book.

We trust that you will find the book both interesting and informative.

Ancillary material for lecturers prescribing the textbook is available on the OUPSA website, www.oxford.co.za. Students may also download the solutions to the end-chapter multiple choice questions from www.oxford.co.za.

Alban Burke

CONTRIBUTORS

Austin, Tracey-Lee MA (Psychology) DLitt et Phil (Psychology): Lecturer: Department of Psychology, University of Johannesburg

Bezuidenhout, Christiaan DPhil (Criminology): Associate Professor: Department of Social Work and Criminology, University of Pretoria

Botha, Karel MA (Clinical Psychology) PhD (Pyschology): Associate Professor: School of Psychosocial Behavioural Sciences, North-West University

Burke, Alban MA (Psychology) DLitt et Phil (Psychology): Department of Psychology, University of Johannesburg

Du Plessis, Edwin MA (Clinical Psychology) PhD (Psychology): Principal Psychologist/ Lecturer: Department of Psychology, University of the Free State

Du Plessis, Larise M. MA (Clinical Psychology): Lecturer: Department of Psychology, University of Johannesburg

Jordaan, Elsabe MA (Clinical Psychology): Lecturer: Department of Psychology, University of Johannesburg

Lake, T. Melanie MA (Clinical Psychology) DLitt et Phil (Psychology): Senior Psychologist: Assessment, Treatment and Rehabilitation Unit, Middlemore Hospital, Auckland, New Zealand

Moletsane, Mokgadi MEd (Educational Psychology) PhD (Educational Psychology): Associate Professor, Department of Educational Psychology, University of the Western Cape

Nel, Juan MA (Clinical Psychology) DLitt et Phil (UNISA): Full Professor: Department of Psychology, UNISA

Pillay, Basil MA (Clinical Psychology) PhD (Med): Head: Department of Behavioural Medicine, School of Nursing and Public Health, College of Health Services, University of KwaZulu-Natal

Ure, Gale MA (Psychology) DLitt et Phil (Psychology) MScMed (Bioethics & Health Law): Mental Health Rehabilitation Standards Manager: Life Esidimeni

Visser, Conrad BScEng (Civil) MB, BCh (Wits); FCPsych(SA): Psychiatrist in private practice, Parktown, Johannesburg

Von Krosigk, Beate MA (Psychology), DLitt et Phil (Psychology): Senior Lecturer: Department of Psychology, UNISA

Vorster, Adri MEd. (Educational Psychology): Lecturer: Department of Psychology, University of the Witwatersrand

1 PSYCHOLOGICAL ASSESSMENT AND PSYCHODIAGNOSTICS

Tracey-Lee Austin

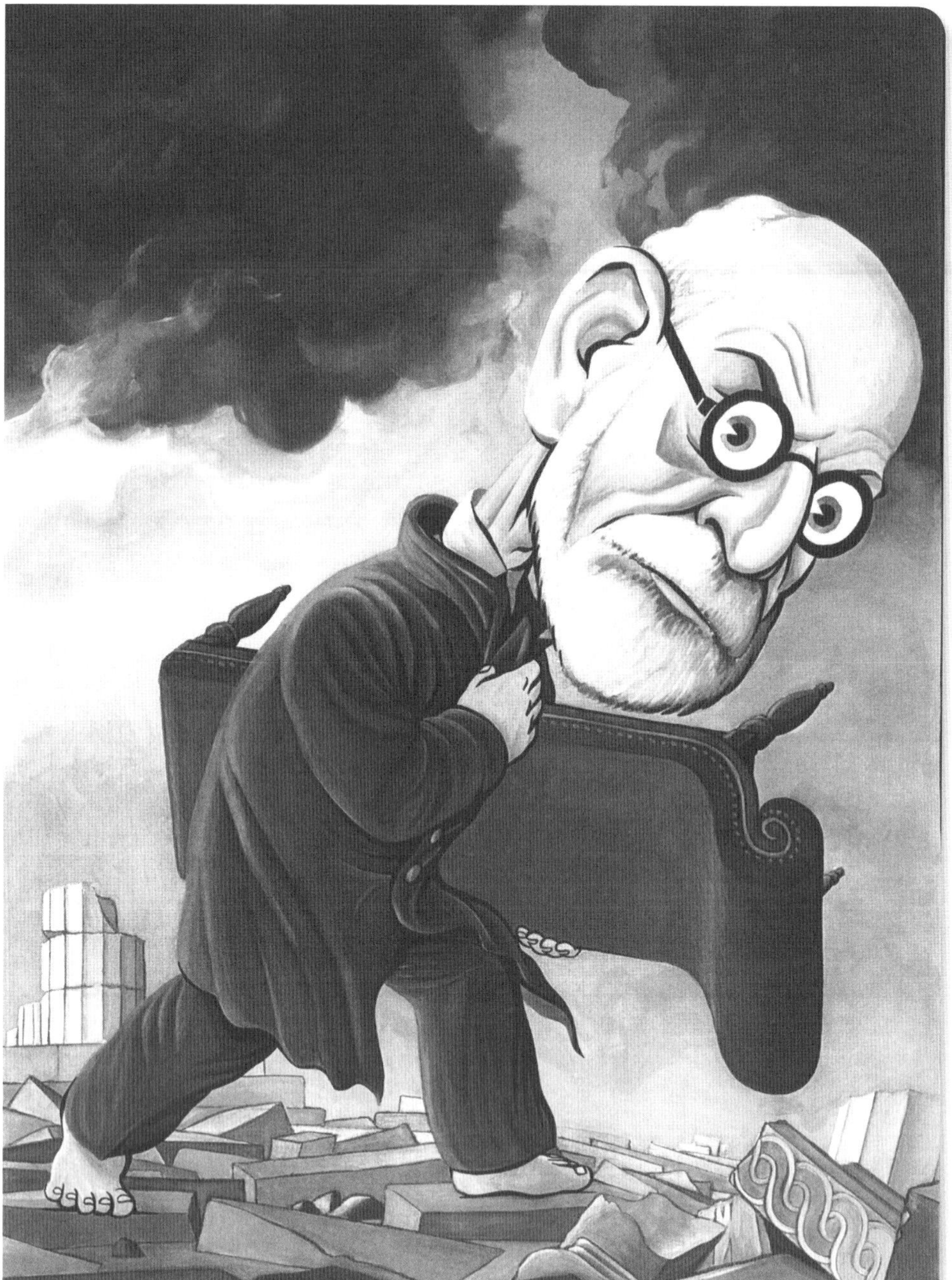

1 CHAPTER OUTLINE

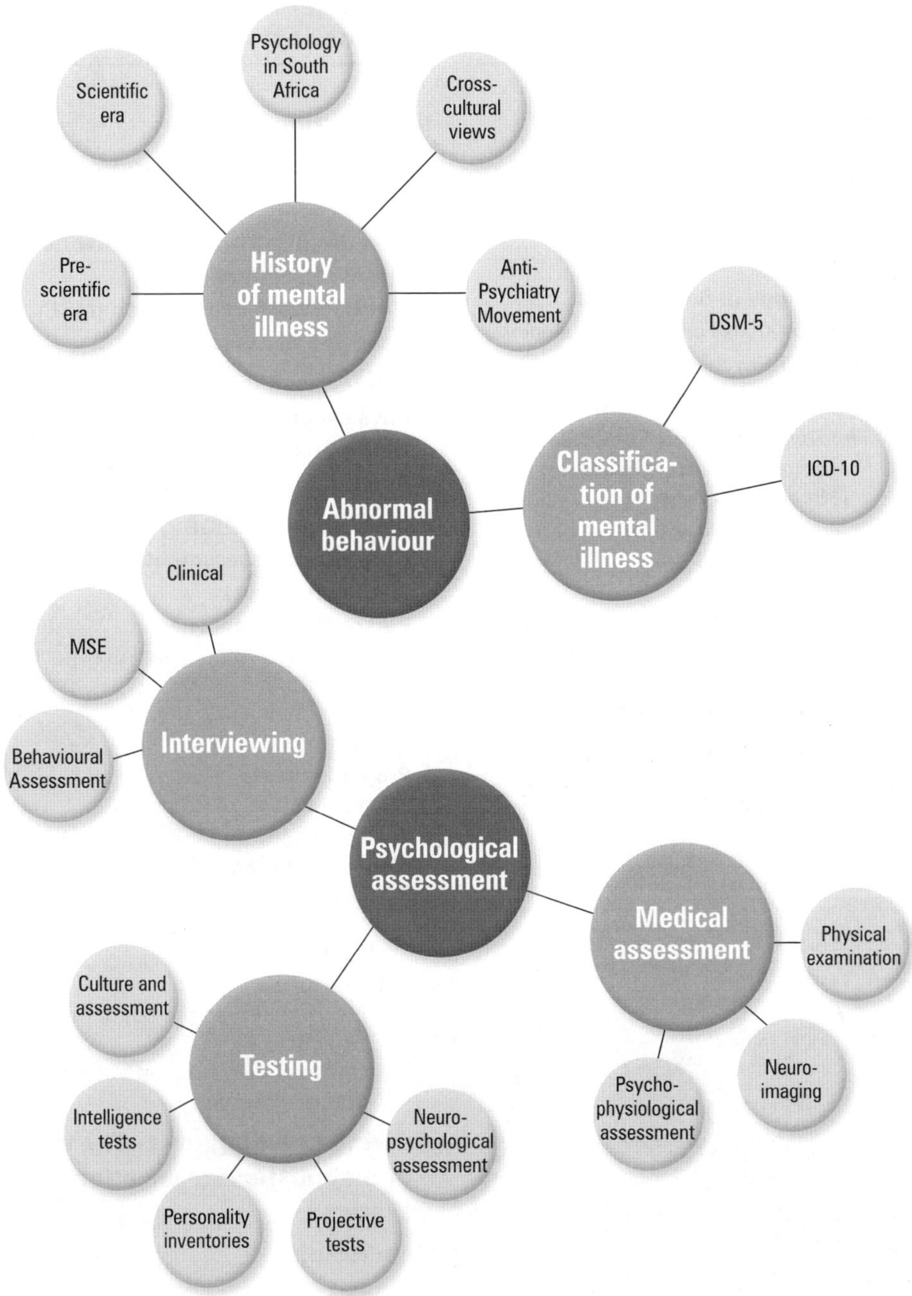

LEARNING OUTCOMES

After studying this chapter you should be able to:

- Explain how abnormal behaviour has been defined using the criteria of statistical deviance, maladaptiveness, and personal distress.
- Briefly review the history of mental illness as it has evolved through a number of eras.
- Describe broader political and sociocultural factors that influence our perceptions of abnormality and normality.
- Describe the classification of mental illness, particularly the use of the *Diagnostic and Statistical Manual of Mental Disorders* and the *International Classification of Diseases.*
- Describe the nature and function of clinical assessment and the concepts that determine the value of assessment (reliability, validity, and standardisation).
- Describe the purpose of the clinical interview, physical examination, and formal behavioural assessment in the evaluation process.
- Compare and contrast projective tests, personality inventories, and neuropsychological tests for the purpose of psychological evaluation.
- Explain how medical techniques such as PET, CAT, and MRI scans are appropriate tools for assessing psychological disorders, including limitations of such methods.
- Explain the nature and purposes of psychiatric diagnosis and how the DSM is used to help therapists and counsellors make an accurate psychiatric diagnosis.

SECTION 1: DESCRIBING AND CLASSIFYING ABNORMAL BEHAVIOUR

INTRODUCTION

Sigmund Freud summarised the forces and processes that all people are exposed to quite eloquently. He saw life as a daily struggle or challenge to cope with, and inevitably there are those who fall victim to life's challenges and who cope in ways that we see to be abnormal or deviant. In this book, we will be exploring the different ways in which abnormal behaviours manifest themselves. You will come to realise that these abnormal behaviours are so diverse and pervasive that they necessitate a subdiscipline in the broader discipline of psychology. Different academics, researchers, and practitioners use different terms to describe this sub-discipline.

The most common descriptions are *psychopathology, psychological disorders, psychiatric disorders, abnormal psychology and abnormal behaviour* (see Box 1.1 for some definitions of these terms). The description of choice often reflects the paradigm or epistemology of the person using it, and often leads to heated debates between academics and practitioners as the term that one uses reflects one's stance on:

- ***How the person who 'suffers', or is 'diagnosed', with a disorder is viewed:*** For example, if you describe this subdiscipline as *psychiatric disorders*, a *patient* is diagnosed with a disorder (*disease/illness*). In the case of the use of the term *psychological disorder*, a *client* copes with adverse life events in such a way that it causes distress for the client and those people directly involved with them.

> **Note:** Although the preferred way of referring to a person who is a recipient of mental health care services is 'mental health care user', many practitioners, depending on their epistemology, refer to such a person as either a patient or a client. These terms will be used interchangeably throughout this book.

- ***The cause(s) of the disorder:*** For example, in the case of *psychiatric disorders*, one would emphasise biological factors, whereas in the case of *psychological disorders*, one would emphasise psychosocial factors.
- ***Treatment:*** In the case of *psychiatric disorders*, one would emphasise medical treatment (e.g. medication, ECT, etc.), whereas in the case of *psychological disorders*, one would emphasise psychological treatment (e.g. psychotherapy, marital therapy, family therapy, etc.).

When writing a book on this topic, it is impossible to accommodate all these different, and often opposing, points of view. For the purposes of this introductory text, the aim is merely to introduce students to the most common disorders; therefore, we will use the terms *abnormal behaviour, psychopathology or psychological disorder* interchangeably.

BOX 1.1: DEFINITION OF TERMS

Abnormal behaviour	Any behaviour that deviates from social and statistical norms and that is maladapative and causes personal distress (Barlow & Durand, 2005).
Psychopathology	Derived from the words psyche, meaning mind or soul, and pathology, meaning disease or illness. In essence, then, the term may be understood as referring to the study of 'mind illnesses' or psychological disorders (Barlow & Durand, 2005).
Psychological disorder	A psychological dysfunction within an individual that is associated with distress or impairment in functioning and a response to this which deviates from the person's culture (Barlow & Durand, 2005).

CASE STUDY

William, a 32-year-old client, has typically been described as 'moody'. He can be very sad and depressed at times, and extremely light-hearted and happy at other times. During his 'down' times, he feels tired and sleeps a lot. He loses his appetite and does not eat. During his 'happy' times, he has a remarkable amount of energy, parties a lot, and is able to get by with very little sleep. He frequently thinks of new ideas and inventions that he is sure will have a major impact on the world. He did very well in school, and graduated with an M.Comm degree. He is employed as an executive for a large corporation. Recently he was bypassed for a promotion at work. Initially, he was very depressed, staying in bed all day for several days. On about the fourth day, he began feeling very exhilarated, and decided to throw a big party. He went shopping and spent R10,000 on party supplies. He then gave the items away, and hired a caterer. At the party, he was very jovial and made sexual advances to many of the women. He left the party with a woman he had never met before. At 03h00, he was picked up by the police under the pavilion of the local soccer stadium, wearing only his underwear and carrying a bottle of vodka. He was alone and talking very loudly and rapidly, in phrases that were difficult to follow. The police brought him into the emergency department, where he was admitted to the psychiatric unit with a diagnosis of manic episode.

The case study of William reflects some of the main features that need to be considered when making a decision about whether a person is indeed suffering from a psychological disorder. In order to make a decision like this, we first need to establish defining criteria that separate such disorders from normal behaviour. These criteria include **statistical deviance**, **maladaptiveness**, and **personal distress**.

- ***Statistical deviance:*** One of the ways in which psychopathology can be defined is by making use of statistical norms of behaviour and experience to determine what is 'normal'. Anything that falls far from the norm would be considered 'abnormal' (Barlow & Durand, 2005). From this perspective, infrequently occurring behaviours, such as violence, public nudity, or hallucinations (such as hearing voices that do not exist) are seen as abnormal or as a sign of mental illness. The shortcoming of this definition, however, is that the norm, or what is considered 'normal' behaviour, will be influenced by our **cultural or social perspectives**. For example, the 'abnormal' behaviours just mentioned, namely, hearing voices and some forms of public nudity, are considered normal in many African cultures and are instrumental in giving cultural meaning to particular life events (Cartwright, 2008).

  Furthermore, just because a particular behaviour is considered to be 'normal', this does not necessarily mean that it is also healthy or socially appropriate. Racially prejudiced attitudes are often the norm in many societies, but it would be incorrect to view these as acceptable. In other words, abnormality and statistical deviance cannot always be equated, and the context in which the individual lives needs to be taken into consideration. Taking this into consideration, a more accurate way of understanding deviance would be to look at the extent to which cultural norms or ideological perspectives have been breached. However, even within a particular cultural context, equating deviance with abnormality is problematic because such a criterion does not distinguish between **positive and negative behaviours** that deviate from the norm. For example, deviations from the norm may be due to characteristics like being a genius or some form of outstanding achievement. These could hardly be viewed as pathological (Cartwright, 2008).

Table 1.1: Some myths about mental illness

Myth	Fact
People with psychological disorders behave in odd or bizarre ways.	The behaviour of mental patients is most often indistinguishable from that of 'normal' people.
Mental patients are unpredictable and dangerous.	A typical mental patient is no more dangerous than a 'normal' person.
Mental disorders are caused by fundamental mental deficiencies and are therefore shameful.	Everyone shares the potential for becoming disordered and behaving abnormally.
Abnormal and normal behaviour are qualitatively different.	Few, if any, abnormal behaviours are unique to mental patients. Abnormality usually occurs when there is a poor fit between behaviour and the situation in which it is enacted.

Source: Cartwright, 2008, p. 453.

- ***Maladaptiveness:*** The degree to which certain behaviours or experiences are maladaptive to the self or others is another way of defining psychopathology. Behaviours that prevent the individual from adapting or adjusting for the good of the individual or group are defined as abnormal. This criterion is grounded in the belief that individuals need to evolve and adapt for the good of the self as well as to ensure the survival of the individual and the broader community. Common indications of psychopathology such as suicide, depression, and fatigue would fit this criterion because they hinder the individual's personal growth and actualisation.

The criterion of maladaptiveness is relative to the particular culture within which it is being examined; for example, in many African countries, there are certain rituals that could be considered to be strange or 'barbaric' to people from other countries. One such example would be trance states (see Chapter 8). Barlow and Durand (2005) quote an example of an East African woman, who heard voices and then killed a goat with her bare hands. If this behaviour is observed out of context, it would seem as if this person suffers from a mental disorder; however, seen within the cultural context, her actions form part of an important ritual. One of the main problems with the criteria of both maladaptiveness and statistical deviance is that they attempt to assess abnormality from a position outside the individual's own experience of the apparent problem. This has led many researchers to prefer the criterion of personal distress over the abovementioned criteria when it comes to defining psychopathology (Cartwright, 2008). You will notice that in this textbook, where possible, sections that describe cross-cultural variations of the disorders have been included in the chapters, in order to sensitise the reader to cultural variations in the presentation of disorders.

- ***Personal distress:*** Psychological disorders are very often accompanied by distress and suffering. In cases where anxiety and depression are the prominent symptoms, people often struggle with intolerable negative thoughts about themselves and their world (Cartwright, 2008). In these instances, it is appropriate that personal distress is considered when deciding what constitutes a mental disorder. However, there are exceptions; for example, people who suffer from personality disorders often do not show overt signs of distress. The absence of distress is, however, not limited to personality disorders. In the case study at the beginning of this chapter, you will have noticed that William, who clearly suffers from a disorder, does not show any overt signs of distress. One could therefore conclude that distress alone is not sufficient to define abnormality. Furthermore, one must also keep in mind the fact that the presence of distress alone does not imply abnormality, as all people can and will experience distress at some stage of their lives. Distress is often a healthy response to adverse life situations (Barlow & Durand, 2005). Examples of normal distress would be grief after the loss of a significant person in one's life, being a victim of a violent crime, or retrenchment.

From the aforementioned it is abundantly clear that distinguishing between normality and abnormality is not as easy as it first seems. This is an issue which has been, and still is, debated in psychology. A further complication in this debate is that cultures, societies, and communities are dynamic and that norms, values, and rituals change over time. What could once have been described as abnormal may be considered to be normal later. For instance, up until quite recently, homosexuality was a diagnosable mental disorder. It is only since 1973 that homosexuality has ceased to be regarded as a mental disorder because there was no clear link to be found between mental disorders, abnormality, and homosexuality (see Chapter 9). Broader political and sociocultural forces have been shown to have a significant impact on how we view mental disorders (Cartwright, 2008).

A BRIEF HISTORY OF MENTAL ILLNESS

The pre-scientific era

Humankind has always been faced with problems with madness and insanity (Porter, 2002). The dominant understanding of mental illness during the pre-scientific era was based on the belief that abnormal behaviour was caused by supernatural forces (Barlow & Durand, 2005).

Evidence of this belief is found in archaeological findings of skulls (dating back to 5000 BCE) that have holes drilled into the cranial region (see Figure 1.1). Presumably, it was thought that by boring a hole in the patient's skull, the evil spirits causing the mental disturbance could be driven out (Cartwright, 2008).

Figure 1.1: Trepanned skull

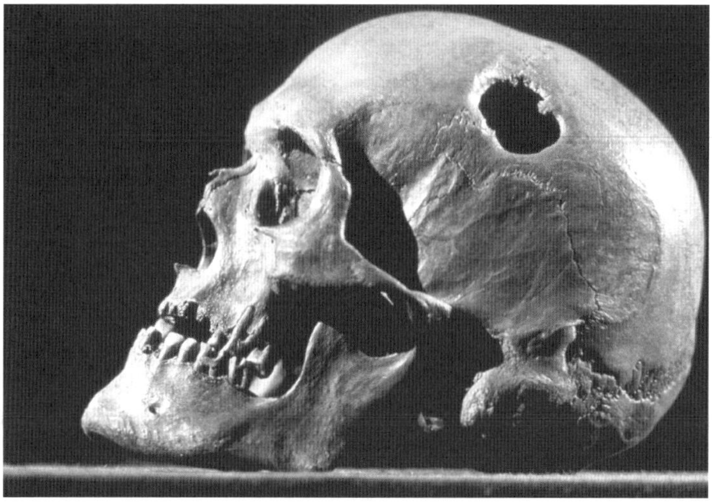

BOX 1.2: ATTITUDES TOWARDS PSYCHOLOGY, PSYCHIATRY, AND MENTAL ILLNESS

Aim: Stones (1996) conducted a study to explore attitudes towards psychology, psychiatry, and mental illness.

Method: Stones (1996) used a self-report questionnaire survey. He conducted his study among a large sample of university students as well as among smaller groups of health care professionals, patients, and the general public.

Results: Some of the main findings of this study included the following:

- The extent of the individual's knowledge of mental illness, and the degree of contact with mental-health professionals, significantly influenced their perception of mental illness.
- Members of the public were found to be more optimistic about the efficacy of psychological treatment than psychologists.
- Although psychologists and other health care professionals were viewed positively, the general public still preferred to consult a friend rather than a psychologist in times of personal distress.

Conclusion: Attitudes towards mental illness and its treatment are influenced by knowledge and understanding of mental illness and its treatment.

Figure 1.2: Hippocrates

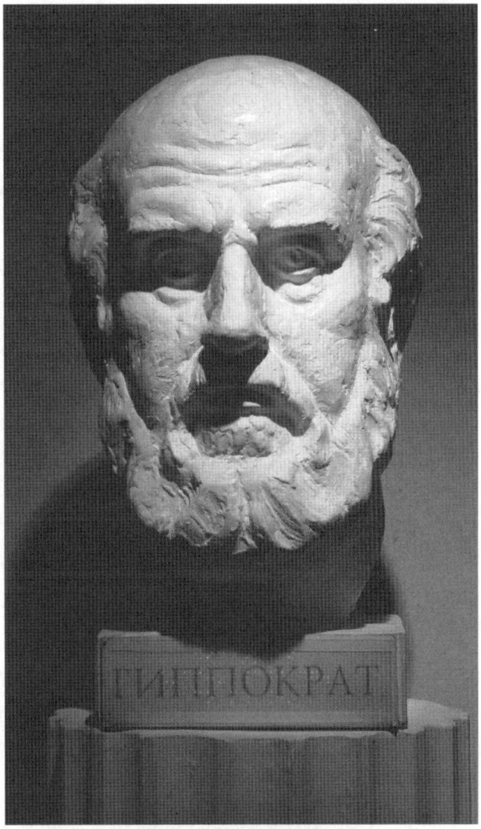

The first sign of a change to a biological view of mental illness can be found in the work of a Greek physician named Hippocrates (460–377 BCE) (Barlow & Durand, 2005) (see Figure 1.2). Hippocrates considered the brain to be the centre of wisdom, consciousness, intelligence, and emotion (Barlow & Durand, 2005). He therefore considered that any changes in behaviour could be ascribed to changes in the brain. However, he did not think that only brain changes were responsible for behaviour changes; he also recognised interpersonal factors as a possible cause. Galen (CE 129–199) later adopted Hippocrates' ideas by ascribing changes in behaviour to imbalances in four essential fluids or humours in the body: blood, phlegm, yellow bile, and black bile (Barlow & Durand, 2005).

Thus, according to Galen, a disproportionate amount of black bile would cause melancholia (a form of depression). Galen would prescribe natural remedies such as solitude, a change in diet, or abstinence from sexual activity, to heal these kinds of problems. Although his understanding of mental illness was later found to be incorrect, his findings marked the rudimentary beginnings of the biomedical approach to understanding psychopathology – this approach emerged centuries later. For this reason, he is often referred to as the 'father of modern medicine'.

During the Middle Ages, instead of building on biological causes of abnormal behaviour as proposed by Hippocrates and Galen, there was a return to ascribing these behaviours to supernatural causes; however, these views were based on more organised forms of religious doctrine (Cartwright, 2008). Mental illness was viewed as a punishment for sins committed, or as a form of demonic possession. The church became the main vehicle through which such 'possessions' could be exorcised. Europe became witness to extensive witch hunts. Anyone who seemed to go against the Christian faith was accused of being possessed by the devil and believed to have various supernatural powers that could cause great harm to others. Many mentally ill people of this era were thought to be possessed by demons and were severely punished or killed as a result (Cartwright, 2008) (see Figure 1.3). Although we may at a first glance deem this view to be very primitive, we must keep in mind that to a greater or lesser extent, many people still see some disorders or afflictions as sins or punishment. Many people still believe that homosexuality is a sin, for example, or that HIV/AIDS is a punishment for 'immoral' behaviour.

Figure 1.3: 'Witches' being burnt at the stake

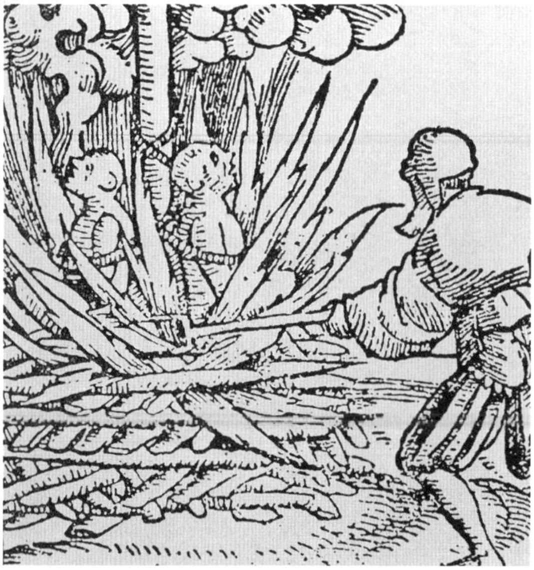

Formal seclusion of mentally disturbed individuals began in the late Middle Ages, when the Church, citing charity, began locking up the so-called 'insane'. The most well-known institution for the insane was established in the religious house of St Mary of Bethlehem (often called 'Bedlam', a term that has come to indicate confusion, disorder, and chaos) in London late in the fourteenth century (Porter, 2002) (see Figure 1.4).

During the Renaissance (1400–1600), patients who were psychologically ill began to be treated more humanely, and ideas related to witchcraft were more openly challenged. Johann Weyer (1515–1588), a German physician, postulated that such individuals were not possessed by the devil but were mentally unstable and therefore could not be held responsible for their actions. In 1584, Reginald Scot published *Discovery of Witchcraft,* in which he contended that so-called 'possessions' were medical illnesses and not visitations from evil spirits (Cartwright, 2008).

Figure 1.4: Bedlam

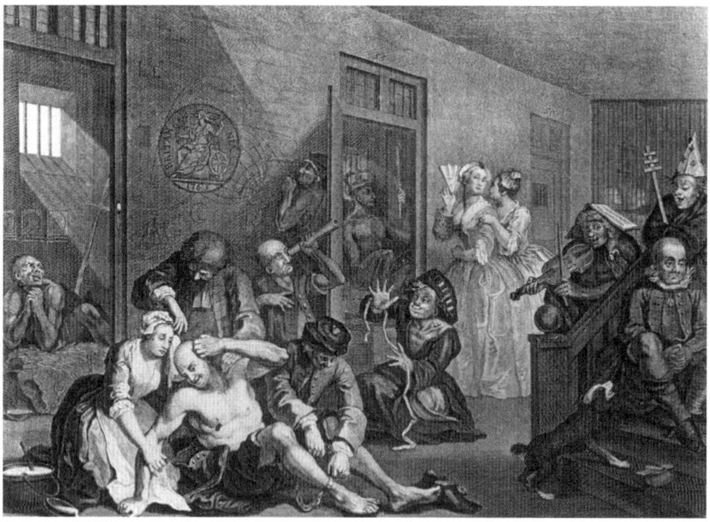

Although the scientific understanding of mental illness began to develop, the institutionalisation of the mentally ill was also on the increase in the sixteenth century. Patients were housed in asylums that became well known for their inhumane treatment of mental patients, as these institutions were more like prisons than hospitals (Barlow & Durand, 2005). The treatment of these patients included restraining them for long periods of time, placing them in dark cells, and subjecting them to torture-like treatments. Patients were also often subjected to electric shocks, bleeding in order to rid the body of 'dangerous' fluids, powerful drugs, and starvation. Late in the eighteenth century, these kinds of treatments were gradually challenged with the emergence of humanitarian reforms across the Western world. In France, Philippe Pinel (1745–1826) put forward the idea that kindness and consideration toward mental patients (moral therapy) was necessary for their recovery (Barlow & Durand, 2005). He argued that their chains should be removed and that, instead of being incarcerated in dungeons, they should be placed in sunny rooms, be permitted to do exercise, and partake in other constructive activities.

Similarly, in England, Tuke (1732–1822) established a country retreat in which patients could rest peacefully and work in a caring and supportive atmosphere (Barlow & Durand, 2005). Many patients were reported to have completely recovered from their mental illnesses once they were treated in a humane fashion. The changes that followed revolutionised the way mental illness was treated during this time. Patients were treated with care and understanding, and gradually, trained nurses and other professionals were introduced to help in the treatment of mental patients.

The scientific era

Towards the end of the nineteenth century, there were many significant factors that started a shift back towards a more biological approach to the causes of mental disorders. One of the main factors was the observation that syphilis (a sexually transmitted disease caused by bacteria infiltrating the brain) produces the same symptoms as a mental disorder, for example delusions of persecution or grandeur (see Chapter 6) as well as other bizarre behaviours (Barlow & Durand, 2005). This encouraged the search for other biological causes that might be associated with mental illness and formed the foundation of modern-day psychiatry. Many other developments, supported and encouraged by John P. Grey, occurred during this era in an attempt to identify, understand, and treat different forms of psychopathology. In 1854, Grey maintained that mental disorders are always caused by physical factors; therefore, these patients should be treated as if they are physically ill (Barlow & Durand, 2005).

In 1883, Emil Kraepelin observed that certain symptoms occurred with specific types of mental disease. Based on this observation, he developed a classification system for a number of disorders, most notably *dementia praecox* (known today as Schizophrenia, see Chapter 6) and manic-depressive psychosis (known today as bipolar affective disorder, see Chapter 5). Kraepelin's views about classification were revolutionary and served as a precursor to the *Diagnostic and Statistical Manual of Mental Disorders* that is currently used to make a diagnosis.

The scientific era has also been characterised by the development of many different psychological theories and treatments (these theories are explained in more detail in Chapter 2). You may or may not have come across these theories in other psychology courses. Many of the theories that we use in the field of abnormal behaviour are typically quite complex, in different ways, and one cannot do justice to them in limited space. It is therefore strongly suggested that you revisit these theories in order to facilitate a better understanding of the different aetiological factors that will be discussed in more detail for each disorder.

In the late nineteenth century, Sigmund Freud designed a theory, named psychoanalysis, which attempted to explain almost all areas of the human psyche. One aspect of his theory also attempted to explain how mental disorders develop. At the basis of this explanation is Freud's understanding of the structure of personality (i.e. the id, ego, and superego), as well as defence mechanisms (Barlow & Durand, 2006). According to Freud, the conflict between the different personality structures, as well as over-reliance on certain defence mechanisms, gives rise to different forms of disorders. You will find more details on this in the descriptions of the different disorders covered in this textbook.

Another important school of thought in the field of abnormal behaviour is behaviourism, which gained prominence in the 1950s. The roots of this school of thought can be traced back to John Watson (1878–1958), who was of the opinion that psychology should follow more stringent scientific research methods, such as those used by the natural sciences (Barlow & Durand, 2006). This opinion emerged in reaction to psychoanalysis and it claims that psychopathology had its genesis in psychological conflict caused by instinctual drives (Cartwright, 2008). Influential theorists like Skinner (operant conditioning) and the South African-born Joseph Wolpe (systematic desensitisation) built on Watson's initial theory. These behaviourists believed that psychopathology could be better understood by the observation of how abnormal behaviour is learned and reinforced by the external environment (Cartwright, 2008; Rachman, 2000).

Numerous other forms of psychological treatments have emerged in the past 50 years, all of them claiming to have a better understanding of the human condition and abnormal behaviour. Existential psychotherapy, primal therapy, cognitive-behaviour therapy, gestalt psychotherapy, logotherapy, and neurolinguistic programming are but a few of the treatments developed in this era (Cartwright, 2008).

Over the years, there has been a great deal of conflict about which treatments are more effective, and this has often led to some treatments being favoured over others without a clear reason being given. Often, the choice of treatment method simply depends on the therapist's chosen theoretical orientation. The choice of different treatment modalities remains an ongoing debate in psychology, and a great deal of research is being compiled to determine if some treatments are indeed more effective than others (Cartwright, 2008).

The introduction of psychotropic (mood-altering) drugs in the 1950s has also been heralded as an important landmark in the history of mental illness. Drugs like lithium, chlorpromazine, and imipramine were hailed as miracle drugs because, for the first time, symptoms associated with mania, psychosis, and depression could be controlled through the use of medication. This made it possible for many patients to be discharged from, or altogether avoid admission to, psychiatric institutions. Many patients were able to maintain normal productive lives under continuing medication. In this way, psychopharmacological treatment was able to provide a cost-effective way of managing patients without having to resort to lengthy stays in psychiatric hospitals (Cartwright, 2008).

Timeline

As the previous sections have shown, the history of mental illness extends over many centuries and features many different people. To help readers grasp the broad sweep of this history, Figure 1.5 presents an overview of important people and events in the history of mental illness.

Figure 1.5: Timeline of the history of mental illness

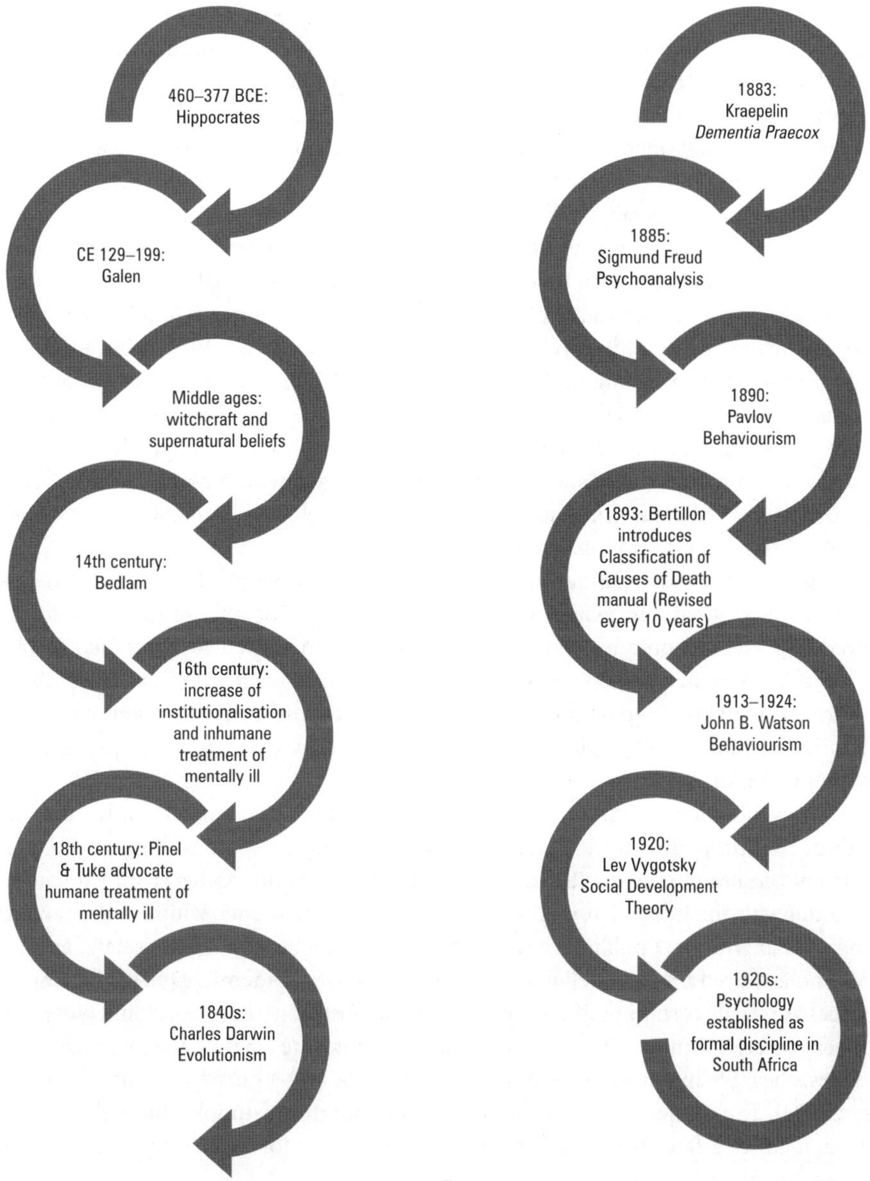

Source: © Austin, 2012

Psychology in South Africa

South Africa, because of its unique geographical location, together with its potential mineral and agricultural wealth, became the scene of ongoing conflicts between various world powers intent on expanding their empires. After its 'discovery' by the Portuguese and a struggle for control between the Dutch and the British, South Africa was 'won' by the British, who set about developing the region. It was mainly the white British colonialists who benefited from South Africa's wealth, whilst white Afrikaners and black South Africans were subjected to poverty. This disenfranchised group created a problem for the ruling class, and in order to solve this problem, the working class was 'divided and conquered' along racial lines (Freund, 1992). Racial exclusion was then adopted by the lower socio-economic white class, who were feeling increasingly threatened by the larger black population (Freund, 1992) and racial segregation was formalised under the leadership of Hendrik Frensch Verwoerd (the father of Apartheid) who obtained his doctorate in psychology at the University of Stellenbosch in 1924 and became prime minister of the Republic of South Africa in 1958 (Scholtz, 1974).

Psychology was first established as a formal academic discipline in South Africa during the 1920s, which was a time of class ordering, labour problems and racial oppression (Foster, 1993). It suited those in power to adopt the dominant social scientific discourse of the time, which was one of racial differences and racial inferiority (Gould, 1981), an idea reinforced by the fact that the psychometric tests being used in South Africa were designed mainly for the white population. These culturally biased tests were used to endorse racial oppression, ill-treatment, substandard education, misdiagnosis, exclusion from various services and opportunities, and neglect. For example, a study conducted by Freeman (1992) found that black patients were more likely to be diagnosed with a psychotic disorder such as Schizophrenia, whereas white patients were more likely to be diagnosed with a mood disorder (see Chapter 2 for more on this).

Treatment was also substandard and primitive for black people, for example, the use of electroconvulsive treatment without the use of anaesthesia or muscle relaxants, as it was believed that black people had less sensitivity to pain compared to white people (Szasz, 1974). Black psychiatric patients also had to sleep on mats on the floor, as it was believed that Africans prefer to sleep on the floor. The rationale for different treatment of psychiatric patients based on race was based on findings from research in anthropology, psychiatry, and psychology (Burke, 2010).

The abovementioned structural conditions of the past, particularly the racial discrimination propounded by the apartheid-era governments, are what underlie most of the current variation in population health in South Africa. South Africa is unfortunately still contending with the legacy left by the colonial and apartheid eras, whilst at the same time having to deal with new public health threats such as the human immunodeficiency virus (HIV) and acquired immunodeficiency syndrome (AIDS) epidemic. Due to the scarcity of resources as well as certain political constraints, the possibility of research in epidemiology has been severely limited. Even though these factors are shared by many developing countries, they are much more prominent in the case of South Africa (Myer, Ehrlich, & Susser, 2004). Thus, it needs to be noted that throughout this textbook, although every effort has been made to establish accurate epidemiological figures for each cultural group, most of the presented figures are estimates.

Additional and cross-cultural views

There are other views and histories of psychopathology that differ from the dominant Western approach (see Table 1.11). In China and India, for example, there are traditions of healing that do not share the Western tradition of trying to separate physical from mental illnesses. In southern Africa, alongside the biomedical or Western perspective of psychopathology, there are other important traditions. Indigenous theories of illness, including theories of psychopathology, commonly see personal problems as being caused by difficulties in social relationships. These relationships may be both with living people and with ancestors or shades, who continue to play an important part in social life even after death. Religious healing is also very common in southern Africa, and some churches, most notably the Zionist Church, practise a form of religion that combines indigenous beliefs with Christianity, often in charismatic forms (Cartwright, 2008).

In addition to psychologists and psychiatrists (of whom there are relatively few on the African continent), people in southern Africa may consult an indigenous healer such as an *isangoma* or *igqira* (indigenous healers), *inyanga* or *ixhwele* (herbalists), or *umprofethi* (prophet in the Zionist church).

The question of whether different forms of treatment are effective, and of how and whether practitioners from different healing traditions can and should work together, is an interesting and complex one, and, partly because of the continuing dominance of Western models in psychology, we do not know enough about these issues (see Swartz (1998) for a further discussion on this topic). Lewis-Fernández and Kleinman (1995) argue that psychosomatic, mind–brain, behavioural health, and psychopathological investigations need to consider the social world in their research paradigms if we are to better understand the sources and consequences of mental illness.

According to Castillo (1998), mental-health practitioners trained in the Western tradition have much to learn from indigenous diagnosticians and therapists in order to design new ways of delivering appropriate care for people from different cultures. Castillo (1998) also suggests a more client-centred approach to mental disorders, in which an individual's context and perspective, emerging from factors such as cultural heritage, socio-economic status, and racial grouping, are important considerations in determining what kinds of treatment might work best in a given situation. This kind of multidimensional approach draws on the strengths of many different models of psychopathology in a way that can best help the patient (Cartwright, 2008). Such an approach is especially useful in the South African context, given the important role that culturally derived understandings of mental illness may play in a practitioner's ability to help a patient. From this perspective, a patient may be diagnosed and medicated for a mental disorder while at the same time being encouraged to consult an indigenous healer, with neither needing to take priority over the other. You will see that in most of the chapters on the different disorders, a South African perspective has been included in order to develop a better understanding of the manifestation of these disorders in different cultures.

The Anti-Psychiatry Movement

Following on from the argument that abnormal behaviour should be viewed from a multi-cultural perspective, yet with the medical model being the dominant discourse in diagnosis and treatment, it is no wonder that a strong movement (the Anti-Psychiatry Movement) resulted in reaction to this. The modern use of the term 'anti-psychiatry' was introduced by David Cooper (1967). The Anti-Psychiatry Movement argued that the construct 'illness' (in its broadest sense) refers to abnormalities in physical functioning and therefore cannot be applied to a psychological disorder that has no signs of physical pathology. Proponents of this movement further argue that doctors tend to view the mentally ill as blameless victims of brain diseases, and that they uncritically accept the idea of structural and physiological bases for mental illness (Double, 1992). This view puts the patient in a very passive role. According to this movement, this has led to the inhumane treatment of patients as though they are objects (Johnstone, 2000). This opposition to the medical psychiatric view leads to an anti-authoritarian position that argues against the use of psychiatric diagnosis, drug treatments, electro-convulsive treatments, and involuntary hospitalisation.

In general, anti-psychiatry has been regarded as simply a passing phase in the history of psychiatry (Tantum, 1991), although, based on observations of recent trends in the popular media, there seems to be a slight resurgence of anti-psychiatry. There are two main reasons that would explain why this movement lost its momentum:

- Some of its main proponents were ultimately more interested in personal authenticity than in carrying through their ideas in practice.
- There were many different and often opposing views within the movement, as is illustrated by the disagreement between Szasz and Laing, who were both proponents of the Anti-Psychiatry Movement. For example, Thomas Szasz (1976) was quite scathing in his censure of Laing, as Laing never denied the reality of mental turmoil, merely contending that so-called 'mental illness' was more understandable than is generally assumed. Szasz (1976), however, was unrelenting in his stance. He stated, for example, that '[it] places psychiatry in the company of alchemy and astrology and commits it to the category of pseudoscience. The reason for this is that there is no such thing as "mental illness"' (Szasz, 1974, p. 1).

CLASSIFICATION OF MENTAL ILLNESS

By now it should be clear that the study of abnormal behaviour is not as simple as it may have seemed to begin with. From the definition of abnormal behaviour, as well as from the history of mental illness, it can be seen that there have been many controversies and debates. These differences and debates have also found their way into the classification of different disorders. It is a typical human characteristic to try to create order out of chaos by classifying observations into categories. This is also a characteristic that underlies science. In line with this, and also arguably in an attempt to make abnormal behaviour more 'scientific', there have been attempts to classify the different disorders according to their (mostly) observable characteristic signs and symptoms.

As with many other domains in the study of abnormal behaviour there are both major and more subtle disagreements in terms of the classification of disorders. The more subtle disagreements have resulted in two main classifications of disorders in current use. The *International Classification of Diseases* (ICD-10) is produced and published by the World Health Organisation (WHO), includes a section on psychiatric conditions, and is used to some extent worldwide. The *Diagnostic and Statistical Manual of Mental Disorders* (DSM), produced and published by the American Psychiatric Association (APA), is solely focused on mental health conditions, and is the main classification tool in the United States. It is currently in its fifth edition (DSM-5, published 2013) and is also used worldwide, perhaps more so than the ICD-10. The ICD system and the DSM are considered roughly on a par with one another, and an explicit concern in the development of the DSM was compatibility with the diagnostic categories and codes of the ICD. South Africa uses both DSM and ICD for different purposes, in that many practitioners in clinical settings prefer to use the DSM, whilst using the ICD for claims from medical aids.

The stated intention of diagnostic manuals is to develop replicable and clinically useful categories and criteria, to facilitate consensus and agreed standards. The DSM-5 does acknowledge aetiology to some extent by using shared aetiology as a criteria for categorising the disorders, whereas the ICD-10 does not incorporate aetiology in any way. Chapter V of ICD-10, the Classification of Mental or Behavioural Disorders, 'is intended for general clinical, educational and service use' (World Health Organisation, 1992, p. 1). The DSM-5 (American Psychiatric Association, 2013, p. xli) is more specific, indicating that 'this edition of DSM-5 was designed first and foremost to be a useful guide to clinical practice'. This includes:

- A means by which the profession **communicates** briefly and clearly within itself (and with other professionals) about clinically recognisable conditions for which it has professional responsibility for diagnosis, care, or research
- To facilitate the objective assessment of the presentation of symptoms in a wide variety of clinical settings
- Information about the likely **outcome** (prognosis) of psychiatric disorders with and without treatment
- What is known of **aetiology** (causes) or patho-physiological processes
- Provision of a structured way in which to understand and diagnose mental disorders.

Despite the intention of these systems to streamline the diagnostic process, the systems are not as atheoretical and problem free as was hoped. Some of the problems with the systems include:

- The diagnostic categories can be considered to be based on particular psychiatric theories and data, and the systems are therefore not truly atheoretical.
- The categories, in many instances, are broad and often specified by numerous possible combinations of symptoms.
- Many of the categories overlap in symptomatology or typically occur together.

Although there are problems with the classification systems, and even though they are widely criticised, and were originally intended only as a guide for experienced clinicians trained in their use, the classification terms are still widely used by clinicians, researchers, administrators, and medical aid providers in many countries.

The Diagnostic and Statistical Manual of Mental Disorders (5th ed.) (DSM-5)

Background and history

As the fields of psychiatry and psychology developed, the list of disorders grew to such an extent that a need arose for a more systematic way of classifying and diagnosing disorders. In 1952, the APA published the first *Diagnostic and Statistical Manual of Mental*

Disorders (DSM-I). Since then, the system has been regularly updated. DSM-III (American Psychiatric Association, 1980), unlike DSM-II, included major revisions. Whereas DSM-II had consisted of a brief 119 pages, DSM-III was 494 pages long and listed 265 distinct subcategories. This number would grow to nearly 400 with the publication of DSM-IV, with each one of these subcategories based on comprehensive research and review by the panel responsible for the revision.

In the late 1970s and beginning of the 1980s, there was a marked shift in psychiatry as an academic discipline. The availability of pharmacological treatments for psychiatric disorders, combined with a desire to remain part of an increasingly scientifically rigorous medical realm, led psychiatry to trade psychoanalytic theory for a new biopsychiatry that largely rejected a disease model rooted in individual biographies, psychological conflict, and psychosocial stressors.

As discussed previously, the Anti-Psychiatry Movement of the 1960s, which critically viewed psychiatry's diagnostic categories as labels constructed by society in order to silence social deviance, created additional pressure on the discipline to define its targets in biological terms. These shifts and debates precipitated a significant change in the DSM classification system. Unlike previous editions, DSM-III was intended to guide psychiatrists actively in assessing and diagnosing patients.

Each diagnosis was thought of not only as stemming from a unique biological cause, but also as being made up of a unique (and determinant) set of symptoms. This represented a marked departure from the psychodynamic view of disease, in which a given set of symptoms, depending as they did on the individual's life history and beliefs, could result from any number of underlying conflicts. DSM-III and DSM-IV have been heavily criticised for their approach to diagnosis, in which the presence of a minimum number of symptoms from a list determines the presence or absence of the disorder in question. Mental disorders do not always fit neatly within the boundaries of a single disorder. Some symptom domains such as anxiety and depression usually involve multiple diagnostic categories. DSM-5 acknowledges this reality by reordering the disorders into a revised organisational structure.

DSM-5 also attempts to address the structural problems of previous editions. In answer to the criticism levelled at the large number of narrow diagnostic categories in the previous editions, DSM-5 makes use of scientific indicators to inform new groupings of related disorders within the existing categorical framework. Ongoing revisions of DSM-5 'will make it a living document, adaptable to future discoveries in neurobiology, genetics and epidemiology.' (American Psychiatric Association, 2013, p. 13).

DSM-5 is organized on developmental and lifespan considerations, beginning with disorders that first manifest in early childhood, followed by disorders that manifest in adolescence and early adulthood, and ending with disorders relevant to adulthood and later life (American Psychiatric Association, 2014).

In contrast to previous editions that made use of a multiaxial system of diagnosis, DSM-5 utilises a nonaxial documentation of diagnosis (previously axes I, II and III), allowing separate notations for key psychosocial and contextual factors (previously axis IV) and disability (previously axis V). This addresses the criticism that previous editions implied that medical conditions were unrelated to behavioural and psychosocial factors.

Table 1.2: Overview of development of the DSM classification system

Year	Revision	Underlying paradigm
1952	APA published the first edition of the DSM (DSM-I), replacing the collection of diagnoses endorsed by the APA in 1933	• DSM-I was heavily influenced by: ▸ psychoanalytic theory and ▸ Adolf Meyer's emphasis on individual failures of adaptation to biological or psychosocial stresses as the cause of psychiatric illness. • The diagnoses enumerated in DSM-I indicate a major enlargement in the ways in which a psychotic illness could be experienced and named.
1968	DSM-II	• The proportion of psychiatrists following psychodynamic tenets rose to a third by the late 1950s, and to half by the early 1970s. • Psychoanalysis and psychodynamics dominated the curriculum of medical schools and residency programs, as well as the orientation of many academic departments, through the mid-1960s. • Like DSM-I, DSM-II presented a psychosocial view of psychiatric illness. • Psychiatric illnesses were reactions to stresses of everyday living, not discrete disease entities that could easily be demarcated from one another or even from normal behaviour or experience. • From this perspective, naming a disease was of much less significance than understanding the underlying psychic conflicts and reactions that gave rise to symptoms.
1980	DSM-III	• Reflected American psychiatry's embrace of a biomedical model of disease, complete with discrete illness categories that were distinct both from one another and from that which qualified as 'normal'. • The whole of medicine had experienced a cultural shift, one that was characterised by: ▸ Reliance on standardised knowledge rather than clinical expertise. ▸ Statistical knowledge based on groups rather than individuals. ▸ An increasingly reductionistic view of disease, in which biology was paramount. • The diagnostic manual that grew out of this transition from psychodynamics to biopsychiatry was explicitly 'atheoretical' with regard to aetiology, but most of the diagnostic categories enumerated in the DSM-III were underpinned by an implicit assumption that biology and not psychological conflict was their primary cause.

Year	Revision	Underlying paradigm
1994	DSM-IV	• DSM-IV built upon the research generated by the empirical orientation of DSM-III. By the early 1990s, most psychiatric diagnoses had an accumulated body of published studies or data sets. • Publications until the end of 1992 were reviewed for DSM-IV, which was published in 1994. • Conflicting reports or lack of evidence were handled by data re-analyses and field trials. • The National Institute of Mental Health sponsored 12 DSM-IV field trials together with the National Institute on Drug Abuse (NIDA) and the National Institute on Alcohol Abuse and Alcoholism (NIAAA). • The field trials compared the diagnostic criteria sets of DSM-III, DSM-III-R, ICD-10 (which had been published in 1992), and the proposed criteria sets for DSM-IV. • The field trials recruited subjects from a variety of ethnic and cultural backgrounds, in keeping with a new concern for cross-cultural applicability of diagnostic standards. • In addition to its inclusion of culture-specific syndromes and disorders, DSM-IV represented much closer cooperation and coordination with the experts from WHO who had worked on ICD-10.
2000	DSM-IV-TR	• DSM-IV-TR does not represent either a fundamental change in the basic classification structure of DSM-IV or the addition of new diagnostic entities. • The textual revisions that were made to the 1994 edition of DSM-IV fall into the following categories: ▸ Correction of factual errors in the text of DSM-IV. ▸ Review of currency of information in DSM-IV. ▸ Changes reflecting research published after 1992, which was the last year included in the literature review prior to the publication of DSM-IV. ▸ Improvements to enhance the educational value of DSM-IV ▸ Updating of ICD diagnostic codes, some of which were changed in 1996.
2013	DSM-5	• Reordering of disorders into a revised organisational structure • Representation of developmental issues related to diagnosis • Integration of the latest scientific findings in genetics and neuroimaging • Consolidating and streamlining the classification of disorders • The addition of a new section highlighting disorders that require further study.

BOX 1.3: ON BEING SANE IN INSANE PLACES

Aim: Rosenhan (1973) conducted a famous study that attempted to explore the validity of psychiatric diagnoses.

Method: A form of participant observation was used in the study whereby eight psychologically healthy individuals were admitted to different psychiatric units after claiming to have been 'hearing voices'. These individuals were instructed by the researcher as to how they should act and what they should say, i.e. they were the research confederates in the study. No other symptoms or problems were discussed with the hospital staff. After gaining admission, all subjects acted their normal selves and no longer claimed to be hearing voices.

Findings: Once the admission to the hospital had taken place, Rosenhan found that no matter what these individuals did, they were perceived as being psychologically ill by the staff in the hospital.

Conclusion: The validity of making a psychiatric diagnosis is questionable as the staff in the hospital failed to distinguish between healthy individuals and those who were genuinely mentally ill.

Source: Rosenhan, 1973.

Despite many criticisms levelled at the DSM classification system, many practitioners, diagnosticians, and researchers find this classification system useful. It must be acknowledged that given the large audience for this system, as well as the wide variety of paradigms and epistemologies that are supported by different people in this audience, it is unlikely that there will ever be a system that will satisfy everybody's opinions. Furthermore, the DSM is not a static system, as there is a constant process of trying to improve on it. The DSM-5 is testimony to the fact that there is a constant attempt to improve on the system as is illustrated by some significant changes to the categorisation and description of the disorders. Even though this fifth edition of the DSM system has attempted to address some of the criticisms, it has already elicited additional criticism from various quarters.

The International Classification of Diseases (ICD-10)

Background and history

In 1893, a French physician, Jacques Bertillon, introduced the Bertillon Classification of Causes of Death at the International Statistical Institute in Chicago. A number of countries adopted Dr Bertillon's system, and in 1898, the American Public Health Association (APHA) recommended that the registrars of Canada, Mexico, and the United States also adopt it. The APHA also recommended revising the system every ten years to ensure the system remained current with medical practice advances. As a result, the first international conference to revise the *International Classification of Causes of Death* convened in 1900, with revisions occurring every ten years thereafter. At that time, the classification system was contained in one book, which included an Alphabetic Index as well as a Tabular List. The book was small compared with current coding texts.

The revisions that followed contained minor changes, until the sixth revision of the classification system (1948). With the sixth revision, the classification system expanded to two volumes. The sixth revision included morbidity and mortality conditions, and its title was modified to reflect the changes: *Manual of International Statistical Classification of Diseases, Injuries and Causes of Death* (ICD). Prior to the sixth revision, responsibility for ICD revisions fell to the Mixed Commission, a group composed of representatives from the International Statistical Institute and the Health Organisation of the League of Nations. In 1948, the World Health Organisation (WHO) assumed responsibility for preparing and publishing the revisions to the ICD every ten years (see Table 1.3).

It was, however, not until the early 1960s that the Mental Health Programme of the World Health Organisation (WHO) became actively engaged in a programme aiming to improve the diagnosis and classification of mental disorders. In order to do so, the WHO convened a series of meetings to review knowledge, actively involving representatives of different disciplines, various schools of thought in psychiatry, and all parts of the world in the programme. As a result of these meetings, research was stimulated on criteria for classification, and reliability of diagnosis. Numerous proposals to improve the classification of mental disorders resulted from this extensive consultation process, and these were used in drafting the eighth revision of the *International Classification of Diseases* (ICD-8). A glossary defining each category of mental disorder in ICD-8 was also developed.

Table 1.3: Historical development of the ICD

Year	Revision
1893	Jacques Bertillon introduces the Bertillon Classification of Causes of Death at the International Statistical Institute in Chicago.
1900	The first international conference to revise the International Classification of Causes of Death convenes.
1910–1940	American Public Health Association revises the system every ten years.
1948	ICD-6: World Health Organisation assumes responsibility for the ICD system. Mental and behavioural disorders are introduced for the first time.
1957	ICD-7
1968	ICD-8
1977	ICD-9
1983–1994	Greater co-operation between DSM-IV and ICD panels in order to bring the two classification systems in line with each other.

Source: ICD–10 Classification of Mental and Behavioural Disorders: Diagnostic Criteria for Research. World Health Organisation (WHO), Geneva, 2007.

As a result of scientific progress in the broader field of medicine, and more specifically psychiatry, the 1970s saw further growth of interest in improving psychiatric classification worldwide. Several major research efforts were undertaken. One of these, which aimed at the development of the Composite International Diagnostic Interview, involved research centres in 17 countries. Another major project focused on developing an assessment instrument suitable for use by clinicians (Schedules for Clinical Assessment in Neuropsychiatry), while a further study was initiated to develop an instrument for the assessment of personality disorders in different countries (the International Personality Disorder Examination). A mutually beneficial relationship evolved between these projects and the work on definitions of mental and behavioural disorders in the tenth revision of the *International Classification of Diseases* (ICD-10). The final result was a clear set of criteria for ICD-10 and assessment instruments which can produce data necessary for the classification of disorders according to the criteria included in Chapter V (F) of ICD-10.

The ICD-10 has also developed alongside the American Psychiatric Association's *Diagnostic and Statistical Manual of Mental Disorders* and although the two manuals seek to use the same codes and diagnostic categories, there are still some differences. The major contribution of the ICD system, and one of the differences between this and the DSM system, is that it attempts to represent the viewpoints of the different psychiatric traditions. Some of the other differences include (see also Table 1.6):

- Whilst the ICD-10 provides description of disorders by means of a multiaxial approach, the DSM-5 no longer uses a multi-axial approach, which is a significant move away from previous editions of the DSM.
- ICD includes personality disorders on the same axis as other mental disorders, unlike the DSM. Since the 1990s, the APA and WHO have worked to bring the DSM and the relevant sections of ICD into concordance, but some differences remain. The WHO is revising its classifications in these sections as part the development of the ICD-11 (scheduled for 2014), and an International Advisory Group has been established to guide this.
- Both the DSM-5 and ICD-10 attempt to be culture sensitive as is illustrated by the fact that Annex 2 of the ICD-10 describes a number of culture-specific disorders (see Table 1.5) and the inclusion of a cultural formation section in Section III of the DSM-5.

Table 1.4: Three axes of ICD-10 classification of mental and behavioural disorders

Axis I	Clinical Diagnosis (mental disorders, physical disorders, and personality disorders)
Axis II	Description of any activity limitations or participation restrictions in specific areas of functioning including: personal care; occupation; family and household; and functioning in the broader social context. Patients who are experiencing functional limitations or restrictions in one or more of these domains generally have more intense treatment needs.
Axis III	Used to describe contextual factors, which are environmental and life style factors relevant to pathogenesis and course of the patient's illness.

Source: ICD–10 Classification of Mental and Behavioural Disorders: Diagnostic Criteria for Research. World Health Organisation (WHO), Geneva, 2007.

Table 1.5: Culture-specific disorders (Annex 2, ICD-10)

Suggested ICD-10 category	Culture-specific disorder	Description	Potentially related syndromes
• Other specified disorders of adult personality and behaviour	Amok (Indonesia; Malaysia)	• Indiscriminate and seemingly unprovoked episode of homicidal or highly destructive behaviour. • Episodes are often followed by amnesia or fatigue and could culminate in suicide. • Often occur without warning, although some are precipitated by a period of intense anxiety or hostility.	• ahade idzi be (New Guinea) • benzi mazurazura (Southern Africa, among Shona and affiliated groups) • berserkergang (Scandinavia) • cafard (Polynesia) • colerina (the Andes of South America) • hwa-byung (Korea) • iich'aa (indigenous peoples of South-Western America)
• Other specified neurotic disorders • Somatoform autonomic dysfunction of the genito-urinary system	Dhat, dhatu, jiryan, shen-k'uei (India; Taiwan)	• Acute anxiety and somatic complaints such as fatigue and muscle pain, related to a fear of semen loss in men or women (also thought to secrete semen). • Precursors are said to include excess coitus, urinary disorders, imbalances in body humours, and diet. • The main symptom is a whitish discharge in urine, interpreted as semen loss.	• *koro* (China) • rabt (Egypt)
• Other specified neurotic disorders • Somatoform autonomic dysfunction of the genito-urinary system	Koro, jinjin bemar, suk yeong (South-East Asia, China, India)	• Acute panic or anxiety reaction involving fear of genital retraction. • In severe cases, men become convinced that the penis will suddenly withdraw into the abdomen; women sense that their breast, labia, or vulva will retract. • Victims expect the consequences to be fatal. • Studies cite factors such as illness, exposure to cold, or excess coitus as precursors, but interpersonal conflict and sociocultural demands reportedly exert greater influence on the condition.	• dhat (India) • rabt (Egypt)

Suggested ICD-10 category	Culture-specific disorder	Description	Potentially related syndromes
• Other specified neurotic disorders • Other specified dissociative or conversion disorder(s)	Latah (Indonesia; Malaysia)	• Exaggerated responses to a fright or trauma. • Responses include involuntary echolalia, echopraxia, or trance-like states. • Studies indicate a neurophysiological response, a hyper-suggestible state, or a mechanism for expressing low self-image.	• amurakh (Siberia) • bah-tsi (Thailand) • imu (indigenous people of Japan) • Jumping Frenchman (Canada) • Lapp panic (Lapps) • mali-mali (Philippines) • pibloktoq (Inuits living within the Arctic Circle) • susto (Mexico, Central and South America) • yaun (Myanmar)
• Moderate depressive episode with somatic syndrome • Neurasthenia • Undifferentiated somatoform disorder	Nerfiza, nerves, nevra, nervios (Egypt; Northern Europe; Greece; Mexico, Central and South America)	• Chronic episodes of extreme sorrow or anxiety. • Associated symptoms include somatic complaints such as head and muscle pain, diminished reactivity, nausea, appetite loss, insomnia, fatigue, and agitation. • Research links the condition to stress, anger, emotional distress, and low self-esteem.	• anfechtung (Hutterites – a religious group) • brain fag (Nigeria) • colerina, pension, bilis (Central and South America) • hsieh-ping (Taiwan) • hwa-byung (Korea) • narahati-e a sab, maraz-e a sab (Iran) • qissaatuq (Inuits living within the Arctic Circle)
• Mixed/other dissociative and conversion disorders	Pibloktoq, Arctic hysteria (Inuits living within the Arctic Circle)	• Prodromal fatigue, depression, or confusion, followed by a 'seizure' of disruptive behaviour. • Other associated behaviours and features include stripping or tearing off clothes, frenzied running, rolling in snow, echolalia, echopraxia, and property destruction. • Most episodes last only minutes and are followed by loss of consciousness, amnesia, and complete remission. • Most researchers link incidents to interpersonal anxieties and cultural stressors.	• amok (Indonesia; Malaysia) • banga, misala (Congo; Malawi) • ebenzi (Southern Africa, among Shona and affiliated groups) • grisi siknis (indigenous people of Honduras) • imu (Ainu) • latah (Indonesia; Malaysia) • mali-mali (Philippines) • nangiarpok, kayak angst, quajimaillituq (Inuits) • ufufuyane (Southern Africa, especially among Zulu and affiliated groups)

Suggested ICD-10 category	Culture-specific disorder	Description	Potentially related syndromes
• Undifferentiated somatoform disorder • Other specified neurotic disorders	Susto, espanto (Central and South America)	• Highly diverse, chronic complaints attributed to 'soul loss' induced by a severe, often supernatural, fright. • In some cases, traumatic events are not personally experienced; individuals may be stricken when others (usually relatives) suffer a fright. • Symptoms often include agitation, anorexia, insomnia, fever, diarrhoea, mental confusion and apathy, depression, and introversion. Studies variously attribute cases to generalised anxiety, and stress resulting from social conflict and low self-esteem.	• lanti (Philippines) • latah (Indonesia; Malaysia) • malgri (aborigines of Australia) • mogo laya (the island of New Guinea) • narahati (Islamic Republic of Iran) • saladera (regions around Amazon river)
• Social phobias • Other phobic anxiety disorders	Taijin kyofusho, shinkeishitsu, anthropophobia (Japan)	• Anxiety or phobia more common among men and young adults. • Cases are marked by a fear of social contact (especially friends), extreme self-consciousness (concern about physical appearance, body odour, blushing), and a fear of contracting disease. • Somatic symptoms include head, body, and stomach aches, fatigue, and insomnia. • Victims, popularly regarded as highly intelligent and creative, may display perfectionist tendencies. • Studies suggest cultural values encourage 'over-socialisation' of some children, producing feelings of inferiority and anxiety in social situations.	• anfechtung (Hutterites) • itiju (Nigeria)

Suggested ICD-10 category	Culture-specific disorder	Description	Potentially related syndromes
• Trance and possession disorders • Mixed dissociative and conversion disorders	Ufufuyane, saka (Southern Africa among Zulu, and affiliated groups; Kenya)	• An anxiety state popularly attributed to magical potions administered by rejected lovers, or spirit possession. • Features include shouting, sobbing, repeated neologisms, paralysis, convulsions, and a trance-like stupor or loss of consciousness. • Most victims are young, unmarried women. Some experience nightmares with sexual themes or rare episodes of temporary blindness. • Attacks, which can continue for days or weeks, may be provoked by the sight of men or foreigners.	• aluro (Nigeria) • phii pob (Thailand) • zar (Egypt; Ethiopia; Sudan)
• Other specified dissociative and conversion disorders • Narcolepsy and cataplexy	Uqamairineq (Inuits living within the Arctic Circle)	• Sudden paralysis associated with borderline sleep states, accompanied by anxiety, agitation, or hallucinations. • Prodromal indicators may include a detectable yet transient sound or smell. • While the condition is usually chronic and can prompt panic, most attacks last only minutes and are followed by complete remission. • Cases are fairly common, and traditionally alleged to result from soul loss, soul wandering, or spirit possession. Studies describe the experience as a dissociative hysterical reaction and possible variant of the narcolepsy-cataplexy syndrome.	• aluro (Nigeria) • old hag (Newfoundland) • phii pob (Thailand)

Source: ICD–10 Classification of Mental and Behavioural Disorders: Diagnostic Criteria for Research. World Health Organisation (WHO), Geneva, 2007.

Comparison and critique

As has been previously mentioned, the format and use of these classification systems are unfortunately not free from criticism. The operationalisation of diagnostic criteria was developed specifically to respond to criticisms of psychiatric classification (Blashfield, 1984). The primary motivation of these standardised, criterion-based definitions was to make diagnosis more consistent and reliable, initially for research (Feighner et al., 1972). Clinically, diagnostic manuals have been developed through editions of DSM-I, DSM-II, DSM-III, DSM-III-R, DSM-IV and currently the DSM-5 (American Psychiatric Association, 2013) and ICD-10 (World Health Organisation, 1992).

However, even the most reliable of diagnostic criteria are not necessarily valid in the sense of measuring what they are supposed to measure. Diagnostic criteria do not solve the dilemma of psychiatric classification. Furthermore, if psychiatric 'illnesses' were indeed unique, identifiable entities, with clear biological causes, the two major classification systems (i.e. DSM and ICD) would classify and describe disorders in exactly the same way (indeed, we would not need more than one system). Table 1.6 reflects the similarities and differences between the DSM and ICD systems and one can see that, in many instances, the differences go beyond only different names for disorders. Due to these differences, you will notice that in each of the chapters of this book where disorders are described, both the DSM and ICD systems are described.

Table 1.6: Comparison of DSM and ICD diagnostic categories

DSM-5 categories	ICD-10 categories
Neurodevelopmental Disorders (Childhood emotional disorders are incorporated under Depressive Disorders, Anxiety Disorders, Obsessive-Compulsive Disorders, Trauma and Stressor Related Disorders, Feeding and Eating, Elimination and Disruptive, Impulse Control and Conduct Disorders)	Behavioural and emotional disorders with onset usually occurring in childhood and adolescence Mental retardation Disorders of psychological development
Neurocognitive Disorders	Organic, including symptomatic, mental disorders
Substance-related and Addictive Disorders	Mental and behavioural disorders due to psychoactive substance use
Schizophrenia Spectrum and other psychotic disorders	Schizophrenia, schizotypal, and delusional disorders
Bipolar and Related Disorders	Mood (affective) disorders
Depressive Disorders Anxiety Disorders Somatic Symptom Disorders Obsessive-Compulsive and Related Disorders Dissociative disorders	Neurotic, stress-related, and somatoform disorders
Feeding and Eating Disorders Sleep/Wake Disorders Sexual Dysfunction and Gender Dysphoria	Behavioural syndromes associated with physiological disturbances and physical factors

DSM-5 categories	ICD-10 categories
Personality disorders Impulse, Disruptive and Control Disorders Conduct Disorders	Disorders of adult personality and behaviour

Source: Reprinted with permission from the Diagnostic and Statistical Manual of Mental Disorders, (DSM), Fifth Edition, American Psychiatric Association (APA), 2013 and ICD–10 Classification of Mental and Behavioural Disorders: Diagnostic Criteria for Research. World Health Organisation (WHO), Geneva, 2007.

The issue at the core of the problem is the meaning of psychiatric diagnosis. Single-word diagnoses do not necessarily help the understanding of a person's problems. The personal meaning of people's distress and the psychological and social origins of their difficulties are obscured by turning them into a simple diagnosis (Johnstone, 2000).

In reaction to the criticism of the two dominant classification systems, a number of different nosologies or schemes of classification have been proposed to replace the current descriptive model of mental disorders. Examples of these include:

- ***The dimensional model:*** Dimensional alternatives have been introduced into DSM-5, however the categorical classification is still prominent throughout the DSM-5. The dimensional approach recognises that mental disorders lie on a continuum with mildly disturbed and normal behaviour, rather than being qualitatively distinct. For example, the personality disorders are increasingly regarded as extreme variants of common personality characteristics. In the dimensional model, a patient would be identified in terms of their position on a specific dimension of cognitive or affective capacity rather than placed in a categorical 'box'.
- ***The holistic model:*** The holistic approach to mental disorders places equal emphasis on social and spiritual treatments, and on pharmacological treatments.
- ***The essential or perspectival model:*** The third and most complex alternative model is associated with the medical school of Johns Hopkins University, where it is taught as part of the medical curriculum. This model identifies four broad 'essences' or perspectives that can be used to identify the distinctive characteristics of mental disorders, which are often obscured by the present categorical classifications. The four perspectives are:
  - ***Disease:*** This perspective works with categories and accounts for physical diseases or damage to the brain which produce psychiatric symptoms. It accounts for such disorders as Alzheimer's disease or Schizophrenia.
  - ***Dimensions:*** This perspective addresses disorders that arise from the combination of a cognitive or emotional weakness in the patient's constitution and a life experience that challenges their vulnerability.
  - ***Behaviours:*** This perspective is concerned with disorders associated with something that the patient is doing (alcoholism, drug addiction, eating disorders, etc.) that has become a dysfunctional way of life.
  - ***Life story:*** This perspective focuses on disorders related to what the patient has encountered in life, such as events that have injured their hopes and aspirations.

In the Johns Hopkins model, each perspective has its own approach to treatment. The **disease perspective** seeks to cure or prevent disorders rooted in biological disease processes;

the **dimensional perspective** attempts to strengthen constitutional weaknesses; **the behavioural perspective** seeks to interrupt the problematic behaviours and assist patients in overcoming their appeal; and the **life story perspective** offers help in 'rescripting' a person's life narrative, usually through narrative therapy.

In retrospect, the history of the development of diagnostic criteria over recent years has been little more than a professional discourse intent on justifying psychiatry. This has narrowed its scope and psychiatry needs to return to a biopsychosocial model, which was becoming more generally accepted by the 1950s before the widespread introduction of psychotropic medication (Wilson, 1993). However, by all indications the trend towards biological psychiatry is actually gaining momentum as is reflected in the changes in the DSM-5. In some instances, it would seem as if the biopsychosocial has been reduced to neurodevelopmental or neurocognitive disorders, not only in the description of the disorders, but also in the way that these disorders are categorised together.

CONCLUSION

Abnormal behaviour can be defined using the criteria of statistical deviance, maladaptiveness, and personal distress. In addition to these criteria, broader political, sociocultural, and historical factors are important in understanding the nature of normality or abnormality. The classification of mental illnesses is a complex task, but this process cannot explain why various psychological problems occur.

In South Africa, it is important that we start embracing a more critical perspective on abnormal behaviour. This not only implies that students in psychology and psychiatry need to be trained from a more critical and culturally sensitive perspective, but also that society as a whole needs to be more educated in terms of what it could and should expect from these professions. In addition, citizens need to be educated about their rights in this regard (see Chapter 14). This would be consistent with the international trend of involving users and user-groups in decision-making and accountability.

Furthermore, there needs to be a more holistic understanding of mental health care users. The lack of a whole-person way of understanding mental health problems originates in medical training which focuses on physical disorder. In particular, reductive causal analyses do not necessarily help us to understand the full range of normal and abnormal human behaviour. In order to achieve this understanding, there needs to be less emphasis on a natural scientific perspective of basic biological processes. Despite the many failings of a positivist approach to abnormal behaviour, its attraction is that it seems to avoid the complexities and uncertainties of psychological and social perspectives. This seduces students and clinicians alike with the idea that experimental natural science is an adequate discourse for a description of what is normal and abnormal, which may lead to their adopting a mechanistic view in their approach to, and treatment and management of, mental health care users.

Despite a positivist or 'scientific' approach to abnormal behaviour, the mechanisms underlying this pathology seem less well understood than is the case for physical conditions. Claims are made for medical techniques which go beyond the evidence. Patients may have needless investigations and be over- or undertreated, or inappropriately treated. In an attempt to bolster professional interests, self-questioning is discouraged in the interests of certainty. Self-reflection is, however, important as it does not necessarily imply dismissing the use of classification systems and medical treatment of disorders, but may lead to a review of the importance of mental health care users' rights as well as the assessment of risk, and a more critical review of treatment modalities that may be more appropriate to the users' needs.

SECTION 2: PSYCHOLOGICAL ASSESSMENT AND PSYCHODIAGNOSTICS

INTRODUCTION

Inherent in the study of psychopathology and in the treatment of psychological disorders is the process of clinical assessment and diagnosis (Kaplan & Sadock, 2007). Clinical assessment is the evaluation and measurement of psychological, biological, and social factors in individuals who present with possible psychological disorders (Kaplan & Sadock, 2007). Diagnosis is the process whereby the clinician determines whether the particular problem with which the individual presents meets all the criteria for a psychological disorder as described in either the DSM-5 (American Psychiatric Association, 2013) or ICD-10 (World Health Organisation, 1993).

To the untrained eye, it would seem relatively unproblematic to make an accurate diagnosis. However, from what you have read thus far, it should be relatively clear that this is not as simple as it first seems. We have already alluded to some of the problems related to diagnostic systems, which form the basis of a diagnosis, but we have also discussed how culture and social forces impact on the experience and presentation of mental disorders. Given this, it is usual for the clinician to begin an assessment by collecting a wide range of information in order to determine where the source(s) of the problem might lie and then to focus on areas that appear to be most relevant. There are three basic concepts that help to establish the value of assessments:

- ***Reliability:*** The degree to which a measurement is **consistent**, that is, two or more assessors will get the same results when using the same assessment tool; this also refers to how stable the results of the assessment are over time.
- ***Validity:*** The degree to which the tool or technique assesses or measures what it is supposed to assess or measure.
- ***Standardisation:*** The process of determining specific **norms** and requirements for an assessment technique to make certain that it is used in a consistent manner across assessment situations. This includes administration instructions, evaluation of the results, and comparison of these with data for large numbers of people (Anastasi, 1988).

There are a number of procedures that can be used during a clinical assessment in order to help the clinician to obtain the information needed to both understand and assist patients. These procedures include a clinical interview, which normally includes a Mental Status Examination (MSE), a physical examination, behavioural observation and assessment, and psychological tests (Kaplan & Sadock, 2007).

BASIC STEPS IN THE DIAGNOSTIC PROCESS

The first step towards making a diagnosis is to ask the patient what is wrong in order to establish the **presenting problem**. Often patients present with more than one problem. If this happens, the diagnostician will rank these from the most important to the least important, and deal with them in sequence from the most to the least important. Then a full history of the presenting condition(s) and other relevant facts should be taken. It must be kept in mind that patients do not verbalise a diagnosis, but they describe their problem in terms of symptoms; thus they give a subjective description of what they feel, experience, and observe of themselves (e.g. feeling depressed, a change in appetite, etc.). During the interview, the diagnostician will focus not only on the content of a patient's history, but also on observable signs (e.g. tone of the patient's voice, eye contact, etc.).

Both the DSM-5 and ICD-10 systems stipulate that the diagnosis of a psychological or psychiatric disorder cannot be made if there is evidence of a medical condition that could explain the problem. It is therefore essential that a **medical examination** be carried out to rule out the possibility of a medical condition. This medical examination would focus specifically on the presenting symptoms. The general physical examination consists of:

- Basic observations, such as the person's gait, skin tone, voice intonation, and ability to hold a normal conversation
- Taking the blood pressure and checking for basic signs of disease such as anaemia or swelling of the legs
- Examining the various organ systems of the body: the heart, lungs, bowels, etc.

It is often also important that a **neurological examination** is performed. This examination gives an understanding of the well-being of the person's central and peripheral nervous systems as well as musculo-skeletal, endocrine, and vascular systems. It is the tool that physicians use to identify structural and psychiatric abnormality.

The next step would be an examination, usually by a psychiatrist or a clinical psychologist, to determine the individual's mental condition. This involves investigating the individual's abilities regarding orientation to time, place, and person (in other words, do they know what the date and time are, where they are, and who they are), attention span, concentration, and memory. Any psychopathology must also be identified, for example, abnormalities in perception of stimuli, thought content, speed of thought, and logical thinking.

Often the abovementioned steps result in only a **provisional** or tentative diagnosis and further investigations such as psychological tests may be conducted in order to refine the diagnosis, or in order to rule out a diagnosis such as mental retardation.

Using all of the available evidence, the diagnostician is then able to make a firm diagnosis (see Figure 1.6). From a list of the possible diagnoses based on the symptoms and signs, the diagnostician identifies the most likely diagnosis (e.g. clinical conditions, personality disorders, as well as physical diseases) through a process of identification and elimination.

INTERVIEWING AND OBSERVATIONS

The clinical interview

The clinical interview is a very important part of the assessment process. It is always the first step of the process and is used by most mental health professionals. It allows the diagnostician to obtain:

- A detailed description of the presenting problem or chief complaint, in other words, the reason for the patient having presented or been brought in
- Detailed history of the patient's life, their current situation (including work, habits, and relationships), and social history
- Information about attitudes, emotions, and current and past behaviour
- Family history
- Information about when the problem started, as well as whether any significant events occurred around the time that the problem started.

Figure 1.6: Triangulation in the diagnostic process

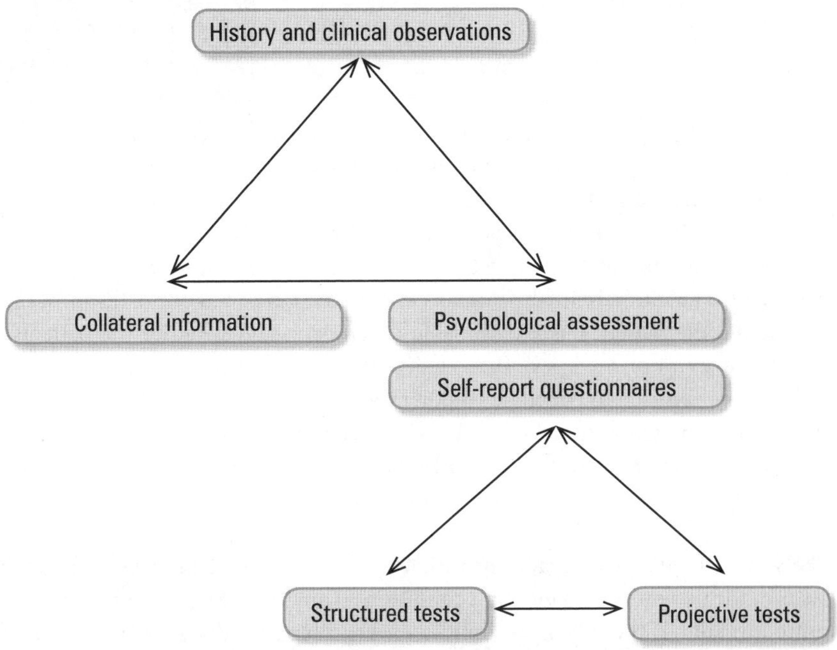

Source: © Burke, 2009.

The Mental Status Examination (MSE) is often used to help organise the information gathered during the clinical interview (Kaplan & Sadock, 2007).

Mental Status Examination (MSE)

The MSE involves a systematic observation of the patient's behaviour and is usually structured and detailed. It is generally performed quite quickly by an experienced interviewer during the course of assessing the patient. The MSE encompasses five categories (Kaplan & Sadock, 2007):

- ***Appearance and behaviour:*** The clinician observes in the patient any overt physical behaviours, dress, posture, appearance, and facial expression. For example, if the patient appears to be listening to or conversing with thin air, this may indicate the presence of hallucinations.
- ***Thought processes:*** The patient's conversation can give a very good indication of their thought processes. One would note the rate and flow of speech (very fast or very slow), as well as continuity of speech (does the patient make sense when talking or are their ideas presented in a disconnected manner?). Attention is also given to the content of the patient's speech. Here one would note the presence of delusions and/or hallucinations.
- ***Mood and affect:*** Mood is subjective, that is, how the patient feels most of the time. Affect is what the clinician observes as the patient speaks (i.e. laughing, frowning, or crying). Here one would note whether the patient's affect is appropriate (i.e. they seem sad when talking about something sad), or whether it is inappropriate (i.e. the patient laughs whilst talking about something very sad). If the patient displays very little or no affect whilst speaking, one would also note this. The affect would then be called 'blunted' or 'flat'.
- ***Intellectual functioning:*** It is possible for a clinician to make a rough estimate of a patient's intellectual functioning simply by talking to them. The clinician would note whether the patient is able to talk in abstractions and understand metaphors (as most of us can do), whether the patient has a reasonable vocabulary, and whether the patient has a good, average, or poor memory. The rough estimate of the patient's intellectual functioning helps the clinician to conclude whether the patient is above or below average intelligence.
- ***Sensorium:*** This term denotes a person's general awareness of their surroundings. Here the clinician would confirm whether the patient knows what the date and time are, and who, and where, they are (orientation to time, person, and place).

HELPFUL HINT:

Mental Status Examination

- A (Appearance and behaviour)
- T (Thought processes)
- M (Mood and affect)
- I (Intellectual functioning)
- S (Sensorium)

The aim of these behavioural observations is to enable the diagnostician to establish which areas of the patient's behaviour and condition (if any) should be assessed in more detail and more formally. If there is a possibility of a psychological disorder being present, then the clinician would be able to hypothesise about which disorder it might be and this in turn would provide more focus for further assessment.

It is important to conduct the clinical interview in an empathic manner that will put the patient at ease and gain their trust, because it is only when the patient feels understood that they are likely to divulge very personal and important information. It is not possible for a clinician to hypothesise about a possible diagnosis if they have only some of the necessary information.

Behavioural assessment

This process makes use of **direct observation** in order to assess formally an individual's thoughts, feelings, and behaviour in a specific context. This process may be more appropriate when a clinician assesses someone who is not old enough or who is unable (due to the nature of their disorder or cognitive deficits) to report their problems and/or experiences (Greene & Ollendick, 2000). This type of assessment can be conducted by going to the patient's workplace or home (or school, in the case of young children), or by setting up a role-play simulation in a clinical setting to observe how the individual might behave in similar situations.

In a behavioural assessment, one would identify the specific behaviour one wants to observe (the **target behaviour**) in order to determine what influences it. One would focus on the antecedent (what happened just before the behaviour), then one would focus on the behaviour itself, and then on the consequences (what happened directly after the behaviour) (Greene & Ollendick, 2000).

EXAMPLE

Behavioural assessment

Mr Grant complains that his daughter is naughty. Upon observing, one would see that Mr Grant asks his daughter to complete her homework (antecedent). His daughter then proceeds to scream and run out of the house to hide in the garden, where she continues to scream at her father (behaviour). Mr Grant tries to placate his daughter and offers her all kinds of treats if she will just do some of her homework (consequence). One can see that the request to do homework triggers the behaviour and the consequence encourages (reinforces) rather than stops the behaviour.

People can also observe their own behaviour using a technique called **self-monitoring** (Haynes, 2000). Here the individual can, for example, record the number of sweets they ate on a particular day and note what occurred before the sweet-eating in order to identify what triggers the sweet-eating behaviour.

Behaviour-rating scales can also be used in order to assess the behaviour and then to assess changes in the person's behaviour. For example, the Brief Psychiatric Rating Scale assesses 18 areas of concern and can be completed by hospital staff (Lezak, 1995).

One needs to note that awareness of being observed (reactivity) can distort any observational data. Any time one observes how people behave, one's presence can cause them to alter their behaviour. The same is true when people observe their own behaviour.

ACTIVITY

Behaviour diary

Pick a certain behaviour that you would like to change, and then monitor it according to the following example.

Example: Not getting enough sleep (insomnia). In this example, it becomes clear how anxiety and behaviour affect the person's sleep pattern. If one keeps a diary such as the one below, it often becomes easy to identify patterns, and possible causes, of behaviour.

	Hours of sleep	Activities before bedtime	Thoughts and feelings when going to bed
Monday	6	Watched television till 23h00. Drank 3 cups of coffee while watching television.	Thinking about Psychology test on Friday
Tuesday	5	Studied until 22h00. Drank 500 ml carbonated cold drink	Worried about test and that I'm not getting enough sleep
Wednesday	5	Studied until 22h00. Drank 500 ml carbonated cold drink	Worried about test and that I'm not getting enough sleep
Thursday	3	Studied until 03h00. Drank 1 l carbonated cold drink, 3 cups of coffee and other energy drinks	Keep worrying that I have not studied enough and keep going through the work in my mind.
Friday	10	Had supper and a hot shower and then went to bed	None – too tired

MEDICAL ASSESSMENTS

Physical examination

It is necessary to recommend a physical examination since many medical conditions can mimic the symptoms of a psychological disorder (see Appendix A). For example, an overactive thyroid can produce symptoms common in most anxiety disorders. It is thus important to rule out a medical condition before making a psychological or psychiatric diagnosis which may lead to an incorrect treatment programme (Kaplan & Sadock, 2007).

Neuro-imaging

This technique allows us to take accurate pictures of the brain's structure and function. When looking at the **structure** of the brain, we look at the size or shape of the various parts and whether there is any damage. When looking at the function**,** we look at metabolic activity and blood flow (Andreasen & Swayze, 1993).

The first technique for examining **brain structure** was developed in the early 1970s and made use of multiple X-rays of the brain taken from different angles. These X-rays are attenuated differentially by tissues of different densities and the degree of attenuation is picked up by detectors. A computer then reconstructs pictures of 'slices' of the brain. This procedure takes about 15 minutes and is called a **Computerised Axial Tomography** (CAT) scan (see Figure 1.7). It is non-invasive and is useful for locating brain tumours and injuries. However, it does involve repeated X-rays and can pose some risk of cell damage (Andreasen & Swayze, 1993).

Figure 1.7: Computerised Axial Tomography (CAT) scan

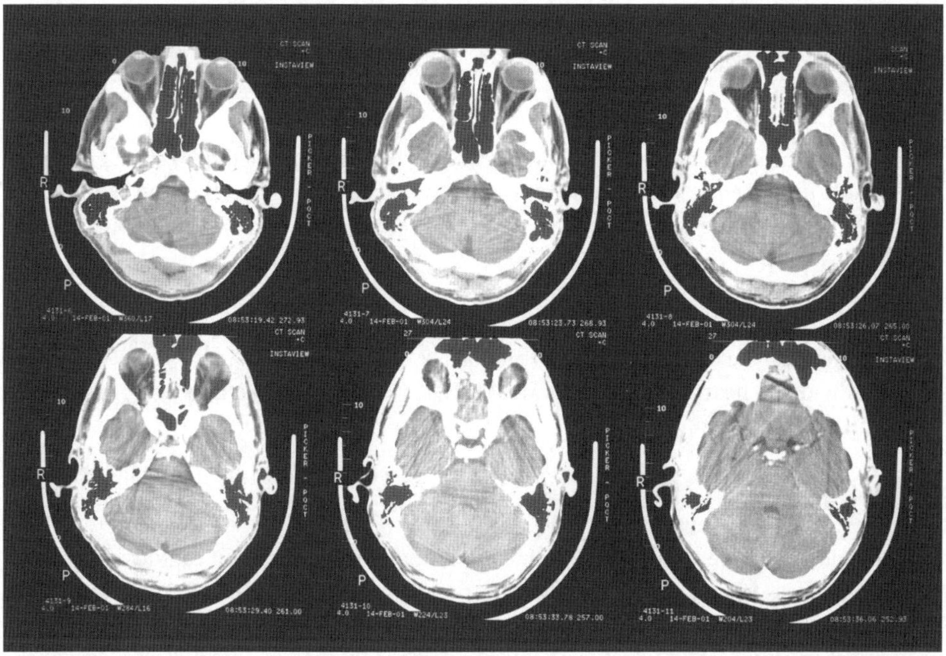

A more recent procedure that gives greater resolution without the risk of X-rays is nuclear **Magnetic Resonance Imaging** (MRI). Here a patient's head is put in a high-strength magnetic field through which radio frequency signals are then transmitted. These signals alter the protons in the hydrogen atoms and the alteration is measured, together with the time taken for the protons to return to normal. This procedure is very expensive and cannot be used if the patient suffers from claustrophobia (Andreasen & Swayze, 1993).

In order to measure **brain function**, several procedures can be used. The first procedure is known as the **Positron Emission Tomography** (PET) scan. Here the individual is injected with a tracer substance attached to radioactive isotopes. This substance then interacts with glucose, blood, or oxygen. When any part of the brain becomes active, the glucose, blood, or oxygen flow to these areas of the brain and detectors can then identify the location of the isotopes. In this way, we can see which parts of the brain are working and which parts are not working. PET scans are useful for supplementing MRI and CAT scans in localising sites of trauma. The PET scan can also be used to identify varying patterns of metabolism that might be associated with different disorders (Andreasen & Swayze, 1993).

Another procedure used to assess brain function is known as **Single Photon Emission Computed Tomography** (SPECT). It is similar to a PET scan, but a different tracer substance is used. It is less accurate than a PET scan; however, it is less expensive than a PET scan and therefore is used more often (Andreasen & Swayze, 1993).

A **functional MRI** (fMRI) is an advanced and very quick technique used to take pictures of the brain at work and to record changes in the brain from one second to the next (Andreasen & Swayze, 1993). An fMRI is a specialised type of MRI scan. It measures the dynamic regulation of the blood flow in the brain, which is related to neural activity in the brain or spinal cord of humans or other animals. It is one of the newest methods of neuro-imaging. It does not expose the patient to radiation, is minimally invasive and widely available and, for these reasons, has come to be the preferred means of brain mapping (Andreasen & Swayze, 1993).

Psycho-physiological assessment

This refers to the measurement of changes in the nervous system that may reflect emotional or psychological events. The measurements can be taken either directly from the brain or from other parts of the body. There are several different ways of measuring these changes (Andrasik, 2000):

- An electroencephalogram (EEG) measures brain wave activity. This can be done while the person is awake or asleep. EEG patterns are often affected by psychological or emotional factors and can be an index of these reactions.
- An individual's heart rate, electrodermal activity (sweat gland activity), and respiration can also be measured.

PSYCHOLOGICAL TESTING

Psychological tests are used to determine emotional, behavioural, or cognitive responses that could be associated with a specific disorder. Generally, the topic of assessment elicits suspicion and confusion in the minds of many due to the tainted history of psychological assessment in South Africa. This is mainly due to the fact that, in the past, very few of the tests were normed on the diverse population in South Africa. This led to the inappropriate use of norms for certain subgroups (Louw & Allen, 1996). The criticism and suspicion of psychological assessment is, in many instances, not unwarranted. The misuse of assessment by both trained and untrained people is significant, and many serious injustices have been, and still are, perpetrated in assessment processes (Saunders, 2008).

Although there are many forms of assessment and many different contexts within which assessment occurs, we will be focusing on testing only in clinical settings (i.e. those settings where one assesses in order to make an accurate diagnosis). In these settings, many different assessment methodologies apply and each of these may require different qualifications and skills. All behavioural and personality-based assessments must be carried out by a registered psychologist with skills and experience in assessment in a cross-cultural context, as this is the nature of the assessment environment in South Africa (Saunders, 2008). Although psychological testing falls mainly in the realm of psychology, many other mental health care professionals (for example, social workers, nurses, and occupational therapists) may make use of some tests. It must be stressed, however, that the use of psychological tests is regulated by legislation, and in some instances it is stipulated that only trained and registered psychologists may use certain tests as specified and legislated by the Health Professions Council of South Africa (HPCSA) (see Appendix A).

One may very well ask why the use of tests is so strictly legislated, but the answer is actually quite simple. Assessment is not an exact science, and tests are not always procedure-bound (that is, sometimes the test instructions do not give specific formulae or techniques). Assessment often requires a great deal of skill and experience to be exercised by a trained expert. If used incorrectly, tests may produce **false negatives** or **false positives** (these concepts will be discussed in more detail later on in this chapter).

According to Saunders (2008), advanced tests in particular, require substantial skill and expertise. These advanced tests include intelligence tests, personality tests, and projective and other diagnostic tests, and they should only be carried out by:

- ***Registered psychologists:*** These are trained professionals, registered with the HPCSA, who are required to use their knowledge and specialist expertise to select, use, and interpret the required assessment instruments. These professionals rely on their knowledge and understanding of the theory of human behaviour.
- ***Psychometrists:*** A psychometrist is a person who has received training in psychology with an emphasis on tests and measurement. The basic function of a psychometrist is to administer and score psychological tests under the direct supervision of an appropriately registered psychologist. Psychometrists are also required to record responses accurately and score tests using appropriate norms. Psychometrists keep note of test behaviour, especially any behaviours which might affect test results. Psychometrists must be competent in the use of a variety of tests in order to assess intelligence, personality, aptitude, achievement, comprehension, memory, perception, and motor skills. They should be aware of ethical issues regarding patient confidentiality, protection of test security, and constraints on dual relationships with patients.
- ***Trained allied professionals:*** Social workers, occupational therapists, and nurses are allowed to be involved in the administrative elements of some instruments. These include test administration and the marking and recording of results. These professionals ought to be trained, supervised, and mentored by a qualified, registered psychologist, due to the fact that the principles and ethics of assessment are the same regardless of what element of competence is being assessed.

Psychological tests have to be reliable as well as valid in order for the results to be of any use to the clinician. There are a number of different types of psychological tests, including intelligence tests, personality inventories, projective tests, and neuropsychological tests.

Culture and assessment

One of the major challenges to psychological testing is the influence of cultural factors on test results. In order to overcome these problems, psychologists aim to construct either culture-free or culture-fair tests (Anastasi & Urbina, 1997). A **culture-free test** is a test that aspires to minimise the effects that culture may have on a person's performance on the test. Although this is the ideal, it seems difficult, if not impossible, to construct a test that is not affected by culture. Furthermore, it is often difficult to determine whether such a test is truly culture-free. A **culture-fair test** is designed to be free of cultural bias, as far as possible, so that no one culture has an advantage over another. The test is designed so as not to be influenced by verbal ability, cultural climate, or educational level. The purpose of a culture-fair test is to eliminate any social or cultural advantages, or disadvantages, that a person may have due to their upbringing. The test can be administered to anyone, from any nation, speaking any language. A culture-fair test may help identify learning or emotional problems (Anastasi & Urbina, 1997).

These tests are designed to assess intelligence, personality, attitudes, interests, and a multitude of other attributes, without relying on knowledge specific to any individual cultural group. They rely largely on non-verbal questions, in order to accommodate English-additional-language speakers. An important issue for assessment of these people is that they are likely to lack familiarity both with the English language and with Western culture. Culture-fair testing is a timely issue, given current debate over bias in intelligence and educational testing. This is so because such testing particularly affects students who can speak and write English, but who are unfamiliar with white, middle-class culture (Anastasi & Urbina, 1997).

Bias in intelligence testing has an historical precedent in early tests which were designed to exclude people from schools, universities, professions, and jobs on the grounds of intellectual abilities. Critics of current tests claim that they discriminate against some ethnic groups in similar ways, in that the tests call for various types of knowledge unavailable to those outside the middle-class cultural mainstream. Although culture-fair tests do reduce differences in performance between Western people and non-Western people who are members of minority groups, the latter still lag behind in the standard tests in predicting success in school, suggesting that in their quest for academic success, members of minority groups must overcome cultural barriers that extend beyond those encountered in IQ tests (Groth-Marnat, 1999).

Intelligence tests

Wechsler considered intelligence to be a global concept involving the ability to act with purpose, to think in a rational manner, and to deal with the environment in an effective way (Groth-Marnat, 1999). Most definitions of intelligence include the following areas: abstract thinking; learning from experience; solving problems through insight; adjusting to new situations; and focusing and sustaining the ability to achieve a desired goal (Groth-Marnat, 1999).

Intelligence Quotient (IQ) tests are very good predictors of academic performance and intelligence tests are quite accurate in predicting future behaviour such as educational achievement, job performance, and earning potential. Intelligence tests also provide clinicians with baseline measures that can be used to determine the degree of change that has occurred in an individual over time, or to determine how the individual compares with other people in a certain area or ability (Groth-Marnat, 1999). However, one needs to be careful not to see the individual simply as their IQ score; people are capable of more cognitive abilities than can be measured on intelligence tests (Frederiksen, 1986). In addition, aspects like emotional intelligence are important for successful functioning in society.

In order to assess intellectual functioning or intellectual disability, the clinician can make use of the **Wechsler Adult Intelligence Scale** (WAIS). The current edition of this test is the

WAIS-III, which has norms for use with South Africans. This instrument contains verbal scales, which measure knowledge of facts, vocabulary, verbal reasoning skills, short-term memory, and abstract thinking ability. The WAIS also contains performance scales, which measure psychomotor ability, ability to learn new relationships, planning ability, and non-verbal reasoning (Tulsky, Zhu, & Prifitera, 2000).

When an individual does not have functional language or is from a culture for which there is no appropriate instrument, one can make use of a non-verbal test such as the **Raven's Standard Progressive Matrices** (RSPM) (Groth-Marnat, 1999). This test emphasises non-verbal tasks and assesses abstract thinking ability and ability to reason, as well as giving an IQ score. Thus, this test can also be used to supplement findings from the WAIS.

Personality inventories

The basic components of personality are called traits, which the DSM-5 defines as enduring patterns of perceiving, relating to, and thinking about the environment and oneself that are exhibited in a wide range of social and personal contexts (American Psychiatric Association, 1994). There is an assumption that if one is able to typify someone's personality, then it will be possible to identify the causes of, as well as predict, that person's future behaviours (Angleitner & Ostendorf, 1994). Linked to this assumption is the notion that a personality disorder (see Chapter 12) is a mental illness with consequences similar to those of other major psychiatric disorders such as Schizophrenia (Angleitner & Ostendorf, 1994).

It is possible to evaluate an individual's personality by a detailed clinical interview (as described above) and by administering a personality test. It is beyond the scope of this section to review the large number of tests that can be used, so we will focus on two that have gained wide acceptance, the **Minnesota Multiphasic Personality Inventory-2** (MMPI-2) and the **Millon Clinical Multiaxial Inventory III** (MCMI-III) (Groth-Marnat, 1999).

Minnesota Multiphasic Personality Inventory-2 (MMPI-2)

The MMPI-2 is a standardised questionnaire that draws out a broad range of self-descriptions that are then scored to give a quantitative assessment of an individual's level of emotional adjustment and attitude toward test-taking (Groth-Marnat, 1999).

The MMPI-2 can be administered to individuals who are 16 years old or older (Groth-Marnat, 1999). The MMPI-2 consists of 567 statements that can be answered as true or false, based on whether or not the individual agrees with the statement. The individual responses are not examined, however; rather, the pattern of responses is evaluated to see whether it resembles patterns from groups of individuals who have specific disorders (Groth-Marnat, 1999. Each group is represented on separate standard scales (Butcher, Graham, Williams, & Ben Porath, 1990). These scales represent measures of personality traits rather than diagnostic categories (Groth-Marnat, 1999) (see Figure 1.8).

The content for most of the questions is quite obvious as it deals with psychological, neurological, psychiatric, and physical symptoms (Groth-Marnat, 1999). Some of the questions are obscure in the sense that the underlying process they are assessing is not intuitively obvious (Groth-Marnat, 1999). The MMPI-2 is extremely reliable when it is interpreted according to standardised procedures, and its validity with a wide range of psychological problems has been attested to by a large number of studies (Butcher, 2000).

Figure 1.8: MMPI-2 profile showing differences between Bipolar Disorder and Schizophrenia

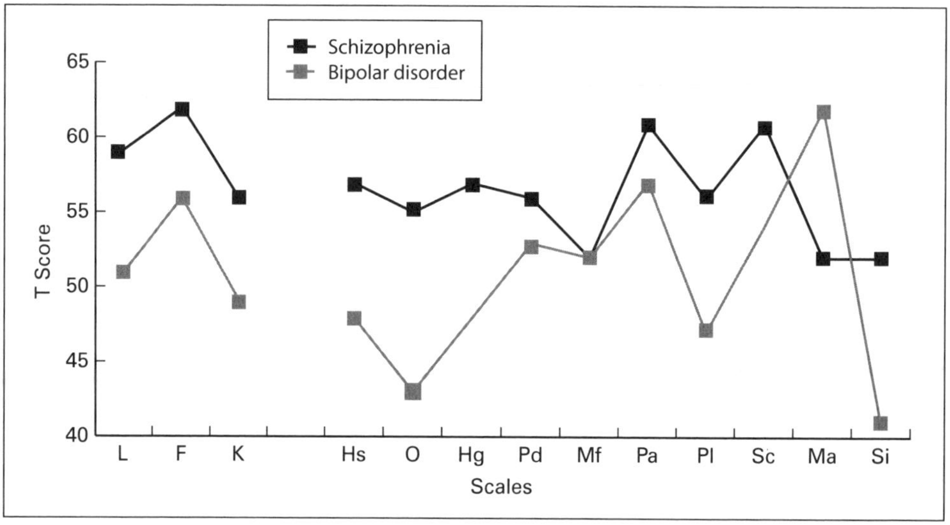

Source: Adapted from Korean Journal of Biopsychiatry.

Millon Clinical Multiaxial Inventory-III (MCMI-III)

The MCMI-III is a standardised self-report questionnaire which comprises 175 statements that can be answered as true or false, based on whether or not the individual agrees with the statement. As with the MMPI-2, it is the pattern of responses that is evaluated in order to determine whether it bears a resemblance to patterns from groups of individuals who have specific disorders. Scoring the instrument produces 28 scales that are divided into five categories, namely, Modifying Indices, Clinical Personality Patterns, Severe Personality Pathology, Clinical Syndromes, and Severe Syndromes (Groth-Marnat, 1999). These scales are closely associated with Millon's theory of personality (Millon, 1969; Millon & Davis, 1996) and the DSM-5.

The MCMI-III can be administered to individuals who are 18 years old or older and it is used to assess a broad range of information related to an individual's personality, emotional adjustment, and attitude towards taking tests. This instrument is distinctive in that it focuses on personality disorders together with symptoms that are normally associated with these disorders (Groth-Marnat, 1999).

The MCMI-III can be used as an alternative to the MMPI-2 or to complement it as both these instruments cover an extensive range of adult pathology (clinical symptomatology and chronic personality patterns). The MMPI-2 focuses on Axis I disorders and the MCMI-III focuses on Axis II disorders (Groth-Marnat, 1999).

Projective tests

Our unconscious processes have the ability to influence psychological disorders (Kaplan & Sadock, 2007). Hence, some way of assessing these unconscious thoughts and feelings was needed, and so assessment measures known as projective tests were developed. Projective tests either present a wide variety of ambiguous stimuli to an individual who is asked to describe what they see, or they ask the individual to draw something. The theory behind these techniques is that people tend to project their own personality and fears onto other people and objects, in this case onto the ambiguous stimuli or drawing, without realising that they are doing so (Watkins, Campbell, Nieberding, & Hallmark, 1995). Although there are many different projective techniques, the most widely used ones include the **Rorschach Inkblot Test**, the **Thematic Apperception Test**, the **Draw-A-Person Test**, and the **Kinetic Family Drawing Test**.

Rorschach Inkblot Test

The test consists of ten cards, each with a bilaterally symmetrical inkblot printed on it (see Figure 1.9). The individual is simply asked to tell the clinician what they see (Groth-Marnat, 1999). The aim of using this technique is to assess the structure of the personality, paying particular attention to how the individual constructs their experience (cognitive structuring) and what meaning they assign to their perceptual experience (Weiner, 1994). The idea behind this instrument is that an individual organises environmental stimuli according to their specific needs, motives, and conflicts. When confronted by ambiguous stimuli, the need for organisation becomes greater. Hence the individual makes use of their own internal ideas, images, and relationships in order to create a response. The manner in which an individual organises their responses to the inkblots is representative of how they will confront any other ambiguous situation. Scoring and interpreting the Rorschach is extremely complex and requires extensive training (Groth-Marnat, 1999).

Figure 1.9: Example of Rorschach-type inkblot

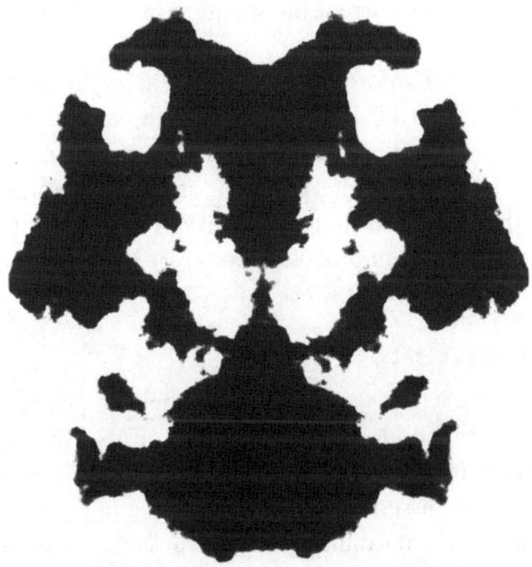

Supporters of the Rorschach Inkblot Test believe that the subject's response to an ambiguous and neutral stimulus can provide insight into their thought processes, but it is not clear how this occurs. There is still considerable controversy around the use of this instrument (Wood, Nezworski, Lilienfeld, & Garb, 2003). The criticisms relating to this are based mainly on quantitative psychometric theory and include, *inter alia,* aspects such as the subjectivity of the interpretation of results, and the reliability (more specifically, the inter-rater reliability) and validity of the test.

The Exner Scoring System has addressed many of these criticisms with an extensive body of research (Exner, 2002). This system of scoring (also known as the 'Comprehensive System') is meant to address problems related to the validity of the test, and has become the scoring system of choice; however, disagreements about test validity remain.

Wood et al. (2003) maintain that, despite the criticisms, there is substantial research supporting the usefulness of some of the scores on this test. For example, there is some evidence that the Deviant Verbalisations scale relates to Bipolar Disorder. Further examples of its usefulness include:

- Several scores correlate well with general intelligence
- Validity has also been shown for detecting such conditions as Schizophrenia and other psychotic disorders, thought disorders, and personality disorders.

One of the major threats to the reliability of the Rorschach is in the detail of the testing procedure, such as:

- Where the tester and subject are seated
- Any introductory words
- Verbal and non-verbal responses to subjects' questions or comments
- How responses are recorded.

Although Exner has published detailed instructions, Wood et al. (2003) cite many instances where the proper prescribed testing and scoring procedures have not been followed.

Thematic Apperception Test (TAT)

This instrument consists of a series of 20 cards, 19 of which have pictures and one of which is blank. The individual is asked to tell a story about what they think is happening in each picture, as well as what the characters might be thinking and feeling (Groth-Marnat, 1999). The purpose of the TAT is to reveal the emotions, sentiments, drives, and conflicts of the individual being assessed (Morgan, 1995). The TAT presents more structured stimuli than the Rorschach and hence tends to elicit more complex and organised responses (Groth-Marnat, 1999). The TAT also looks at the individual's current life situation rather than the underlying personality structure (Morgan, 1995).

The findings on the TAT can provide valuable information supplementary to other psychological test results, due to the fact that the TAT is able to elicit rich, varied, and multifaceted information, as well as personal data that the individual may consciously resist divulging (Groth-Marnat, 1999). Owing to the fact that interpretation of the TAT stories is more qualitative than quantitative, and therefore also quite subjective, it is difficult to determine this instrument's reliability. The reliability improves, however, if one uses the quantitative scoring methods that are available (Murstein, 1972).

Neuropsychological assessment

One very important area in clinical practice is the screening for, and assessment of, possible neuropsychological impairment or brain dysfunction (Goldstein, 2000). This type of screening might be necessary when an individual has suffered some kind of head injury and the extent of damage to the brain needs to be assessed. This may be done in order to determine eligibility for workman's compensation, a disability grant and/or compensation from the Road Accident Fund. There are other situations where a neuropsychological screening or assessment might be useful. These would include: determining whether an individual is suffering from depression or organically based dementia, determining why an individual is performing badly at work or school, working with someone who has been abusing drugs or alcohol, and so forth.

When preparing to do a neuropsychological assessment the clinician has two options. One option is to administer one of the existing, standardised batteries such as the **Luria-Nebraska Neuropsychological Battery** or the **Halstead-Reitan Neuropsychological Battery** (Lezak, 1995), both of which offer a complex and comprehensive battery of tests to assess a variety of skills. Alternately, they can compile their own battery of neuropsychological tests based on the functions that they want to assess.

The Luria-Nebraska Neuropsychological Battery (LNNB)

The LNNB is based on Luria's theory of higher cortical functioning (Luria, 1966). Luria's examination techniques were originally organised into a battery by Christensen and, subsequently, items from this battery were selected by Golden based on whether they were able to discriminate between normal individuals and neurologically impaired patients (Golden, 1981). The LNNB produces eleven scores, namely: Motor Functions, Rhythm, Tactile Functions, Visual Functions, Receptive Speech, Writing, Reading, Arithmetic, Memory, and Intellectual Processes; optional scales are Spelling and Motor Writing (Lezak, 1995).

In order to determine whether or not there is brain damage, an individual's score on each of the battery's eleven clinical scales is compared to a critical level appropriate for that person's age and education level. For example, if the individual has five to seven scores above the critical level, they most likely have some sign of neurological impairment. If they have eight or more scores above the critical level, this indicates a clear history of neurological disorder (Lezak, 1995).

There is controversy surrounding the LNNB's reliability and validity. The LNNB has been criticised by some researchers on the grounds that it tends to overestimate the degree of neuropsychological impairment (i.e. it gives false positives); in other cases, it has failed to detect neuropsychological problems (i.e. it gives false negatives) (Adams, 1984). Another criticism is that the Intellectual Processes scale has not been found to correspond well with other measures of intelligence, for example, the Wechsler Adult Intelligence Scale (WAIS) (Crosson & Warren, 1982). Other research, however, has found the LNNB to be a useful measure for distinguishing between brain-damaged individuals and non-brain-damaged individuals with psychiatric problems (Lezak, 1995).

The Halstead-Reitan Neuropsychological Battery (HRNB)

The Halstead-Reitan Neuropsychological Battery (HRNB) began as a battery of seven tests that were apparently able to discriminate between individuals with frontal lobe lesions, individuals with other lesions, and normal individuals (Lezak, 1995). The HRNB is able to evaluate a wide range of nervous system and brain functions, including: visual, auditory, and tactual input; verbal communication; spatial and sequential perception; the ability to analyse information, form mental concepts, and make judgments; motor output; and attention, concentration, and memory (Lezak, 1995). The battery also provides useful information regarding the cause of damage (for example, closed head injury, alcohol abuse, Alzheimer's disorder, stroke, etc.), which part of the brain was damaged, whether the damage occurred during childhood, and whether the damage is getting worse, staying the same, or getting better. Information regarding the severity of impairment and areas of personal strengths can be used to develop plans for rehabilitation or care (Lezak, 1995). The HRNB consists of the Category Test, the Tactual Performance Test, the Rhythm Test, the Speech Sounds Perception Test, the Finger Tapping Test, the Trail Making Test, and the Aphasia Screening Test (Lezak, 1995).

Due to its complexity, the HRNB needs to be administered by a professional examiner and interpreted by a trained psychologist. Test results can be affected by the examinee's age, education level, intellectual ability, and, to some extent, gender or ethnicity, which should always be taken into account. Owing to the fact that the HRNB is a fixed battery of tests, some unnecessary information may be gathered, or some important information may be missed. Overall, the battery requires five to six hours to complete. There is controversy surrounding the HRNB's reliability and validity, and the battery has also been criticised because it does not include specific tests of memory; rather, memory is evaluated within the context of other tests (Lezak, 1995).

False positives, false negatives, and malingering

For any assessment strategy, one has to bear in mind that there may be times when the test results indicate a problem when there is no problem (**false positives**) and times when the results indicate that there is no problem when actually some difficulty does exist (**false negatives**). False results are particularly worrying when one is assessing for brain dysfunction because important medical problems that need to be treated might go unnoticed (Boll, 1985). Because neuropsychological tests are mainly used as screening devices, they should be paired with other assessments in order to improve the likelihood that problems will be identified.

Complicating the process of diagnosis, there will also be times when a person deliberately falsifies their results in the hope that a problem will be diagnosed so that they can gain something (**secondary gain**). This may include getting out of court appearances, receiving monetary compensation, receiving attention from relatives, and so forth (Kaplan & Sadock, 2007). When malingering is suspected, the clinician can make use of the Rey 15-item test and the Forced Choice test, both of which are good indicators of Malingering (Lezak, 1995) (see also Chapter 8).

Arriving at a diagnosis: The use of diagnostic classification systems

The ultimate goal of an assessment would be to arrive at a **multiaxial diagnosis** by using either the DSM or ICD classification systems. The purpose of the aforementioned techniques is both to generate a list of signs and symptoms and to rule out other disorders that could better explain the symptoms with which the person is presenting. This list can then be compared with the diagnostic criteria of either the DSM or ICD classification systems. There are, however, some important points to remember when one arrives at the point of making a diagnosis:

- Both classification systems specify the minimum number of symptoms that need to be present. If the minimum **number of symptoms** is not present, one cannot make the diagnosis (see Figure 1.10).

- In conjunction with the above, both systems specify the minimum **duration of the symptoms** (how long these symptoms must be present before the diagnosis can be made). Once again, if the symptoms have not been present for the minimum time, one cannot make the diagnosis (see Figure 1.10).
- In many cases, there are overlaps between the symptoms in disorders, or a person may display symptoms of more than one disorder. In these cases, the diagnostician will make a **differential diagnosis**, that is, the diagnostician will list all the possible disorders.
- Often the differential diagnosis will include disorders that naturally occur together. We refer to these as co-morbid disorders.
- The classification systems also list the epidemiology of disorders (ages of onset, gender, and cultural statistics), as well as the prognosis (expected outcome or course of a disorder).
- The final diagnosis, which is made on the multi-axial system (as described previously in this chapter) is used to communicate information about the person to other professionals, and this information informs professionals about the treatment or management of the person, as well as the expected course and outcome of the disorder.

Figure 1.10: The interaction between number of criteria and duration of symptoms

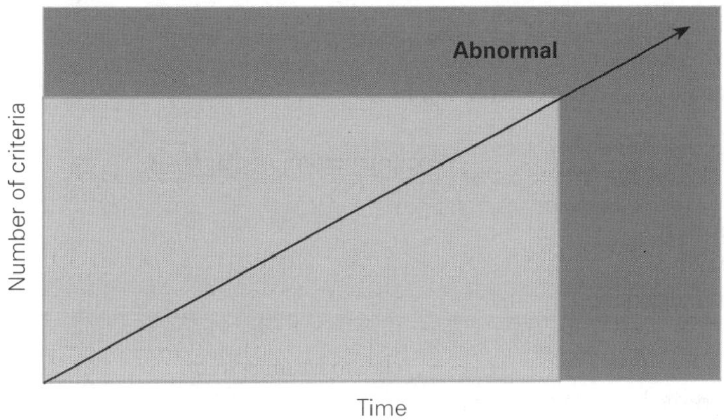

Source: © Burke, 2009.

CONCLUSION

The assessment and diagnostic process involves complicated, and often time-consuming, procedures. It is also not a purely mechanistic process in which a set series of steps are followed. It requires a certain amount of investigative and deductive reasoning, technical skills, and sensitivity to the person's cultural and social background. It is for this reason that only qualified psychologists and medical professionals may make a diagnosis. A diagnosis is important to inform the professionals about treatment and prognosis; however, a diagnosis (especially a misdiagnosis) may also cause a lot of harm. It is therefore important that diagnosticians abide by a strong set of ethical rules (see Chapter 14).

MULTIPLE-CHOICE QUESTIONS

1. According to the criteria of statistical deviance, a behaviour is abnormal when it deviates from:
   a) previous family patterns
   b) the norms of a specified social or cultural group
   c) maladaptiveness
   d) personal distress

2. DSM-5 makes use of ____________ to inform new groupings of related disorders within the existing categorical framework.
   a) brain scans
   b) scientific indicators
   c) educated guesswork
   d) social indicators

3. DSM-5 is organised on:
   a) developmental and lifespan considerations
   b) medical considerations
   c) socio-economic considerations
   d) personality structure considerations

4. DSM-5 utilises a ____________ documentation of diagnosis.
   a) axial
   b) categorical
   c) nonaxial
   d) non dimensional

5. DSM-5 is based on a ____________ classification system.
   a) dimensional
   b) categorical
   c) prototypical
   d) psychoanalytic

6. Which of the following factors is typically NOT part of a clinical assessment?
   a) Psychological
   b) Social
   c) Biological
   d) Astrological

7. In terms of psychological assessment, which of the following describes the concept of validity?
   a) Two or more 'raters' get the same answers.
   b) An assessment technique is consistent across different measures.
   c) Scores are used as a norm for comparison purposes.
   d) An assessment technique measures what it is designed to measure.

8. Which of the following describes an intelligence test?
   a) It determines the possible contribution of brain damage to the person's condition.
   b) It uses imaging to assess brain structure and/or function.
   c) It assesses long-standing patterns of behaviour.
   d) It ascertains the structure and patterns of cognition.

9. As part of a psychological assessment, a mental status exam is used to find out how a person thinks, feels, and behaves; its primary purpose, however, is to determine:
   a) if a psychological disorder might be present.
   b) what type of treatment should be used.
   c) which medication would be most effective.
   d) whether the individual also has a medical condition.

10. Use of the Rorschach test has long been considered controversial because of all of the following concerns EXCEPT:
    a) the test is based on psychoanalytic theory.
    b) there is little or no data regarding its reliability or validity.
    c) the inkblots have been changed many times since the test was developed.
    d) until recently there were no standardised procedures for administering the test.

PARAGRAPH AND ESSAY QUESTIONS

1. Choose a behaviour that you consider abnormal. Using the criteria of maladaptiveness, statistical deviance, and personal distress, consider which criterion best fits the chosen behaviour.

2. Why do we need a classification system for mental illness?
   a) How does the DSM-5 differ from the DSM-IV?
   b) Describe how the DSM and ICD classifications differ.
   c) Describe the major objectives and procedures of clinical assessment.

2 WESTERN AND AFRICAN AETIOLOGICAL MODELS

Karel Botha and Mokgadi Moletsane

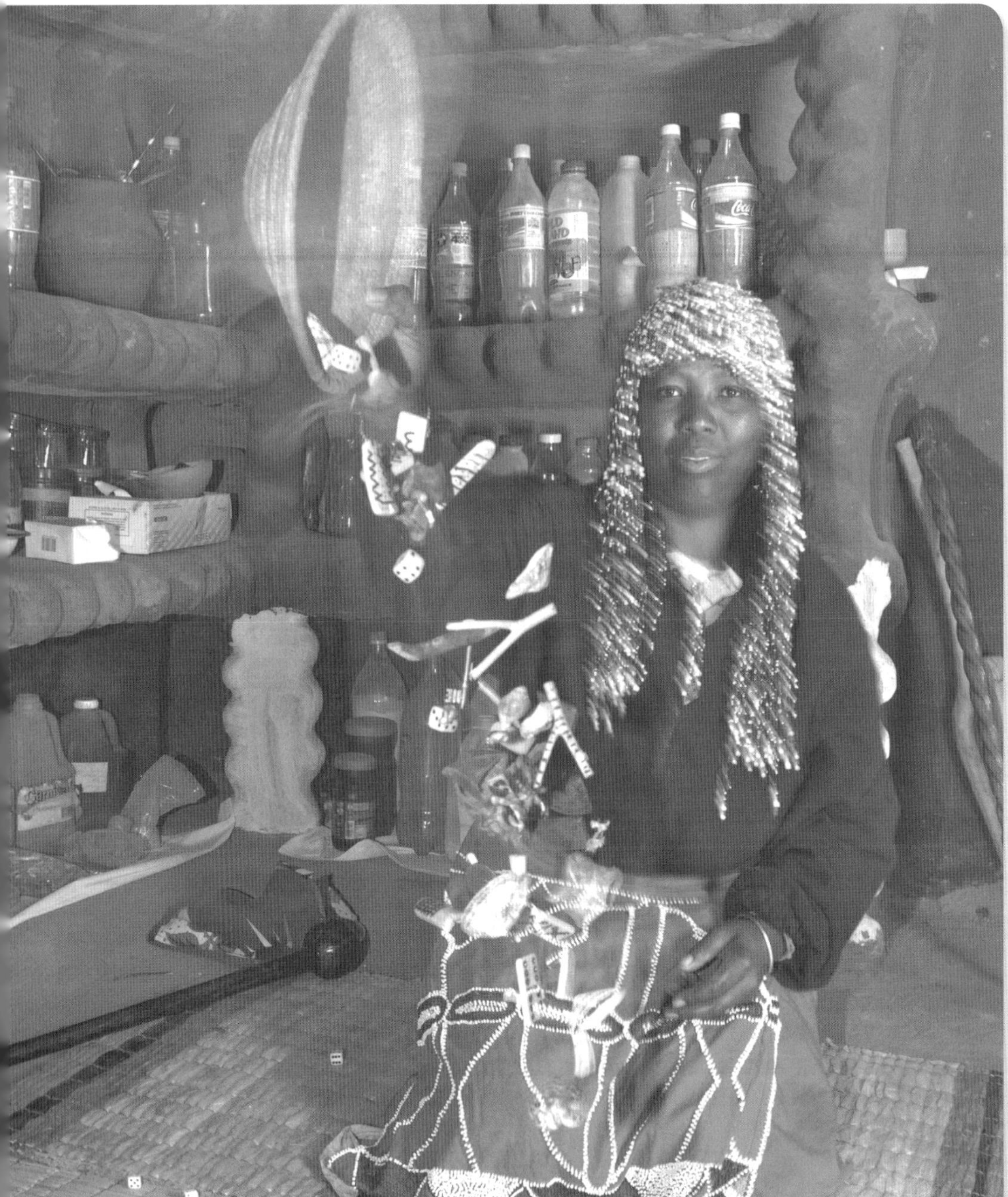

2 CHAPTER OUTLINE

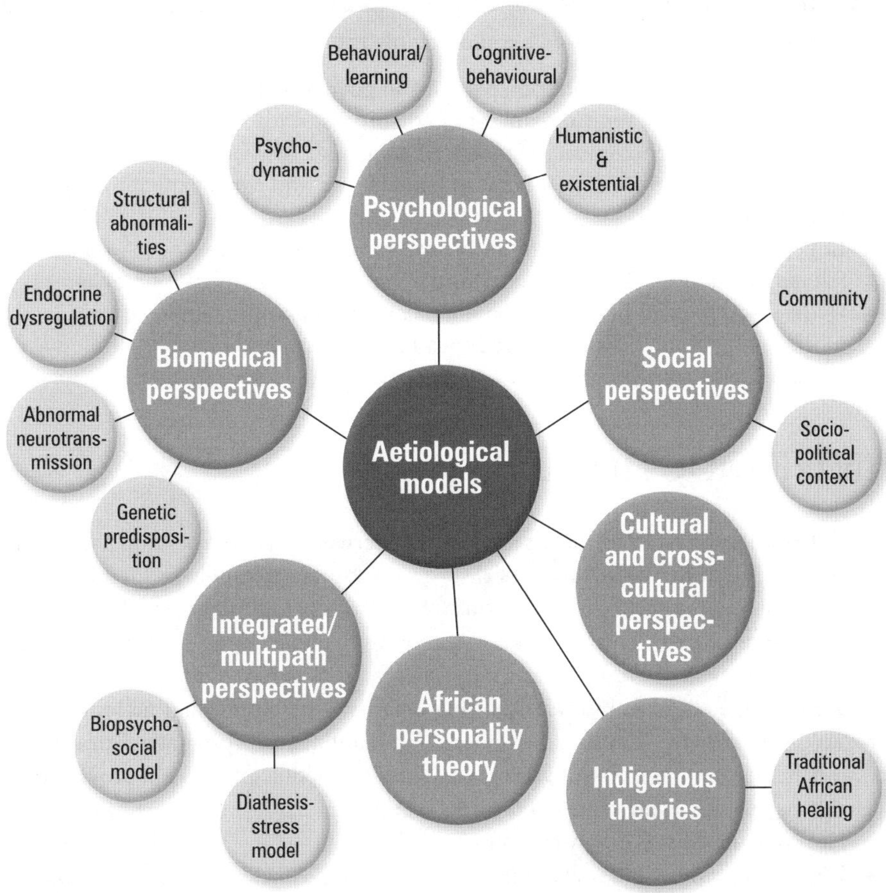

LEARNING OUTCOMES

After studying this chapter, you should be able to:

- Review some of the current perspectives in psychopathology.
- Explain the role of neurotransmitters in disorders.
- Describe the psychological defence mechanisms.
- Understand the importance of cultural awareness and sensitivity in the field of psychology.
- Critically analyse and interpret the African personality model.
- Explain indigenous African understandings of the aetiology of mental illness.
- Understand the use of the biopsychosocial model and the diathesis-stress model as multidimensional approaches to understanding psychopathology.

INTRODUCTION

A central question in abnormal psychology concerns why people develop psychological disorders. The study of the causes of disorders is known as aetiology, literally meaning the study of origination or causation. This is an extremely important area of knowledge in psychology, psychiatry, and medicine, as it helps us to understand what factors contribute to the development of a disorder and how these factors operate. Understanding aetiology thus guides the clinician in understanding a patient's symptoms and making decisions regarding treatment. In a broader sense, it may influence preventative measures and thus help to prevent the onset of disorders. However, aetiology does not provide us with direct answers about the causes of disorders, because:

- Human behaviour is highly complex.
- Disorders are more often than not caused by multiple factors.
- Causal factors change over the lifespan.
- Different causal routes exist for the same disorder (the principle of 'equifinality').
- The same causal route may develop into different disorders.

There are a number of reasons why the study of the aetiology of disorders is important. These include:

- Treatment and management of disorders is often, if not always, informed by the aetiology of the disorder.
- A better understanding of aetiology can also inform categorisation and classification of disorders. An example is that DSM-I and DSM-II were both structured around aetiology, rather than clinical picture (see Chapter 1), and it seems DSM-5 will also classify disorders based on aetiology to a greater extent than in previous editions.
- Studies of aetiology stimulate further research. You will notice that for many disorders, the causes still elude us or are still not fully understood. Examples would include Bipolar Disorders (see Chapter 5) and Autism (see Chapter 13).

When studying the aetiological models in this chapter, it is important to remember that not any one of these models is better than the others, as in most cases each model offers explanations from different perspectives.

Given the fact that psychiatry dominates the discourse in abnormal behaviour, we can expect that the medical model will dominate both the classification and explanations of the aetiology of disorders. Throughout the book, we will investigate the biomedical explanations of the causes of disorders, but focussing on these factors only would provide a limited and one-dimensional view of psychopathology. Jaspers (1962) argues that it is essential to understand abnormal behaviour in its totality. This statement implies that one has to go further than 'mere' biological descriptions, in that one must also investigate all of the factors that contribute to the clinical picture and to the development and maintenance of disorders. For this reason, it is important to describe both macro (e.g. psychodynamic, cognitive-behavioural, behavioural, and humanistic) and micro (uni- and multivariate) psychological understandings of disorders.

One could argue that both the medical and psychological explanations focus quite strongly (to varying extents) on intrapersonal factors, and may exclude external factors. You will notice, however, that for most disorders there are also external factors that influence the development of these disorders. It is therefore important to consider social factors, such as socio-economic, socio-political, and cultural factors; failing to do so will lead to a very superficial understanding of abnormal behaviour. Indeed, one of the aims of this book is to familiarise readers with a cross-cultural, (southern) African view of abnormal behaviour. You will notice that this theme is included in all the chapters; however, in order to understand how these explanations fit into the descriptions of the different disorders, it is imperative to understand the broader African view of abnormal behaviour which will be described in this chapter.

BIOMEDICAL PERSPECTIVES

The biomedical model claims that all mental illnesses have a biological cause. Modern neuro-imaging methods have enabled relatively non-invasive *in vivo* studies of brain structure and function. There are many studies which report abnormalities in shape, size, and function in multiple anatomical regions of the brain, particularly related to the so-called 'neuropathology' of the different disorders; however, structural and functional cerebral abnormalities in most of these disorders are at best subtle rather than gross (Chua & McKenna, 1995). Unfortunately, from this perspective, other factors such as social pressures, type of parenting, or additional environmental factors are seen as secondary in the precipitation of mental disorders (Cartwright, 2008). Biological abnormalities are understood to occur mainly in four different areas: genetic predisposition, abnormal functioning of neurotransmitters, endocrine dysregulation, and structural abnormalities in the brain.

Genetic predisposition

We inherit our genetic predisposition from our parents. Genes, or chemical units, are arranged in a specific order along chromosomes and they are responsible for determining things such as the physical appearance (e.g. eye colour, hair colour) and the sex of an individual. Most of us have 46 chromosomes. Some researchers have found that abnormalities in genetic makeup can predispose some individuals to particular mental illnesses. A great deal of the research in this area has been done on twins because of the genetic makeup they have in common (Cartwright, 2008). It has been found, for instance, that monozygotic twins (twins with the same genetic makeup), whose mother has a mental disorder, have a greater likelihood of both developing mental illness. However, this is not the case with twins who do not share exactly the same genetic makeup (dizygotic twins). Cartwright (2008), citing the works of Gottessman (1991), McGuffin and Katz (1993), and McGue (1993), argues that there is evidence that genetic predisposition plays a role in the development of mental illnesses such as Schizophrenia (see Chapter 6), mood disorders (see Chapter 5), and alcoholism (see Chapter 10).

A common mistake is to simply blame genetic transmission when mental illness seems to run in families. Twin studies and adoption studies are regarded as 'natural experiments' which enable an estimate to be made of the extent to which traits are familial because of shared genes, shared environment, or a combination of both. In recent years, a confusing and apparently contradictory array of studies has reported links with various genes in Schizophrenia (Moldin, 1997). In contrast, the identification and cloning of genes and the clarification of chromosomal abnormalities have led to progress in understanding the molecular biology of genetic neuropsychiatric disorders. For example, in Huntington's disease, the abnormality of triplet repeat on chromosome four has been demonstrated (see Chapter 7).

Multigene (polygenetic) models of inheritance are still commonly regarded as the best model of familial transmission of Schizophrenia (Tsuang, Stone, & Faraone, 2000). There is speculation that the mapping of the human genome will help to develop better treatments for psychiatric illness, and to make discrimination against people with mental disorders a thing of the past (McGuffin & Martin, 1999). However, despite the hype, accurate prediction may never be possible because of the complexity of the genetics of common disorders (Holtzman & Marteau, 2000). Scepticism about the current over-enthusiasm for genetic explanations is required.

Abnormal functioning of neurotransmitters

Neurotransmitters are chemical substances in the brain and are responsible for the communication of nerve impulses among the brain cells (Cartwright, 2008). An increase or decrease in certain neurotransmitters, like dopamine and serotonin, has been found to be associated with a number of psychiatric illnesses (see Table 2.1).

Table 2.1: Summary of role of neurotransmitters in disorders

Neurotransmitter	Pathology
Dopamine	• Over-secretion seems to play a role in Schizophrenia. • Dopamine hypothesis was initially derived from observations that drugs that block dopamine receptors have anti-psychotic results, AND that drugs that stimulate dopamine activity induce psychotic symptoms in people who do not suffer from Schizophrenia. • It seems as if over-secretion is not limited only to Schizophrenia, but is present in all disorders where psychotic symptoms may be present. • It is also implicated in the pathophysiology of mood disorders, where dopamine activity may be low in depression and high in mania.
Serotonin	• Depression is associated with too little serotonin and mania with too much serotonin. • According to the permissive hypothesis, serotonin seems to work in conjunction with norepinephrine, where low levels of serotonin permit abnormal levels of norepinephrine to cause depression and mania.
Norepinephrine	• Norepinephrine in conjunction with serotonin may play a role in the pathophysiology of depression. • The interrelationship between these two neurotransmitters is still unclear.
Gamma Amino Butyric Acid (GABA)	• GABA may play a role in the pathophysiology of anxiety disorders.
Acetylcholine	• The most common association is between degeneration of cholinergic neurons and dementia. • It may also be involved in mood and sleep disorders.

Source: Kaplan, Sadock, & Grebb, 1994.

Theories of neurotransmitter dysfunction arose following the introduction of psychotropic drugs at a time when few neurotransmitters had been discovered. Despite the subsequent discovery of a vastly more complex neurotransmitter network, psychiatrists still use such simplistic notions as a 'chemical imbalance', when they explain mental illness in their everyday management of patients. For example, the dopamine hypothesis of Schizophrenia (dopamine overactivity in schizophrenic brains) arose because neuroleptic drugs, such as chlorpromazine, appear to act via an inhibition of dopamine receptors.

However, measurements of dopamine metabolites *in vivo*, or of the transmitter and its receptors in post-mortem brain tissue, do not provide unequivocal evidence of a hyperactivity of dopaminergic neurotransmission in the disease, which may be because it is difficult to disentangle the iatrogenic effects of the drugs themselves (Reynolds, 1989).

Moreover, many of the newer drugs do not appear to work by dopamine antagonism, raising the question of the nature of atypical antipsychotic medication.

Endocrine dysregulation

According to Kaplan et al. (1994), there seems to be abnormal regulation of the neuro-endocrine axes in some disorders such as mood disorders and Schizophrenia (see Table 2.2). The link between endocrine functioning and the pathophysiology of disorders is, however, still unclear as it is difficult to determine whether endocrine dysregulation is the cause of disorders, or whether the dysregulation is merely due to abnormal brain functions. Kaplan et al. (1994) maintain that the latter may be more accurate, for two reasons:

- The neurotransmitters that are implicated in disorders are also the primary regulators of the neuro-endocrine axes. If this is the case, the implication is that dysregulation of neurotransmitters precedes the dysregulation of hormones.
- Once a disorder is successfully treated, hormonal functioning returns to normal, which seems to imply that endocrine dysfunctions are part of the symptomatology of the disorder, rather than a predisposition or cause of such a disorder.

Table 2.2: The link between selected hormonal axes and disorders

Hormonal axis	Pathophysiology of disorders
Adrenal	This axis responds to stress by increasing the secretion of cortisol which help us adapt to stress.
Thyroid	Absence of thyroid hormone in early infancy leads to mental retardation (cretinism). Administration of thyroid hormone has a brief mood-elevating response in depression.
Growth	Growth hormone dysregulation may be implicated in mood disorders and Schizophrenia.
Prolactin	Release of prolactin is dependent on dopamine release and therefore may be implicated in psychotic disorders
Melatonin	Involved in the regulation of circadian rhythms and has been implicated in the pathophysiology of depression.

Source: Adapted from Kaplan et al. 1994, p.145.

Structural abnormalities

Adolf Meyer (1951/2) was fond of seeing his philosophical approach to psychiatry, with its emphasis on the person, as an advance over the mechanistic approach of the nineteenth century. However, his work was largely neglected as the biomedical discourse in describing and explaining disorders became progressively more dominant. It seems as if reducing a person to merely a brain makes disorders easier to describe and treat, with the result that the philosophical debate around the relationship between mind and brain has dwindled.

The discovery, however, that the adult brain is capable of extensive reorganisation has necessitated a radical revision of traditional notions of anatomical fixity, and has sparked interest and research into the concept of brain plasticity (Castillo, 1998; Eisenberg, 1995). Research has also moved beyond the role of neurotransmitters to the role of neuromodulators and it is becoming abundantly clear that the brain is biochemically able to modify its own responsiveness to incoming stimuli. This implies that the human brain seems to be socially constructed in the literal sense that brain cyto-architecture itself is fashioned by input from the social environment.

Traditionally, structural abnormalities occurring in the brain have also been associated with various disorders. It has been well established that different parts of the brain regulate different aspects of human functioning (see Chapter 7). For instance, it has been found that the limbic system serves to regulate emotional reactions like fear, aggression, and sexual expression. Thus, injuries to these parts of the brain could impair a person's emotional control (Cartwright, 2008). Structural abnormalities in the brain may be caused by a wide variety of factors and may result in a number of disorders (see Chapter 7).

PSYCHOLOGICAL PERSPECTIVES

It is particularly in the field of abnormal behaviour that opposing theoretical paradigms meet head to head. At the one extreme, we have the medical paradigm that maintains that the causes of most of the disorders are biological or physiological in nature. This theoretical approach bases its argument on the fact that there is increasing evidence of the heritability of disorders as well as the efficacy of pharmacological treatments of disorders. At the other extreme, we have the theorists who believe that all disorders are caused by psychosocial factors. The approach in this textbook is that there is room for both these arguments; therefore, it is necessary to investigate psychological theories of disorders.

Psychodynamic approaches

Contemporary psychodynamic approaches are derived from Freud's theory of psychoanalysis. Those who work from a psychoanalytic point of view believe that the way in which we relate to others and ourselves is largely influenced by internal forces that exist outside consciousness. Freud believed that sexual and aggressive instincts, and the associated thoughts and feelings, become repressed and unconscious once they are perceived to be forbidden by society. Freud believed that although such thoughts and feelings are forced into the unconscious, they are still able to exert partial control over the individual by expressing themselves through symptoms. He viewed the formation of psychological symptoms as a compromise between the expression of forbidden wishes and their total repression (Cartwright, 2008).

Freud viewed the personality as being divided into three parts: the id, the ego, and the superego. He used the term 'id' to refer to instincts and drives, the term 'ego' to refer to the part of the psyche that attempts to control the expression of the id, and the term 'superego' to refer to a person's conscience and the ability to distinguish between right and wrong. Freud believed that the formation of these mental structures was strongly influenced by early childhood experiences and the quality of the child's relationship with their parents (Cartwright, 2008).

According to Cartwright (2008), this paradigm understands psychopathology to occur for two main reasons. Firstly, psychological disorders emerge when conflict between the id, the ego, and the superego give rise to distressing symptoms. Secondly, mental disorders emerge when deficiencies in the ego hinder the individual's ability to repress instinctual drives. In both cases, the individual makes use of psychological defence mechanisms (see Table 2.3) in an attempt to ward off excessive psychological pain and repressed fears.

Table 2.3: Examples of psychological defence mechanisms

Defence mechanism	Description
Displacement	One way to avoid the risk associated with feeling unpleasant emotions is to displace them, or put them somewhere other than where they belong. You may be angry with a lecturer for a poor mark but be unable to express it, so you go home and get angry with your mother instead. This is an example of displacement.
Sublimation	Sublimation is the healthy redirection of an emotion. For example, when receiving a bad mark, you may choose to direct more energy into your studies rather than getting angry with your mother.
Projection	Projection is something we all do. It is the act of taking something of ourselves and placing it outside us, onto others. Sometimes we project positive and sometimes negative aspects of ourselves. Sometimes we project things we don't want to acknowledge about ourselves (for example, 'I have not made a mistake; it is you who are critical of me and everything I do').
Intellectualisation	Intellectualisation involves removing the emotion from emotional experiences, and discussing painful events in detached, uncaring, sterile ways. Individuals may know all the words that describe feelings, but have no idea what they really feel like.
Denial	Denial is the refusal to acknowledge what has happened, is happening, or will happen (for example, when a man's wife is having an affair but he says she is not).
Repression	Repression involves unconsciously putting painful thoughts and memories out of our minds and forgetting about them.
Suppression	Suppression involves consciously trying to put painful thoughts and memories out of our minds and forget about them.
Reaction-formation	When we have a reaction that is too painful or threatening to feel (such as intense hate for someone with power over us), we turn it into the opposite (intense liking for that person). Another example of reaction-formation would be if you were behaving very badly towards someone because you really liked them.

Source: Cartwright, 2008, p. 462.

In contemporary psychodynamic thinking, the fundamental ideas remain the same as in the original psychoanalytic theory: human actions and experiences are seen to be strongly influenced by unconscious processes (Frude, 1998). However, the psychodynamic model has developed in many diverse ways over the years (Frude, 1998). For instance, the work of Melanie Klein (1882–1960) emphasises the importance of internalised object relations in the development of the personality. Internal objects are essentially mental representations that are formed when significant others (or external 'objects') are 'internalised' by the individual, adding to the nature of the personality. Object-relations theorists believe that early relationships, particularly with the mother (or primary caregiver), shape the personality and lay the foundation for other relationships in the person's life (Cartwright, 2008).

Early trauma and/or deprivation are also understood to be key factors in the development of psychopathology. An example of this approach is the attachment theory of John Bowlby (1980), who emphasised bonding between a caregiver and a child, and the long-term effects that the quality and nature of this bond have on relationships (Frude, 1998).

In this way, contemporary psychodynamic approaches, such as the object-relations approach, emphasise the role that emotional relationships and the surrounding environment play in the formation of the personality. The contemporary approaches place less emphasis on the role of instinctual drives than the traditional Freudian approach (Cartwright, 2008).

Behavioural/learning perspectives

The behavioural perspective is mainly influenced by the experimental work of Pavlov, Watson, and Skinner. The fundamental viewpoint is that behaviour is learned through a number of different processes and mechanisms, like habituation, sensitisation, conditioning, and modelling. Habituation refers to the process whereby a person ceases to respond to a stimulus after repeated presentations. It is thus a gradual adaptation to a new situation or stimulus. Although it has an adaptive function, it may also cause maladaptive behaviour, for example, drug addiction. Habituation does not require the person to be aware of the process; it may occur naturally and unconsciously.

Sensitisation, in contrast, refers to an extreme response to a stimulus that holds significant consequences. It is a learning process wherein we become sensitive to pain, sound, smell, and other senses. While sensitisation is a good adaptive learning process of an organism, it can also lead to maladaptive process when the organism is 'sensitised' with harmful stimuli, for example, fear or anxiety.

The process through which a person manages these two opposite influences is called conditioning. Classical conditioning refers to the learning process in which an individual initially associates a stimulus with another (neutral) stimulus, and later responds to the associated stimulus in its absence. For example, when you react nervously to the neighbour's aggressive dog (stimulus), your response is expected and therefore unconditioned (unlearned). However, when another neutral stimulus is paired with the unconditioned stimulus, it may elicit a conditioned response. For example, if the only time you see the dog is when the neighbour opens a screeching garden gate (neutral stimulus) to take it for a walk, you could start to act nervously whenever you hear the screeching gate, even if the dog is not in sight. Your nervous reaction is now conditioned by the screeching gate.

Another example is Posttraumatic Stress Disorder (PTSD) (see Chapter 4) which is often characterised by classically conditioned responses to stimuli such as sounds present at the time of the traumatic event (Charney, Deutsch, Krystal, Southwick, & Davis, 1993). This is why PTSD sufferers tend to avoid situations that remind them of their traumatic experience.

Operant conditioning refers to how an individual gradually learns to achieve a specific goal. A critical factor in this type of conditioning is reinforcement, which can either be obtained by a positive stimulus or reward, or by avoidance of a negative stimulus. If you avoid going outside every time you hear the neighbour's screeching gate, you soon learn that in doing so you don't have to confront the dog. By avoiding the negative stimulus, you are conditioned to stay indoors whenever you hear the screeching gate.

Finally, modeling, based on the work of Albert Bandura, refers to learning that takes place through observation alone, without directly experiencing an unconditioned stimulus or a reward. Through a number of experiments, Bandura demonstrated that children learn and imitate behaviours they have observed in other people through a process of (i) attention – noticing something; (ii) retention – remembering what was noticed; and (iii) reproduction – producing an action that is a copy of what was noticed. From this point onwards, other processes like conditioning may play a role that changes the probability of the behaviour being executed again.

Thus, according to the behavioural perspective, dysfunctional behaviour develops because an individual learns ineffective or dysfunctional responses or fails to learn appropriate, adaptive behaviour. A number of therapeutic approaches, based on the behavioural perspective have been developed, for example, behaviour modification, behaviour therapy, systematic desensitisation, and biofeedback.

Cognitive-behavioural perspective

Central to the cognitive-behavioural perspective is the idea that mental disorders are caused by aspects of the content of thoughts (e.g. biases in thinking) as well as information-processing factors (e.g. biases in perception, cognitive distortions, etc.). There are many variations of this theory, for example, the theories of helplessness (Seligman, 1975) and hopelessness (Beck, 1972), as well as the rational-emotive theory of Ellis (1995). These theorists believe that irrational beliefs and automatic thoughts are primarily responsible for the development of psychopathology (Beck, 1972; Ellis, 1995; Glasser, 1984).

This perspective may explain some types of disorders better than others (see, for example, Chapters 4 and 5). An example would be Beck's (1976) cognitive theory of depression. He suggested that negative automatic thoughts (for example, 'nobody likes me') trigger a negative process that includes cognition, affect, and behaviour. After developing such distorted thoughts, a person would look for ways to confirm these thoughts through adopting negative behaviours (for example, not learning for a test or behaving badly in class). These would, in turn, impact on the person's emotions, making him or her feel more depressed. This sets up a vicious cycle as the more depressed the individual feels, the more negatively they perceive themselves, the world, and the future. This is commonly referred to as the 'cognitive triad' of depression (Beck, 1976). Chapter 5 in this textbook illustrates how cognitive factors play an important role in the development and maintenance of mood disorders.

Humanistic and existential perspectives

A so-called third force in psychology emerged during the middle of the twentieth century, opposing the determinism of both the psychodynamic and behaviourist approaches. This force consists of two broad approaches, the humanistic and existential perspectives.

The principal figures in developing a humanistic approach to psychology were Carl Rogers and Abraham Maslow. The humanistic perspective believes in a person's free will and their ability to choose how to act in different contexts. According to Rogers, each human being lives in a world of his or her own creation and has a unique perception of the world, also known as their phenomenal field (Gross, 2010). It is this perception of external reality that shapes life, and not the external reality itself. The most significant element within the phenomenal field is the sense of self, which, according to Rogers, is constantly in the process of forming and reforming. Maslow, in turn, saw self-actualisation at the peak of a hierarchy of human needs. According to the humanistic perspective, a fully functioning person has achieved self-actualisation, whereas psychopathology develops when a person is blocked from realising his/her potential.

The existential perspective emphasises the uniqueness of each individual, the quest for values and meaning, and the existence of freedom for self-direction and self-fulfilment (Butcher, Mineka, & Hooley, 2010). Although it also emphasises free will and the ability to choose, it is less optimistic than the humanistic approach as it indicates that the socio-political context is often alienating and dehumanising. Rollo May specifically pointed out that the growth in science and technology - think in terms of today's digital age, the internet and social networks – poses a social and emotional threat to the individual, which if not managed constructively, may easily develop into anxiety and eventually, psychopathology. Ronald Laing was another existentialist, who as a psychiatrist, was against what he called the dehumanising science of psychiatry and the focus on medication as a form of treatment.

SOCIAL PERSPECTIVES

Community psychology perspective

Psychologists who are actively involved in the community define community psychology in many ways. Community psychology is defined by Orford (1992, in Pillay, 2003) as understanding people within their social worlds. Trickett's (1996, in Pillay, 2003) definition includes theory, research, and intervention as important components in locating individuals within communities in their sociocultural context while Edwards (1998, p. 70, in Pillay, 2003) defines community psychology as 'psychology of, with and for the people'.

Community psychology focuses on preventing rather than treating dysfunction. According to some writers, sensitivity to under-represented groups, such as those previously disadvantaged, is critical in understanding the community perspectives. Louw and Edward (1993) have criticised the way most South African psychology students are trained according to an American-European model of education and they argue that this needs to be seriously considered by institutions which train psychologists. This concern is echoed by many writers (e.g. Pillay, 2003) who call for training that focuses on prevention and mass intervention and thus prepares mental health care workers to function in the South African community.

Based on the definitions stated above, community psychologists would argue that broad social factors need to be considered if we are to fully understand the development of psychological problems. This would include factors such as the socio-economic status of the community, access to resources, and the nature of social interaction within the community. All these factors impact on the mental health of the individual. From this perspective, problems like violence and sexual abuse cannot be understood unless the social context of the community is also considered.

Community psychology is therefore interested in understanding psychopathology from within the context of the community. As Ahmed and Pretorius-Heuchert (2001, p. 19) state, 'this means that community psychology regards whole communities, and not only individuals, as possible clients. There is an awareness of the interaction between individuals and their environments, in terms of causing and alleviating problems'. Thus, the emphasis here lies on the importance of the social, political, and cultural context in understanding, identifying, and treating psychological problems (Cartwright, 2008).

Many authors (e.g. Castillo, 1998) argue that an individual's actions always take place within a cultural context. How someone experiences distress or makes sense of psychological problems depends on deeply ingrained cultural beliefs and practices. Castillo (1998) maintains that we cannot truly explain a person's normal behaviour (or what is considered in some cultures to be abnormal behaviour) if we do not have an understanding of that individual's cultural background.

For example, Cartwright (2008) cites the examples of Zulu- and Xhosa-speaking communities, where *ukuthwasa* is a psychological state associated with an ancestral calling to become an indigenous healer. Individuals experiencing this condition endure states of emotional turmoil and hear voices (of the ancestors calling the individual to become an indigenous healer) which from a typical Western psychiatric perspective would be considered to be symptoms of Schizophrenia (see Chapter 6). They also experience bouts of depression and mania (i.e. symptoms of a mood disorder; see Chapter 5). If we view this behaviour in isolation (i.e. without taking the person's cultural beliefs into account), we run the risk of making an incorrect diagnosis. This would mean that the individual would not receive the most appropriate treatment.

This should not be taken to mean that mental illness is non-existent in non-Western communities (see Table 2.4). A number of studies using epidemiological research have indicated that psychiatric disorders do exist in non-Western communities (e.g. Asuni, Schoenberg, & Swift, 1994; Swartz, 1998). Understanding how mental illness is experienced and treated in different cultures is also inextricably linked to appreciating concerns about access to treatment (Castillo, 1998). We know, for instance, that indigenous healers from within a particular community are able to reach communities in ways that Western forms of medicine cannot (Swartz, 1998). As well as helping patients gain better access to treatment, community psychologists concern themselves with the prevention of mental illness (and other social problems) by facilitating social change and empowerment in the community.

Table 2.4: Four myths about mental illness in non-Western countries

Mental illness does not exist in developing countries.
Mental illness is not recognised as pathological in non-Western communities.
Mental illness is accepted in non-Western communities in an unstigmatised manner.
All mental disorders can be cured by indigenous healers.

Source: Cartwright, 2008, p. 463.

Another community aspect relates to violence and trauma. Reports indicate that post-apartheid South Africa has extremely high rates of violent crime, sexual violence, and domestic abuse. For example, some surveys have found that South Africa has among the highest incidences of murder, armed robbery, and intimate partner violence (Kaminer, Grimsrud, Myer, Stein, & Williams, 2008). These authors examined the relative risk for Posttraumatic Stress Disorder (PTSD) associated with political, domestic, criminal, sexual, and other forms of assault in the South African population. They found that over one-third of the South African population has been exposed to some form of violence. Among men, political detention, torture, criminal assault, and childhood abuse were the forms of violence most strongly associated with a diagnosis of PTSD, while rape and intimate partner violence had the strongest association with PTSD among women.

Given these problems, community psychologists in South Africa see their role as extending beyond the traditional consulting room to include such diverse practices as consciousness-raising, advocacy, and social upliftment (Gibson & Swartz, 2008). They position themselves in identification with the concerns of the socially and politically disadvantaged members of any society and have the potential to challenge social phenomena that lie at the heart of human unhappiness. Gibson and Swartz (2008) further argue that community psychologists must attempt to resist pathologising and medicalising human problems. According to them, the problems are inevitably intertwined with a particular social or political environment.

Importance of the socio-political context

The previous section has suggested that the discipline of community psychology developed largely out of a need to challenge oppressive forces in society (Seedat, Duncan, & Lazarus, 2001). For this reason, community psychologists are sensitive to the fact that socio-political factors impact on our mental health. Apartheid, for instance, clearly had a tremendous impact on the way that members of the oppressed black population of South Africa perceived themselves. Racist attitudes and policies depicting black South Africans as stupid, lazy, and primitive may have caused many to think negatively of themselves and identify themselves as inferior to the white population, many of whom in turn considered themselves to be superior to all other races.

Many research reviews and reports (Dommisse, 1987; Foster, Freeman, & Pillay, 1997; Holdstock, 1981; Lambley, 1980; Nzimande, 1986; Swartz, 1987; Van der Spuy & Shamley, 1978) highlight the discriminatory and abusive effects of apartheid. Mental health care during the apartheid era was conducted within the discriminatory context of apartheid laws, and Lazarus (1988) described the mental health system as inadequate, inaccessible (particularly for rural communities), inappropriate, and discriminatory. The imbalance in mental health provision is further evident in that the population of psychologists in South Africa remains predominantly white and middle class (see Chapter 14).

In addition, the nature of the mental health services has been criticised for being Eurocentric in its derivation, value base, and orientation (Lazarus, 1988; Naidoo, 1996; Wouters, 1993). The focus on individual curative therapy may not be culturally appropriate or comfortable for all sectors of South African society, especially for those cultures that are more group-oriented (collectivist) (Naidoo, 1996). Psychology in South Africa has been preoccupied with the individual dynamics of psychopathology with its associated practice of individual therapy. But this approach has ignored social determinants of human behaviour and has not examined or confronted the underlying structural societal conditions. This resulted in psychology being seen as maintaining and perpetuating an oppressive economic–political system (Bulhan, 1985; Dawes, 1985; Lazarus, 1988), and psychologists being labelled as the servants of power and more specifically as 'servants of apartheid' (Webster, 1986). Although much has changed in recent years, it is important for the profession to be self-reflective and critical about its approaches and practices.

When one deals with people in a therapeutic context, cultural awareness and sensitivity are of paramount importance. In a multicultural society like South Africa, one would expect that the mental health profession would reflect the demographic characteristics of the country; however, as described above, in South Africa, during the apartheid years, psychologists and psychiatrists were mainly white. These professionals were often far removed from the cultural milieu of their black patients and were often unable even to speak the language of their patients.

In addition to the above, it must be noted that the field of psychological assessment has been plagued by discrimination and exploitation of minority groups. Although scientific studies of behaviour gained momentum towards the end of the nineteenth century (Louw & Edwards, 1993), it was only in 1920, when professors from different universities in South Africa attempted to develop a group intelligence test for South African learners, that this trend reached South Africa. Huysamen, (1980, in Kekae-Moletsane, 2004) states that in 1924, a committee was appointed by the Department of Mines and Industries of the Union of South Africa to develop an intelligence test. As a result, the South African Group Intelligence Test was developed and was published in 1930.

After the introduction of apartheid policies, psychological tests were developed based on racial groupings. The post-apartheid state inherited this system of separate tests designed for racially defined groups. Disappointingly, however, very few of these tests have been standardised for all South Africans, which implies that discrimination still continues to a greater or lesser extent. Given the lack of locally appropriate measures, tests meant for a Westernised population are still used for other cultural groups today, although test users are then obliged to include a caveat specifying that the results may have been influenced by cultural differences. However, this does not necessarily compensate for the reduction in reliability and validity when the cultural appropriateness of those tests remains questionable.

According to Kazarian and Evans (1998, in Kekae-Moletsane, 2004), there is a lack of adequate measures of culture in psychological assessment. Furthermore, there has been a growing concern over the failure of mental health professionals to adequately meet the needs of a culturally diverse society. One of the contributing factors to this, according to Louw and Edwards (1993) is that South African students in psychology are trained mainly according to an American-European model of education. The model is problematic in that it does not address the psychological challenges of the majority of South Africans. Louw and Edwards (1993) further mention that this training is applicable mainly to whites and middle-class black South Africans. However, external pressures are mounting via various professional boards to mobilise psychologists and test developers into actively addressing the problem (Professional Board for Psychology, 1998).

Cross-cultural challenges may also extend to diagnosis, which may be racially skewed. In a study by Freeman (1992) in which 669 records in 17 community clinics were examined, the distribution of diagnoses shown in Table 2.5 and Figure 2.1 was reported.

Table 2.5: Comparison of diagnosis along racial lines

	Black		White		Total	
	N	%	N	%	N	%
Schizophrenia	308	68	41	19	348	52
Mood disorder	41	9	89	41	127	19
Other	104	23	86	40	194	29
Total	453	100	216	100	669	100

Source: Freeman, M. Providing mental health care for all in South Africa – structure and strategy. Johannesburg: Centre for Health Policy, University of the Witwatersrand: 1992, p. 32.

Kale (1995) offers three possible explanations for these differences:

- Black patients are unlikely to receive psychiatric treatment unless they have a serious disorder.
- Black patients are more likely to be diagnosed with Schizophrenia simply because it is believed to be more common among them.
- Black people may not seek psychiatric help possibly due to social prejudice.

Figure 2.1: Distribution of diagnoses along racial lines

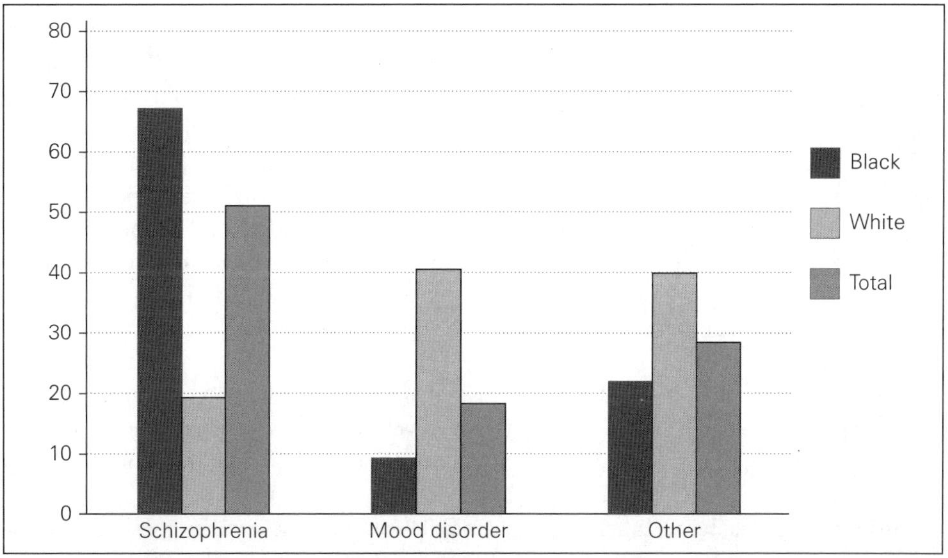

Source: Freeman, M. Providing mental health care for all in South Africa – structure and strategy. Johannesburg: Centre for Health Policy, University of the Witwatersrand: 1992, p. 32.

There could be various explanations for the trends pointed out by Kale (1995). One of the main reasons could be cultural insensitivity of the clinician. Making an accurate diagnosis (see Chapter 1) relies on intricate processes and an understanding of the finer nuances of languages and culture. Cultural insensitivity could arguably lead to a crude diagnostic process in which a clinician may make a diagnosis based on only a few obvious symptoms (for example, hearing voices in the case of *ukuthwasa*), leading to misdiagnosis. Furthermore, access to mental health services, especially in rural areas, is limited, which may lead to 'minor disorders' (such as anxiety and depression) not being recognised or treated (see Chapter 14).

CULTURAL AND CROSS-CULTURAL PSYCHOLOGY IN SOUTH AFRICA

The word 'culture' has been used many times in this book up to this point. This is because culture is an extremely important construct in defining, describing, and explaining abnormal behaviour. Dana (2000) states that culture is not like any other variable because it comprises the context for the operation of all the other variables. In his model, Dana (2000) maintains that culture has provided a centralised role in understanding behaviour. Culture refers to the way much of our behaviour is shared and learned behaviour is transmitted from one generation to the next.

Psychologists have for some time argued that behaviour can be viewed as a function of the interaction between people and their environment. Culture plays an important role in many prominent macro-theories of human development, such as ecological systems theory, sociocultural theory, social learning theory, and the eco-cultural model. In each of these models, psychological outcomes, both positive (see Chapter 3) and negative, are influenced by culture in highly complex and interactive ways.

Cultural psychology as a subdiscipline began with the study of the behaviour of people in widely diverse and previously unfamiliar cultures that were conspicuously different from the investigator's own culture. It rapidly evolved into the systematic exploration of the different experiential histories of people reared in different cultures. Essentially, the current field of cultural psychology represents recognition of the cultural specificity of all human behaviour, through which basic psychological processes may result in highly diverse performance, attitudes, self-concepts, and world views in members of different cultural populations.

Cultural differences can become cultural handicaps when the individual moves out of the culture or subculture in which he or she was reared and endeavours to function, compete, or succeed within another culture. However, it is these very contacts and interchanges between cultures that often stimulate the advancement of civilisations (Anastasi & Urbina, 1997).

The contribution of culture is being increasingly recognised and integrated in all fields of psychology from research and theory on lifespan development, social behaviour, emotion, or thinking, on the one hand, to the practice of industrial/organisational, clinical or counseling psychology, on the other (Anastasi & Urbina, 1997).

Given the fact that humans are extremely mobile and that, due to many social forces (e.g. wars, emigration, etc.), they move to and settle in different societies and communities, there are very few, if any, societies that have not become culturally diverse. It is therefore safe to assume that mental health professionals across the world will be in regular contact with people who are from different cultures. If they are to deal effectively with these people they will need special skills. According to Kazarian and Evans (1998, in Kekae-Moletsane, 2004), skills and knowledge for multicultural assessment include:

- Recognising cultural diversity
- Understanding the role of culture, ethnicity, and race in the socio-political and economic development of diverse ethnic and cultural populations
- Understanding the significant impact of socio-economic and political factors on the psychosocial, political, and economic development of groups
- Helping clients to understand, maintain, and/or resolve their own sociocultural identification
- Understanding the interaction of culture, gender, and sexual orientation on behaviour and needs.

One of the main hurdles in dealing with people from different cultures is ethnocentrism. Ethnocentrism refers to judging other people from within one's own cultural perspective. All people are to a greater or lesser extent ethnocentric; however, a problem arises when one views one's own culture as superior to other cultures. Typically, ethnocentric individuals will judge other people relative to their own particular ethnic group or culture, basing this on language, behaviour, customs, and religion. Cross-cultural psychology, according to Berry, Poortinga, Segall, and Dasen (2002), attempts to reduce the ethnocentrism of psychology described above by:

- Recognising the limitations of our current knowledge
- Seeking to extend our data and theory through the inclusion of other cultures
- Reducing the culture-bound nature of the discipline.

ACTIVITY

Suppose you are a psychologist in a multicultural society such as South Africa. Explain and discuss the necessary skills and knowledge for multicultural assessment that you need to acquire in order to better serve clients from different cultural backgrounds.

A typical example of ethnocentrism is the tendency in Western medicine to discredit the methods of the traditional African healer. However, some psychologists and psychiatrists who have studied and worked closely with traditional healers have developed empathetic understandings of their methods, and acknowledged the healing that they achieve (Buhrmann, 1986; Edwards, 1982; Kottle, 1988, all in Louw & Edwards, 1993). Large numbers of black people in South Africa consult traditional healers. They have as much faith (if not more) in traditional healers as they have in Western medicine. Most South African psychologists maintain that healthy cooperation between psychologists and traditional healers ought to exist. A comprehensive understanding of some types of psychopathology is found among the traditional healers in African societies.

According to Moodley and Sutherland (2010), traditional healing methods in Africa include the following practitioners: indigenous doctors, herbalists, religious healers, etc. Their healing practices are now re-emerging alongside modern Western clinics in several large metropolitan cities. Moodley and Sutherland (2010) further maintain that shamanism is one of the many practices that are used for maintaining the psychological health and well-being of society.

AFRICAN PERSONALITY THEORY

According to African culture, a person exists because of other people. In Sotho it is commonly known that '*Motho ke motho ka batho ba bangwe*', which means, a person is a person because of other people while in Zulu, it is expressed as '*Umuntu ngumuntu ngabantu*'. These phrases demonstrate the importance of collective identity in African cultures (Moletsane, 2011). Thus, for example, if a person does something good, the credit goes to the community not to the individual.

Africans believe that there is a powerful being which supersedes all of us. This supreme power is invisible and can be seen as God or more than one god. According to Bojuwoye (2003), God is the supreme being and the ultimate source of life energy.

Below this supreme being are the ancestors, as indicated in Figure 2.2. Ancestors are people who have died but whose spirits are still alive and are among the living. The ancestors are watching and protecting their living relatives. It is believed that the ancestors play a crucial role in people's lives by communicating with God on behalf of the living. The ancestors use dreams, signs, or traditional or spiritual healers to deliver the messages from God (or the gods) to those who are alive. Holdstock (1982, in Louw & Edwards, 1993) states that the relationship with the ancestors (and through the ancestors, with God) permeates all beings.

In Figure 2.2, the person is represented as 'the body'. The outer layer of the body is like a cover or container of the human's body. The body needs to be active in order to be in a good physical shape. There are other levels of functioning, such as the physiological, which focuses

Figure 2.2: African model of personality

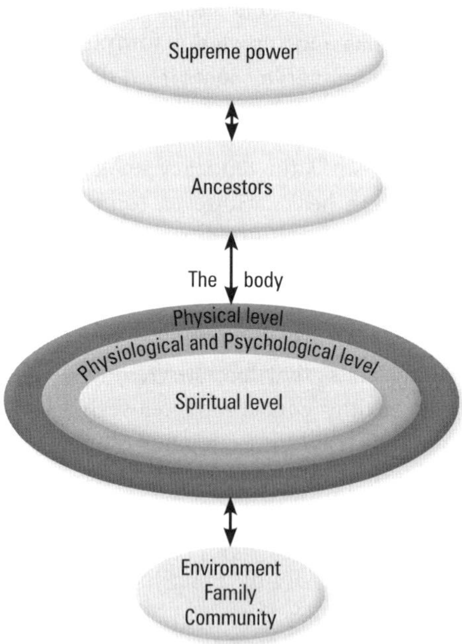

Source: Moletsane, 2011.

on the body's physiological functioning and the psychological, which focuses on the stability of a person's mind. The physiological and psychological levels of a person are important; for the body to survive and to be healthy, it needs good nutrition and a stable mind.

The spiritual part is the inner part or the seed of a person. The spirit is regarded as the seed because it does not die even after the body has died. Sow (1977, in Berry et al., 2002) also regards the inner layer as the 'spiritual principle', which represents a soul that can never perish. It can leave the body during sleep and during trance states (see Chapter 8) and leaves definitively upon death. Sow (1977, in Berry et al., 2002) further states that the spiritual principle does not give life to the body; rather, it has an existence of its own, belonging to the sphere of the ancestors and representing that sphere in each person.

Every person has a connection or relationship with their environment; hence, people adapt to their own environment. If people do not adapt to their environment, they get sick. This happens because their state of equilibrium is weak. The arrows in Figure 2.2 represent the firm connections between the gods or the supreme power, the ancestors, a person, the environment, the family, and the community. This bond or connection also represents the state of equilibrium. Thus, the state of equilibrium is represented by the lines that join the different levels together. If the different levels are held together firmly (the levels being the supreme power; ancestors; physical, physiological and psychological; and spiritual), then there is a state of equilibrium in a person's life. In that state, a person is healthy and happy, or satisfied with life in general. This can be because the ancestors are satisfied that he or she has a strong bond and good relationships with his or her family or he or she takes good care of the elderly people in the family, etc. On the other hand, if one or more (or all) of the levels is/are not held firmly, then the person is in a state of disequilibrium. While in a state of disequilibrium, the person is unhappy and gets sick often because the relationships or bond between the levels is weak. For example, amongst others, this can happen when a person has angered the ancestors by not performing rituals.

The African personality model described above helps to provide an explanation of the aetiology and treatment of illness and mental disorder (see also Table 2.6). Thus, illnesses and disorders happen when the lines of connection are disturbed. In order to diagnose the illness or disorder, one has to establish where in these lines of connection the disturbances have occurred.

According to Sow (1977, in Berry et al., 2002), a rupture of the connection between a person and their ancestors leads to serious chronic psychotic states, a rupture of the connection between a person and their family leads to organic illness, while a disequilibrium in the connection between a person and their community leads to more benign organic and psychosomatic illnesses as well as neurotic states. Once the site and nature of the rupture have been identified, the person's equilibrium can then be restored by means of therapy or other indigenous ways of healing. Thus, healing occurs when there is resolution of conflict with community, family, and/or ancestors because by doing so, the connection lines will become firm again and the connection will not be disturbed.

ACTIVITY

Mandla's mother passed away recently. He feels guilty because he feels he did not give his mother enough support while she was still alive. His mother suffered a stroke and on several occasions Mandla refused to transport her to the hospital for regular check-ups, saying that he was too busy. He used to go to parties with friends and now that his mother is no longer alive, he feels bad that he did not give her all the support she deserved and he did not take the chance to tell her that he loved her. Mandla is now experiencing severe headaches and sleepless nights. He often dreams about his mother being angry with him.

Based on Mandla's scenario, explain:

- The consequences of disequilibrium and rupture of connection between Mandla and his mother, who has passed away
- The reason why firm connection and good relationship between different levels of the African personality model are crucial for a person's health.

Nsamenang (2001, in Berry et al., 2002) states that, contrary to the modern psychology views that regard the individual as autonomous, the African view regards a person as co-existing with the community, with the world of spirits, and the environment. The existence of an indestructible and powerful force which continues to exist in the world of spirits after death is emphasised in Africa. Personhood is a manifestation of this vital force through a body. Thus, respect for the person is vital; for example, greetings are extremely important. The amount of time spent when greeting a person is not considered to be a waste of time and effort, but it reflects the social value attached to the greetings. The greetings include asking people about the health and well-being of their families. The high value placed on greetings implies a high regard for person being greeted. Nsamenang (1991, in Berry et al., 2002, p. 107) further describes how in Africa 'a man [sic] is not a man on his own' but is rooted in the community in which and for which he exists. The importance of the community is reflected in the saying 'Seek the good of the community and you seek your own good; seek your own good and you seek your own destruction'.

ACTIVITY

Explain the importance of greetings and why time spent when greeting a person is not considered to be a waste in African culture.

INDIGENOUS THEORIES OF HEALTH AND ILLNESS

Traditional beliefs and practices concerning illness and health are still widely followed especially in rural areas of South Africa (Louw & Edwards, 1993). These beliefs and practices form a coherent system that has maintained individual and social equilibrium for generations. Since the traditional healers are easily available and represent the same cultural group as the clients, they are trusted and perceived as well trained. Also, for the unemployed and poor, modern medicine is unaffordable and not easily accessible. In addition, some of the older people in African communities, who are not traditional healers, acquired knowledge of indigenous healing from the past generations and are therefore familiar with traditional prevention, diagnosis, prognosis, and medicine. They are usually wise older women and men who give advice to the community members. They can be regarded as indigenous community counsellors. Out of these traditional beliefs and practices has come an African understanding of aetiology. The study conducted by Moletsane (2011) highlights these African aetiological explanations (see Table 2.6). When assisting clients from an African cultural background, it is crucial to have an understanding of these aetiological explanations.

Table 2.6: Indigenous African aetiological explanations

Cause of illness	Explanation
Boloi (*Sesotho*) or *ubuthakathi* (*isiZulu*): to be bewitched	It can be described as sorcery/witchcraft or use of super-power to harm or even kill someone, usually an enemy.
Go roula (*Sesotho*)	A widow has to wear black clothes for 12 months to show that she is mourning for her husband. This only applies to wives, not husbands. If this practice is not properly followed, it can cause illness.
Sefifi/senyama (*Sesotho*) or *isinyama* in *isiZulu*	A widow is regarded as contagious as she has 'senyama' or 'sefifi' which means bad luck due to her husband's death. The bad luck can be cured if the widow and the youngest child in the family are cleansed by bathing with a herb concoction as recommended by the traditional healer or a traditional community counsellor after the death of her husband. A person who is menstruating or who had sex that day is also regarded as having 'sefifi'. Such people are not allowed to enter the same room as a new-born baby or a sick person because they might pass their bad luck or illness to the baby or aggravate the condition of the sick person.
Makgome (*Sesotho*)	After the death of the husband, a widow is prohibited from having a sexual relationship with anyone. Widows are supposed to abstain from sexual activities for a period of one year. If this practice is ignored, they can cause serious illness to themselves and to anyone who has sexual contact with them.
Go tlola (*Sesotho*) or *Ukudlula* in *isiZulu*	When a widow fails to abstain from sex during the mourning period, this can cause compulsion neurosis (the uncontrollable impulse to perform stereotyped irrational acts).
Go lahla maseko/setso (*Sesotho*) or *ukulahla amasiko* in *isiZulu*	This is the failure to perform the traditional practices. For example, due to Western cultural influence, people might not believe in African rituals. This might anger the ancestors which will cause ill-health or other types of problems in a person's life.

Cause of illness	Explanation
Ba fase ba re furaletse/ ba fase ba re lahlile (*Sesotho*) or *abaphansi ba si fulathele* (*isiZulu*)	This means the ancestors have turned their backs against a person. Usually happens when people experience problems either with relationships, work, finance, health, etc., and they then think that ancestors are angry with them.
Go thwasa (*Sesotho*) or *ukuthwasa* (*isiZulu*) (calling)	The calling by the ancestors to become a traditional healer. If ignored, it can cause illness or even death.
Sejeso (*Sesotho*) or *isidliso* (*isiZulu*)	Growth or pain in the stomach due to sorcery/witchcraft
Tokolosi (*Sesotho*) or *tokoloshe* (*isiZulu*)	Witchcraft through an animal-like witch. The witches can send 'tokolosi' to take part in bewitching another person.
Letswalo (*Sesotho*) or *uvalo* (*isiZulu*)	Anxiety attributed to witchcraft or sorcery.
Go gatiswa/mohlala (*Sesotho*) or *umeqo* (*isiZulu*)	A disorder attributed to stepping on a concoction of herbs of sorcery. This can cause pain and swollen feet for the person who stepped on the concoction.
Mafofonyane (*Sesotho*) or *amafufunyane* (*isiZulu*)	Spirit possession as a result of witchcraft or sorcery.

Source: Adapted from Moletsane, 2011.

Traditional African healing model

According to Lesolang-Pitje (2003), South Africa in the post-apartheid era recognises traditional healing as part of the health system (see also Chapter 14). The process of consultation with traditional healers' associations started in 1995. According to Bojuwoye (2003), traditional healers are acknowledged for their extraordinary knowledge of histories, religions, philosophies, institutions, and other bodies of knowledge and language of their culture. They are experts in the use of their cultural languages to accurately construct, explain, and communicate what is culturally believed to be fundamentally true about the world people live in. Bojuwoye (2003) further states that traditional healers are reputed to have clairvoyance and astounding abilities to read clients' minds and to ensure their health.

ACTIVITY

Tshidi's husband has passed away. Explain how you understand the indigenous African cultural practices associated with bereavement.

As described in earlier sections, many traditionally oriented Africans consult traditional healers when they have health or emotional problems (Madu, 2003). Traditional Africans believe that a sickness, especially one which is emotional or psychological in nature, originates from a disruption in the connections between people, the gods, and the ancestors. In response to these disruptions, traditional healers work with clients and their families and not on an individual basis with the client alone. Traditional healers also work with gods and ancestors in the healing process.

According to Bojuwoye (2003), traditional African health care delivery approaches are said to be active and directive. The process moves through three main stages which include establishing a relationship; identification and discussion of the problem; and the problem-solving stage. Certain principles guide the decisions, choices, and actions which take place in these stages. Some of them are:

- ***The principle of education or information:*** The traditional healer helps the patient understand the different elements contained in the universe, for example, the connection between the different levels that constitute a person according to African personality theory (see Figure 2.2). This helps the patient understand how their illness or misfortune may be caused by their state of disequilibrium (see Figure 2.2).
- ***The principle of interconnectedness or the phenomenal world:*** This principle is found in the African world view which states that people are interconnected. For instance, if a mother is sick or not happy, her situation will affect other people such as family members, neighbours, colleagues at work, etc.
- ***The principle of social contact and interpersonal relationship:*** This principle ensures harmony within the universe. Problems are dyadic in nature and using relationships to address some of them may be a good strategy. Activities such as ritual ceremonies are regarded as important for interpersonal growth.
- ***The principle of personal empowerment:*** By performing rituals a person is empowered. If a person is empowered, the power is transferred to other people. For example, if one is healthy and positive about life, the positive energy spreads to people around him or her.
- ***The principle of psychological arousal:*** During the ritual ceremony, through the vigorous exercise of singing and dancing, the spirits are lifted and this process arouses people psychologically and emotionally. It is a space where people can express their emotions.
- ***The principle of ritualistic support:*** Participating in vigorous body movements during the ritual ceremony is therapeutic. During these ceremonies, people are made aware that they are not alone but their problems and grief are shared with others.

These therapeutic components do not necessarily follow a sequence but can be applied interchangeably during sessions. Traditional healing models are holistic and treat the 'whole' person, employing interventions targeted at all forces responsible for ill health including both symptoms and causes of ill health (Bojuwoye & Sodi, 2010). Furthermore, traditional healing is comprehensive and concerned with illness prevention, health promotion, and/ or cure (Bujowoye & Sodi, 2010).

INTEGRATED PERSPECTIVES

As indicated in the introduction to this chapter, psychological disorders are most often caused by multiple factors acting in complex and dynamic ways. The biopsychosocial model and diathesis-stress model discussed here provide us with broad theoretical frameworks that allow a number of different perspectives to be used thus demonstrating the multidimensional nature of psychopathology.

The biopsychosocial model

According to this perspective (see Figure 2.3), behaviour is too complex to be understood from one perspective only. It takes the view that psychological disorders are caused by multiple biological, psychological, and social factors in interaction with each other.

Figure 2.3: The biopsychosocial model

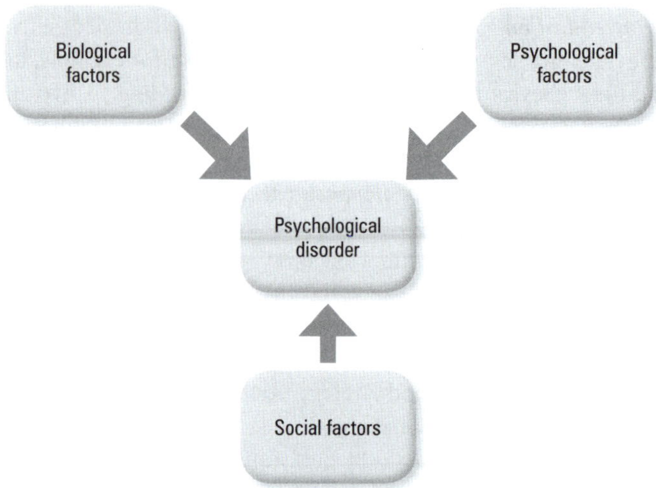

For example, Isaac is diagnosed with depression. Biologically, a contributing factor could be his neurophysiological vulnerability to producing unhealthy levels of stress hormones when experiencing stress. On a psychological level, Isaac has observed that his parents are extremely negative and avoidant when things go wrong and so he has developed irrational beliefs regarding uncertainty (e.g. 'I can't cope with uncertainty'). On a social level, Isaac, who is part of a minority group, has been discriminated against in his school, which has contributed to a feeling of helplessness. Thus, factors from all three dimensions interact to contribute to his depression.

The diathesis-stress model

The diathesis-stress model was first introduced by Meehl (1962). He suggested that some people inherit or develop biological predispositions (diathesis) to psychopathology. In this situation, mental disorders will not emerge until environmental stressors or biological stressors become intense enough to convert predispositions into actual psychological disorders (see Figure 2.4).

Figure 2.4: The diathesis-stress model

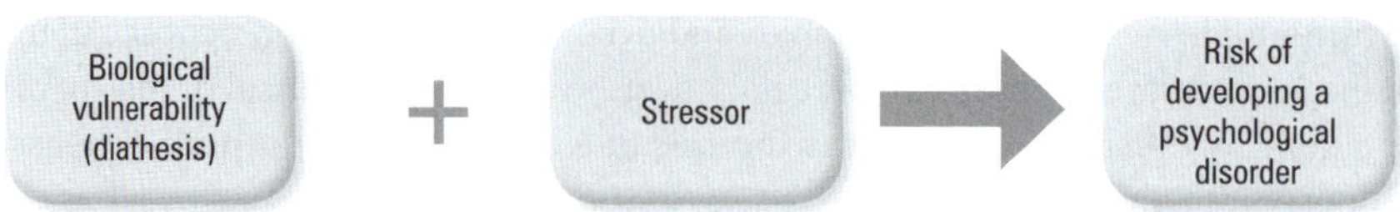

Thus, there is an interaction between the diathesis (a biological predisposition to a disorder) and a stressor, which together causes a disorder to develop. A biological predisposition on its own is therefore usually not sufficient to develop a psychological disorder. For example, when a person has a biological vulnerability to developing depression, this may lie dormant until the person is exposed to a significant stressor, for example, a traumatic divorce. Only then is the predisposition to develop depression triggered and actualised. This also explains why not all people develop disorders after experiencing stressors (they do not have a biological predisposition), or why all people with biological predispositions do not develop a disorder (they have not been exposed to a significant stressor). There are exceptions, however; in some cases, the biological predisposition is so strong that a disorder develops without a stressor. Also, without a predisposition, a strong enough stressor may lead to the development of a psychological disorder.

CONCLUSION

In South Africa, it is important that we start embracing a more critical perspective on abnormal behaviour. This not only implies that students in psychology and psychiatry need to be trained from a more critical and culturally sensitive perspective, but also that society as a whole needs to be better educated in terms of what it could and should expect from these professions. In addition, citizens need to be educated about their rights in this regard (see Chapter 14). This would be consistent with the international trend of involving users and user groups in decision-making and accountability.

Furthermore, there needs to be a more holistic understanding of patients. The lack of a whole-person way of understanding mental health problems originates in medical training which focuses on physical disorder. In particular, reductive causal analyses do not necessarily help us understand the full range of normal and abnormal human behaviour. In order to achieve this understanding, there needs to be less emphasis on a natural scientific perspective of basic biological processes. Despite the many failings of a positivist approach to abnormal behaviour, its attraction is that it seems to avoid the complexities and uncertainties of psychological and social perspectives. This seduces students and clinicians alike with the idea that experimental natural science is an adequate discourse for a description of what is normal and abnormal, which may lead to their adopting a mechanistic view in their treatment of patients.

In South Africa, we also need to go a step further due to our culturally diverse society. Cultural beliefs and the traditional African way of living in South Africa are not well known to most mental health professionals, especially those socialised within Western culture. It is imperative that when psychological interventions (any type of therapy, counselling, diagnosis, or psychological test) are conducted with indigenous African people, that the psychologist concerned be familiar with these traditional African cultural beliefs and ways of living. In that way, the risk of misdiagnosis will be reduced, if not eliminated, and clients will be appropriately and ethically treated.

MULTIPLE-CHOICE QUESTIONS

1. The chemicals that allow transmission of signals between neurons are called:
   a) re-uptake inhibitors
   b) hormones
   c) neurotransmitters
   d) genes

2. From a psychoanalytic perspective psychopathology occurs when:
   a) conflict between the id, the ego, and the superego gives rise to distressing symptoms
   b) deficiencies in the ego hinder the individual's ability to repress instinctual drives
   c) instinctual drives take over the superego
   d) both a and c

3. You have failed your last psychology test but you put this out of your mind while you study for your next test. Which defence mechanism are you using?
   a) reaction-formation
   b) denial
   c) projection
   d) repression

4. The goals of community psychology include the following:
   a) prevention (rather than just treatment) of mental illness
   b) understanding of people within their social worlds
   c) understanding psychopathology from within the context of community
   d) all of the above

5. Which of the following is NOT a myth about mental illness in non-Western countries?
   a) All mental disorders can be cured by indigenous healers.
   b) Mental illness is not recognised as pathological in non-Western communities.
   c) Mental illness is accepted in non-Western communities in an unstigmatised manner.
   d) Mental illness does not exist in non-Western countries.

6. Which of the following is a consequence of apartheid?
   a) The population of psychologists in South Africa is predominantly black, middle-class, and male.
   b) Psychologists serve predominantly black patients.
   c) The mental health needs of black South Africans and the disadvantaged community have been largely neglected.
   d) All of the above are consequences of apartheid.

7. Which of the following is incorrect in terms of the skills and knowledge required for multicultural assessment?
   a) ability to recognise cultural uniformity

b) ability to help clients to understand, maintain, and resolve their own sociocultural identification
c) understanding of the interactive effects of culture, gender, and sexual orientation on behaviour and needs
d) none of the above

8. Ethnocentrism refers to:
a) misjudging other people within from one's own cultural system
b) judging other people from within their own cultural system
c) judging other people from within one's own cultural system
d) b and c

9. According to African personality model, a rupture between the person and their ancestors leads to:
a) organic illness
b) a serious chronic psychotic state
c) a mild psychotic state
d) none of the above

10. Collective identity is important in African culture. *Motho ke motho ka batho ba bangwe* means:
a) A person is a person because of other people.
b) A person is not a person because of other people.
c) A person is a person because of his or her family.
d) A person is a person because of God.

PARAGRAPH AND ESSAY QUESTIONS

1. Explain the importance of cultural awareness and sensitivity in therapy. Give practical examples.

2. Traditional beliefs and practices are still respected, especially in rural areas. Describe the causes of illness and their explanation according to the indigenous African aetiological explanation.

3. Critically explain and analyse the African personality theory, emphasising the importance of the firm connections between different levels.

4. Analyse the challenges faced by mental health professionals in a multicultural and multilingual South Africa and give your own recommendation as to how they can better serve their clients in a diverse society.

5. Explain the ways in which socio-political factors can have an impact on our mental health, according to community psychologists

3 ABNORMAL PSYCHOLOGY FROM A MENTAL WELLNESS PERSPECTIVE

Karel Botha and Edwin du Plessis

3 CHAPTER OUTLINE

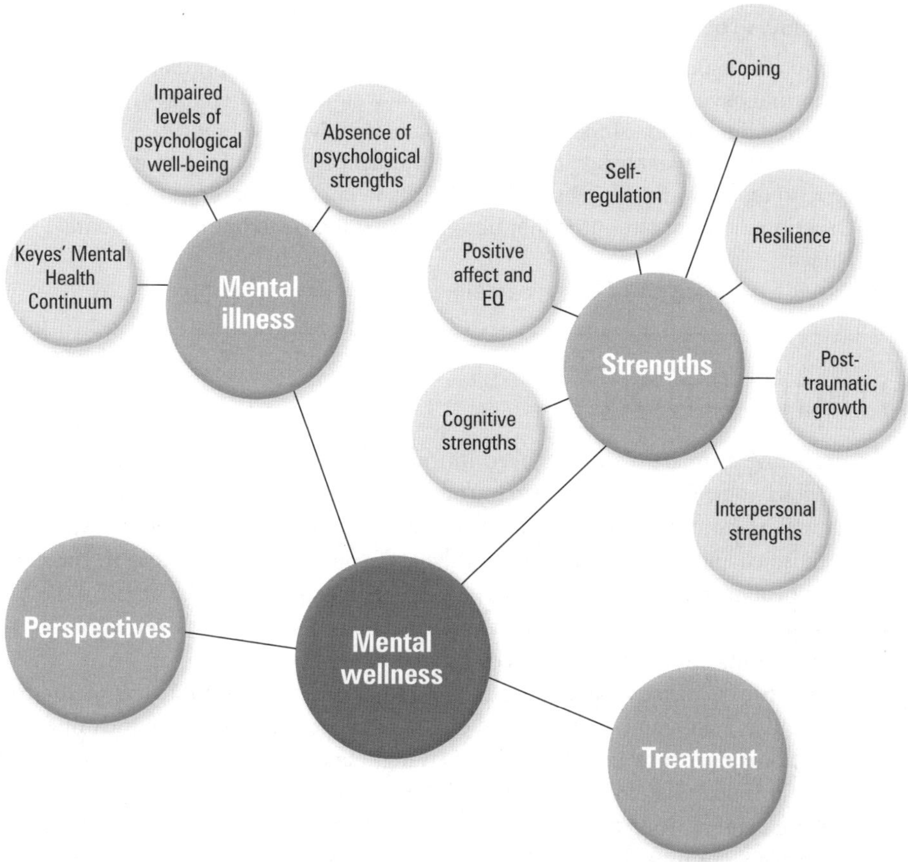

LEARNING OUTCOMES

After studying this chapter you should be able to:

- Demonstrate understanding of what we can benefit from approaching abnormal psychology from a psychological well-being perspective.
- Describe the history of mental wellness and positive psychology.
- Explain mental wellness in terms of the mental health continuum, impaired psychological well-being, as well as deficits in character strengths.
- Describe different strengths that buffer against the development of mental illness.
- Provide an overview of different wellness-based psychotherapies.

INTRODUCTION

In the preceding chapters, you have been introduced to the definition and description of abnormal behaviour. You have also been introduced to the diagnostic process and diagnostic labels, as well as various models that explain how a disorder may develop. When reading through those chapters, two aspects should have become clear, firstly, that in the typical description of abnormal behaviour, there seems to be an emphasis on the negative (i.e. what is or has 'gone wrong) and, secondly, that abnormal behaviour develops over time and that the course and outcome may be influenced by a number of factors.

Focusing only on negative factors leads to a rather one-dimensional view of abnormal behaviour, and as Seligman (2005) pointed out, psychology is not only the study of disease, weakness, and damage, but also the study of strength and virtue. This chapter, in contrast to the rest of this textbook, focuses on mental illness from a strength-and-wellness point of view. The aim is to improve your understanding of abnormal psychology, emphasising the strengths available to individuals and communities in adversity, how these strengths may prevent pathology, promote psychological well-being, and finally, how a strengths-based approach may be used in treating abnormal behaviour. First, let us discuss some reasons why we need to look at abnormal psychology from a wellness perspective:

- ***Normality and abnormality are not different in kind:*** Maddux (2005) states that both adaptive and maladaptive psychological functioning are acquired and maintained through the same processes, and differ in degree rather than in quality. Supporting this idea, Manderscheid et al. (2010) remind us that mental health and mental illnesses can both cause and be influenced by positive or negative social determinants of health, for instance, income, housing, stress, early childhood experiences, education level, social support, and access to resources. Therefore, Wood and Tarrier (2010) argue that it is not logical to study either negative or positive functioning in isolation. This is because any designation of a characteristic as positive or negative is simplistic and inaccurate, because any trait can be positive or negative, depending on the situation.
- ***Abnormal psychology is limited and narrows our focus:*** According to Maddux (2008), clinical psychology, with its focus on abnormal behaviour, has to a large extent narrowed our focus onto what is weak and defective about people to the exclusion of what is strong and healthy. Although clinical psychology has produced many successes in treating

psychopathology, and has built an extensive understanding of mental illness, Ryff and Singer (1998) believe that psychology should be more than a 'repair shop' for broken lives. In this regard, Wright and Lopez (2005) argue that it is a common error in professional psychology to make important decisions based primarily on the deficiencies of the person instead of giving serious consideration to his or her deficits and strengths. Being problem oriented, the clinician easily concentrates only on pathology and dysfunction, to the neglect of discovering available strengths that could be drawn upon in problem-solving efforts.

- ***Understanding strengths may help us to understand and treat mental disorders:*** In support of the growing perception that psychotherapy should be more about amplifying strengths than repairing weaknesses, there is an increasing interest in building human strengths in different psychotherapeutic strategies. For example, Ruini and Fava (2004) proposed that psychological well-being needs to be incorporated into the definition of recovery, while Seligman (2008) believes that the promotion of well-being may be one of the best ways to alleviate mental disorder. These authors support the belief that absence of well-being creates vulnerability to adversity and that the route to long-term recovery lies in facilitating the positive, rather than on exclusively treating the negative.

Even though these reasons are primarily theoretically motivated, they make an important statement that needs to be explored further. To start with, we will now explore the concept of psychological well-being.

EXAMPLE CASE

Imagine that you are a clinical psychologist with a strong focus on abnormality only, in other words, with what is wrong with clients. A 30-year-old client, John, experienced shock and fear when he was a victim of a hijacking and has been referred to you. By taking a one-sided perspective focussing on abnormality only, there is a risk that you (i) are biased into thinking that something must be wrong with John; and (ii) focus on signs and symptoms that confirm the diagnosis of, say, Posttraumatic Stress Disorder. The possibility exists, however, that John's behaviour is a natural, healthy response to the trauma, and/or that his response to the trauma fits a category in the DSM called Additional Conditions that May be a Focus of Clinical Attention. This category describes conditions that led to contact with the mental health care system, but without sufficient evidence to justify a diagnosis of a mental disorder. Taking this abnormality perspective risks a missed opportunity or, at best, limited ability to recognise and facilitate the strengths John might have.

A BRIEF HISTORY OF MENTAL WELLNESS AND POSITIVE PSYCHOLOGY

The scientific study of human strengths and mental wellness is not a new venture. Questions about what makes life fulfilling and meaningful were raised by early philosophers like Socrates, Aristotle, and Plato, long before psychology became a discipline. William James, in the late 1800s, made a significant contribution to the science of psychology in general, but also to a first understanding of positive functioning in particular (Hefferon & Boniwell, 2011). Most of the prominent early psychologists (see Table 3.1) described human potential to some extent, despite the fact that they mainly focused on abnormal behaviour. According to Abraham Maslow, for example, a person is healthy and shows mental wellness when their potential is actualised, rather than blocked.

Table 3.1: Some early psychologists' views on human strengths

Psychologist	Concept of mental wellness
Gordon Allport	Maturity
Carl Jung	Balance
Carl Rogers	The fully functioning person
Erich Fromm	Productivity
Abraham Maslow	Self-actualisation
Viktor Frankl	Self transcendence

Source: Adapted from Peterson, 2006b, p. 36.

In 1958, the psychologist Marie Jahoda was amongst the first to attempt to operationalise psychological well-being, when she listed six criteria she argued were needed to establish positive mental health (Compton, 2005). In addition, Baumgardner and Crothers (2010) note that the humanistic movement, led by Maslow and Rogers, criticised traditional psychology for primarily focusing on negative aspects of human behaviour. They saw human nature as basically positive, and proposed that the goal of psychology should be to study and promote the achievement of productive and healthy lives.

In a world-wide explosion of interest and research on psychological well-being during the 1990s, significant contributions were made by South African researchers like Strümpfer (1995) who extended Antonovsky's construct salutogenesis (the origins of health) to fortigenesis (the origins of strengths), and by Wissing and Van Eeden (1997), who proposed the term fortology (the study of strengths). However, these terms were not adopted and in 1998, Martin Seligman (then president of the APA) made a plea for a major shift in psychology's focus to what became known as 'positive psychology'. Seligman's intention was that this would broaden the scope of psychology to promote the study and understanding of healthy human functioning.

Positive psychology is defined in a number of ways. However, the following definition is particularly relevant to this chapter as it emphasises the integration between positive and negative aspects of human functioning. According to Linley, Joseph, Harrington, and Wood (2006, p. 8), positive psychology is 'the scientific study of optimal human functioning, which aims to redress the imbalance in psychology integrating the positive aspects of human functioning and experience with our understanding of the negative aspects of human functioning and experience'.

Positive psychology studies what people do right and how they manage to do it (Compton, 2005). However, it complements, rather than replaces, our understanding of how positive and negative life events and emotions are interconnected (Baumgardner & Crothers, 2010). Wong (2011) indicates that positive psychology has effectively changed the language and landscape of mainstream psychology and it continues to grow exponentially in terms of teaching, research, and applications.

DIFFERENT PERSPECTIVES ON MENTAL WELLNESS

Generally, mental wellness or psychological well-being has been conceptualised within the positive psychology approach from two related, but different traditions, namely hedonic and eudaimonic well-being. Hedonic well-being relates to subjective experiences of pleasure and life satisfaction, and most work in this regard has focused on the concept of happiness. Diener (2000) indicates that happiness is a form of subjective well-being, which he defined as life satisfaction, characterised by the subjective presence of positive affect, and a relative absence of negative affect.

HELPFUL HINT

- **Hedonic well-being is about happiness, pleasure, and life-satisfaction.**
- **Eudaimonic well-being is about meaning, purpose, and engagement.**

Seligman (2008), in formulating the conceptual framework for positive psychology, broke the term 'happiness' down into three quantifiable aspects. The first, positive emotion (the pleasant life), reflects the emphasis on understanding the determinants of happiness as a desired state. The other two aspects relate more to eudamonic well-being, characterised by meaning, purpose, and the realisation of one's potential. In this regard, Seligman (2008) describes happiness as being a result of engagement (the engaged life) which refers to active and meaningful involvement in activities and relationships with others and purpose (the meaningful life) which is about going beyond our own self-interests and preoccupations and being involved in something larger than oneself.

Carol Ryff's work on eudaimonic well-being is probably the most influential. According to her, positive functioning consists of six basic elements, which together she calls psychological well-being (Ryff & Keyes 1995). Each element is important in the striving to become a better person and to realise one's potential. The six elements are:

- ***Self-acceptance:*** a positive and accepting attitude toward aspects of self in past and present
- ***Purpose in life:*** goals and beliefs that affirm a sense of direction and meaning in life
- ***Autonomy:*** self-direction as guided by one's own socially accepted internal standards
- ***Positive relations with others:*** having satisfying personal relationships in which empathy and intimacy are expressed
- ***Environmental mastery:*** the capability to manage the complex environment according to one's own needs
- ***Personal growth:*** the insight into one's own potential for self-development.

The work of Ryff, and many others, focuses mainly on optimal functioning in terms of individual fulfillment. However, Keyes (1998) has argued that it is also important to study the optimal social functioning of individuals in terms of their social engagement and societal embeddedness. He provided a conceptual analysis of social well-being that consists of five dimensions which describe a person who is functioning optimally in society. These dimensions are social coherence, social acceptance, social actualisation, social contribution, and social integration. According to Keyes (1998), well-being thus consists of emotional well-being (happiness/hedonic well-being), psychological well-being (the six dimensions by Ryff), and social well-being.

In support of international findings, the South African researchers Wissing and Van Eeden (2002) indicate that psychological well-being is multifaceted, and encompasses facets of self, as well as intrapersonal, interpersonal, social, and contextual domains in various spheres of life such as intimate relationships, work, and recreation. These authors identified a general psychological well-being factor, consisting of satisfaction with life, positive affect balance, and a sense of coherence (the extent to which an individual perceives life as comprehensible, manageable, and meaningful). More recently, Wissing and Temane (2008) and Khumalo, Wissing, and Temane (2008) explored the nature of psychological well-being in an African context, as cultural factors may influence the manifestation of psychological well-being. Both studies supported the applicability of current psychological well-being models to the African context, but also suggested that relatedness, a sense of community, and interpersonal trust and integrity in group contexts seem to be more important to black South Africans, while competency and agency may be more important to white South Africans.

Apart from the few approaches to psychological well-being mentioned here, other notable perspectives include flow theory (Csikszentmihalyi, 1990), self-determination theory (Ryan & Deci, 2000), and the broaden-and-build theory of positive emotions (Fredrickson, 2005). However, these will not be discussed in depth in this chapter. In the next section, we will focus on three perspectives which specifically help us to see abnormal psychology in a different, perhaps new, light.

MENTAL ILLNESS FROM A WELL-BEING PERSPECTIVE

In this section, we will describe three different well-being perspectives on mental illness.

Mental illness according to Keyes' Mental Health Continuum

Keyes (2002) proposed a mental health continuum in which mental health is viewed as a complete state consisting of the presence and/or absence of mental illness and mental health symptoms. Later, Westerhof and Keyes (2010) described this as a two-continuum model where one continuum indicates the presence or absence of mental health, and the other shows the presence or absence of mental illness. Both are related but distinct dimensions, so that the absence of mental illness does not equate to the presence of mental health, or vice versa. Thus, for each individual, there is at any point in time, an independent indication on both these continua of the level of mental health and mental illness. Four levels of well-being are identified in this way (see Figure 3.1):

Figure 3.1: The mental health continuum

		Mental health	
		High	**Low**
Mental illness	High	Struggling	Floundering
	Low	Flourishing	Languishing

Source: Adapted from Keyes & Lopez, 2005, p. 50.

These four levels of well-being can be described as follows:

- ***Flourishing:*** Characterised by high levels of mental health, as well as the absence of recent mental illness. People in this category are in a state of complete mental health.
- ***Languishing:*** Those without mental illness, but who also have low levels of well-being, are in a state of incomplete mental health.
- ***Struggling:*** Those who have a mental illness, but who also present with aspects of well-being, are in a state of incomplete mental illness.
- ***Floundering:*** Those who present with mental illness as well as an absence of well-being are in a state of complete mental illness.

According to Keyes and Lopez (2005), the ability to diagnose complete and incomplete states of mental illness and health may lead to more effective prevention and treatment programmes. For example, incomplete mental health (languishing) may be a 'way station' at which individuals find themselves prior to the onset of depression, or a place where many people are left following traditional psychotherapeutic treatment. Preventatively, the diagnosis of languishing among youth may be used to identify individuals who require interventions to elevate well-being and prevent development of mental illness.

In a group of South African adolescents from various ethnic backgrounds, Van Schalkwyk and Wissing (2010) found 42% to be flourishing, with 53% moderately mentally healthy, and 5% languishing. Thus, nearly 60% are not functioning optimally. Lower psychological well-being was characterised by meaninglessness, impaired relations, identification with dysfunctional outsiders, self-incompetence, destructive behaviours, negative emotions, and helplessness. The adolescents understood and experienced 'flourishing' as purposeful living, being a role-model, having positive relations, self-confidence and self-liking, a constructive lifestyle, constructive coping, and positive emotions.

Mental illness as impaired levels of psychological well-being

Ruini and Fava (2004), in developing Well-being Therapy (WBT) (see later in chapter), provide an interesting perspective on mental illness. Their approach is motivated by the observation that, among others, Ryff's model of psychological well-being provides a useful description of specific impairments of patients with mood disorders. In support of the idea that well-being and distress are not mutually exclusive, and that well-being could thus not be attained simply from the removal of distress, they had to demonstrate impaired levels of psychological well-being in a clinical population to justify therapeutic efforts aimed at increasing psychological well-being.

Rafanelli and colleagues (Ruini & Fava, 2004) found patients with anxiety and mood disorders displayed significantly lower levels in all six dimensions of Ryff's psychological well-being model compared to healthy subjects. Individuals are therefore at risk of mental illness when they show impaired levels of the six dimensions in the following way (Ruini & Fava, 2004, p. 376):

- ***Impaired self-acceptance:*** Feels dissatisfied with self; is disappointed with what has occurred in past life; is troubled about certain personal qualities; wishes to be different from what he or she is.
- ***Impaired purpose in life:*** Lacks a sense of meaning in life; has few goals, lacks a sense of direction, does not see purpose in past life; has no outlooks or beliefs that give life meaning.
- ***Impaired autonomy:*** Over-concerned with the expectations and evaluation of others; relies on judgment of others to make important decisions; conforms to social pressures to think or act in certain ways.
- ***Impaired positive relations with others:*** Has few close, trusting relationships with others; finds it difficult to be open and is isolated and frustrated in interpersonal relationships; is not willing to make compromises to sustain important ties with others.
- ***Impaired environmental mastery:*** Difficulties in managing everyday affairs; unable to change or improve surrounding contexts.
- ***Impaired personal growth:*** A sense of personal stagnation; lacks a sense of improvement or expansion over time; bored and uninterested with life; unable to develop new attitudes or behaviours.

This framework provides us with a new way of looking at mental illness. For Ruini and Fava (2004), the most important benefit is that it provides a clear goal for WBT, which is to move impaired levels of psychological well-being to optimal levels of functioning.

Mental illness as the absence, opposite, or exaggeration of psychological strengths

Park, Peterson, and Seligman (2004, p. 603) define character strengths as 'positive traits reflected in thoughts, feelings, and behaviours'. They exist in degrees and can be measured as individual differences. As an initial step toward specifying important positive traits, the Values in Action (VIA) Classification of Strengths was developed to complement the *Diagnostic and Statistical Manual of Mental Disorders* (DSM) (see Chapter 1) by focusing on what is right about people (Peterson, 2006b). The VIA categorises and describes 24 character strengths with reference to six broad virtue classes, namely, wisdom, courage, humanity, justice, temperance, and transcendence.

Peterson (2006b) indicates that the VIA classification identifies ways of doing well, and by implication, it also identifies ways of doing poorly. As all character strengths are on a continuum between deficiency and excess, disorders may thus be generated from both of these, thus adding another dimension to the understanding of abnormal psychology. The classification is therefore approached from the existence of strengths and disorders in degrees along a continuum ranging from *opposite* through *absence* to *strength* and finally *exaggeration*. Table 3.2 shows the six virtues, with one example each of a character strength, and Peterson's (2006b) classification thereof in terms of psychological disorders:

Table 3.2: Adapted version of the VIA: A well-being and mental illness perspective

Psychological well-being		Psychological disorder		
Virtue	**Character strength**	**Absence**	**Opposite**	**Exaggeration**
Wisdom: Cognitive strengths	e.g. Creativity	Conformity	Triteness	Eccentricity
Courage: Emotional strengths	e.g. Persistence	Laziness	Helplessness	Obsessiveness
Humanity: Interpersonal strengths	e.g. Kindness	Indifference	Cruelty	Intrusiveness
Justice: Civic strengths	e.g. Citizenship	Selfishness	Narcissism	Chauvinism
Temperance: Self-control strengths	e.g. Self-regulation	Self-indulgence	Impulsivity	Inhibition
Transcendence: Meaning strengths	e.g. Hope	Present orientation	Pessimism	Pollyannism

Source: Adapted from Peterson, 2006b, p. 39.

Absence of the strength creativity is *conformity*, for example. According to Peterson (2006b), this is probably not a significant problem for any given individual; however, for an entire group or society it means stagnation. The opposite of creativity, *triteness*, or unoriginality, Peterson (2006b, p. 41) indicates is a disorder as it is an 'aesthetic offence' and causes people to blindly follow fads. Finally, exaggeration of creativity, *eccentricity*, is in essence referring to a person who is out of touch with the reaction of others. Peterson refers to exhibitionism as an example, but one could just as well include Schizotypal and Histrionic Personality Disorders (see Chapter 12).

Another good example would be the character strength of persistence. The absence of persistence, *laziness*, is probably not a disorder in itself, but may put people at risk later on of developing disorders. Its opposite, *helplessness*, may be associated with mood disorder (see Chapter 5), while exaggeration of persistence, *obsessiveness*, may be associated with Obsessive-Compulsive Disorder (see Chapter 4).

According to Peterson (2006b), this approach creates a new language from which we can better understand psychological disorders. For example, when we examine depression in terms of its association with such difficulties as disinterest, indifference, helplessness, isolation and loneliness, pessimism, and alienation, then we can readily understand when and why depression is a psychological problem.

STRENGTHS THAT PROTECT AGAINST MENTAL ILLNESS

The previous section put abnormal psychology in a different light, and helped us to better understand the complex relationship between mental illness and mental wellness. Although a large number of strengths/protective factors are described in the literature, this section focuses on how a selected few cognitive, emotional, and interpersonal strengths buffer/protect against the development of mental illness.

Cognitive strengths: Optimism, hope and mindfulness

Many forms of psychopathology are related to cognitive dysfunctions. Anxiety and mood disorders, for instance, are often precipitated and maintained by pessimism, irrational beliefs, hopelessness, and mindlessness. Optimists, in contrast to pessimists, are people who expect good things to happen to them (Carver & Scheier, 2005). They have high levels of expectancy – a sense of confidence about the attainability of a goal, even when things are difficult. Optimism and pessimism are basic qualities of personality, and influence people's subjective experiences when confronting problems, as well as the actions people engage in to try to deal with these problems. Optimists tend to be more hopeful; they believe, according to Snyder, Rand, and Sigmon (2005), that they can find pathways to desired goals and become motivated to use those pathways. The motivational component in hope is agency, which is the perceived capacity to use one's pathways so as to reach desired goals.

Another cognitive strength is mindfulness, which refers to paying attention to the world around us in a way that allows openness and flexibility (Langer, 2005). It is the ability to refine one's perspective in the face of new circumstances, thus keeping multiple perspectives about the same phenomenon 'alive' at any given moment. Mindfulness includes qualities like *non-judging* (the ability to recognise that things are not inherently equal to how we judge them), *patience* (the ability to allow events to unfold in their own time rather than always pushing, wishing, or working to make things happen according to our present desires), and *non-striving* (the ability to let go of preconceived ideas of what should happen) (Kabat-Zinn, 1990). Langer (2005) indicates that mindfulness is the opposite of mindlessness, a state of consciousness marked by little awareness of what is going on in the present moment, in which a person is governed by rule and routine, habit, and automatic behaviour.

Cognitive strengths protect against the development of psychopathology in a number of ways. Optimists, for example, are more proactive in that they take active steps to ensure the positive quality of their future. They also use more problem-centered coping, and, when this is not a possibility, they turn to strategies such as acceptance, humour, and positive reframing (Carver & Scheier, 2005). Kasayira and Chireshe (2010) indicate that individuals affected by poverty and HIV/AIDS in sub-Saharan Africa who ascribe more positive meaning to their situation, for instance, by construing it as creating opportunities for personal growth, report higher levels of psychological well-being and lower levels of depressed mood. Hope enhances confidence, effective future thinking, and flexibility in finding alternative goals when goal blockages are experienced (Snyder at al., 2005). In a South African study, Maree, Maree, and Collins (2008) found that hope, among others, fosters energy to pursue goals. Finally, mindfulness helps in dealing with uncertainty as it helps the individual to accept that things change and that change need not be feared. When uncertain, mindfulness leads to engagement with the task at hand (Langer, 2005).

Positive affect and emotional intelligence

Our evolutionary heritage and life learning have given us the capacity to experience a rich array of emotions. We can feel sad, happy, anxious, surprised, bored, exhilarated, scared, disgusted, or disappointed, to name just a few emotions (Baumgardner & Crothers, 2009). The exact number of basic human emotions varies from seven to ten depending on the theorist; however, the various lists show a fair amount of agreement (Compton, 2005; Ekman, 1993). Positive psychologists typically measure people's emotional experience in terms of both the positive and negative affective dimensions. This two-dimensional assessment and summary follows from research suggesting that despite their diversity, if we evaluate emotions by their psychological and physiological effects, we see that emotions come in two basic forms, namely positive and negative affect (Baumgardner & Crothers, 2009). Positive affect refers to emotions such as cheerfulness, joy, contentment, and happiness while negative affect refers to emotions such as anger, fear, sadness, guilt, contempt, and disgust.

Emotions can serve a very useful function if 'used' properly (Compton, 2005). The ability to use emotions wisely might be considered a type of intelligence. Over the past few decades, a number of theorists have developed the concept of emotional intelligence (Compton, 2005). Emotional intelligence involves the ability to monitor one's own and others' feelings and emotions, to discriminate among them, and to use the information to guide one's thinking and actions (Salovey & Mayer, 1990). People who are high in emotional intelligence have the ability to use their emotions wisely, and they appear to have a deeper understanding of their emotional lives (Salovey, Mayer, & Caruso, 2002), and are as a consequence, happier and more successful in their lives (Chamorro-Premuzic, Bennett, & Furnham, 2007; Murphy & Janeke, 2009).

Several studies have pointed out that a higher level of emotional intelligence correlates with more adaptive ways of coping (Salovey, Bedell, Detweiler, & Mayer, 1999; Salovey, Stroud, Woolery, & Epel, 2002), contributes to the achievement of better academic results (Parker, Summerfeldt, Hogan, & Majeski, 2004; Van der Zee, Thijs, & Schakel, 2002), is associated with better interpersonal relations (Mayer, Caruso, & Salovey, 1999), and is a protective factor in both physical and mental health (Austin, Saklofske, & Egan, 2005; Tsaousis & Nikolaou, 2005).

Self-regulation

According to Vohs and Baumeister (2004) and Baumeister, Vohs, and Tice (2007), every major personal and social problem, including drug addiction, eating disorders, excessive spending, crime and violence, emotional problems (like depression), underachievement in work and school, procrastination, and sexually transmitted diseases, involves some kind of failure of self-regulation. Self-regulation is defined by Maes and Karoly (2005, p. 269) as 'a systematic process of human behaviour that involves setting of personal goals and steering behaviour toward the achievement of established goals'. It includes 'self-corrective adjustments, originating within the person, that are needed to stay on track for whatever purpose is being served' (Carver, 2004, p. 10).

Self-regulation unfolds in at least three phases (see Figure 3.2):

Figure 3.2: A simplified, generic model of the self-regulation process

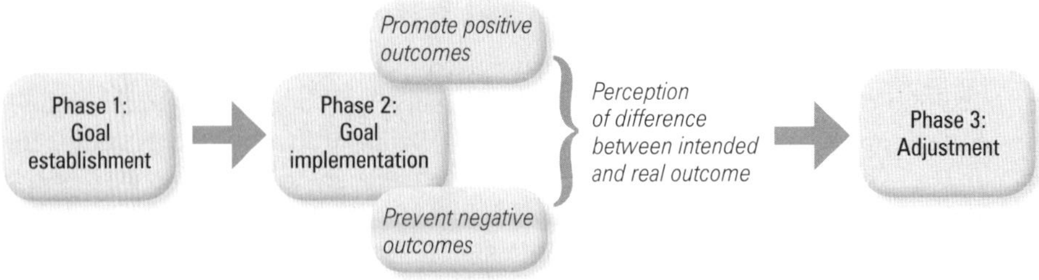

Source: © Botha, 2012.

In the first phase, goal establishment gives direction to how goals are put into action. During this phase, motivational aspects like self-efficacy beliefs and intrinsic motivation play a vital role in establishing goals that will be easier to self-regulate. In the second phase, during goal implementation, the individual aims to promote positive outcomes and prevent negative outcomes. To do this, he or she needs to focus attention on the task at hand, control and regulate internal and external distractions, and monitor his or her own behaviour by comparing it with personal goals and standards in an effort to get feedback about the success of one's behaviour. Finally, if a difference between an intended and real outcome is anticipated, or actually occurs, the individual needs to make appropriate adjustments. According to Brandtstädter and Rothermund (2002), adjustment is possible through adaptive flexibility, the ability to flexibly switch between different means of reaching a goal, whether persevering, changing, or even disengaging from a goal, depending on what would be most appropriate or effective in any given situation.

Kuhl, Kazén, and Koole (2006) state that self-regulation is an immensely adaptive capacity, as effective self-regulation fosters health-promoting behaviours, positive psychological well-being, and high job performance. This adaptive capacity has been supported by a number of South African studies, for example, in (i) black South African students, in which self-regulation correlates positively with positive affect and subjective well-being (Khumalo et al., 2008); (ii) children in the Durban area, who regulate themselves in an attempt to adopt a position of care and concern for those who are living with HIV (Bhana, 2008); and (iii) street youths in the Free State and Gauteng who cope by being able to regulate themselves by adjusting their behaviour, for example, by demonstrating respect for the community's values, even if different from their own, and asking forgiveness when appropriate (Malindi & Theron, 2010).

Coping

The ability to cope with the stress associated with daily living plays an important role in determining the mental wellness of an individual. Coping can be defined as 'constantly changing cognitive and behavioural efforts to manage specific external and/or internal demands that are appraised as taxing or exceeding the resources of a person' (Lazarus & Folkman, 1984, p.141). These cognitive and behavioural efforts are directed at mastering, tolerating, reducing, and/or minimising environmental and internal demands and conflicts that strain an individual's resources (Schafer, 2000). Lazarus and Folkman (1984) have proposed that the way individuals appraise situations they are faced with largely determines the level of stress they experience. Coping, however, is not just related to the demands of the situation, but is also determined by the extent of the resources available to a person (Compton, 2005; Frydenburg, 1997).

There are a large number of coping styles which can be grouped into three subtypes: (1) those in which a person attempts to change negative emotions, (2) those in which a person attempts to change the situation that caused the stress, and (3) those that just seek to avoid the problem. These are called emotion-focused coping, problem-focused coping, and avoidance, respectively (Compton, 2005). According to Lazarus and Folkman (1984, p.150), emotion-focused coping is 'directed at regulating emotional responses to problems'. The goal is to release the tension, forget the anxiety, eliminate worry, or just release the anger. Research suggests that emotion-focused coping might be effective in the initial stages of coping; however, the beneficial effects of these strategies are usually short-lived, with levels of renewed anxiety and stress returning as stressful circumstances persist (Reineke, 2006).

Another coping style, problem-focused coping, involves the use of realistic strategies that could make a tangible difference in the situation that causes stress (Compton, 2005). The use of problem-focused coping strategies has been reported to increase the likelihood of positive outcomes, which then allows individuals to be hopeful and improve their levels of motivation and satisfaction (Lewis & Frydenburg, 2002). Examples of problem-focused coping strategies include situational coping, self-restructuring, and accessing social support. These types of coping strategies are associated with good problem-solving skills, cognitive and behavioural restructuring, seeking help or advice and information regarding the problem, and establishing plans and steps that should be taken to deal with a stressful situation (Wong, Reker, & Peacock, 2006).

Of course, in many instances, people combine the above two types of coping. For instance, if a person consistently takes work problems home to their spouse, but the discussions help the person to decide on a course of action that could change the situation, then he or she has combined emotion-focused and problem-focused coping to help solve the problem.

Lastly, another way of dealing with stressors is to simply use avoidance (Compton, 2005). Here, a person attempts to run away from stress, refuses to confront difficulties presented by life events, or attempts to deny their impact and importance. Under most circumstances this strategy is not very adaptive.

Cultural and gender differences may also influence the type of coping used. Possible differences between the coping strategies employed by individuals from collectivist cultures and those from more individualist cultures have been noted (Hashim, 2003; Mann et al., 1998). People from mainly individualistic cultures are more inclined to demonstrate more active forms of coping such as emotion-focused and problem-focused coping, while people from collectivist cultures are more inclined to utilise avoidant coping (Hashim, 2003; Mann et al., 1998). Although very little research is available with regard to ethnic differences and coping within the South African context, George (2009) reported a higher usage of avoidance coping strategies amongst black and coloured adolescents than white adolescents.

Frydenburg (1997) found that boys (more than girls) use avoidance as a coping mechanism. Boys tend to get involved in alternative activities, such as sport to reduce their stress and in this way they suppress or ignore the problem more than girls do. Girls, however, are more inclined to use social support, rely on others for approval, and appraise events as more complex and negative so they are more affected by stressful situations than boys (Frydenburg, 1997; Frydenburg, 2008; Seiffge-Krenke, 2006). In a South African study involving adolescents, Wissing, Claassens, and du Toit (1998) found that female participants more often used emotion-focused coping strategies such as seeking social support and emotional discharge to deal with stress.

Resilience

Adverse life events such as family violence, the loss of a loved one, traumatic experiences and sexual molestation often result in mental health problems. However, what is surprising is that many of the individuals exposed to these adverse life events turn out to be quite well adjusted (Baumgardner & Crothers, 2009). After a brief period of disturbance, some people quickly return to competent and healthy functioning. Like a rubber band that is stretched, but does not break, resilient individuals are able to regain their composure and confidence, and move forward with their lives.

As suggested above, the underlying concept of resiliency is the belief that some people emerge from stressful conditions as competent, well-adapted individuals (Peterson, 2006a; Phan, 2006). Masten (2001) defines resilience as a phenomenon characterised by good outcomes in spite of serious threats to adaptation or development. Similarly, Ryff and Singer (2003, p. 20) define resilience as 'maintenance, recovery, or improvement in mental or physical health following challenge'. Resilience is often operationalised as the positive end of the distribution of developmental outcomes in a sample of high-risk individuals. Risk and resiliency research is traditionally part of the field of developmental psychopathology. In other words, resilience is a construct that emerged from the field of child and adolescent psychology, and which surfaces here as the contrast of psychopathology (Masten, 2001; Phan, 2006).

It is important to note that the descriptions of resilient responses or resilient individuals are judgment calls (Baumgardner & Crothers, 2009). For a judgment of resilience to be made, a person must first face a significant threat or risk that has the potential to produce negative outcomes. Without a demonstrated risk, there is no resilience. The second part of resilience requires judgment of a favourable or good outcome. The standards for judging outcomes may be defined by the normative expectations of society for the age and situation of the individual. Finally, as suggested above, Masten (2001) notes that some researchers have defined resilience as an absence of problem behaviours or psychopathology following adversity. Children of alcoholic, mentally ill, or abusive parents may be judged resilient if

> **HELPFUL HINT**
>
> **Three types of coping**
>
> - Emotion-focused
> - Problem-focused
> - Avoidant.

they do not develop substance abuse problems, suffer mental illness, become abusive parents themselves, or show symptoms of poor adjustment.

Studies suggest various adaptive systems as explanations of resilience, focussing on processes acting at multiple levels from childhood to old age, which promote and protect human development across the lifespan (Carrey & Ungar, 2007; Lerner, 2006; Masten & Obradovic, 2006).

Post-traumatic growth

A growing body of empirical literature reveals that many people find meaningful life lessons, a renewed appreciation for life, and increased feelings of personal strength as a result of traumatic experiences (see Affleck & Tennen, 1996; Nolen-Hoeksema & Davis, 2002; Tennen & Affleck, 2002, for reviews). Previously, this area of study has been referred to as benefit-finding, positive changes, growth from adversity, thriving, and psychological growth (Lechner, 2009; Tennen & Affleck, 2002) but this phenomenon is now known as post-traumatic growth (Hefferon & Boniwell, 2011). Drawing on the work of the existential psychiatrist Viktor Frankl (1976), post-traumatic growth captures the main theme of research showing the potential for growth and enhancement that may result from personal suffering (Baumgardner & Crothers, 2009). Frankl argued that a will to find meaning was a basic motivational force in people's lives. He thought that people need an overarching sense of purpose, meaning, and direction to sustain them through life's journey.

A meaningful life is expressed in people's goals and ambitions that, in turn, direct their energy towards the future. When traumatic experiences shatter or disrupt these goals and purposes, life may be perceived as meaningless. Under such conditions, people are highly motivated to restore a sense of meaning and purpose to their lives. Such circumstances present opportunities for personal growth as people develop and commit themselves to new goals, ambitions, and purposes that re-establish their sense of meaning and direction (Baumgardner & Crothers, 2009).

Between the initial traumatic event and the subsequent experience of post-traumatic growth, the individual needs to engage in appropriate cognitive work (Triplett, Tedeschi, Cann, Calhoun, & Reeve, 2011). Thus, a significant factor in the path from cognitive threat to growth is assumed to be the degree to which the person engages in repeated thinking about the event. Meaning-making seems to be an important aspect of this process. Meaning-making refers to an active process of reappraisal and revision of how an event might be interpreted or what it might signify (Baumeister & Vohs, 2002).

Researchers have focused on two forms of meaning-making following a traumatic event: making sense of the event and finding benefits or positive outcomes from the event (Nolen-Hoeksema & Davis, 2002). Sense-making refers to making the event comprehensible in terms of a person's assumptions or beliefs about how the world operates (Baumgardner & Crothers, 2009; Janoff-Bulman, 1992). The second form of meaning-making is called benefit-finding (Baumgardner & Crothers, 2009). This involves finding benefits or positive outcomes in trauma and loss. Research consistently finds that people report positive benefits from adversity. For example, Nolen-Hoeksema and Davis (2002) found that six months after losing a loved one to terminal illness, 73% of bereaved people reported at least some positive outcomes. Eighteen months later, 77% reported some benefit from their loss.

Interpersonal strengths

One of the most important risks for the development of abnormal behaviour relates to interpersonal deficits, for instance, lack of effective interpersonal skills, aggression, revenge, unresolved conflict, neglect, and abuse. In this section, we will briefly discuss altruism, empathy, humility, and forgiveness as interpersonal strengths.

Altruism is a form of prosocial behaviour intended to benefit others. It is motivated by internal motives such as concern for others or by internalised values, goals, and self-rewards rather than by the expectation of concrete or social rewards or the avoidance of punishment (Eisenberg & Ota Wang, 2003). The source of altruistic motivation, according to Batson, Ahmad, Lishner, and Tsang (2005, p. 496), is empathy, defined as 'an other-oriented emotional response elicited by and congruent with the perceived welfare of someone else'. It is interesting to note that transpersonal patterns of empathy also appear in rock art and the San people's history (Edwards, 2010). In the Nguni culture, this deep social empathic process is known as *umuntu ngu umuntu ngabantu*, which literally means 'a person is a person through others'. This expression, generally known as *ubuntu*, refers to humane care, dignity, and cultured humanity, developed through processes of mutuality, humanisation, socialisation, and communal spirituality (Edwards, 2010).

Related to altruism and empathy is the capacity of individuals for tolerance and understanding of people different from themselves – a capacity necessary for peaceful coexistence and cooperation among people from various cultures and racial or ethnic backgrounds (Eisenberg & Ota Wang, 2003). Critical ingredients and prerequisites of tolerance and understanding are humility and forgiveness. Tangney (2005) indicates that humility is:

- The ability to keep one's talents and accomplishments in perspective
- To have a sense of self-acceptance
- An understanding of one's imperfections
- To be free from both arrogance and low self-esteem.

Tangney (2005) further emphasises that humility is an increase in the valuation of others, rather than a decrease in the valuation of oneself. Indeed, Tangney argues that, to a certain extent, humility is the opposite of narcissism (a pathological form of self-focus – see Chapter 12), while it also inhibits anger and aggression, and fosters forgiveness.

McCullough and Van Oyen Witvliet (2005, p. 446) define forgiveness as 'an approach whereby people suppress their natural negative responses to transgressors and become increasingly motivated to enact positive ones instead'. According to Van Dyk (2008), given our country's history of conflict and violence, there is a great need for forgiveness between ethnic and racial groups. McCullough and Van Oyen Witvliet (2005) argue, however, that the tendency to retaliate or seek retribution after being victimised is deeply ingrained in the biological, psychological, and cultural levels of human nature. This is costly, Van Dyk (2008) indicates, as lack of forgiveness is related to, among others, higher levels of depression and health complaints; obsessions with power, stereotypes, and paranoia; lower self-esteem; and power struggles. It makes sense, therefore, that one of the aims of the Truth and Reconciliation Commission in South Africa was healing through forgiveness, preventing further pathology developing from the adverse consequences of apartheid.

TREATMENT FROM A WELLNESS PERSPECTIVE

In traditional clinical psychology, the primary goal has been symptom reduction in mental illness, whereas from a wellness perspective, symptom reduction should only be one component in treatment (Keyes & Lopez, 2005). The objective in positive psychology treatment is to promote levels of well-being or build upon a person's existing strengths. More specifically, Joseph and Linley (2004) argue that the positive psychotherapist's task is to facilitate the client's inherent tendency towards actualisation. Moreover, if psychological problems are seen as deficits in the tendency toward actualisation, the therapist, in working to facilitate the actualising tendency, is both helping to alleviate problems and to promote well-being. In this way, ill-being and well-being are understood as a continuum of experience rather than as distinct categories. Joseph and Linley (2004) recognise, however, that the medical approach need not be rejected altogether, and some disorders should still be treated within the medical field by psychiatrists.

A number of psychotherapeutic models have been developed from the positive psychology perspective. For example, solution-focused therapy (De Shazer & Berg, 1997) places the focus on solutions rather on problems. Within a collaborative therapist-client relationship, strengths that have been used to solve similar problems in the past are rediscovered and realistic goals for newer healthy behaviours are set. The focus is thus clearly on what is right in the person's functioning, and what works, rather than on what is wrong.

Positive psychotherapy (Peseschkian, 1997, in Compton, 2005) hypothesises that each person has inherent but underutilised capabilities for dealing with problems. The task of the therapist is to assess the person's abilities, possibilities, and problems and to enhance a person's underutilised strengths and capabilities.

Hope therapy (Lopez, Floyd, Ulven, & Snyder, 2000) is based on the idea that hope is characterised by pathways thinking (see earlier in this chapter). The aim is thus to help people to identify and develop clear goals; to facilitate the belief that they have the capacities and resources to reach those goals; to identify numerous paths to those goals; and to summon the energy and commitment to reach those goals.

Finally, **well-being therapy** (WBT) (Ruini & Fava, 2004) is a structured, directive, short-term psychotherapeutic strategy based on Ryff's model of psychological well-being. The purpose of WBT is to move people from impaired to optimal functioning in the six dimensions of psychological well-being (Ruini & Fava, 2004). For example, if we take the well-being dimension *purpose in life*, the aim is to move the client from lacking a sense of meaning and goal-directedness in life to having goals, aims and objectives for living, and a sense of directedness, meaning, and purpose in life. WBT's effectiveness may be based on two distinct clinical phenomena: (i) an increase in psychological well-being may have a protective effect in terms of vulnerability to chronic and acute life stresses (cf. Ryff & Singer, 1998); and (ii) the inverse correlation between positive and negative affects contributes to the fact that changes in well-being may induce a decrease in distress and vice versa. Therefore, an increase in psychological well-being may decrease residual symptoms that direct strategies like cognitive therapy or pharmacology would be unlikely to affect. It is important, however, to remember that WBT is still at a developmental stage, and more validation studies are required to further elucidate its specific role in clinical and health psychology.

CONCLUSION

Although there is some critique that positive psychology is nothing more than a trend with a short lifespan, Baumgardner and Crothers (2010) indicate that positive psychology has generated a large amount of research and theory, and achieved scientific respectability to promote the study and understanding of healthy human functioning. According to Peterson (2006b), positive psychology does have something to say about abnormal psychology, specifically in providing a lens of normality through which to view abnormality. Peterson (2006b) proposes that as positive psychology is about the presence of strengths, the absence of these strengths should be used as the hallmark of 'real' psychological disorder. In support of Seligman (2006), who proposed that positive psychology is not intended as a replacement for clinical psychology, Peterson (2006b) further indicates that this approach might expand what clinical psychologists most helpfully do.

In this regard, both Maddux (2008) and Wood and Tarrier (2010) propose a new approach to abnormal psychology, called positive clinical psychology, which should:

- Be more integrated and reject the illness ideology
- Predict disorders above and beyond the presence of negative characteristics
- Promote resilience in non-clinical populations
- Foster positive characteristics to treat clinical disorder
- Have the potential to rapidly expand the knowledge base of clinical psychology.

In conclusion, we would like to support Sheldon and King (2001, p. 216) who said that 'positive psychology is an attempt to urge psychologists to adopt a more open and appreciative perspective regarding human potentials, motives and capacities'.

MULTIPLE-CHOICE QUESTIONS

1. According to Martin Seligman, psychology is not just the study of disease, weakness, and damage, but also:
   a) the study of relationships
   b) the study of mental illness
   c) the study of strength and virtue
   d) the study of human beings

2. Generally, well-being has been conceptualised within the positive psychology approach from two related, but different traditions, namely:
   a) wisdom and courage
   b) hedonic and eudaimonic
   c) coping and resilience
   d) psychoanalytic and clinical

3. Which of the following is NOT an example of a protective factor against the development of mental illness?
   a) optimism
   b) emotional intelligence
   c) denial
   d) resilience

4. Emotional intelligence involves the ability to:
   a) know what other people are thinking before they do
   b) monitor one's own and others' feelings and emotions, to discriminate among them, and use the information to guide one's thinking and actions
   c) set personal goals and steer behaviour toward the achievement of established goals
   d) none of the above

5. According to the theory on coping described in this chapter, three types of coping styles can be identified. They are:
   a) emotion-focused coping, problem-focused coping, and avoidant coping
   b) emotion-focused coping, behaviour-focused coping, and denial-focused coping
   c) emotion-focused coping, relationship-focused coping, and solution-focused coping
   d) none of the above

PARAGRAPH AND ESSAY QUESTIONS

1. Discuss the six basic elements of positive functioning as proposed by the work of Carol Ryff.

2. Compare and contrast the different forms of coping. Make sure to note similarities and differences.

3. Describe the different psychotherapeutic models that have been developed from the positive psychology perspective. Provide a brief description, as well as the specific aim, of the different models.

4 ANXIETY, OBSESSIVE-COMPULSIVE AND TRAUMA RELATED DISORDERS

Melanie Lake

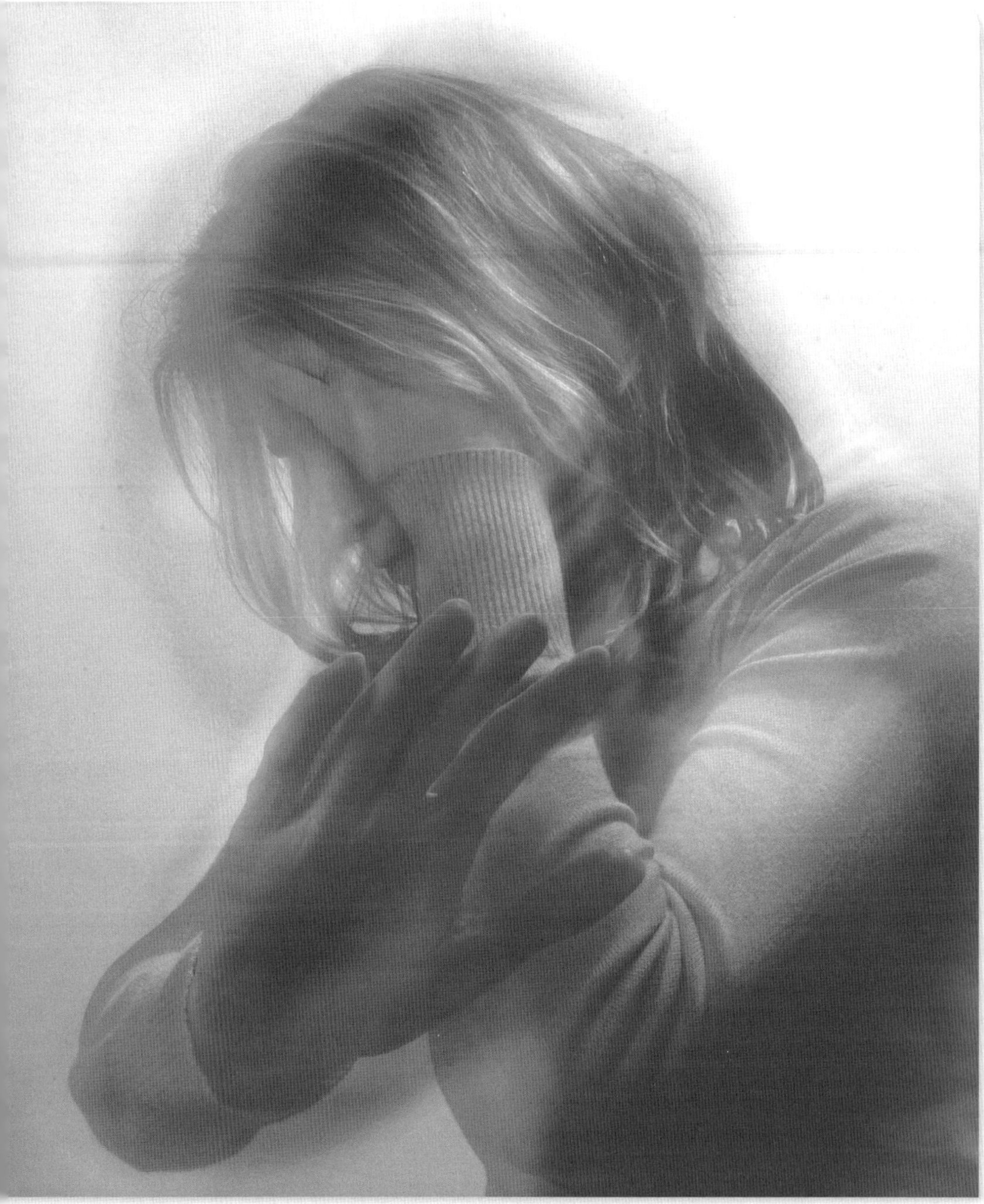

4 CHAPTER OUTLINE

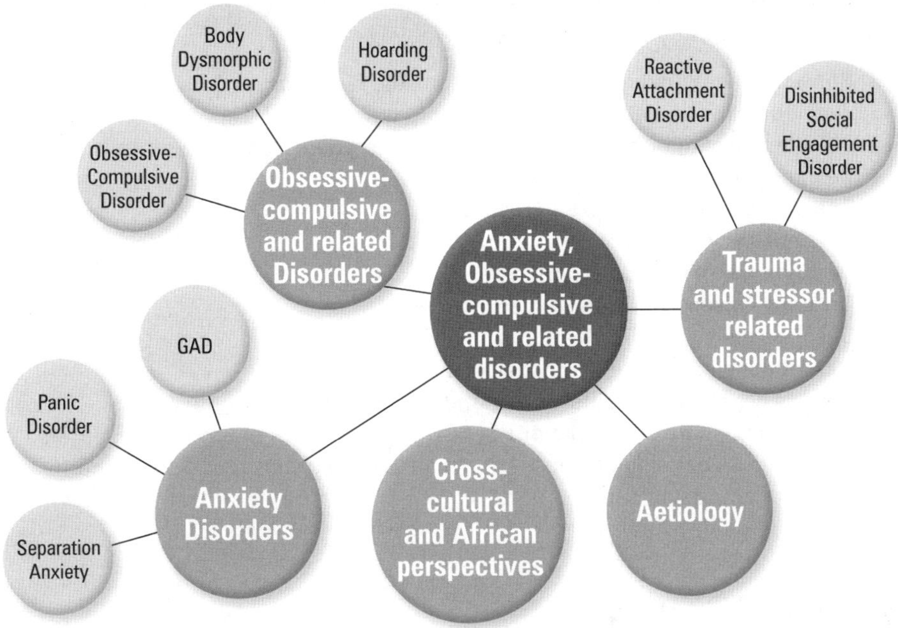

Introduction

Fear, anxiety and stress

Fear

Anxiety

Stress

History of anxiety and panic disorders

Clinical picture

Section 1: Anxiety Disorders

Separation Anxiety Disorder

- Specific Phobias
- Social Anxiety Disorder

Panic Disorder

- Agoraphobia

Generalised Anxiety Disorder

Section 2: Obsessive-Compulsive and related disorders

Obsessive-Compulsive Disorder

Body Dysmorphic Disorder

Hoarding Disorder

- Trichotillomania (Hair-Pulling Disorder)
- Excoriation (Skin-Picking Disorder)

Section 3: Trauma and stressor related disorders

Reactive Attachment Disorder

Disinhibited Social Engagement Disorder

- Posttraumatic Stress Disorder (PTSD)
- Acute Stress Disorder

Cross-cultural and African perspectives

Aetiology

Biological perspectives

- Genetics
- Neurochemistry
- Brain structure and functioning

Psychological perspectives

- Psychodynamic models
- Humanistic models
- Behavioural models
- Cognitive models
- Personality and temperament

Psychosocial stressors

Familial perspectives

Sociocultural perspectives

Integrated perspectives

Conclusion

LEARNING OUTCOMES

After studying this chapter you should be able to:

- Show a general understanding of the anxiety disorders, and be able to distinguish the anxiety disorders from the other mental disorders.
- Be able to distinguish the different anxiety disorders from each other.
- Describe the history of the anxiety disorders.
- Describe Generalised Anxiety Disorder.
- Describe the panic disorders.
- Describe the phobic disorders.
- Describe Obsessive-Compulsive Disorder.
- Describe the stress disorders.
- Describe the additional diagnoses of anxiety.
- Discuss cross-cultural differences, and more specifically South African particulars, in terms of variations in the presentation of the anxiety disorders.
- Formulate an aetiological model of the anxiety disorders and discuss the integrated model of aetiology.

INTRODUCTION

In previous editions of the DSM, the anxiety disorders (e.g. Generalized Anxiety Disorder, Panic Disorder and Phobias), obsessive-compulsive disorders and stress related disorders were all grouped together in one category, Anxiety Disorders. In the DSM-5, these disorders are now split into three distinct categories; however, the sequential order of these chapters in DSM-5 reflects the close relationships (the presence of anxiety) between them. The anxiety and stress related disorders make up the most common categories of mental disorders. They are often the principal diagnosis or the 'reason for visit' of a new patient to a psychologist or psychiatrist. People who experience anxiety and stress related disorders may be left with compounded problems. The costs of general health care for those with anxiety problems are estimated to be double that of the non-anxious (Barlow, 2004). The prescription drugs given to treat anxiety disorders are also considered to be the most widely used.

In terms of epidemiological data, the anxiety and stress related disorders are considered to be the most commonly occurring form of psychological disturbance (Craske, 2003). Moreover, patients with an anxiety disorder have been found to have a co-morbid mental disorder in 74% of cases. The co-morbid conditions most often found with these disorders are the mood disorders, another anxiety disorder, substance use-related disorders (Conway, Compton, Stinson, & Grant, 2006), somatoform disorders, and the personality disorders (Grant et al., 2005). These disorders are also common in people with an Intellectual Disability (ID) level of cognitive impairment (Reid, Smiley, & Cooper, 2011). Stressful life events are associated with the onset of anxiety related disorders in all people, but particularly so in ID adults, whose anxiety was often found to be precipitated by a recent history of life events and by a lack of day-time employment.

ACTIVITY

See the online version of the Social Readjustment Rating Scale (SRRS), with results given in Life Change Units (LCUs). The SRRS goes some way towards quantifying the eustress and distress related to recent life events, as discussed below.

Source: http://www.mindtools.com/pages/article/newTCS_82.htm

A gender bias is observed in anxiety diagnoses, with women suffering disproportionately from anxiousness, and being at greater risk for developing anxiety disorders across all of the age groups, when compared to men (Barlow, 2004; Craske, 2003). The prevalence rates of anxiety disorders tend to decline with age, but anxiety remains very common, especially in women (Byres, Yaffe, Covinsky, Friedman, & Bruce, 2010). In Byres et al.'s (2010) study, anxiety disorders were as high as, if not higher than, mood disorders, in populations of older community-dwelling adults and the rates of co-existing mood-anxiety disorder were also high.

Figure 4.1: Understanding the difference between problematic anxiety and worry that is still 'within normal limits' is important in psychology.

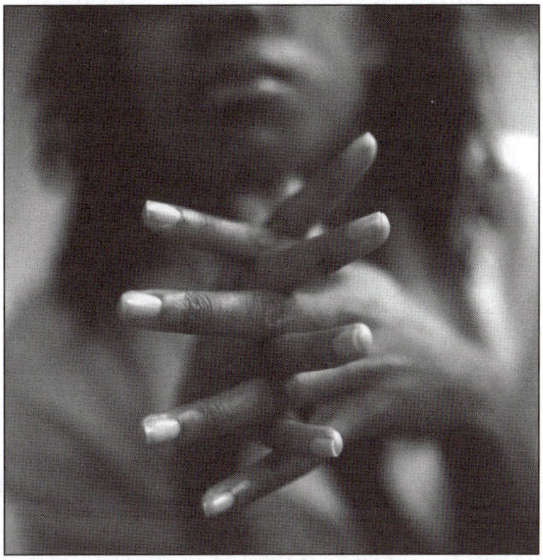

To better understand anxiety that reaches the level of disordered behaviour, we need to understand how it can also be functional in daily life. For example, experiencing a reasonable amount of anxiety during your driver's licence test is normal and may even help you to function optimally. Feeling worried and anxious about your first job interview tomorrow morning can, likewise, be expected and may not do any harm. Anxiety can serve both a protective and a useful function in that it can motivate us to adapt to or plan for the future (Barlow, 2004). Fear can serve an essential biological survival function through preparing us to escape or fight back when faced with danger. In truly threatening circumstances, an organism will benefit from the mobilisation of physical and cognitive resources in preparation for a concentrated action or reaction. Even the panic response of 'freezing up' has been acknowledged for its survival value in certain situations.

Most of the symptoms of the anxiety related disorders are subjective experiences (emotions and cognitions) and a patient would need to report the presence and severity of psychological phenomena such as worry, apprehension, fear, or derealisation to a mental health practitioner. Cognitively, a central feature of anxiety disorders is the preoccupation with threat and danger (Beck, 2005a). Perceptually, a person's hypervigilance to physical symptoms, which are then interpreted as dangerous, fuels this vicious cycle of fear.

Worry, or anxious apprehension, is very common in people with anxiety related disorders (Olatunji, Wolitzky-Taylor, Sawchuk, & Ciesielski, 2011) as is worry across several domains, and high incidences of 'meta-worry'. Meta-worry, or worry about being worried, is well discussed in the Rational Emotive Behaviour Therapy (REBT) writings of Albert Ellis. He considered meta-worry (or any form of distress about being distressed) to be an important treatment target that needs addressing before the presenting anxiety can be dealt with.

CASE STUDY

Maria's employer thinks of her as 'very shy and self-conscious' but this really refers to Maria's apprehensive avoidance of talking about herself. Maria has unusual obsessions and compulsions, which she realises are unreasonable, and that she keeps very private. Maria may be excessively concerned about her symptoms, and believe that others will dislike her when they discover how anxious she is and what she worries about. If this is meta-worry, how do you think Maria's psychologist would need to start working with her in order to best be able to help?

When anxiety becomes excessive, impairs general functioning, or causes significant distress, we can say that it is dysfunctional. An anxiety disorder may also result when the symptoms of fear continue to be experienced long after the legitimately fear-producing situation had passed.

This can be summed up by saying that the fears of people with anxiety disorders are:

- Severe and distressing, and ultimately reduce quality of life
- Chronic or sufficiently frequent in order to impair functioning
- Out of proportion to the reality of danger or the threat of danger.

FEAR, ANXIETY AND STRESS

The constructs of fear, anxiety and stress are often erroneously used interchangeably, but they are in fact three distinct constructs. These constructs actually define the parameters for the different anxiety and stress related disorders.

Fear

Fear is a psychological phenomenon closely related to anxiety. Fear is best defined as a present-oriented mood state, with strong negative affect, that motivates one to escape or avoid danger or threat (Barlow & Durand, 2005). For example, if you are walking in your suburb and see a large, vicious-looking dog down the road, your experience of fear will probably cause you to move away quickly. In this way, fear in response to the real threat of danger has an important survival function. Our nervous system is designed to function well up to a point, and a 'true alarm' in terms of fear is mostly functional (Beck, 2005a).

The sudden activation of the sympathetic nervous system will cause an immediate 'alarm response' (fight or flight response) meant to prepare one both physically and mentally for self-defence or escape. Fear is a normal and essential emotional state, albeit an intensely unpleasant one. It is, however, precisely this unpleasantness that motivates one to get out of danger, and thus reduce the intense negative affect. With adaptive levels of fear, the alarm response will subside once the danger or threat passes. With maladaptive levels of anxiety, people's fear persists even once a threat has passed and they may experience excessive anticipatory anxiety about the future.

An episode of fear can be seen to impact across the human systems: physiologically (sweating), cognitively (anticipation), affectively (terror), behaviourally (inhibition), and motivationally (wish to escape). These well-known signs and symptoms alert us to the presence of intense fear (Beck, 2005a). Many of these signs are listed as criteria for a Panic Attack (see Table 4.4). People who experience insufficient fear and anxiety may, in fact, have problems with functioning. The low levels of arousability found in people exhibiting Antisocial Personality Disorder (see Chapter 12) are linked to the fearlessness and stimulation-seeking behaviours that cause many of their symptoms (Nolen-Hoeksema, 2007).

Anxiety

Anxiety is a future-oriented mood state, again accompanied by strong negative affect; it is also a normal emotional state that can be functional within certain limits (Barlow & Durand, 2005). Most often, anxiety concerns some future event that is very important or that may be difficult. A functional level of anxiety about an upcoming entrance examination, for example, may involve thinking about all possible ways in which it might turn out, so-called 'scenario testing', which results in a person being very well prepared.

It may be said that 'evolution favours anxious genes' (Beck, 2005a, p. 4) and that generations of people have been selected for their responsiveness to anxiety in situations of true threat. A dysfunctional level of anxiety, however, could result in a different person feeling so wound-up and overwhelmed by the prospect of the abovementioned examination that they avoid going altogether and miss out on a much-wanted opportunity.

Anxiety has psychological components that are both affective and cognitive. The negative affect is experienced in feelings of fear, distress, apprehension, and uneasiness. Related to these unpleasant emotions may be preoccupying thoughts about imminent danger, a perception of powerlessness in the face of danger, and intense watchfulness or hypervigilance as one expects, and attempts to detect, danger. Frequently, these processes have an escalating effect on the experience of anxiety. As a result of the intense unpleasant emotions, the person finds signs of psychophysiological arousal in him- or herself, and believes these to be evidence of some threat or danger that must be real, which results in further arousal. It can be said that anxiety has a compounding, self-aggravating effect that may worsen the experience of its symptoms unless the individual breaks this cycle with calmed emotions (relaxation) or more rational thoughts (cognitive monitoring). Many people who experience incapacitating anxiety report that they are unable to control it, however, and they may need anxiolytics (anti-anxiety medications) to manage their symptomatology.

The anxiety disorders are best understood as 'false alarms', as a person responds with fear and anxiety when there is no truly life-threatening or dangerous situation. When a generally harmless situation (speaking in public) or stimulus (riding an elevator) produces sufficient fear or anxiety in a person such that he or she experiences intense distress, cannot function normally, or avoids the situation or stimulus excessively, then an anxiety disorder is most likely present. This category of disorder often has a debilitating effect on people's lives, preventing them from doing, enjoying, or even trying out many activities that the non-anxious take for granted. Moreover, certain anxiety disorders may impair an individual's capacity to perform necessary activities such as taking public transport daily or functioning in a job that requires interaction with people.

Anxiety has both psychological and physical components, with apprehension about future threat or danger, and somatic symptoms of tension, being typical signs. The psychological symptoms (both emotional and cognitive) and somatic symptoms are frequently accompanied by behavioural symptoms that also assist us in identifying anxiety disorders. Examples of these are given in Table 4.1.

Table 4.1: Typical emotional, cognitive, somatic and behavioural symptoms of anxiety

Emotional	Cognitive	Somatic	Behavioural
Restlessness Irritability Sense of dread Terror	Worry, ruminations Poor concentration Anticipating harm Fear of losing control or dying Hypervigilance	Adrenaline secretion Increased heart rate Increased perspiration Deep, quick respiration Dilated pupils Dilated peripheral blood vessels Widened bronchioles Muscle tension Goosebumps Decreased salivation, stomach acid	Freeze up Escape (flight) Aggression (fight) Avoidance Decreased appetite

You will almost certainly have experienced some of the typical physical symptoms of anxiety in your life. Researchers Freeston et al. (1996) had non-clinical subjects complete a Generalised Anxiety Disorder (GAD) questionnaire and found that a number of them experienced certain physical symptoms that resemble GAD. It was concluded that the DSM-IV contained some items that are regularly endorsed even by those who do not have anxiety disorders; therefore, the physical symptoms that are currently in the DSM should be weighed more heavily in the diagnosis of GAD, in order to differentiate between this disorder and 'ordinary' worrying.

Stress

One way of defining stress is the reaction(s) of an organism to any demand such that they feel they cannot cope. However, people are most likely to perceive such demanding life events as qualitatively positive or negative. Hans Selye (Cooper, 2005) introduced the concepts of 'eustress' for the former and 'distress' for the latter condition. However, the stress medicine field does tend to focus its research efforts on the negative events or distress reported by participants. Empirical findings have shown that the relationship we see between life events and illness is mainly due to the effects of negative events.

Fear and the 'alarm response' mentioned above are considered to be the first phase of the stress response and the General Adaptation Syndrome (GAS) as theorised by Hans Selye (Barlow, & Durand, 2005). Phase two of the GAS is called 'Resistance' and is characterised by coping actions, while Phase three is called 'Exhaustion' and refers to the point at which chronic stress and damage can be seen. Ongoing and unmanageable stress has an unfortunate negative effect on the immune system and plays a role in the psychological causation or maintenance of certain physical disorders which are then addressed by health psychology.

HISTORY OF ANXIETY AND PANIC DISORDERS

Until recent times, the anxiety disorders were regarded predominately as the expression of emotion (such as terror or anxiety) that was out of control (Beck, 2005a). The emphasis was clearly placed on emotion as the dramatic central feature of the conditions that we will discuss in this chapter. Theorising about anxiousness and the anxiety disorders has also focused on a search for its causes (Barlow, 2004). Since the time of Freud, the definitions and distinctions of fear and anxiety have been based on the presence or absence of cues. The missing piece of the puzzle was that of cognitions, which have recently, however, taken the forefront in much theorising around anxiety.

Phobias are considered to be very specific kinds of intense fear that typically mobilise avoidance behaviours. This term for fear, 'phobia', derives from the Greek *phobos*, which literally means 'flight' (Beck, 2005a). This word originates from the name of a mythological Greek deity, Phobos, who was purportedly able to inspire great fear (and panic) in his enemies. Hippocrates (460–377 BCE), the ancient Greek physician often referred to as the 'father of medicine' (see Chapter 1), wrote two of the earliest recognisable clinical descriptions of specific phobias, one of nightfall and one of cats. Cicero and Demosthenes were described as having some form of stage fright before overcoming their fears and going on to be renowned orators. Another well-known figure, Augustus Caesar (63 BCE–14 CE), supposedly had a phobic fear of the dark.

From these ancient times, the clinical descriptions of phobias have not changed much (Beck, 2005a). Celsus, believed to be a Greek philosopher and writer in the first and second centuries, is believed to have coined the term 'hydrophobia'. This term describes an aversion to water, a common symptom of the end stages of rabies. Non-medical writings, such as those of religious writers and philosophers, contain accounts of phobias (including demon phobias and theophobias) from the thirteenth century onwards. Even Shakespeare's play *The Merchant of Venice* (in 1596–1598) includes mention of people who have a phobia of cats. From historical accounts, we are able to assume that the mathematician Pascal (1623–1662) suffered from the condition that we now know as Agoraphobia.

It took until the late nineteenth century for 'phobia' to enter the psychiatric literature, however. In 1870, the neurologist Moriz Benedickt described a condition similar to Agoraphobia in his patients in Vienna, Austria. He used the German term *Platzschwindel*, from the German for 'place dizziness' (Balaban & Jacob, 2001; Hinton, Nathan, Bird, & Park, 2002). Soon thereafter, the psychiatrist Carl Westphal coined another German term, *agoraphobie* in 1871 (Callard, 2006; Sinnott, Jones, & Fordham, 2006), from the Greek words *agora* meaning 'open space' or *ageiren* meaning 'to assemble' and *phobia* for 'fear'. In this year, Westphal clinically described three cases of Agoraphobia and the condition became known as a named disorder. The term became known in English from 1873 onwards, taken from Westphal's original usage, and meaning a 'fear of open spaces'.

Beck (2005a) claims that the term 'panic' can be found in general usage from as early as 1603. Swingler (2007) adds that the term can be found specifically in medical literature from 1866 onwards. A similar clinical picture is found in De Costa's 1871 reference to 'irritable heart', a common, panic-like condition observed in soldiers of the American Civil War. Danish explorers of Greenland in the early 1900s reported a panic-like condition they called 'kayak angst' amongst the Inuit (Eskimo) seal hunters. An afflicted hunter would unexpectedly and suddenly begin to experience somatic and psychological symptoms similar to those we rely on today in diagnosing a Panic Attack.

The term 'panic' is derived from the name of the mythological Greek deity, Panikos, also known as Pan (Beck, 2005a). Legend has it that Pan was half-man and half-goat, and a fearsome sight to behold. He was regarded by the Greeks as being the god of the woods and shepherds, and he regularly got up to mischief. One story holds that he would descend daily at midday to frighten the animals, their shepherds, and the nearby nymphs (Swingler, 2007). One such nymph, Syrinx, was purportedly terrified and froze, becoming the reed from which Pan cut his famous pipes. Another story tells that Pan would lie in wait under bridges for unsuspecting travellers on the road. As they passed by, he would leap out and utter a scream so blood-curdling as to petrify his victims, some of whom might even die of fright. Regardless of which legend was believed, the Greeks regarded Pan as the cause of any sudden and groundless fear, thus the link to Panic Disorder.

Previously viewed as a form of 'free-floating' anxiety, Panic Disorder was not always considered a distinct anxiety disorder (Craske & Barlow, 2007). The lack of clear conceptualisation around Panic Disorder could be seen in the non-specific psychological treatment approaches followed, which included relaxation, cognitive restructuring, and pharmacotherapy. In 1980, however, the DSM-III recognised Panic Disorder Without Agoraphobia (PD) and Panic Disorder With Agoraphobia (PDA) as distinct disorders within the greater anxiety category.

As mentioned before, the previous editions of the DSM grouped all the anxiety related disorders together, and although these disorders do share a component of anxiety to a greater or lesser extent, the differences between anxiety disorders, obsessive-compulsive disorders and trauma and stressor related disorders are distinct enough to warrant three separate categories.

CLINICAL PICTURE

Figure 4.2 provides an outline of the three categories of anxiety and stressor related disorders. The clinical pictures of most of these disorders will be discussed in three separate sections, i.e. Section 1: Anxiety Disorders, Section 2: Obsessive-Compulsive and Related Disorders and Section 3: Trauma and Stressor Related Disorders.

Figure 4.2: Categories of anxiety obsessive-compulsive and trauma/stressor related disorders

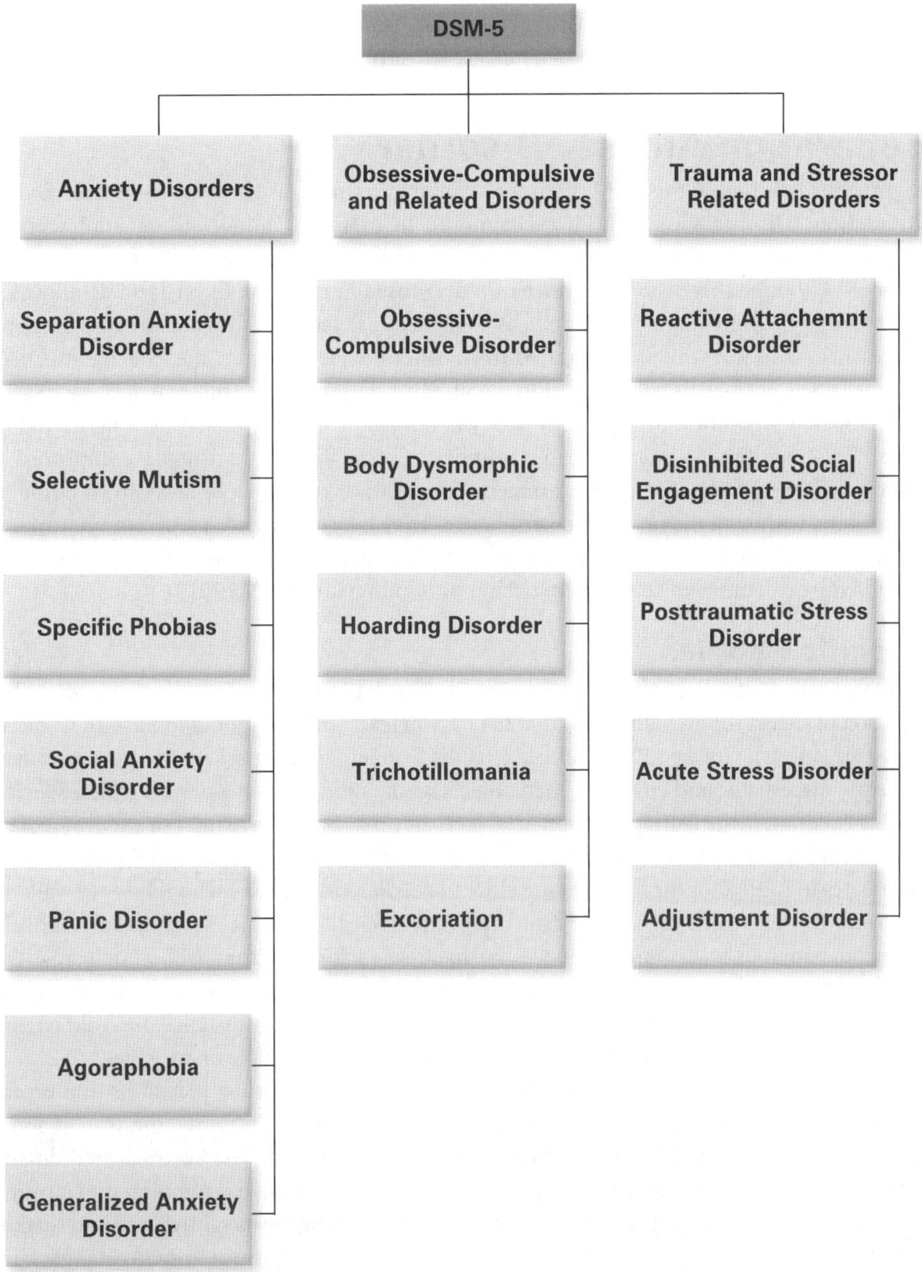

SECTION 1: ANXIETY DISORDERS

This category includes disorders that share features of excessive fear and anxiety and related behavioural disturbances (APA, 2013). They differ from each other in terms of the triggers that induce this fear and anxiety as well as in terms of behavioural consequences and cognitive antecedents.

Separation Anxiety Disorder

In previous editions of the DSM disorders that are common in children were classified in the section "Disorders Usually First Diagnosed in Infancy, Childhood, or Adolescence", however, in the DSM-5 many of the disorders that were in this category were moved to other sections. Although this disorder is primarily diagnosed in children, the criteria do allow for this this diagnosis to be made in adults as well. The core feature of this disorder is extreme distress when an individual is separated from other people to whom she / he are attached. The distress is not necessarily limited to a real, physical separation, but may also be related to anticipated separation or persistent worry about losing a major attachment figure (APA, 2013). The disorder also manifests in a number of behavioural and physical sympsroms. A person suffereing from this disorder may be reluctant, or refuse, to go away from home or being alone without a major attachement figure. They may experience recurrent nightmares (related to separation) and physical symptoms (e.g. headaches, stomach aches, etc,), the latter being evident when separetaion occurs or is anticipated (APA, 2013).

Specific Phobias

Formerly called 'simple phobias', the Specific Phobias typically refer to a clearly recognisable situation or object (often inanimate) that the person fears (unlike Agoraphobia with its many feared situations). Craske (2003) defines Specific Phobias as the marked and persistent fear of clearly discernable and circumscribed objects or situations. When a person with a Specific Phobia encounters the feared situation or object, they may experience intense and immediate anxiety that could reach the levels of a full-blown Panic Attack. For example, someone who never goes to the doctor for fear of being close to needles, or someone who refuses to walk on the beach for fear of encountering a crab, may have a Specific Phobia. Such a person is likely to become anxious and apprehensive at the mere suspicion that they will come across the specific situation or object, and will often make a concerted effort to avoid any contact with it. It is not unheard of for a person with a severe phobia of snakes, for instance, to avoid paging through wildlife magazines for fear of seeing a photograph of a snake on its pages.

Beck (2005a) contends that many fears are innate and that they played an important protective function in the early years of human development. Certainly, the fear of some situations or objects has held survival value for human beings and has been selected during evolution (Barlow, 2004). It is, for instance, adaptive to fear and avoid jumping into a rough sea alone (especially if you are a non-swimmer) or picking up brightly coloured snakes (which are likely to be poisonous). However, with repeated exposure to many dangers, an adaptive mechanism may develop. Firefighters who have trained to fight fires, for example, may experience less anxiety than would other people, even in 'high risk' situations. This may be linked to the heavy reliance on behavioural and cognitive-behavioural treatments favoured for anxiety (Craske & Barlow, 2007).

Figure 4.3: These firefighters may become 'tough-minded' over the years or may have gone through Stress Inoculation Training at work.

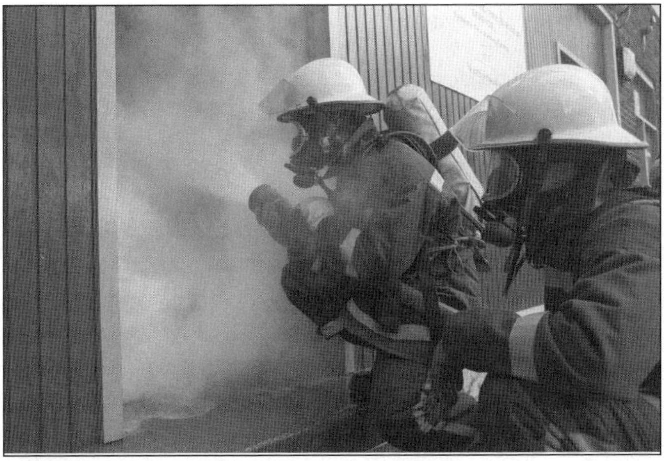

Table 4.2: Diagnostic criteria for Specific Phobia as adapted from the DSM-5 and ICD-10

DSM-5	ICD-10
A. Marked fear or anxiety about a specific object or situation (e.g. flying, heights, animals, receiving an injection, seeing blood). Note: In children, the fear or anxiety may be expressed by crying, tantrums, freezing, or clinging. B. The phobic object or situation almost always provokes immediate fear or anxiety. C. The phobic object or situation is actively avoided or endured with intense fear or anxiety. D. The fear or anxiety is out of proportion to the actual danger posed by the phobic object or situation and to the sociocultural context. E. The fear, anxiety, or avoidance is persistent, typically lasting for six months or more. F. The fear, anxiety, or avoidance causes clinically significant distress or impairment in social, occupational, or other important areas of functioning.	• A disorder in which anxiety is provoked only, or predominately, in certain highly specific situations. • These situations may include proximity to particular animals, heights, thunder, darkness, flying, closed spaces, dentistry, or the sight of blood or injury. • The specific phobic object or situation is then characteristically avoided or endured with dread. • The triggering situation is often discrete. • Contact with the triggering situation can evoke panic attacks.

DSM-5	ICD-10
G. The disturbance is not better explained by symptoms of another mental disorder, including fear, anxiety, and avoidance of situations associated with panic-like symptoms or other incapacitating symptoms (as in agoraphobia); objects or situations related to obsessions (as in obsessive-compulsive disorder); reminders of traumatic events (as in posttraumatic stress disorder); separation from home or attachment figures (as in separation anxiety disorder) or social situations (as in social anxiety disorder).	

Source: Reprinted with permission from the Diagnostic and Statistical Manual of Mental Disorders (DSM), Fifth Edition, American Psychiatric Association (APA), 2013 and ICD–10 Classification of Mental and Behavioural Disorders: Diagnostic Criteria for Research. World Health Organisation (WHO), Geneva, 2007.

The maladaptive fears characteristic of phobias are typically unreasonable or excessive (Beck, 2005b). Adults are able to recognise that their phobic fears are out of proportion to the potential threat of the situation or object, or that they are simply illogical, while children will not necessarily have insight into this. However, this 'danger value' tends to dominate a phobic person's appraisal of a situation (not objectivity) and they are likely to estimate greater harm from the situation or object as they approach it.

Specific Phobia may affect as many as 10% of all people, making it one of the most common disorders, and yet only about 10% of those with a Specific Phobia will seek professional help. Most Specific Phobias develop during childhood. The Specific Phobias are divided into four categories, and when diagnosing this disorder, one must specify the type of situation or object feared. The categories focus on specific types of animals or insects (animal type), specific human-made structures or public transport (situational type), specific situations or events in nature (natural environment type), and the specific circumstance of seeing an injury or blood (blood-injection-injury type).

Common examples of feared objects or situations are:

- ***Animal type:*** dogs, mice, snakes, spiders, moths, worms
- ***Situational type:*** driving in a car, flying in an airplane, elevators, tunnels, bridges, enclosed spaces
- ***Natural environment type:*** heights, water, thunder, lightning
- ***Blood-injection-injury type:*** blood, injection needles, medical practitioners, hospitals, someone else's injury.

People with a Specific Phobia typically experience sympathetic nervous system arousal that causes an alarm response and resultant physiological changes such as increased heart rate, blood pressure, respiration, and perspiration as described above. They react to the phobic situation (e.g. airplane) or object (e.g. mouse) as if it were a truly life-threatening danger that they have to be prepared to either fight or flee. People with a blood-injection-injury type phobia, however, exhibit different and unusual physiological reactions. They typically experience marked decreases in heart rate and blood pressure when encountering their feared situation or object and very often faint as a result. This does seem counterproductive if the fear or anxiety component of these disorders is a false alarm of preparation for better survival responses.

Figure 4.4: An animal type Specific Phobia may lead people to avoid environments, such as the bush, where they are likely to encounter a feared object.

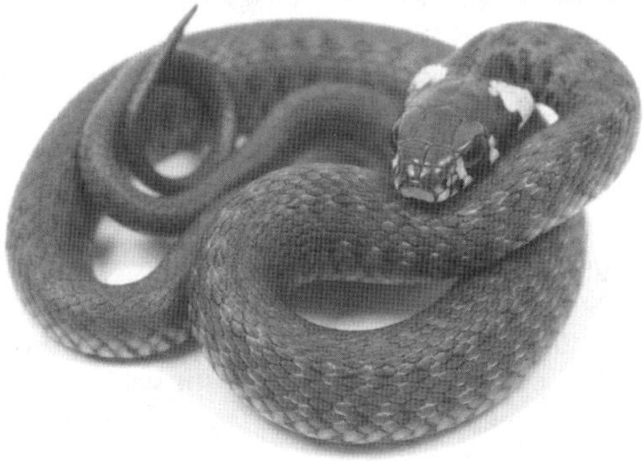

Social Anxiety Disorder

Social Anxiety Disorder is not the fear of a specific situation or object, but rather the fear of scrutiny and evaluation by others or being embarrassed in front of others. It is defined as an excessive fear of social performance situations in which embarrassment is feared (Craske, 2003). For most people, being judged or embarrassed in social situations (especially in front of important others) is an unpleasant experience. Having to speak in public or perform an activity while being closely watched or evaluated is also not a favoured activity for most. However, those who have this disorder exhibit more than moderate nervousness and may experience a full-blown Panic Attack in a social performance situation. They have also been found to believe that everyone judges and criticises the performance skills of others (Turk, Heimberg, & Magee 2007).

The socially anxious individual strongly wishes to avoid being observed or judged by others but, if this should occur, they are likely to experience anxiety, increased perspiration, heart palpitations, trembling and shaking, dizziness, and confusion. People with Social Anxiety Disorder may avoid doing simple things such as eating or drinking with others, writing in front of others, or even using public toilets. The more complex the social task at hand, however, the more likely it is for the phobia to impair performance.

Socially anxious people often believe that others will be able to notice the signs of their anxiety (although these are mostly more subjective than observable) and will judge them for it. For these reasons, behavioural and cognitive-behavioural arguments exist for group therapy treatment of this disorder. Chen et al. (2007) reported that group CBT was an acceptable treatment for Social Anxiety Disorder and that it offers a similar degree of symptom reduction for Japanese as it does for Western patients. In a South African study, Nortje, Posthumus, and Moller (2008) found that, compared to a wait-list control condition, both an 'integrated cognitive restructuring plus exposure' treatment model and an 'exposure alone' model resulted in significant improvements for individuals experiencing Social Phobia. Both of these were delivered in group treatment modalities and their efficacy may underline the importance of managing avoidance and increasing exposure to the feared social setting.

Table 4.3: Diagnostic criteria for Social Anxiety Disorder as adapted from the DSM-5 and ICD-10

DSM-5	ICD-10
A. Marked fear or anxiety about one or more social situtations in which the individual is exposed to possible scrutiny by others. Examples include social interactions (e.g. having a conversation, meeting unfamiliar people), being observed (e.g. eating or drinking), and performing in front of others (e.g. giving a speech). Note: In children, the anxiety must occur in peer settings and not just during interactions with adults. B. The individual fears that he or she will act in a way or show anxiety symptoms that will be negatively evaluated (e.g. will be humiliating or embarrassing; will lead to rejection or offend others). C. The social situations almost always provoke fear or anxiety. Note: In children, the fear or anxiety may be expressed by crying, tantrums, freezing, clinging, shrinking, or failing to speak in social situations. D. The social situations are avoided or endured with intense fear or anxiety. E. The fear or anxiety is out of proportion to the actual threat posed by the social situation and to the sociocultural context. F. The fear, anxiety, or avoidance is persistent, typically lasting for six months or more. G. The fear, anxiety, or avoidance causes clinically significant distress or impairment in social, occupational, or other important areas of functioning. H. The fear, anxiety, or avoidance is not attributable to the physiological effects of a substance (e.g. a drug of abuse, a medication) or another medical condition. I. The fear, anxiety, or avoidance is not better explained by symptoms of another mental disorder, such as panic disorder, body dysmorphic disorder), or autism spectrum disorder. J. If another medical condition (e.g. Parkinson's disease, obesity, disfigurement from burns or injury) is present, the fear, anxiety, or avoidance is clearly unrelated or is excessive.	• A disorder in which anxiety is provoked only, or predominately, in the situation of possible scrutiny by other people. • Certain social situations are then characteristically avoided or endured with dread. • More pervasive social phobias are usually associated with fear of criticism and low self-esteem. • Secondary manifestations may include: blushing, hand tremor, and nausea. Patient is sometimes convinced that these signs are the primary problem. • Symptoms may progress to panic attacks.

Source: Reprinted with permission from the Diagnostic and Statistical Manual of Mental Disorders (DSM), Fifth Edition, American Psychiatric Association (APA), 2013 and ICD–10 Classification of Mental and Behavioural Disorders: Diagnostic Criteria for Research. World Health Organisation (WHO), Geneva, 2007.

Whereas some Specific Phobias may go almost unnoticed and result in minimal disruption in a person's life (a man who fears lizards can live in the city, on the twenty-ninth floor, and avoid the country), the effects of Social Anxiety Disorder are not easy to hide or manage in some cases. Those with Social Anxiety Disorder may engage in 'safety behaviours' when in a social situation, in order to avoid the negative outcome of having their anxiety noticed (Turk et al., 2007). Paradoxically, these compensatory acts may in fact heighten anxiety levels and accompanying shaking, for instance. This disorder can markedly impair one's social and educational or occupational functioning, as these areas of life almost always expose one to interaction with, and dependence on, others. It typically runs a chronic course, and is often co-morbid with other anxiety disorders and mood disorders. The disorder is relatively common, somewhat more so amongst women than men, and yet most people with Social Anxiety Disorder will not seek professional help. Age of onset is most often during either early childhood or adolescence.

This disorder should be distinguished from the other anxiety disorders such as Panic Disorder, Agoraphobia, and Separation Anxiety Disorder. It also shares features with Body Dysmorphic Disorder, Autism Spectrum Disorders, and Schizoid Personality Disorder. A comprehensive diagnosis should specify whether or not the social anxiety is 'generalised', which would be the case if the individual's fears include most social situations as opposed to one or only a few situations. An individual with generalised Social Anxiety Disorder may have a severe fear of initiating or maintaining conversations, attending parties, dating, participating in small groups, and speaking to authority figures. In a less severe form, another group of individuals only moderately fears a variety of social situations, while a third group fears only public speaking. There may be an additional diagnosis to be made of Avoidant Personality Disorder (see Chapter 12).

Figure 4.5: As the symptoms of Panic Attack are often mistaken for medical conditions such as heart attack, medical teams often identify patients with Panic Disorder.

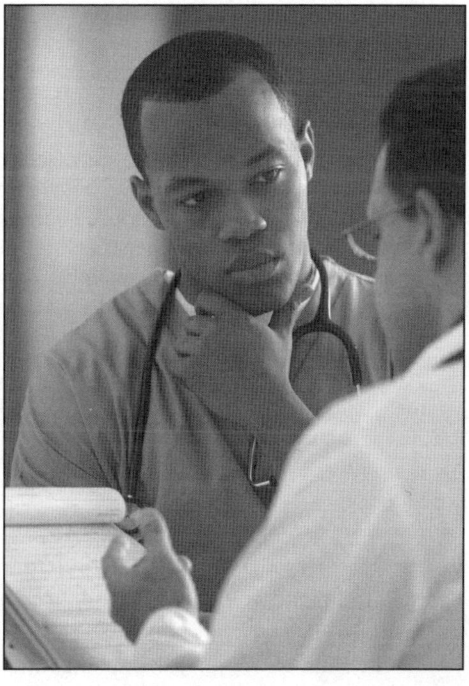

Panic Disorder

Frequently occurring Panic Attacks can be considered a disorder in their own right, called Panic Disorder. However, panic can also be a part of many other anxiety disorders. Panic Attacks may also occur as isolated events for people who do not have a diagnosable anxiety disorder. When facing a severely traumatic event or during times of intense stress, such people may experience panic and find it very unpleasant. Once the situation has passed, they return to normal functioning and probably change nothing else in their lives. Panic Attacks do not have their own diagnostic code and are not diagnosable if they are one-off or infrequent occurrences (Craske & Barlow, 2007).

Table 4.4: Diagnostic criteria for Generalised Anxiety Disorder as adapted from the DSM-5 and ICD-10

DSM-5	ICD-10
A. Excessive anxiety and worry (apprehensive expectation), occurring more days than not for at least six months, about a number of events or activities (such as work or school performance). B. The individual finds it difficult to control the worry. C. The anxiety and worry are associated with three (or more) of the following six symptoms (with at least some symptoms having been present for more days than not for the past six months: Note: Only one time is required in children. (1) Restlessness or feeling keyed up or on edge. (2) Being easily fatigued. (3) Difficulty concentrating or mind going blank. (4) Irritability. (5) Muscle tension. (6) Sleep disturbance (difficult falling or staying asleep, or restless, unsatisfying sleep). D. The anxiety, worry, or physical symptoms cause clinically significant distress or impairment in social, occupational, or other important areas of functioning. E. The disturbance is not attributable to the physiological effects of a substance (e.g. a drug of abuse, a medication) or another medical condition (e.g. hyperthyroidism). F. The disturbance is not better explained by another mental disorder (e.g. anxiety or worry about having panic attacks in panic disorder, negative evaluation in social anxiety disorder [social phobia], contamination or other obsessions in obsessive-compulsive disorder, separation from attachment figures in separation anxiety disorder, reminders of traumatic events in posttraumatic stress disorder, gaining weight in anorexia nervosa, physical complains in somatic symptom disorder, perceived appearance flaws in body dysmorphic disorder, having a serious illness in illness anxiety disorder, or the content of delusional beliefs in schizophrenia or delusional disorder).	• A disorder in which the manifestation of anxiety is the major symptom. • The anxiety is generalised and persistent, and not restricted to, or even strongly predominating in, any particular environmental circumstances (i.e. it is 'free-floating'). • The dominant symptoms are variable, but include: complaints of persistent nervousness, trembling, muscular tensions, sweating, light-headedness, palpitations, dizziness, and epigastric discomfort. • Fears that the patients or a relative will shortly become ill or have an accident are often expressed. • Depressive and obsessional symptoms, and even some elements of phobic anxiety, are often present, provided that they are clearly secondary or less severe.

Source: Reprinted with permission from the Diagnostic and Statistical Manual of Mental Disorders (DSM), Fifth Edition, American Psychiatric Association (APA), 2013 and ICD–10 Classification of Mental and Behavioural Disorders: Diagnostic Criteria for Research. World Health Organisation (WHO), Geneva, 2007.

Just as fear serves a crucial function for survival, so too does panic (Barlow, 2004). Pathological panic would refer to instances when this ancient alarm system is accompanied by inappropriate and dysfunctional learning that results in cognitive and emotional problems. Thus, we may speak of panic functioning as either a 'true alarm' or a 'false alarm', at different times and depending on circumstances. Panic or fear in response to a real danger or life-threatening event is functional and successfully mobilises us in a 'fight or flight response'. It is only as a 'false alarm' that panic will be considered disordered. Panic is a complex biopsychosocial process that can be recognised as powerfully physiological and psychological from the list of criteria given in Table 4.5, as well as social, when one considers the extent to which it is a learned or conditioned anxiety response.

Table 4.5: The criteria for a Panic Attack as adapted from the DSM-5

DSM-5
A. Recurrent unexpected panic attacks. A panic attack is an abrupt surge of intense fear or intense discomfort that reaches a peak within minutes, and during which time four (or more) of the following symptoms occur: Note: The abrupt surge can occur from a calm state or an anxious state. (1) Palpitations, pounding heart, or accelerated heart rate. (2) Sweating. (3) Trembling or shaking. (4) Sensations of shortness of breath or smothering. (5) Feelings of choking. (6) Chest pain or discomfort. (7) Nausea or abdominal distress. (8) Feeling dizzy, unsteady, light-headed, or faint. (9) Chills or heat sensations. (10)Paresthesias (numbness or tingling sensations). (11)Derealisation (feelings of unreality) or depersonalization (being detached from oneself). (12)Fear of losing control or 'going crazy'. (13)Fear of dying. Note: Culture-specific symptoms (e.g. tinnitus, neck soreness, headache, uncontrollable screaming or crying) may be seen. Such symptoms should not count as one of the four required symptoms. B. At least one of the attacks has been followed by one month (or more) of one or both of the following: (1) Persistent concern or worry about additional panic attacks or their consequences (e.g. losing control, having a heart attack, 'going crazy'. (2) A significant maladaptive change in behavior related to the attacks (e.g. behaviors designed to avoid having panic attacks, such as avoidance of exercise or unfamiliar situations). C. The disturbance is not attributable to the physiological effects of a substance (e.g. a drug of abuse, a medication) or another medical condition (e.g. hyperthyroidism, cardiopulmonary disorders). D. The disturbance is not better explained by another mental disorder (e.g. the panic attacks do not occur only in response to feared social situations, as in social anxiety disorder; in response to circumscribed phobic objects or situations, as in specific phobia; in response to obsessions, as in obsessive-compulsive disorder; in response to reminders of traumatic events, as in posttraumatic stress disorder; or in response to separation from attachment figures, as in separation anxiety disorder).

Source: Reprinted with permission from the Diagnostic and Statistical Manual of Mental Disorders (DSM), Fifth Edition, American Psychiatric Association (APA), 2013.

Panic attacks are, furthermore, specified as those that are either cued, uncued, or predisposed (Halgin & Whitbourne, 2007). Cued Panic Attacks are considered to be situation bound in that the person will have a Panic Attack every time they are exposed to the specific stimulus or cue in the environment (or sometimes on only anticipating exposure to it). Uncued Panic Attacks are considered to be quite unexpected and the person's Panic Attack will typically arise 'out of the blue'. These are the most difficult to live with or manage, as can well be imagined, and are the type most associated with Panic Disorder and the development of Agoraphobia. With situationally predisposed Panic Attacks, the person merely has a tendency to respond with a Panic Attack in a particular situation or when faced with a cue; it will not happen every time.

Panic Disorder is said to exist when an individual experiences recurrent, unexpected Panic Attacks and the accompanying, persistent apprehension about possible recurrence or the consequences of having another attack (Craske, 2003). It is when Panic Attacks become frequent, and unprovoked by a stressful situation, that the panicked person's fear or anticipation of subsequent attacks may cause them to change aspects of their behaviour or life as a result of this worry. A diagnosis of Panic Disorder would be given to such an individual. The Panic Attacks may occur irregularly and grouped into shorter periods of time, or more regularly but with longer inter-episode periods. People with Panic Disorder may have more minor experiences of panic in between discrete, full-blown Panic Attacks.

Panic Disorder develops most commonly in people between late adolescence and the mid-thirties (Nolen-Hoeksema, 2007). The disorder tends to run a chronic course. Many people who receive a diagnosis of Panic Disorder will also co-morbidly experience chronic generalised anxiety, depression, and alcohol abuse. Panic Disorder may also co-occur with recurrent suicidal ideation and suicide attempts, although Todder and Baune (2007) report that this may be directly due to pharmacological treatment with specific antidepressants. When diagnosing Panic Disorder, it is important to first exclude the common or overt confounders of the clinical picture, such as substance (e.g. caffeine) intoxication or a general medical condition (e.g. hyperthyroidism).

Due to the physiological symptoms of Panic Disorder, many people who experience Panic Attacks may assume that they are in a physical crisis such as having a heart attack, a stroke, or a seizure. Many believe that they have a life-threatening illness and that they are going to die during the attack. General medical practitioners frequently send patients home (hopefully along with a referral to a psychologist) with the reassurance that what appeared to be a heart attack was in fact a Panic Attack. During a Panic Attack, many people also fear that they are going crazy or will lose control. These frightening psychological phenomena may cause them to feel ashamed or unwilling to share the event with anyone. As a result, many cases of Panic Disorder go unreported, undiagnosed, and untreated, with the most likely result being aggravation of the condition or the co-morbid development of other disorders or problems.

Agoraphobia

Agoraphobia most commonly develops as an avoidance response to the fear of future Panic Attacks and occurs in people who have a history of panic (Craske, 2003). Agoraphobia is most often the fear of any places in which one would not easily be able to escape or get help in the case of an emergency. Most frequently, this 'emergency' is another Panic Attack. The person can fear a wide variety of situations, including busy and crowded places such as shopping malls, wide open spaces such as an empty stadium, and restricted or enclosed spaces such as elevators and train compartments. Agoraphobic fears frequently include clusters of situations such as being alone outside the home, standing in a queue, or using public transport.

Figure 4.6: An open setting such as a shopping mall can be a trigger for Agoraphobia.

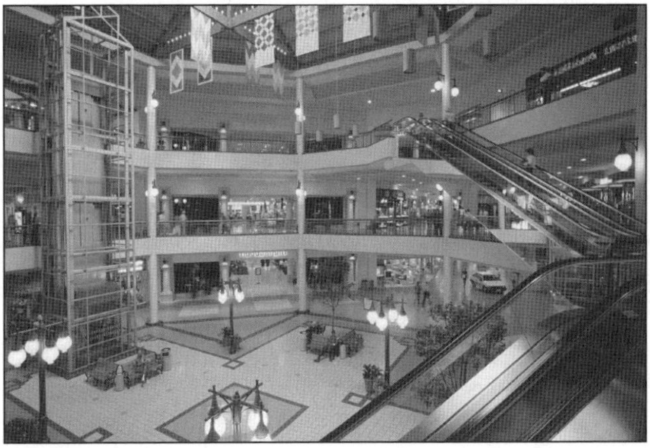

Panic Disorder may be considered an acquired fear of certain bodily sensations (Craske & Barlow, 2007). As a result of the fear and anticipation of subsequent Panic Attacks, an individual may develop Agoraphobia and change their behaviour and life in such a way as to avoid the feared situations. An extreme case of Agoraphobia may limit a sufferer to their home, or even to specific parts of a house or apartment (e.g. their bedroom) that are considered safe or under control. In this way, Agoraphobia can be a very disruptive, distressing, and debilitating condition. Some people with the disorder may turn to substance use or abuse as a means of minimising or masking the symptoms that they experience. The role of cognitions and expectations in this disorder is very important, and may point the way for developments for enhancing its psychological treatment. Furukawa, Watanabe, Omori, and Churchill (2007) concluded that the act of taking a placebo pill enhanced the effectiveness of cognitive-behavioural therapy (CBT) in their meta-analysis of randomised controlled trials of Panic Disorder treatment.

Table 4.6: Diagnostic criteria for Agoraphobia as adapted from the DSM-5 and ICD-10

DSM-5	ICD-10
A. Marked fear or anxiety about two (or more) of the following five situations: (1) Using public transportation (e.g. automobiles, buses, trains, ships, planes). (2) Being in open spaces (e.g. parking lots, marketplaces, bridges). (3) Being in enclosed places (e.g. shops, theaters, cinemas). (4) Standing in line or being in a crowd. (5) Being outside of the home alone. B. The individual fears or avoids these situations because of thoughts that escape might be difficult or help might not be available in the event of developing panic-like symptoms or other incapacitating or embarrassing symptoms (e.g. fear of falling in the elderly; fear of incontinence).	• The essential feature is recurrent attacks of severe anxiety (panic). • The panic attacks are not restricted to any particular situation or set of circumstances and are therefore unpredictable. • The dominant symptoms include: sudden onset of palpitations, chest pain, choking sensations, dizziness, and feelings of unreality (depersonalisation or derealisation). • There is often a secondary fear of dying, losing control, or going mad.

C. The agoraphobic situations almost always provoke fear or anxiety. D. The agoraphobic situations are actively avoided, require the presence of a companion, or are endured with intense fear or anxiety. E. The fear or anxiety is out of proportion to the actual danger posed by the agoraphobic situations and to the sociocultural context. F. The fear, anxiety, or avoidance is persistent, typically lasting for six months or more. G. The fear, anxiety, or avoidance causes clinically significant distress or impairment in social, occupational, or other important areas of functioning. H. If another medical condition (e.g. inflammatory bowel disease, Parkinson's disease) is present, the fear, anxiety, or avoidance is clearly excessive. I. The fear, anxiety, or avoidance is not better explained by symptoms of another mental disorder – for example, the symptoms are not confined to specific phobia, situational type; do not involve only social situations (as in social anxiety disorder); and are not related exclusively to obsessions (as in obsessive-compulsive disorder), perceived defects or flaws in physical appearance (as in body dysmorphic disorder), reminders of traumatic events (as in posttraumatic stress disorder), or fear of separation (as in separation anxiety disorder). Note: Agoraphobia is diagnosed irrespective of the presence of panic disorder. If an individual's presentation meets criteria for panic disorder and agoraphobia, both diagnoses should be assigned.	

Source: Reprinted with permission from the Diagnostic and Statistical Manual of Mental Disorders (DSM), Fifth Edition, American Psychiatric Association (APA), 2013 and ICD–10 Classification of Mental and Behavioural Disorders: Diagnostic Criteria for Research. World Health Organisation (WHO), Geneva, 2007.

It is possible for Agoraphobia to occur in people who do not have Panic Attacks, but it most frequently accompanies some level of panic experience or severe social phobia. It should be coded as either of the specific anxiety disorders in which it occurs. These are Panic Disorder With Agoraphobia and Agoraphobia Without History of Panic Disorder.

The ICD-10 describes Agoraphobia as follows: a fairly well-defined cluster of phobias, including fears about leaving home; entering shops, crowds, or public places; or travelling alone in trains, buses, or aeroplanes. Craske and Barlow (2007) give examples of Agoraphobia-inducing places such as malls, queues, theatres, public transport, and crowds, or the converse of being all alone. Panic Disorder is a frequent feature of both present and past episodes of Agoraphobia. Agoraphobia may be considered a behavioural response (avoidance) to anticipation of the bodily sensations of a Panic Attack. This conceptualisation is supported by experimental, clinical, and longitudinal research (Craske & Barlow, 2007). Avoidance of the phobic situation is often prominent, and some people with Agoraphobia experience little anxiety because they are able to avoid their phobic situations. Depressive and obsessional symptoms, as well as social phobias, are also commonly present as subsidiary features.

Women are about twice as likely as men to be diagnosed with this disorder. The teenage and early adulthood years represent the most frequent modal ages of onset. These conditions are also frequently co-morbid with another mental disorder; depression, another anxiety disorder, and substance use-related disorders are the most common.

Generalised Anxiety Disorder (GAD)

CASE STUDY

Lindiwe is a 25-year-old woman, studying and living at her Pretoria university campus. She presented to her GP recently with low mood, numerous physical complaints, and difficulty sleeping. The GP noticed that Lindiwe was restless and on edge in the consultation, and that she complained about excessive worry, related to a variety of things including her elderly mother and all other family members back at home, her residence and her room mate, the interest rates on her loans, the student job that she had held for one week, her ex-boss and co-workers, as well as the future in general. It seemed that Lindiwe had not done anything to address her concerns despite certain obvious solutions or help offered at the Student Counselling Centre and campus bank. The GP considered that Lindiwe was not easy to reassure and it seemed that her anxiety persisted in the face of evidence against her worries.

Lindiwe saw a clinical psychologist on her GP's advice and completed the Beck Anxiety Inventory (recording a high score), had two long interviews, and consented to have the psychologist call her Aunty Primrose. This aunty was the best person to talk to as she 'knew everyone in the family'and Lindiwe had lived with her for her high school years. Lindiwe added that her aunty was 'not a worrier' and was knowledgeable about health as she was a nurse. Of note, Aunty Primrose was married into the family and not genetically related to Lindiwe.

Aunty Primrose gave a long history of anxious avoidance of normal childhood activities in Lindiwe, who agreed that she could not remember a time when she had not worried. Lindiwe's mother was apparently also a compulsive worrier, and Aunty Primrose felt that that side of the family was very alike in terms of general apprehensiveness and physical symptoms that she believed were related to anxiety.

Despite really liking her niece and encouraging her to stop worrying over the years, it seemed to Primrose that Lindiwe was unable to control her anxiety levels. With this history, collateral information, psychometric results, and Lindiwe's presentation, the psychologist felt that a diagnosis of Generalised Anxiety Disorder could be made. They planned to begin treatment sessions and refer Lindiwe to a psychiatrist for assessment as well. The two professionals would work together with Lindiwe to address her condition.

Figure 4.7 Anxious and depressed mood frequently share a similar presentation.

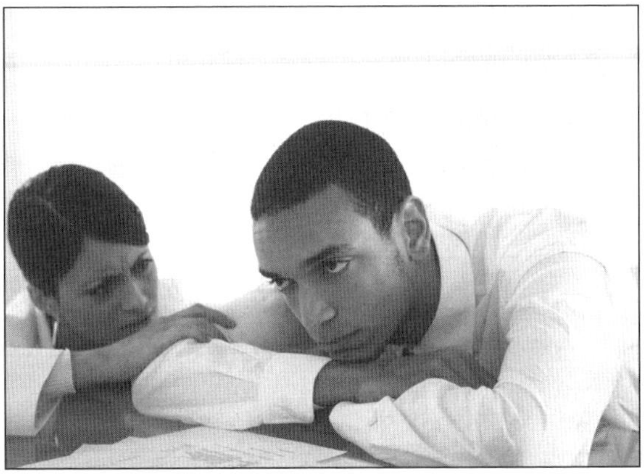

Unlike the acute and focused fears of a Panic Attack or a Specific Phobia, Generalised Anxiety Disorder (GAD) is characterised by chronic and diffuse anxiety. GAD can be defined as excessive and uncontrollable worry, about a number of life events, accompanied by bodily symptoms of physical tension and heightened vigilance (Craske, 2003). People with GAD tend to feel anxious in almost all situations, and for almost all of the time. They may worry about major matters in life, such as academic or occupational performance and the health or welfare of loved ones, as well as minor issues, such as the dirty dishes in the kitchen and being short-changed by 50 cents. The object of their worry is not focused and specific, and is thus very difficult to avoid or escape. It is as if the worry of a person with GAD goes with them wherever they go and can simply jump from one to another of many different things.

Experiencing such chronic anxiety, and feeling unable to control the amount or the cause of one's worry, will understandably be exhausting. People diagnosed with GAD also experience a number of the physiological symptoms of anxiety. They may feel restless and irritable, and have chronic muscle tension, difficulty concentrating, disturbed sleep, and possible physical problems such as nausea. People with GAD are also easily fatigued and often tired, which may be a result of sleep disturbances and other symptoms such as muscle tension.

GAD is a common anxiety disorder that runs a chronic course, and affects somewhat more women than men (Barlow, 2004; Craske, 2003). Being female, middle-aged, widowed/separated/divorced, and of a low income bracket were found to increase risk in a USA general population prevalence study (Grant et al., 2005). GAD has a high rate of co-morbidity, most often with a mood disorder, another anxiety disorder, or a substance-use disorder.

The typical age of onset for GAD is early, usually during the years of childhood or adolescence, and many people with the disorder report having been very anxious and tense for as long as they can remember (Kessler, Keller, & Wittchen, 2001) (see the case study of Lindiwe).

It is important to be able to distinguish amongst the mental disorders that share aspects of their respective clinical pictures. The term syndrome is used for clusters of disorder symptoms that often occur together. GAD can be considered a syndrome with a number of symptoms, some of which may overlap with the symptoms of other clinical disorders. Rickels and Rynn (2001) point out that certain symptoms considered cardinal for the diagnosis of GAD (such as worry, rumination, and, especially, the somatisation criteria) are also present in other disorders, for instance Major Depressive Disorder or MDD (see Chapter 5). A closer look at the diagnostic criteria shows how GAD has certain symptoms distinct from, but also some shared symptoms with, MDD (see Figure 4.8).

Figure 4.8: Similarities and differences between Generalised Anxiety Disorder and Major Depressive Disorder

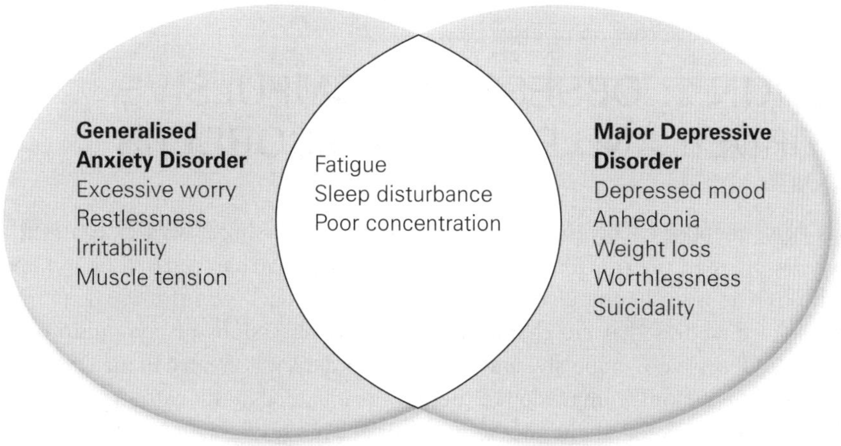

Source: © Burke, 2009.

However, Kessler et al. (2001) report that the symptoms of GAD form an empiric cluster that argues for the disorder's status as an independent condition. They add that the environmental determinants, socio-demographic predictors, and clinical course of GAD differ from that of MDD. Depressed patients who completed the Penn State Worry Questionnaire (PSWQ) for Chelminski and Zimmerman (2003) had lower worry levels than patients with GAD but similar to patients with other anxiety disorders. Patients with 'pure' GAD had the highest scores for worry whereas the control group, as would be expected, had subclinical levels of 'normal' worry.

Ruscio et al. (2005) evaluated the DSM-IV-TR criterion of 'excessive worry' as required for a diagnosis of GAD. In contrast, the ICD-10 does not have this as a required criterion (Wittchen, Kessler, Zhao, & Abelson, 1995). Many more people (approximately 40%) would be diagnosable with GAD if clinicians were to follow the latter diagnostic criteria.

The findings of the Ruscio et al. (2005) study challenged the validity of the excessive worry requirement, and made it possible for us to consider a somewhat milder presentation for some patients. Kessler and Wittchen (2002) also investigated the requirement of anxiety symptoms being present for six months and suggest that generalised anxiety symptoms for a shorter period of time may be as seriously impairing as the full syndrome. The diagnostic criteria for Overanxious Disorder of Childhood are the same as those given for GAD (see Table 4.2) except that Criterion C requires only one of the six possible items in children.

The proposed changes to Anxiety Disorders in DSM-5 are quite substantial. The first of these includes establishing separate categories for 'Anxiety Disorders', 'Obsessive-Compulsive and Related Disorders', and 'Trauma and Stressor-Related Disorders'. The splitting of disorders into these categories has not only meant that some disorders have been moved around to new categories, but it has also given rise to the creation of a whole host of new disorders.

Other significant changes relate to the Panic Disorders. In DSM-IV, Panic Attacks were recognised as a disorder; however, this will no longer be the case in DSM-5. In previous editions of DSM, Agoraphobia could only be diagnosed within the context of Panic Disorders (i.e. Panic Disorder With or Without Agoraphobia); however, in DSM-5 Agoraphobia will be recognised as a disorder on its own.

SECTION 2: OBSESSIVE-COMPULSIVE DISORDER AND RELATED DISORDERS

As has been mentioned before, Obsessive-Compulsive Disorder was categorised as an Anxiety Disorder in the previous DSM's. This disorder was characterised by the presence of both obsessions and compulsions, however, this approach was restrictive as there are a number of disorders that are characterised by only obsessions or compulsions. A new category, i.e. Obsessive-Compulsive and Related Disorders, was created in the DSM-5 and all disorder with obsessions, compulsions or both, were included in this category. The disorders in this category are related to one another in terms of a range of diagnostic validators, as well as the clinical utility of grouping these disorders. Obsessive-Compulsive Disorder has been moved from Anxiety Disorders to this category, and a number of new disorders have been introduced in this category, for example hoarding disorder and excoriation (skin-picking) disorder, and other disorders such as trichotillomania and Body Dysmorphic Disorder has been moved from Somatoform Disorders (in the DSM-IV-TR) to Obsessive-Compulsive and Related Disorders.

Obsessive-Compulsive Disorder

Obsessive-Compulsive Disorder (OCD) can be defined as the experience of obsessions or compulsions, which are often very time consuming and cause significant distress or impair global functioning (Craske, 2003). In the DSM-5 diagnostic criteria for the disorder, Criterion A stipulates that either obsessions or compulsions must be present, although usually both are present. Obsessions and compulsions are defined by the following criteria for the purposes of making this diagnosis:

- ***Obsessions*** are persistent, intrusive, and anxiety-provoking thoughts, images, or impulses that the person feels unable to control, and yet can recognise as being inappropriate or irrational. For this reason, the thoughts and behaviours of people with OCD are not considered psychotic, although they may appear bizarre, as these people are still in contact with reality. Typical symptoms of obsessions include:

- Recurrent and persistent thoughts, impulses, or images that are experienced, at some time during the disturbance, as intrusive and inappropriate, and that cause marked anxiety or distress.
- The thoughts, impulses, or images are not simply excessive worries about real-life problems.
- The person attempts to ignore or suppress such thoughts, impulses, or images or to neutralise them with some other thought or action. The person recognises that the obsessional thoughts, impulses, or images are a product of his or her own mind and not imposed from outside (as with thought insertion).

- ***Compulsions*** are the repetitive mental acts or behaviours that the individual feels compelled to perform. Thereafter, the person may feel relieved from the obsessions or the anxiety that they produce (Craske, 2003). Typical symptoms of compulsions include:
  - Repetitive behaviours (e.g. hand washing, ordering, or checking) or mental acts (e.g. counting, praying, or repeating words silently) that the person feels driven to perform in response to an obsession, or according to rules that must be applied rigidly.
  - The behaviours or mental acts are aimed at preventing or reducing distress or preventing some dreaded event or situation; however, they either are not connected in a realistic way with what they are designed to neutralise or prevent, or are clearly excessive.

This disorder is potentially disruptive and even debilitating. The subjective experience of anxiety and distress from the OCD and the impairment to an individual's global functioning are sufficient to warrant its classification as a disorder. Cognitive-behavioural psychologists have believed that 'normal' obsessional intrusive thoughts (OITs) and clinical obsessions existed on a continuum relative to one another, but this assumption has been criticised (Garcia-Soriano, Belloch, Morillo, & Clark, 2011). Fairly normal OITs occur in both community and OCD populations, with the most frequent relating to contamination, doubts and checking, symmetry and order, superstition, aggressive, sexual, religious, immoral, and repugnant thoughts.

Table 4.7 Diagnostic criteria for Obsessive-Compulsive Disorder as adapted from the DSM-5 and ICD-10

DSM-5	ICD-10
A. Presence of obsessions, compulsions, or both: Obsessions are defined by (1) and (2): (1) Recurrent and persistent thoughts, urges, or images that are experience, at some time during the disturbance, as intrusive and unwanted, and that in most individuals cause marked anxiety or distress. (2) The individual attempts to ignore or suppress such thoughts, urges, or images, or to neutralize them with some other thought or action (i.e. by performing a compulsion).	• The essential feature of this disorder is recurrent obsessional thoughts or compulsive acts. • Obsessional thoughts are ideas, images, or impulses that enter the patient's mind again and again in a stereotyped form. • Obsessions are almost invariably distressing and the patient often tries, unsuccessfully, to resist them. • Obsessions are recognised as own thoughts, although they are involuntary and often repugnant.

Compulsions are defined by (1) and (2): (1) Repetitive behaviours (e.g. hand washing, ordering, checking) or mental acts (e.g. praying, counting, repeating words silently) that the individual feels driven to perform in response to an obsession or according to rules that must be applied rigidly. (2) The behaviours or mental acts are aimed at preventing or reducing anxiety or distress, or preventing some dreaded event or situation; however, these behaviours or mental acts are not connected in a realistic way with what they are designed to neutralise or prevent, or are clearly excessive. Note: Young children may not be able to articulate the aims of these behaviours or mental acts. B. The obsessions or compulsions are time-consuming (e.g. take more than one hour per day) or cause clinically significant distress or impairment in social, occupational, or other important areas of functioning. C. The obsessive-compulsive symptoms are not attributable to the physiological effects of a substance (e.g. a drug of abuse, a medication) or another medical condition. D. The disturbance is not better explained by symptoms of another mental disorder (e.g. excessive worries, as in generalized anxiety disorder; preoccupation with possessions, as in hoarding disorder; hair pulling, as in trichotillomania [hair-pulling disorder]; skin picking, as in excoriation [skin-picking] disorder; stereotypies, as in stereotypic movement disorder; ritualized eating behaviour, as in eating disorders; preoccupation with substances or gambling, as in substance-related and addictive disorders; preoccupation with having an illness, as in illness anxiety disorder; sexual urges or fantasies, as in paraphilic disorders; impulses, such as in disruptive, impulse-control, and conduct disorders; guilty ruminations, as in major depressive disorder; thought insertion or delusional preoccupations, as in schizophrenia spectrum and other psychotic disorders; or repetitive patterns of behaviour, as in autism spectrum disorder).	• Compulsive acts or rituals are stereotyped behaviours that are repeated again and again. • Compulsions are not inherently enjoyable, nor do they result in the completion of inherently useful tasks. • Compulsions function to prevent some objectively unlikely event, often involving harm to or caused by the patient, that he or she fears might otherwise occur. • The patient usually recognises that this behaviour is pointless or ineffectual, and repeatedly makes attempts to resist. • Anxiety is almost invariably present. • If compulsive acts are resisted, the anxiety gets worse.

Source: Reprinted with permission from the Diagnostic and Statistical Manual of Mental Disorders (DSM), Fifth Edition, American Psychiatric Association (APA), 2013 and ICD-10 Classification of Mental and Behavioural Disorders: Diagnostic Criteria for Research. World Health Organisation (WHO), Geneva, 2007.

Clinically significant obsessions typically focus on similar content, but are distressing and much more disruptive. They can focus on dirt and contamination (such as concerns about germs entering one's house), repeated doubts (such as continuous worrying that one has not switched off the iron), aggressive impulses (such as hurting one's child), sexual thoughts (such as intrusive pornographic images), and impulses to do something that goes against one's values and morals (such as swearing at one's grandparents). People with OCD do not usually go on to do any of the things that they obsess about. Instead, the thoughts, images, and impulses alone provoke a great deal of anxiety and, possibly, guilt.

Most people with severe obsessions also perform compulsions which they are convinced will somehow erase or neutralise the obsessions or the anxiety that they produce. Compulsive behaviours may become so repetitive and extreme as to be debilitating or dangerous. Checking compulsions (such as returning to the garage dozens of times to ensure that the car is locked) can take up a great deal of a person's time. Cleaning compulsions (such as hand washing) may become harmful as some people wash so many times a day that they induce bleeding. These compulsions do succeed in calming the anxiety that accompanies obsessions, but only temporarily. The obsessions and anxiety typically return and require a repeat of the compulsive behaviours.

Some compulsions have a logical link to the obsessions they are tied to, as with obsessional doubts and compulsive checking. Other combinations appear to be the result of 'magical thinking', as with a compulsion to touch all doors in the house seven times to ward off the obsessive fear of harm befalling one's family. OCD will typically run a chronic course if not diagnosed and treated. OCD often begins at a young age, and children frequently hide their obsessions and compulsions such that their symptoms may go undetected for a long period of time.

The content of the obsessions or compulsions in OCD will not be restricted to another Axis I disorder, if one is present. For instance, these include:

- Preoccupations with food in an eating disorder or drugs in a substance abuse disorder
- Preoccupation with physical appearance in Body Dysmorphic Disorder
- Hair-pulling in the presence of Trichotillomania
- Preoccupation with having a serious illness in Hypochondriasis
- Sexual urges or fantasies in a paraphilia
- Guilty ruminations in the presence of a major depressive disorder.

Body Dysmorphic Disorder

Could the late Michael Jackson, renowned for repeatedly undergoing facial surgery have suffered from Body Dysmorphic Disorder? First recognised more than a century ago, and named Dysmorphophobia by Emil Kraepelin, the condition was considered a 'compulsive neurosis', a conceptualisation endorsed by Pierre Janet. Freud also described the condition in the 'Wolf-Man', who had had morbid concerns about his nasal structure and appearance. Before the publication of DSM-III in 1980, most of the literature on Body Dysmorphic Disorder originated from Europe and Japan. As sufferers may request cosmetic surgery, much research on the condition emanates from the worlds of dermatology and plastic surgery. In the previous DSM, Body Dysmorphic Disorder was included under the banner of somatoform disorders. Apart from the concern about something bodily, this condition is quite unlike Somatisation Disorder or Pain Disorder, therefore this disorder was relocated to the Obsessive-Compulsive and Related Disorders category.

Table 4.8: Diagnostic criteria for Body Dysmorphic Disorder as adapted from DSM-5

DSM -5 BODY DYSMORPHIC DISORDER
A. Preoccupation with one or more perceived defects or flaws in physical appearance that are not observable or appear slight to others. B. At some point during the course of the disorder, the individual has performed repetitive behaviours (e.g. mirror checking, excessive grooming, skin picking, reassurance seeking) or mental acts (e.g. comparing his or her appearance with that of others) in response to the appearance concerns. C. The preoccupation causes clinically significant distress or impairment in social, occupational, or other important areas of functioning. D. The appearance preoccupation is not better explained by concerns with body fat or weight in an individual whose symptoms meet diagnostic criteria for an eating disorder.

Source: Reprinted with permission from the Diagnostic and Statistical Manual of Mental Disorders, (DSM), Fourth Edition, Text Revision, American Psychiatric Association (APA), 2000.

Body Dysmorphic Disorder primarily concerns the preoccupation with a perceived bodily abnormality. Facial features are the most common focus of concern, but more than one body region can elicit attention. Concerns can be specific or vague. Mirror checking or avoidance, repetitive grooming, and attempts to hide deformities are common compulsive features. Concerns about a perceived bodily deformity can reach delusional intensity. It is interesting to note than men and women share many of the clinical features such as disliked body areas, types of repetitive behaviours, etc., however men are more likely to have genital preoccupations and women more likely to have a comorbid eating disorder (APA, 2013). Depression and anxiety are common in the history and mental state examination, and psychosocial dysfunction can be severe. Suicide attempts are not uncommon. Common co-morbid conditions are major depression and anxiety disorders. Perfectionist, schizoid and narcissistic personality traits are also found. An insidious onset is characteristic and it runs a chronic course with fluctuating symptoms (Hales, 2008; Sadock & Sadock, 2000).

Other disorders with disturbances in body image must be considered: Anorexia Nervosa, Gender Identity Disorder, non-dominant parietal lesions, and psychotic conditions. In addition, major depression, Obsessive-Compulsive Disorder, Narcissistic and Obsessive-Compulsive Personality Disorders warrant consideration. In Malaysia, a *koro*-sufferer is preoccupied that his penis is shrinking. Once shrunk to the extent that it has disappeared into his abdomen, death will ensue (American Psychiatric Association, 2000). Although exposure to cold and excessive coitus have been implicated as causes, *koro* is also associated with interpersonal conflicts and sociocultural demands. *Jinjin bemar* and *suk yeong* are similar conditions found in India and China respectively.

Concerns about physical appearance, the dimensions, positioning and proportions of body features, and the quality of physical entities like facial texture and colour, are common. Most teenagers successfully negotiate preoccupations with appearance.

Concern about physical appearance is adaptive and can confer survival advantage. In humans, like other animals, mate selection is significantly influenced by visual factors like proportions, symmetry, and surface texture, attributes believed to communicate good stock and absence of disease.

Globally, a multibillion-rand industry has developed around the enhancement and preservation of beauty. In Western and Westernised societies, cosmetic surgery is an established reality. But, cosmetic modification of physical appearance is not limited to Western cosmetic surgery. In Thailand, Myanmar, China, and amongst the Ndebele in South Africa, cosmetic elongation of the female neck is desirable and achieved by means of the successive insertion of rings. Similarly, binding of the female foot in China and Japan, common even during the twentieth century, is considered a form-enhancing practice. Foot binding results in gross orthopaedic deformity and dysfunction. The stiletto is not dissimilar and also causes substantial foot pathology as well as problems with the knees, hips, and back.

Worldwide, many cultures desire the lightening of dark skin. In South Africa, skin- lightening is a mature industry. Skin-lightening preparations, particularly those containing hydroquinolone as the bleaching agent, can cause a permanent and unsightly blotchy skin-pigmentation known as exogenous ochronosis. Removal of the upper incisor teeth is considered attractive by aboriginal peoples in Australia and Papua New Guinea. Shaving, a bewildering array of skin conditioners, glosses, perfumes, and colognes, nail extensions, lacquer, nose rings, haute coiffure, and haute couture attest to humankind's quest to enhance natural beauty.

HELPFUL HINT
Body Dysmorphic Disorder: Rules of thumb

- **Preoccupation with an imagined bodily defect**
- **Repetitive behaviours aimed at hiding or modifying imagined defect**
- **Reassurance not helpful**
- **Belief can reach delusional intensity.**
- **Areas of bodily focus, in descending order of frequency: hair, nose, skin, eyes, head, shape and size of face, overall build, lips, chin, abdomen, waist, teeth, legs and knees, breasts and pectoral muscles, ears, cheeks, buttocks, penis, arms and wrists, neck, forehead, facial muscles, shoulders, hips.**

Sources: Hales, 2008; Phillips, McElroy, Keck, Pope, & Hudson, 1993; Sadock & Sadock, 2000.

Hairdressers and other astute observers in the beauty industry not infrequently remark that trade picks up during periods of economic downturn and social upheaval. In animals, grooming behaviours become pronounced when under threat, particularly when the threat is unrelenting, for example, feather-plucking in the parrot family and paw-licking in dogs. Human grooming is no different. When faced with uncertainty, individuals feverishly strive to improve physical appeal so as to increase their chances to mate.

Epidemiological studies have demonstrated the co-occurrence of Body Dysmorphic Disorder with Obsessive-Compulsive Disorder and Social Phobia. In Japan, *taijin kyofusho*, considered an expression of Social Phobia, involves the preoccupation with having bad breath and offensive body odour.

Hoarding Disorder

In the DSM-IV hoarding was listed as one of the possible symptoms of obsessive-compulsive personality disorder and it was noted that extreme hoarding may occur in obsessive-compulsive disorder. However, reviewing available data seemed to indicate that there are sufficient symptoms to warrant a separate disorder and not just a variant of obsessive-compulsive disorder or another mental disorder. The core feature of this disorder is a persistent difficulty discarding or parting with possessions due to a perceived need to save the items and distress associated with discarding them (APA, 2013). The hoarding is excessive to such an extent that that the resulting clutter "...impairs basic activities such as: moving through the house, cooking, cleaning, personal hygiene, and even sleeping" (APA, 2013, p.250). Hoarding disorder may have unique neurobiological correlates, but is not diagnosed if the disorder is the direct consequence of a degenerative disorder (e.g. frontotemporal lobar degeneration or Alzheimer's disease) (APA, 2013). People with this disorder often have comorbid disorders such as major depressive disorder, social anxiety disorder, generalized anxiety disorder or OCD.

Trichotillomania (Hair-Pulling Disorder)

The essential feature of this disorder is the recurrent pulling out of one's hair, which may be from any area of the body where hair grows. These sites may vary over time and typically occurs in brief episodes during the day. The disorder may endure for months and years and is associated with both distress and social and occupational impairment (APA, 2013). Not only could the disorder lead to irreversible hair growth, but also associated physical problems (e.g. carpal tunnel syndrome, shoulder, back and neck pain, and trichophagia) (APA, 2013). The disorder seems to have a genetic vulnerability to this disorder and it is commonly associated with OCD.

Excoriation (Skin-Picking) Disorder

Excoriation (skin-picking) disorder is newly added to DSM-5, with the essential feature of this disorder being picking at one's own skin. The skin picking is not limited to a particular body site and people with this disorder may pick at healthy skin or at minor skin irregularities (e.g. pimples, calluses, scabs, etc.). It often involves rituals (e.g. searching for particular kind of scab, pulling, examining, playing or swallowing the skin after it has been pulled) and is often triggered by an emotional state (e.g. anxiety, boredom, etc.) There seems to be a genetic vulnerability to this disorder and it is often associated with OCD and OCD-related disorders (APA, 2013).

SECTION 3: TRAUMA AND STRESSOR RELATED DISORDERS

The ICD-10 states that the stress disorders differ from other disorders in that they are identifiable on the basis not only of symptoms and course, but also of the existence of a specified causative influence (an exceptionally stressful life event producing an acute stress reaction). Along the same line, the DSM-5 states that this group of disorders are characterised by exposure to a traumatic or stressful event, and this is stated explicitly as a diagnostic criterion (APA, 2013). In previous editions of the DSM the trauma and stressor related disorders were categorised as Anxiety Disorder, probably because many people display fear or anxiety when they are confronted with a stressor or threat. However, many people who have been exposed to a stressor display anhedonic, dysphoric, aggressive or dissociative symptoms (APA, 2013). It is because of this wide array of possible symptoms, that are not limited to fear or anxiety symptoms, that this group of disorders have been moved out of the category of Anxiety Disorders and now have their own category.

Reactive Attachment Disorder

This disorder is one that is limited to infancy (at least 9 months old) or early childhood (evident before the age of 5 years). The disorder is the result of extremes of insufficient care such as social neglect or deprivation, repeated changes of primary care givers or contexts where there are limited opportunities to form stable attachments. This results in a consistent pattern of inhibited, emotionally withdrawn behaviour toward adult caregivers such as not seeking comfort when distressed or not responding to comfort when provided. The child also exhibits persistent social and emotional disturbances such as limited responsiveness, limited positive affect and periods of unexplained irritability, sadness or fearfulness (APA, 2013). It is generally accepted that children with this disorder have the capacity to form attachments; however, due to their environments they have not been given the opportunity to do so (APA, 2013). The main cause of this disorder is serious neglect, however, what is of note is that not all children that are exposed to extreme neglect, develop this disorder (APA, 2013).

Disinhibited Social Engagement Disorder

In this case a child actively approaches and interacts with unfamiliar adults in an impulsive, incautious, and overfamiliar way. As was the case with the previous disorder, this disorder also seems to be the result of of extreme neglect before the age of 2 years (APA, 2013). This disorder, which is also limited to children, can almost be described as the inverse of Reactive Attachment Disorder (RAD).As opposed to RAD, children with this disorder readily approach strangers without fear and with excessive familiarity. This familiarity includes a readiness to hug and accept comfort, food or toys from an unknown person (APA, 2013). As is the case with RAD, serious social neglect is a diagnostic requirement for this disorder, but again, not all seriously neglected children develop this disorder. Although unconfirmed, it seems as if children who develop this disorder may have a neurobiological vulnerability to this disorder (APA, 2013).

Posttraumatic Stress Disorder (PTSD)

The diagnosis of Posttraumatic Stress Disorder (PTSD) requires, primarily, that a person has been exposed to a traumatic event that led to a response of intense fear, helplessness, or horror. A traumatic event could refer to direct or vicarious exposure to actual or threatened death, serious injury or sexual violence (APA, 2013).

The diagnosis of PTSD further requires that a person presents with a set of symptoms following exposure to a traumatic event as described above (Craske, 2003). The person would have to meet a certain minimum number of each of the following three categories of symptoms:

- Re-experiencing the traumatic event
- Avoiding associated stimuli, or emotional numbing and detachment
- Hypervigilance and chronic arousal.

A large number and range of events can serve as traumas in producing PTSD symptoms. Events may be natural disasters (e.g. floods), 'human-made' traumas such as interpersonal aggression (e.g. rape), or accidents (e.g. a mining disaster). Moreover, such traumas may be found both in very rare (e.g. being taken hostage) and more common events (e.g. motor vehicle accidents). Research has investigated the scope of traumatic events that may precipitate PTSD or Posttraumatic Stress Symptoms (PTSS), and an interesting study reports the significant rates of PTSD found in fathers during the acute stage following a child's diagnosis with a chronic disease or unintentional injury (Ribi, Vollrath, Sennhauser, Gnehm, & Landolt, 2007).

Undergoing certain medical procedures can be traumatic and Schelling (2002) studied a population of patients who received intensive care unit (ICU) treatment along with the administration of stress hormones such as cortisol, epinephrine, and norepinephrine for medical reasons. The majority of them reported traumatic memories of their stay in ICU. The memories contained little factual detail but described respiratory distress, pain, nightmares, and anxiety. Schelling found, however, that there was a complex, and at times protective, interaction between the administration of certain stress hormones and PTSD development.

In a sample of women who survived intimate partner violence (IPV), PTSD was found to be significantly associated with their shame, guilt, distress, and guilt cognitions (Beck et al., 2011). Johnson, Zlotnick, and Perez (2011) described HOPE, an effective CBT intervention for the shelter setting for women victimised by IPV. The treatment was found to significantly lower the symptom severity of emotional numbing, effortful avoidance, and arousal, as well as reduce the likelihood of re-abuse over a six month follow-up period.

Edwards (2005c) discusses the numerous psychological factors that play a role in the development and maintenance of PTSD and its symptomatology. Such emotionally distressing and problematic processes include guilt, shame, grief, anxiety, dysfunctional or distorted cognitions, and various cognitive, affective, and behavioural avoidance mechanisms, which may interfere with the emotional processing of the traumatic event. Elhai et al. (2011) describe the symptoms that PTSD and Major Depressive Disorder (MDD) share, suggesting that they are highly correlated and that there may be a single, underlying PTSD-MDD symptom dimension.

ACTIVITY

Consider Vusi, who was a passenger in a terrible bus accident that killed eleven people. He reports that he experienced intense fear during the event and believed that he was going to die. For many months thereafter, Vusi experienced distressing dreams about the event while trying to avoid thinking or talking about what had happened. He also had intense psychological and physiological distress when travelling along the same street, and tried to avoid public transport altogether. Vusi's roommate noticed that Vusi had experienced disturbed sleep since the accident and had lost interest in activities that he had once enjoyed, such as music and his part-time DJ work. Would Vusi qualify for a diagnosis of PTSD with this presentation?

Contrary to general public impression, most people who experience a traumatic event will *not* go on to develop PTSD. Edwards, Sakasa, and van Wyk (2005) examined the proportion of people who do go on to develop PTSD following trauma relative to those who do not. This study highlighted the importance of understanding the variables associated with resilience, such as personality factors, developmental factors, social support, and gender, as these are believed to play a role in protection against pathology and recovery.

Figure 4.9: Our understanding of Posttraumatic Stress Disorder has been advanced through many studies of soldiers, who remain at risk of this disorder.

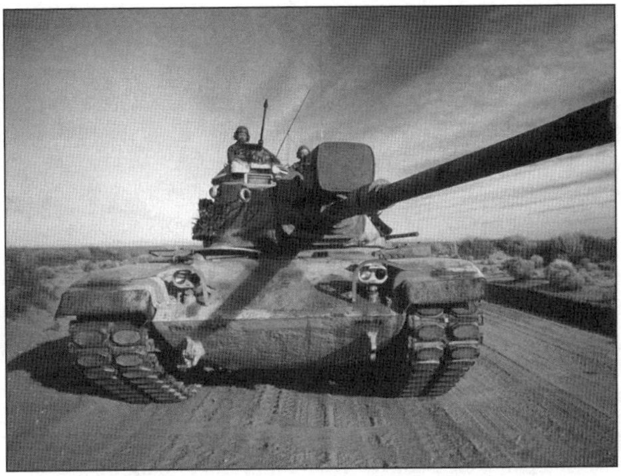

Psychological research primarily describes the deleterious effects of trauma exposure. Taking a different focus, Pietrzak et al. (2010) examined post-traumatic growth (see Chapter 3) in a population of war veterans. Post-traumatic growth refers to subjective definitions of positive change that can result from exposure to major life crises and trauma. Of note, 72% of the veteran sample studied endorsed a significant degree of positive change, particularly in terms of changed life priorities as well as being better able to appreciate each day and handle difficulties. Hierarchical regression analysis revealed that greater unit member support and effort or perseverance were significantly associated with post-traumatic growth, suggesting that appropriate interventions may help to promote it.

Certain people exposed to trauma may present with some PTSD symptoms, but find that these are manageable or that they resolve spontaneously and these people continue to function normally despite the disturbance. Nonetheless, Raja, Onofri, Azzoni, Borzellino, and Melchiorre (2008) found that PTSD was the most prevalent of the mental disorders to be clinically diagnosable in a group of subjects exposed to a disaster. PTSD symptoms can present in both children and adults, although the clinical picture may be somewhat different for children.

Table 4.9: Diagnostic criteria for Posttraumatic Stress Disorder as adapted from the DSM-5 and ICD-10

DSM-5	ICD-10
A. Exposure to actual or threatened death, serious injury, or sexual violence in one (or more) of the following ways: (1) Directly experiencing the traumatic event(s). (2) Witnessing, in person, the event(s) as it occurred to others. (3) Learning that the traumatic event(s) occurred to a close family member or close friend. In cases of actual or threatened death of a family member or friend, the event(s) must have been violent or accidental. (4) Experiencing repeated or extreme exposure to aversive details of the traumatic event(s) (e.g. first responders collecting human remains; police officers repeatedly exposed to details of child abuse). **Note:** Criterion A4 does not apply to exposure through electronic media, television, movies, or pictures, unless this exposure is work related. B. Presence of one (or more) of the following intrusion symptoms associated with the traumatic event(s), beginning after the traumatic event(s) occurred: (1) Recurrent, involuntary, and intrusive distressing memories of the traumatic event(s). Note: In children older than 6 years, repetitive play may occur in which themes or aspects of the traumatic event(s) are expressed. (2) Recurrent distressing dreams in which the content and/or affect of the dream are related to the traumatic event(s). **Note:** In children, there may be frightening dreams without recognizable content. (3) Dissociative reactions (e.g. flashbacks) in which the individual feels or acts as if the traumatic event(s) were recurring. (Such reactions may occur on a continuum, with the most extreme expression being a complete loss of awareness of present surroundings.) **Note:** In children, trauma-specific reenactment may occur in play. (4) Intense or prolonged psychological distress at exposure to internal or external cues that symbolize or resemble an aspect of the traumatic event(s).	• Disorder arises as a delayed or protracted response to a stressful event or situation (brief or long in duration) of an exceptionally threatening or catastrophic nature, likely to cause pervasive distress in almost anyone. • Typical features include: ▸ Episodes of repeated reliving of the trauma (in intrusive memories, 'flash-backs', dreams, or nightmares). ▸ Persisting background of a sense of 'numbness' and emotional blunting (detachment from other people, unresponsiveness to surroundings, anhedonia) as well as avoidance of activities and situations reminiscent of the trauma. ▸ A state of autonomic hyperarousal and hypervigilance (enhanced startle reaction and insomnia). • Anxiety and depression are commonly associated with the above signs and symptoms, and suicidal ideation is not infrequent. • Onset follows the trauma with a latency period that may range from a few weeks to months. • Course is fluctuating, but recovery can be expected in the majority of cases. • In a small proportion of cases, the condition may follow a chronic course over many years, with eventual transition to an enduring personality change.

DSM-5	ICD-10
(5) Marked physiological reactions to internal or external cues that symbolize or resemble an aspect of the traumatic event(s). C. Persistent avoidance of stimuli associated with the traumatic event(s), beginning after the traumatic event(s) occurred, as evidenced by one or both of the following: (1) Avoidance of or efforts to avoid distressing memories, thoughts, or feelings about or closely associated with the traumatic event(s). (2) Avoidance of or efforts to avoid external reminders (people, places, conversations, activities, objects, situations) that arouse distressing memories, thoughts, or feelings about or closely associated with the traumatic event(s). D. Negative alterations in cognitions and mood associated with the traumatic event(s), beginning or worsening after the traumatic event(s) occurred, as evidence by two (or more) of the following: (1) Inability to remember an important aspect of the traumatic event(s) (typically due to dissociative amnesia and not to other factors such as head injury, alcohol, or drugs). (2) Persistent and exaggerated negative beliefs or expectations about oneself, others, or the world (e.g. 'I am bad', 'No one can be trusted', 'The world is completely dangerous', 'My whole nervous system is permanently ruined'. (3) Persistent, distorted cognitions about the cause or consequence of the traumatic event(s) that lead the individual to blame himself/herself or others. (4) Persistent negative emotional state (e.g. fear, horror, anger, guilt, or shame). (5) Markedly diminished interest or participation in significant activities. (6) Feelings of detachment or estrangement from others. (7) Persistent inability to experience positive emotions (e.g. inability to experience happiness, satisfaction, or loving feelings). E. Marked alterations in arousal and reactivity associated with the traumatic event(s), beginning or worsening after the traumatic event(s) occurred, as evidenced by two (or more) of the following:	

DSM-5	ICD-10
(1) Irritable behaviour and angry outbursts (with little or no provocation) typically expressed as verbal or physical aggression toward people or objects. (2) Reckless or self-destructive behaviour. (3) Hypervigilance. (4) Exaggerated startle response. (5) Problems with concentration. (6) Sleep disturbance (e.g. difficult falling or staying asleep or restless sleep). F. Duration of the disturbance (Criteria B, C, D, and E) is more than one month. G. The disturbance causes clinically significant distress or impairment in social, occupational, or other important areas of functioning. H. The disturbance is not attributable to the physiological effects of a substance (e.g. medication, alcohol) or another medical condition	

Source: Reprinted with permission from the Diagnostic and Statistical Manual of Mental Disorders (DSM), Fifth Edition, American Psychiatric Association (APA), 2013 and ICD–10 Classification of Mental and Behavioural Disorders: Diagnostic Criteria for Research. World Health Organisation (WHO), Geneva, 2007.

Acute Stress Disorder

In DSM-IV-TR, Acute Stress Disorder had the same symptoms as Posttraumatic Stress Disorder (PTSD), but a shorter period of time following the trauma was specified. In the DMS-5, Acute Stress Disorder would start immediately after the trauma, but the symptoms should persist for at least three days and up to one month of experiencing the traumatic event but last no longer than four weeks. In addition, the criteria for the diagnosis differ significantly from those of PTSD (See Table 4.10).

Table 4.10: Diagnostic criteria for Adjustment Disorders as adapted from the DSM-5

DSM-5 ADJUSTMENT DISORDERS
A. The development of emotional or behavioural symptoms in response to an identifiable stressor(s) occurring within three months of the onset of the stressor(s). B. These symptoms or behaviours are clinically significant, as evidenced by one or both of the following: (1) Marked distress that is out of proportion to the severity or intensity of the stressor, taking into account the external context and the cultural factors that might influence symptom severity and presentation.

DSM-5
ADJUSTMENT DISORDERS

(2) Significant impairment in social, occupational, or other important areas of functioning.

C. The stress-related disturbance does not meet the criteria for another mental disorder and is not merely an exacerbation of a preexisting mental disorder.

D. The symptoms do not represent normal bereavement.

E. Once the stressor or its consequences have terminated, the symptoms do not persist for more than an additional six months.

CROSS-CULTURAL AND AFRICAN PERSPECTIVES

People's cultures play an important role in the manifestation of anxiety symptoms, in their conceptualisation of the phenomenon, and in whether or not it is considered problematic by them and those around them. As will be seen below in the section on aetiology, sex role socialisation may lead men and women to respond differently to symptoms of distress and to be either more or less likely to report these. Similarly, cultural norms that surround different groups may also explain the variability in presenting with a disorder, admitting to symptoms, and being distressed by symptoms. In psychology, culture can be taken to refer broadly to the traditional and communicated meanings and practices, common values, beliefs, and behaviours within groups who share an identity (Squire, 2000). How psychological events are interpreted within a patient's cultural framework (as more significant or neutral, more qualitatively positive or negative) will also have an impact on the presentation.

Psychology has historically taken a positivist approach to understanding people. It has also been largely 'disinterested in the diverse forms of psychological experience represented in ethno-racial and cultural studies' (Gone, 2011). If the discipline is to remain relevant, psychologists will need to consider more appropriate paradigms and methods of inquiry. To this end, Cauce (2011) believed that psychology would be strengthened by drawing on both qualitative and quantitative methods when investigating psychosocial issues especially as they affect diverse populations.

Figure 4.10 Imagine that the young women are American psychology students visiting South Africa and consider the amount of cultural knowledge they would need to gain to be able to work here.

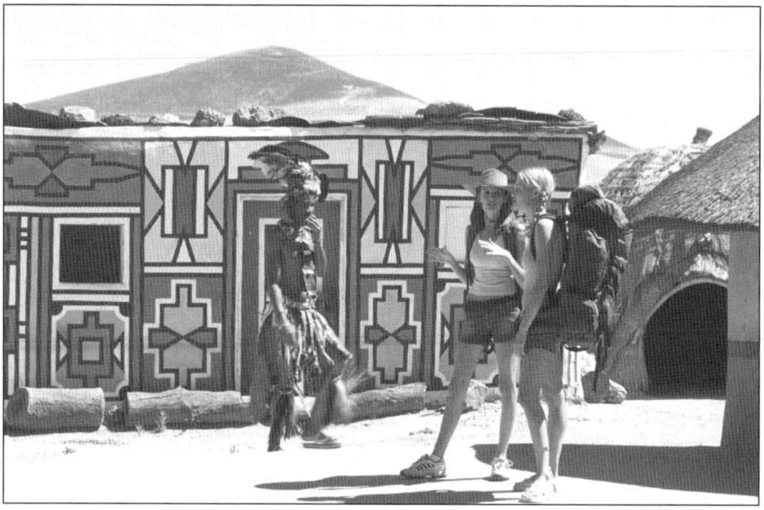

In terms of understanding such diverse populations as exist, for example, in South Africa, we often talk of collectivist versus individualist cultural perspectives. This differentiation may be important to consider in discussing cultural differences in mood disorders and anxiety. For example, collectivist individuals often have a strong fear of rejection whereas individualist people may be more prone to loneliness. Torelli and Shavitt (2011) considered that people with 'vertical/hierarchical' individualist cultural values were more likely to stereotype others, whereas people with 'horizontal' collectivist cultural values were more likely to strive to learn the individualist needs of others.

In line with international trends, the anxiety disorders are reported to be the most common of the mental disorders in South Africa. Locally, concern has been expressed about the assumed universality of the PTSD diagnosis cross-culturally (Edwards, 2005a). Edwards (2005c) is confident, however, that South African practitioners have access to current evidence-based treatment approaches and he goes on to identify the importance of developing skill at adapting these best practices to local cultures and situations.

South Africa has little data on the prevalence and incidence of anxiety disorders across the various cultural groups of its people. South East Asian countries, similarly, have little epidemiological data on anxiety disorders (Lim et al., 2005) and this may be due to factors which also play a role in the South African picture. The South East Asian region is also considered 'multi-ethnic', has a collectivist culture, and is known to have low rates of professional help-seeking for mental health issues. The above authors studied GAD in Singaporean individuals and found increased prevalence of the condition in older people, in those who had experienced one or more threatening life events, and who had co-morbidities (specifically, three or more other conditions). Interestingly, both the lowest and highest socio-economic status Singaporean groups were most associated with GAD, with uniquely different types of events affecting each. This suggests that GAD is not only a disorder of socially disadvantaged persons in Singapore and this trend may warrant investigation in South Africa as well.

Taku (2011) found that there were both cultural and individual differences for the type and amount of post-traumatic growth reported by subjects from different cultures. For instance, United States participants reported greater post-traumatic growth on the commonly-defined factors, such as having experienced growth on factors such as 'Relating to Others' and 'New Possibilities'. Japanese participants, on the other hand, considered themselves to have experienced more personal growth that was individually defined. It may be that both cultural orientations emphasised the kinds of personal growth that were less naturally occurring for them.

ACTIVITY

Imagine that you see Reshmi for a first session at your psychology practice in a major South African city to assess her presenting complaint of social anxiety and what sounds like moderate depressive symptoms. You know that her family is Hindu, live in far Northern KwaZulu-Natal, and that she has come to the city for work. What more do you need to know about Reshmi in order to understand how her cultural values are likely to impact on her experience of these problems, professional help-seeking, and support from her family/community?

Malik (2000) argues that the Western values dominating psychological knowledge introduce severe limitations when doing cross-cultural research (Squire, 2000). In addition, Hinton et al. (2002) debate the meaningfulness of the epidemiological rates of Panic Disorder in a cross-cultural study with Cambodian subjects using methods developed in the West to describe this phenomenon. They contend that psychology will need to take note of a detailed ethnography of the (possibly different) symptoms, cues, and cognitions that are relevant to different cultural groups and contexts, rather than simply assuming Western understandings of health and illness are universally applicable.

In South Africa, McDermott (2005) confirms that, in order to be most effective, practitioners need to respond to abnormal behaviour in patients by using assessment and treatment frameworks that acknowledge both Western and indigenous constructions of meaning. It is important that these integrative efforts contribute to developing a foundation of locally contextualised and applicable scientific knowledge in psychology, as well as uniquely African theory in psychotherapy (Edwards, 2005c; McDermott, 2005). In South Africa, such research is ongoing, especially in terms of the preferred psychotherapeutic responses to individuals and communities exposed to traumatic events (Eagle, 2005; Van Wyk & Edwards, 2005).

In multicultural settings such as South Africa, clinicians need to be aware of cultural and ethnic contributions to psychological problems when treating diverse patient populations. It is also important, in attempting to make sense of abnormal behaviour, to know the extent of a particular patient's degree of involvement with their culture of origin. In certain cultures, people may report local pathologies that express patterns of behaviour reflecting predominant cultural beliefs and themes that date back for centuries, and these would be considered 'culture-bound syndromes' in the DSM-5. This term refers to recurrent patterns of abnormal behaviour that are limited to specific cultural groups or societal areas (see Table 1.11 in Chapter 1).

The 'idiom of distress', *amafufunyana*, is considered a serious disorder amongst African people. Sufferers reportedly exhibit extreme agitation, and they may break possessions, become extremely tired, lose appetite, speak in tongues, and have command hallucinations, disturbed sleep, nightmares, and episodes of angry outbursts. Beuster (1997) describes this condition as a mixed syndrome, with diverse symptoms including those typical of anxiety, mood, psychotic, and conduct disorders. It is also sometimes reported as a form of mass hysteria. The anxiety-based symptoms include general nervousness, tension, and obsessive-compulsive behaviours. African traditional healers (*isangoma* for Zulus or *igqira* for Xhosas) explain that people with this condition have been invaded and possessed by evil spirits as a result of witchcraft. In terms of traditional African cosmology, such external and personalised factors would often be considered the causes of abnormal behaviour (Beuster, 1997).

In contrast to beliefs around *amafufunyana*, *ukuthwasa* is believed in South African indigenous culture to be the calling by the ancestors to study and practice African traditional healing, and is mostly viewed positively. In terms of the clinical diagnostic system of the DSM-5, the presentation of this condition includes symptoms characteristic of anxiety, psychotic, dissociative, somatoform, and impulse-control disorders. The more positive connotations of the culture-specific phenomenon of *ukuthwasa* and the negative associations with the culture-bound syndrome *amafufunyana* may play a role in the reporting of symptoms and treatment compliance. Possible misdiagnoses within the anxiety, mood, and psychotic disorder categories may be made by clinicians who lack an awareness of the relevant traditional African belief systems and cultural contexts (Beuster, 1997). Identification of cases as *amafufunyana* and *ukuthwasa* are believed, however, to correlate with a distinction between familial and sporadic cases of Schizophrenia.

Ongoing research into the local prevalence of anxiety disorders, as well as the unique presentation of culture-bound syndromes in South Africa, is indicated. This is not exclusively a local need, and internationally there is an appreciation of the importance of indigenous knowledge in psychopathology. The whole developing world will need to respond to the high burden of anxiety disorders in its various populations. The prevalence of anxiety disorders in many cultures is not known, in large part due to the lack of culture-sensitive assessment practices and psychiatric symptom questionnaires that are validated in indigenous languages (Ahmer, Faruqui, & Aijaz, 2007). Khan et al. (2007) report on their use of the validated Urdu version of the Hospital Anxiety and Depression Scale (HADS) and conclude that there is a need for further studies into the scope of anxiety disorders in Pakistan. Within more uniformly Westernised societies such as the United States, the previously reported ethnic differences between African and Caucasian Americans with regard to anxiety symptoms are no longer found in some studies (Reinhardt & Rogers, 1998) and we may speculate that they are reducing.

The high levels of crime, violence, and accidents in South Africa have a special bearing on anxiety disorders that develop in response to trauma exposure. McDermott (2005) confirms the alarming rate in South Africa of violent trauma and domestic abuse, as well as HIV/AIDS-related deaths. Reviews of the frequency of traumatic events (Eagle, 2005) and the corresponding prevalence of reported PTSD symptoms in the South African population highlight these problems as urgent psychological concerns (Edwards, 2005b). PTSD is a serious public health concern for the local populace, unfortunately affecting both adults and children (Leibowitz-Levy, 2005) across all societal levels.

Figure 4.11 Unfortunately, high crime statistics leave people at greater risk of experiencing stressors or traumas likely to play a role in the development of psychological difficulties.

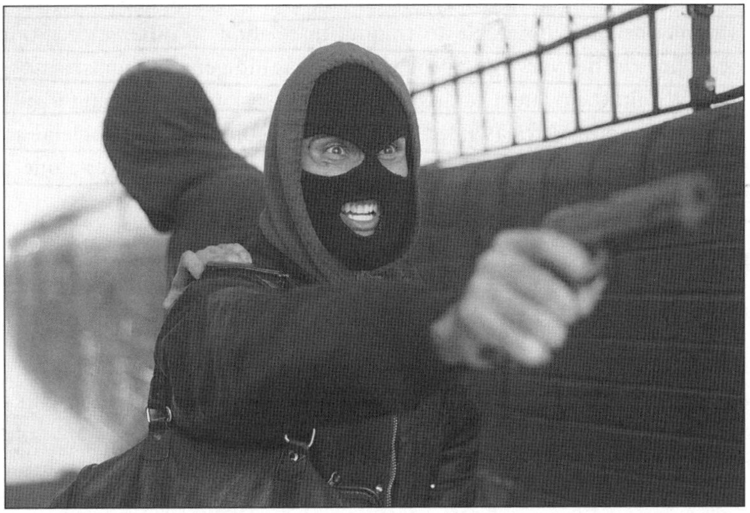

Sexualised violence against women in South Africa is a recognised national problem (Earl-Taylor & Thomas, 2003). The People Opposing Women Abuse (POWA) (2007) statistics showed that one in two women have a chance of being raped in their lifetime. In South Africa, a woman is raped every 26 seconds, most often by armed rapists and most often as a gang rape as opposed to a rape by an individual rapist. The sexual debut statistics for adolescent girls are also alarming, with between one-third and two-thirds of township teenage girls studied reporting that their first sexual experience was rape or forced sex. The incidence of rape relative to age in South African girls was found to peak at ages eight to eleven years, taking the problem into the younger years. Indeed, in South Africa, the sexual abuse of children and infants is widespread and a serious problem (Earl-Taylor & Thomas, 2003). Current statistics report that 1 in 4 girls and 1 in 5 boys under the age of 16 years have been sexually abused, and that a child is raped every 24 minutes in South Africa (POWA, 2007).

POWA (2007) offers a description of Rape Trauma Syndrome (RTS), a form of PTSD that often affects rape survivors. RTS is reported to have a spectrum of physical, emotional, cognitive, and behavioural symptoms very close to that of PTSD. POWA does, however, attempt to normalise the symptoms of RTS as a response to sexualised trauma. Labe (2005) discusses the case of a young South African woman who developed entrenched PTSD after the trauma of repeated rape and who was hospitalised and treated with psychotherapy a year later. This researcher confirms the role that earlier traumas, losses, and significantly disturbing life events played in the patient's idiosyncratic vulnerability to developing PTSD.

South Africa's high number of road accidents also add to the potential rates of pathological response to trauma, as in Karpelowsky and Edwards' (2005) case study of a young, South

African man presenting with Acute Stress Disorder following a number of motor vehicle accidents that directly involved him and his family.

Opinion differs on repetitive trauma and its tendency to lead to either compounded vulnerability or the development of resilience. In some instances, township children have been found to be more vulnerable to repeated exposure to trauma. On the other hand, other children, who were not emotionally overwhelmed (by experiencing intense helplessness) by even severe traumas, were found to have increased resilience. The belief that South African black people may be less vulnerable to trauma in relation to other race groups, due to stronger social support networks and processes such as indigenous rituals, is not supported by experience. Within the context of this elevated local risk for developing PTSD, Edwards (2005a) emphasises South Africa's need for political, economic, and societal solutions to this situation. However, these trauma rates are not limited to South Africa alone, and would better be viewed as a problematic feature of life all over Africa.

AETIOLOGY

From an integrative point a view, mental health practitioners consider many hypotheses on the aetiology or causation of anxiety disorders. The biological, psychological, and social factors believed to contribute to the development of an anxiety disorder can be viewed as working together to play certain roles in each illness. Some factors are considered to be predisposing, that is, referring to the tendency or vulnerability to develop a disorder at some time if other conditions, often stressors, are also present. Someone may inherit a genetic predisposition to an anxiety disorder that never develops, however, especially if they have certain protective factors that counteract its expression or if their circumstances never expose them to great stressors, for instance.

Life stressors are frequently considered to be potentially predisposing and precipitating factors within anxiety disorders. This means that stressors may make a person vulnerable to developing an anxiety disorder in the future, or that they may be sufficient to precipitate (or bring about) the expression of a disorder now. The 'diathesis-stress model' in mental disorders considers the two components, a diathesis or vulnerability and a stressor, both of which are necessary in order to lead to the development of a disorder. Common life stressors that are considered relevant in the aetiology of many mental disorders are poverty, experiencing or witnessing violence, poor parenting, and losing a loved one to death. A full multiaxis diagnosis of a patient's anxiety disorder and other problems would include any psychosocial life stressors that were found to be present or to play a role in the development of the disorder.

After the presentation of an anxiety disorder, certain factors may serve a maintaining function that then keeps the disturbance in place or even aggravates the symptoms that an individual experiences. Maintaining factors may again be those psychosocial and environmental stressors mentioned above, or include personal, familial, and social or cultural factors that prevent the person's condition from improving and thus keep them ill. Maintaining factors in mental illness may also prevent an individual from seeking treatment. In Social Anxiety Disorder, for instance, the individual may fear the focus and assessments of a mental health practitioner and avoid reporting any problems. The tendency for people with an anxiety disorder to develop another mental illness, often a mood disorder, may function in this way. A person who has experienced Generalised Anxiety Disorder over many difficult years may develop a Major Depressive Disorder as well and withdraw even further from people, thereby exacerbating their isolation and receiving even less support from others or health services.

The aetiology of anxiety disorders can be considered from a variety of perspectives. The following section will discuss both biological and psychological perspectives. Biological perspectives include genetic, neurochemical, and brain structure issues, while psychological perspectives will include psychodynamic, humanistic, behavioural, and cognitive models, as well the role of personality and temperament in the aetiology of anxiety disorders.

Biological perspectives

Genetics

Genetics appears to play a role in the development of many anxiety disorders. Both Panic Disorder and phobias appear at least partly to develop due to genetics, as shown by family history studies and twin studies (Hettema, Neale, & Kendler, 2001). It is believed that the general tendency towards anxiety is much more clearly heritable as it may lead to a temperament that heightens the risk of developing an anxiety disorder.

A significant South African example of research into the genetic aetiology of OCD is that of Niehaus et al. (2001). It is believed that the catechol-o-methyl transferase (COMT) gene may play a role in the causation of OCD. The above researchers assessed the risk for OCD that this COMT polymorphism may contribute in the relatively genetically homogenous population of South African Afrikaners. This study found that the H/L (high activity/low activity) alleles in the COMT gene were significantly more common than expected in the OCD patient group. These important results emphasise the need for further aetiological studies on this and other disorders in genetically homogenous populations (Stein, 2006). The '"Genetics of Anxiety Disorders Research Project" in South Africa aims to identify factors contributing to the development of these disorders locally' (Lochner, 2003).

Neurochemistry

Poor regulation of the neurotransmitter norepinephrine has been implicated in Panic Disorder symptoms (Charney, Paraherikas, & Gill, 2000). This dysregulation may be especially pronounced in the locus ceruleus, an area of the brain stem believed to be related to panic attacks. Other neurotransmitters, especially serotonin, gamma amino butyric acid (GABA), and cholecystokinin (CCK), are also believed to play a role in this disorder (Bell & Nutt, 1998). The efficacy of selective serotonin reuptake inhibitors (SSRIs) in treating OCD, for instance, has suggested that the disorder might be related to the functioning of brain serotonin systems (Van Dyk, Klompmakers, & Denys, 2010). Research on serotonin suggests that, at different times, both deficiency and excessively high levels of serotonin in key brain areas may cause Panic Disorder. Barlow (2004) adds that dopaminergic pathways are also linked to the brain systems that support the fundamental emotions of fear and anxiety.

The limbic system in the brain, which is involved in the physiological, emotional, and behavioural responses to threat, has been implicated in the experience of diffuse, anticipatory anxiety (Gorman, Papp, & Coplan, 1995). Poor locus ceruleus regulation may then lower the threshold for activation of the limbic system and the experience of chronic anxiety. People with Panic Disorder may have an over-reactive autonomic nervous system, which causes their 'alarm' (fight or flight) response to be activated unnecessarily. The physiological symptoms of the alarm response may be induced by having someone hyperventilate or ingest strong coffee. In someone prone to panic attacks, these procedures alone can initiate an alarm response without a fear stimulus being present.

The inhibitory neurotransmitter GABA has also been implicated in the development of GAD, with the assumption that people with this disorder have insufficient GABA or GABA receptors on neurons (Charney, 2004). This would result in excessive neuronal firing, especially in the limbic system, and resultant symptoms of chronic and diffuse anxiety.

Brain structure and functioning

Research into the diathesis-stress model of aetiology indicates that early stressful life events appear to alter brain function permanently (Barlow, 2004). This is particularly of concern in South Africa with the number of children being affected by HIV/AIDS. A significant impact may be made on the corticotrophin-releasing factor (CRF) neurons and the developing HPA axis, which results in a changed level of responsiveness to future psychological stressors.

As far as the possible neural substrate of Body Dysmorphic Disorder and how its manifestation is shaped by societal expectations are concerned, the manifestations of the condition are overwhelmingly biased towards visual appraisal of bodily features. The preoccupation about the bodily shortcoming possesses a distinctly obsessive quality and implicates serotonergic systems. Support for serotonergic involvement is found in the modest success achieved with agents augmenting serotonergic function like clomipramine, fluoxetine, and citalopram. Functional neuro-imaging studies have demonstrated similarities between Body Dysmorphic Disorder and Obsessive-Compulsive Disorder. Social influences, like prevailing attitudes towards beauty and desirability, create an environment where vulnerable individuals focus on a perceived bodily imperfection to the exclusion of other mental activities and behaviours.

A recent study from California demonstrated excessive activation in the left-hemisphere and amygdala when patients with Body Dysmorphic Disorder viewed faces of other people. The implication is that, in a subgroup of patients, abnormal visual processing may underlie the condition: attention is focussed on specific details at the expense of appreciation of the whole. This assertion is further supported by neuropsychological evidence of disturbed figure-ground processing (Feusner, Townsend, Bystritsky, & Bookheimer, 2007).

Psychological perspectives

Psychodynamic models

Freud's well-known theory of the development of phobias argues that unconscious anxiety is displaced onto a symbolic or even neutral object. Freud also put forward an explanation for OCD, stating that obsessions are unconscious conflicts that create so much anxiety for the person that they can only be approached indirectly. The compulsions that the person performs would be the more acceptable thoughts or behaviours onto which the conflict anxiety is displaced. However, these theories are limited to the principles of psychoanalytic theory and have no ready support from treatment evidence (Nolen-Hoeksema, 2007). Freud (1917) also developed a theory of GAD which explains that a person whose defence mechanisms are no longer able to contain either the id impulses or the neurotic or moral anxiety caused by these impulses would be anxious all the time. When one greatly fears the expression of id impulses or finds no acceptable means of expressing them, GAD may be the psychopathological result.

Humanistic models

The Humanistic theory of Carl Rogers offers an explanation for the development of chronic anxiety and depressive symptoms. When people grow up with only the conditional positive regard of others, and develop resultant internal conditions of worth, they may believe that they fail to win the approval of others and/or do not meet their own harsh standards of an ideal self (Corsini & Wedding, 2005). The Existential theorists would explain that GAD develops from not confronting the existential issues of life (such as the finality of death and meaninglessness of life), which omission leads to existential anxiety and an 'inauthentic life' (Corsini & Wedding, 2005).

Behavioural models

Behavioural theories successfully explain the development of phobias from the learning theory principles of classical and operant conditioning. Classical conditioning would explain the development of a phobia from the pairing of an object or situation with a fear-producing stimulus. Operant conditioning may then reinforce this learning as the phobic person experiences a reduction in anxiety (negative reinforcement) through the avoidance of the feared object or situation, thereby maintaining the fear (Mowrer, 1939). However, many people with a Specific Phobia can report no frightening event that triggered the fears. It may also be sufficient for a person to observe someone else experience extreme fear in response to an object or situation for vicarious or observational learning to lead to the development of a phobia (Bandura, 1969).

Due to the role of fear-inducing stimuli, exposure-based psychological interventions have, historically, been considered effective and have become the established treatments for anxiety. Treanor (2011) argued that 'mindfulness' and 'acceptance-based' psychotherapeutic approaches, similarly, show some promise in treating certain anxiety disorders. Based on literature reviews, Treanor concluded that mindfulness positively impacts on exposure and facilitates extinction learning.

ACTIVITY

Read more about the newer approaches in psychotherapy, 'Mindfulness' and 'Acceptance and Commitment Therapy' or ACT, in the blog on Mindfulness and Acceptance for Anxiety (http://mindfulness-and-anxiety.blogspot.com/) and the ACT website (http://www.actmindfully.com.au/acceptance_&_commitment_therapy).

The concept of 'prepared classical conditioning' refers to the evolutionary selection for the rapid conditioning of fear (that had survival value) in response to certain objects or situations. Thus, humans tend to fear snakes, spiders, and heights more often than harmless stimuli (Mineka, 1985). The most effective treatments for the Specific Phobias are behavioural exposure and skill training approaches. This suggests that behavioural models in aetiological explanation may be essential in our understanding of this disorder. Craske (2003) adds that the associative pathway allows us to explain how specific stimuli can become particularly threatening. Phobias can develop via direct traumatic association (although seldom by single trial conditioning), through vicariously observing others (who are traumatised or modelling distress), and through information transmission (of frightening accounts).

Cognitive models

Cognitive theory would explain that Social Phobia develops from the negative beliefs and cognitive biases by which social situations and the self are evaluated. People whose beliefs include excessively high expectations of their social functioning and the assumption that others judge them harshly may be more likely to be hypervigilant for criticism and rejection. They may exercise biases in attention towards 'negative' cues and interpret these in self-defeating ways (Heinrichs & Hofman, 2001). People with Social Phobia have been found to perceive social interactions as more competitive than do the non-anxious, to overestimate the visibility of their anxiety, and to have their negative predictions feed back into a perpetuating cycle of anxiety (Turk, Heimberg, & Magee, 2007). Individuals who following social situations, engage in post-event processing that is coloured by more negative self-perceptions and regret-based cognitions, were found to be likely to experience higher levels of social anxiety (Makkar & Grisham, 2011). Individuals who undertook a more formal and group-based act such as making a speech (as opposed to having a conversation) were found to be more likely to engage in negative, detailed, and self-focused reviewing of the event. Those with more negative assumptions in their self-related cognitions were also predicted to engage in more post-event processing.

The development of GAD may similarly hinge on cognitions that focus on threat. Consciously, a person may have a number of maladaptive beliefs that lead to negative assumptions, especially around issues of control (Matthews & MacLeod, 2005). Automatic thoughts regarding threat and its consequences may develop and result in hypervigilance, over-reaction to situations, and resultant anxiety. Even the unconscious cognitions of people with GAD may focus on signs of impending threats and remain vigilant in an attempt to detect them.

Some people who have a biological vulnerability to developing Panic Disorder also have accompanying psychological factors. For example, people prone to Panic Attacks may exhibit the cognitive processes of:

- Closely attending to physical sensations
- Negatively misinterpreting these physical sensations
- Catastrophic thinking that exaggerates the symptoms and negative consequences of the symptoms (Craske & Barlow, 2001).

These cognitive biases may increase both the person's subjective experience of anxiety and their sympathetic nervous system activity. Those prone to Panic Attacks are also higher on anxiety sensitivity (the catastrophic misinterpretation of certain bodily sensations) (Noda et al., 2007) and interoceptive awareness (a heightened awareness of bodily cues for panic) (Craske & Waters, 2005). Beliefs that panic symptoms are uncontrollable and the lack of a 'safe person' nearby may also exacerbate Panic Attacks (Carter, Hollon, Carson, & Shelton, 1995).

Cognitive theories argue that OCD obsessions develop through rigid, moralistic thinking (Rachman, 1997). Negative intrusive thoughts and rigid ritualistic behaviours may be common for many people, especially when distressed. Difficulty tolerating uncertain or ambiguous situations may be related to pathological doubt, a prominent feature of OCD (Tolin, Abramowitz, Brigidi, & Foa, 2003). This so-called intolerance of uncertainty is thought to feature particularly in people who have checking compulsions. This has implications for increasing tolerance in those with OCD via cognitive-behavioural therapy.

Personality and temperament

A person prone to phobias may have been born with a temperament which contributes to this disorder's development. This is seen in the higher rates of Specific or Social Phobia in children who are socially and behaviourally inhibited (i.e. excessively shy and timid) and who also receive parenting that exacerbates their anxiety (Craske & Waters, 2005). They may also be overly sensitive to anxiety and exhibit less tolerance of this psychological phenomenon than would another person. Negative affectivity and threat-based styles of emotion regulation may explain individual differences between people in vulnerability to disorders (Craske, 2003). Thus, two individuals may react differently to the same trauma or transfer of traumatic information, depending on their own temperaments.

Psychosocial stressors

The ICD-10 states that, although less severe psychosocial stressors and 'life events' may precipitate the onset, or contribute to the presentation, of a very wide range of mental disorders, their aetiological importance is not always clear. In each case, the aetiological role of stressors will be found to depend on individual, and often idiosyncratic, vulnerabilities. Stressors will be found to be neither necessary nor sufficient to explain the occurrence and form of the disorder.

In contrast, the stress disorders (Acute Stress Disorder and Posttraumatic Stress Disorder) are thought to arise as a direct consequence of acute, severe stress or continued trauma, according to the ICD-10. The stressors here are the primary and over-riding causal factor and the disorder would not have occurred without their impact. The stress disorders can be regarded as maladaptive responses to severe or continued stress, in that they interfere with successful coping mechanisms and therefore lead to problems in global functioning.

In both Acute Stress Disorder and Posttraumatic Stress Disorder, individual vulnerability and coping capacity play a role in the occurrence and severity of maladaptive stress reactions. In PTSD, factors such as personality traits or a history of neurotic illness may predispose an individual to the development of the syndrome, or the aggravation of its course, through lowering susceptibility thresholds. These factors are, however, neither necessary nor sufficient to explain its occurrence. It is believed that individual proximity to the traumatic event is directly related to the risk of developing PTSD. Raja at el. (2008) found partial confirmation for this hypothesis in a recent study of an Italian street disaster. The same study also found that exposure to episodes of trauma can cause long-lasting psychiatric morbidity.

Familial perspectives

A child may inherit a genetic predisposition towards anxiety and a sensitive temperament, but this is typically not sufficient to result in an anxiety disorder unless the parenting that the child receives also exacerbates their anxiety (Craske & Waters, 2005). Within a family setting, it is possible for a person to observe someone else experience extreme fear in response to an object or situation such that observational learning occurs (Bandura, 1969). For instance, a child may see his or her mother be extremely afraid of the dark and thus reluctant to venture out at night and learn to respond with fear to this situation.

Sociocultural perspectives

Where group differences exist between populations with different disorders, some theorists use social and cultural models to explain the presentation of certain disorders. Environmental demands may differ between groups such that they are either variously more predisposed to, or more protected from, certain disorders than other groups. People in disadvantaged groups, who may be of lower socio-economic and educational status, are more likely to have a stressful environment such as an unsafe neighbourhood, and to experience chronic and pervasive anxiousness (Manson et al., 1996). People in a country that is experiencing a war, political oppression, or, even, rapid social changes may be at a greater risk of exhibiting anxiety symptoms and developing anxiety disorders. Women are more likely than men to become the victims of physical and sexual abuse, a factor that increases their risk for developing most of the anxiety disorders (Burnam, Stein, Golding, & Segal, 1988). The risk of victimisation for women increases with very low incomes and being recently divorced, and may contribute to chronic anxiousness.

Social and cultural norms that surround different groups, and that differ between the genders, may also explain the difference between people when it comes to presenting with a disorder, admitting to their symptoms, and being distressed by their symptoms. Women are many times more at risk for developing most of the anxiety disorders, a skew in prevalence that is attributed to a number of cultural and social theories. The historically lower status of women in society may have lent them less social power, developed in them a sense of being defenceless and thus vulnerable, and caused them to adopt subservient and passive roles in their relationships with men in order to win their love and protection.

Sex role socialisation may lead men and women to respond differently to symptoms of distress. Men may be socialised to view the expression of anxiety as unacceptable (and thus they confront and 'extinguish' their fears), to view symptoms as medical problems (and thus they seek and receive early and effective treatment), and to view substance use for managing symptoms as acceptable (and thus they try to 'self-medicate' to cope).

A sign of one's culture and the times will be found in the dominant social discourses active around an individual, as per postmodern theory in psychology. Smith (2010) argued for the usefulness of short-term psychodynamic therapy for the treatment of anxiety and Panic Disorder, and commented on the absence of such an approach in the UK's National Institute of Clinical Excellence (NICE) guidelines. Smith linked anxiety aetiology to the theory of brief dynamic therapy, especially the so-called symptom-context method, which understands symptoms as meaningfully related to the narrative context in which they emerge. This suggests that social discourses about anxiety disorders co-create the experience of distress in an individual. That is, that an individual who has spoken about and accepted the 'construct' of panic is more likely to recognise and call his or her distress panic.

ACTIVITY

See the NICE (http://guidance.nice.org.uk/Topic/MentalHealthBehavioural) website for an example of the UK's best practice guidelines for various mental health conditions. These guidelines are particularly evidence-based and tend to recommended CBT above most others.

Integrated perspectives

Barlow (2004) suggests that the anxiety disorders should be viewed from a biopsychosocial perspective and understood as having an integrated aetiology. The dysregulation of neurotransmitters alone is not able to account adequately for the anxiety disorders. Instead, the following factors are all likely to interact, in order to result in the presentation of anxiety disorders:

- ***Biological factors*** (e.g. genetic vulnerability, accompanied by neurochemical imbalance)
- ***Psychological factors*** (e.g. maladaptive psychological constructs in terms of interpretations, attributions, and meanings)
- ***Social factors*** (e.g. dysfunctional learned responses or conditioning).

In the integrated diathesis-stress model of Panic Disorder, it is believed that a biological predisposition to an overactive alarm response interacts with the person's catastrophic cognitions about physiological symptoms to produce Panic Attacks and further hyper-vigilance for symptoms (Craske & Barlow, 2001; Craske & Waters, 2005). Craske and Barlow's (2007) 'triple vulnerability theory' is a good example of the importance of using an integrated perspective in aetiology. They refer to the interaction of three vulnerability factors: genetic contributions, generalised psychological vulnerability, and early learning experiences that focus anxiety on specific concerns, and see these as necessary in the development of chronic Panic Disorder. In Social Phobia, some people report that their disordered response to social situations was precipitated by early humiliating experiences, while others report having felt a lifelong discomfort in social situations.

CONCLUSION

Within the spectrum of anxiety disorders, it is apparent that changes in the classification of individual conditions have been, and still are, a part of the nature of our clinical knowledge. As we better understand and more clearly describe these mental disorders, so too will we see shifts in the diagnosis and prevalence data reported for those who struggle to live with anxiety conditions. It is difficult to achieve consensus on the classification of these disorders, especially when we take into consideration the multiple influences that cultural and ethnic factors have on disorder presentation, and while we still use the possibly limited Western conceptualisations of psychopathology that follow the medical model.

Furthermore, we cannot safely assume that we fully understand the causes of these disorders. Indeed, our body of aetiological knowledge has changed and grown in every successive decade, and it will probably continue to do so as a function of advances in medical technology and psychological research. We will need to meet the challenges of the future in psychopathology by developing broader explanatory models to account for the development of the various anxiety disorders. An acceptance of the integrated approach to aetiology will in all likelihood remain the best practice in researching and understanding disorder predisposition, precipitation, presentation, and maintenance. Furthermore, a biopsychosocial model that acknowledges risk and vulnerability factors, as well as the protective and resilience factors that prevent the development of pathology or aid in recovery, is indicated. This is especially the case if we are to respond to our knowledge of abnormal behaviour from a strengths-based and recovery-focused position.

MULTIPLE-CHOICE QUESTIONS

1. Which of the following statements about would not be considered true for people with an anxiety disorder?
   a) Severe distress which ultimately results in the reduction of the quality of life.
   b) Chronic anxiety, or sufficiently and frequent anxiety is enough to lead impaired functioning.
   c) Simple reaction of 'fight or flight' as a survival function
   d) Disproportionate reaction to the possibility danger of a threat.
   e) The symptoms of fear continue to be experienced long after the legitimately fear-producing situation had passed.

2. Worry and ruminations are considered to be ___________ symptoms of anxiety
   a) Emotional
   b) Cognitive
   c) Somatic
   d) Behavioural
   e) None of the above

3. Obsessions are:
   a) Persistent, nonintrusive, normal thoughts
   b) Normal impulses, but abnormal responses
   c) Inappropriate behaviour
   d) Nearly excessive worries
   e) Persistent, intrusive, and anxiety provoking thoughts

4. Compulsions are:
   a) Mental actual behaviours of the individual can decide to perform, or not to perform
   b) Repetitive mental act or behaviours of the individual feels compelled to perform
   c) Behaviours or mental acts that increase distress
   d) Behaviours that realistically connected to the preceding thought
   e) None of the above

5. The South African culture-bound syndrome amafufunyana is:
   a) To include physical symptoms but are largely psychological in presentation
   b) Culture-specific, descriptive terms used by Zulu- and Xhosa-speaking South Africans
   c) An 'idiom of distress'
   d) Described as a mixed syndrome, with diverse symptoms including those typical of anxiety, mood, psychotic, and conduct disorders
   e) All of the above

PARAGRAPH AND ESSAY QUESTIONS

1. Distinguish between fear and anxiety, as well as between 'normal' and 'pathological' anxiety.

2. Define Generalised Anxiety Disorder. Compare and contrast GAD with the other anxiety disorders.

3. Give an integrated explanation of the aetiology of Generalised Anxiety Disorder.

5 MOOD DISORDERS

Alban Burke

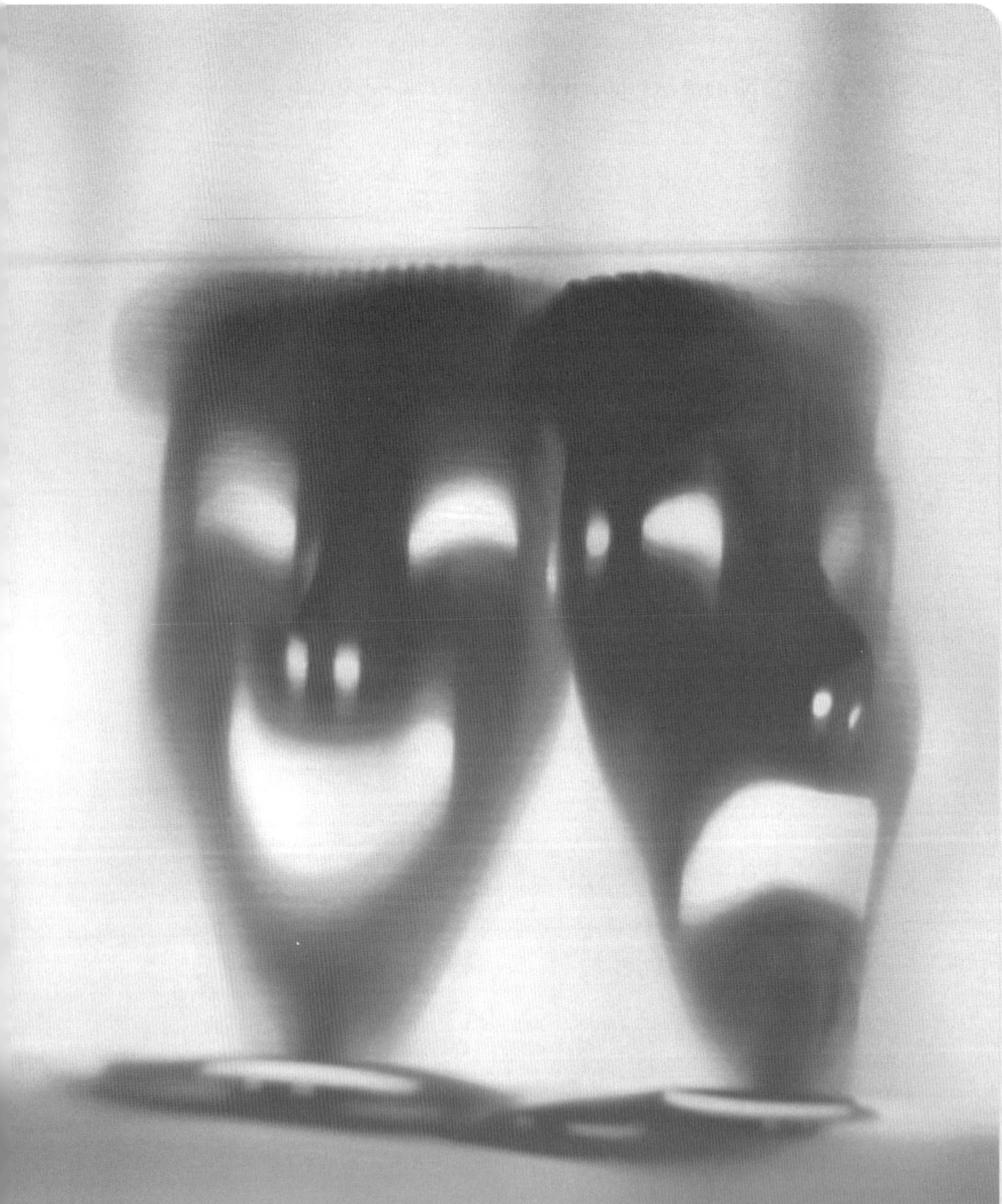

5 CHAPTER OUTLINE

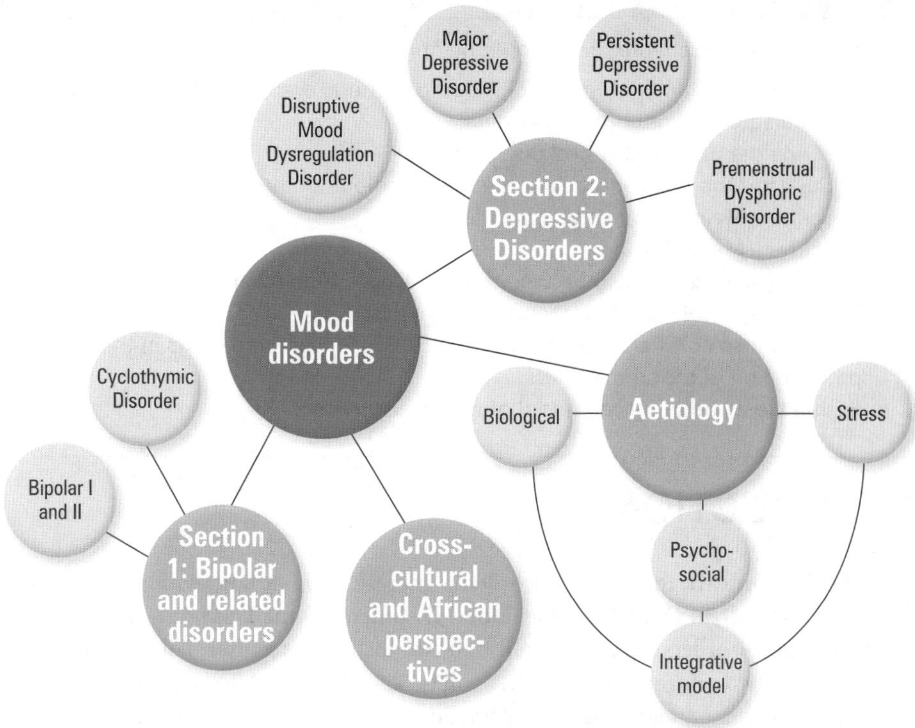

Introduction
History of mood disorders
Epidemiology
Life course
Clinical picture
Section 1: Bipolar and related disorders
- **Bipolar I and Bipolar II Disorders**
  - Cognitive symptoms
  - Somatic symptoms
  - Behavioural symptoms
  - Emotional symptoms
- **Cyclothymic Disorder**

Section 2: Depressive Disorders
- **Disruptive Mood Dysregulation Disorder**
- **Major Depressive Disorder**
  - Cognitive symptoms
  - Somatic symptoms
  - Behavioural symptoms
  - Emotional symptoms
  - Perceptual symptoms
- **Persistent Depressive Disorder (Dysthymia)**
- **Premenstrual Dysphoric Disorder**

Cross-cultural and African perspectives
Aetiology of mood disorders
- **Biological factors**
  - Genetics
  - Brain structures
  - Medical Illness
  - Neurochemicals
  - Endocrine system
- **Stress**
- **Psychosocial factors**
  - Childbirth
  - Loss and rejection
  - Social support
  - Personality and temperament
  - Behaviour
  - Cognition
- **Integrative Model**

Conclusion

LEARNING OUTCOMES

After studying this chapter you should be able to:

- Show a general understanding of mood disorders, and be able to distinguish mood disorders from other disorders.
- Describe the history of mood disorders.
- Understand the problems relating to the nosology of these disorders.
- Describe a Major Depressive Episode.
- Describe a Manic Episode.
- Describe, and distinguish between, Major Depression (Unipolar Depression), Dysthymia, Bipolar Disorder, and Cyclothymia.
- Identify cross-cultural, more specifically South African, variations in the presentation of mood disorders.
- Formulate an aetiological model of mood disorders.

INTRODUCTION

Traditionally depressive and bipolar disorders were seen to be variations of mood, and were categorised together in DSM-IV-TR as Mood Disorders. In the DSM-5, however, Bipolar and Depressive Disorders have been split into two distinct categories. For the purposes of this chapter the two categories of disorders will be discusses collectively as mood disorders, as they share the component of mood. Distinctions between the two categories will however be made in the discussion of the clinical pictures.

Mood disorders are the most common disorders and, in many instances, especially in developing countries, they are amongst the most under-treated group of disorders. The human suffering and the risk of suicide that accompanies these disorders make it imperative that they are diagnosed accurately, to ensure effective treatment (Bielski & Friedel, 1977). At first glance, this group of disorders seems to be relatively simple and it may seem the classification systems are over-inclusive. On closer inspection, it becomes clear that these disorders are complex both in their nosology and in their aetiology.

As clinical and biological research on mood disorders became more advanced, a more complex picture of mood disorders started to emerge as is reflected in the classification of mood disorders in both the DSM-5 and ICD-10. In this chapter, we will be exploring these disorders, which include Major Depression, Bipolar Mood Disorders, Dysthymia, and Cyclothymia.

At first glance, many people would assume that they know what 'mood' refers to and many would assume that a mood disorder refers to depression or anxiety (i.e. anything to do with emotions, feelings, or mood). This would be wrong to a greater or lesser extent, but this is not unexpected. Swartz (1998) refers to a study in Britain in 1988 by Leff, in which it was found that English patients generally have trouble distinguishing between anxiety, depression, and anger. These findings should come as no surprise as the word 'mood' is often used (and misused) in colloquial terms to refer to a wide variety of human emotional states. You have probably heard people referring to someone as being 'moody' (irritable/emotionally labile), in a 'bad mood' (angry) or even in a 'good mood' (happy). This difficulty in interpreting emotional states becomes more complicated when we consider different cultures, and the ways in which they may or may not refer to certain mood states.

Psychology and psychiatry rely on finer differentiations of emotion, as this enables a more detailed description of normal and abnormal emotions as well as a more detailed explanation of human functioning. However, the gap in understanding between professionals and the general public seems to be getting wider. It is therefore imperative that when a professional works with a person, they should be culturally sensitive, failing which a communication gap between the two may lead to a poor outcome. Table 5.1 provides some guidelines as to the meanings of the words that are used in the context of mood disorders.

Table 5.1: Common terms used to refer to mood

Term	Description/Definition
Emotion	In its most general definition, can be considered to be a complex psychophysical process that: • Arises spontaneously, rather than through conscious effort, and • Evokes either a positive or negative psychological response, as well as • Physical expressions, and • These responses are often involuntary.
Feeling	Conveys information about situations, on both conscious and subconscious levels.
Affect	The scientific term used to describe a person's mood as displayed in their behavioural response. You will notice in psychopathology that there is often reference to 'blunted' affect (reduction in emotional reactivity) or 'labile' affect (unstable display of emotion). The ICD-10 typically uses the term affect, e.g. Bipolar affective disorder.
Mood	Differs from emotions in that moods are considered to be sustained emotional states that are less specific and intense, longer lasting and less likely to be triggered by a particular stimulus or event. The DSM-5 typically uses mood, e.g. depressed mood.

You will notice in Table 5.1 that the descriptions encompass *normal* human states and furthermore that emotions, feelings, and affect could be considered to be transient (reactive, external expression of emotions) states, whereas mood is a more prolonged and sustained internal emotional state. It therefore becomes clear that the term *mood disorder* is more apt for this category of disorders than an *emotional* or *affective disorder*. Before we can really understand mood disorders, it is important to first define and describe what is meant by a mood disorder (see Box 1).

BOX 1: DEFINITION OF MOOD DISORDERS

A **mood disorder** can be defined as a disorder where a person feels depressed and/or elated, and outwardly shows signs (affect) of depression and/or mania for a significant period of time, and which is severe enough to impair normal functioning, and which occurs in the absence of a clearly identifiable stressor or trigger.

It is easy to understand mood disorders when one keeps a few key factors in mind:

- ***There are two extreme poles in mood disorders:*** On the one end, we have extreme **dysphoria** (Major Depressive Episode), and on the other, extreme **euphoria** (Manic Episode), as illustrated in Figure 5.1. In mood disorders, there is always an episode of depression. In those cases where there is only depression, we refer to those categories as **unipolar** mood disorders, and in those cases where we have an episode of depression and mania we refer to those categories as **bipolar** mood disorders (see Figure 5.2). Episodes of mania are always linked to depressive episodes and never exist on their own (Carson & Carson, 1984); therefore, one would never find a unipolar manic disorder.

Figure 5.1: The two poles of mood disorders

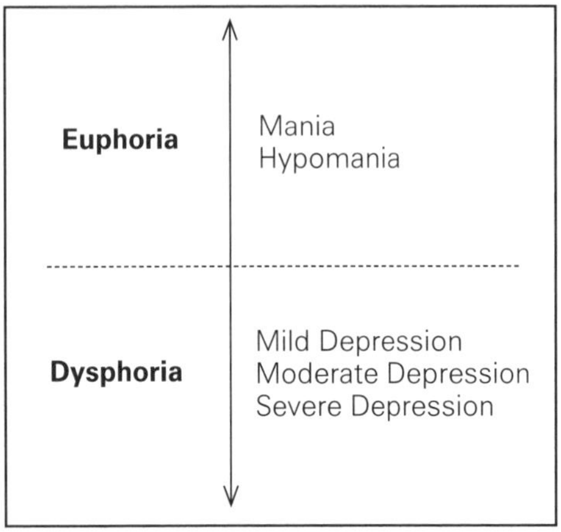

Source: Adapted from Carson & Carson, 1984.

- ***The severity of the symptoms:*** Many people experience such feelings or emotions as sadness, unhappiness, or disappointment, almost on a daily basis, as this is part of normal human existence. Often these emotions are the result of setbacks in life such as academic failure, relationship difficulties, financial problems, or the loss of a loved one. Under these circumstances, a person's normal functions (e.g. appetite, sleep, and motivation) may be affected, but this usually changes back to normal within a reasonable period of time. In many instances, though, these feelings, and the resultant changes in behaviour and functioning, are not triggered by clearly identifiable events, or may be abnormally prolonged following adverse events. It is only once a person's daily functioning is impaired due to the severity of the symptoms that one would make the diagnosis of a mood disorder. However, even the different diagnostic categories of mood disorders make provision for the severity of the symptoms. Parker (2006) states that both the DSM-5 and ICD-10 use the severity of symptoms to classify the different disorders. However, he warns against this approach as the cut-off points are so vaguely defined that this may lead to either the over- or under-diagnosis of these disorders. Examples of differences are Major Depression versus Dysthymia or Bipolar Disorder versus Cyclothymia.
- ***The duration of the symptoms:*** The duration of symptoms differs from one mood disorder to another. In the case of Major Depression, the symptoms must have been present for a two-week

period, whereas in the case of Dysthymic Disorder, the symptoms (of lesser severity than Major Depression) must be present for a period of two years. This also holds true for the distinction between Bipolar and Cyclothymic Disorders. In the case of Bipolar Disorder, the symptoms of mania must have been present for a period of one week. Cyclothymia, which is a less intense version of Bipolar Disorder, is a disorder where periods of hypomania and depression must have been present for a period of two years. Using the duration of the symptoms alone may not yield an accurate diagnosis. In this regard, Kendler and Gardner (1998) found little empirical support for the DSM-IV-TR requirements for two weeks' duration, five symptoms, or clinically significant impairment for a diagnosis of Major Depression.

Figure 5.2: Bipolar and Depressive Disorders in DSM-5

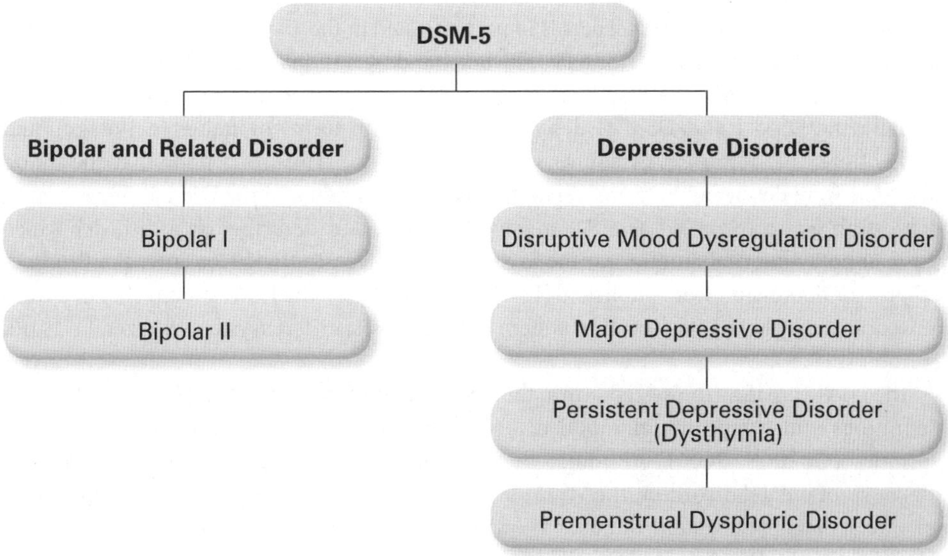

HISTORY OF MOOD DISORDERS

According to Solomon (2001), depression has been around since humankind developed self-conscious thought; however, the first documentation of disorders that would later be classified as mood disorders can be traced back to ancient times. The earliest written accounts of depression were recorded in ancient texts of the Mesopotamian era. Depression also appears in the writings of medical scholars from the ancient Greek and Roman civilisations and the early Greeks were seemingly the first to coin the terms melancholia and mania (Klein, Shankman, & McFarland, 2006). Since then, the history of mood disorders, especially depression, has been characterised by various theories about its causes and classification. These have ranged from biological humours, religious and spiritual failings, early loss, unconscious conflicts, irrational cognitions, and genetics, to neurotransmitter and neuropsychological abnormalities (Sweeney & Maas, 1978).

It is interesting to note that throughout history, the descriptions and causes of mood disorders have stayed relatively consistent over time, although they may have been refined as science has progressed. The term 'depression' was first used in the early 1600s, but did not replace the use of the word melancholia until the mid 1800s. The bipolar disorders (i.e. those disorders which are characterised by both mania and depression) were first identified in the 1850s. Initially, this disorder was named a manic-depressive disorder but it has undergone a number of name changes through the centuries. The attempts to classify disorders in a more scientific way culminated in the first classification of disorders in the *Diagnostic and Statistical Manual of Mental Disorders* (DSM) in 1952 (see Chapter 1). Subclassification of bipolar disorder was first proposed in 1957 by the German psychiatrist, Karl Leonhard, who also introduced the concept of bipolar (for those with manic and depressive episodes) and unipolar (for those with depressive episodes only) disorders. In 1968, both the newly revised classification systems ICD-8 and DSM-II termed the condition 'manic-depressive illness'.

The complexity of mood disorders is in part reflected in the way they have been described in the DSM from DSM-I to DSM-IV-TR, but the descriptions of the disorders have also changed due to changes in discourse of the DSM system over this time (see Chapter 1). Initially, the DSM-I and DSM-II described disorders in terms of causes (aetiology), and at this time, the dominant discourse was psychoanalytic. Thus, one finds that the mood disorders were described in terms of psychoanalytical causality. In the DSM-II, for example, depression was categorised as a 'Depressive Neurosis', and described as a disorder which was caused by internal conflicts or the loss of a love object. In the 1970s, after the Feighner criteria for depression were published (Feighner et al., 1972), the DSM system changed from an aetiologically based classification system to a diagnostic criteria system (Spitzer, Endicott, & Robins, 1978).

The DSM classification system, from the DSM-III onwards, not only provides operational definitions and symptoms of mood disorders, but also includes the clinical severity of episodes (Goldney, 2006). Although the DSM is an influential, international tool for diagnosis of mental disorders, the World Health Organisation (WHO) has not adopted it as an official diagnostic system, but uses its own classification system, namely the *International Classification of Diseases* (ICD). Although there are minor differences between the two systems with regard to mood disorders, there seems to be a significant congruence between the two systems (Goldney, 2006). The extent of overlap is such that authors such as Paykel (2002) argue that these differences are so small that ultimately a single system could be used for clinical and research purposes. Goldney (2006) is of the opinion that the debate surrounding the classification of mood disorders will never really be resolved to everyone's satisfaction, but predicts that the next advance in this regard will probably be characterised by a move away from 'clinical phenomenological descriptions' to 'biological markers'.

The DSM-5, which was published in 2013, introduced a new era in the classification of mood disorders. One of the major changes was dividing mood disorders into two separate chapters, i.e. Depressive Disorders and Bipolar and Related Disorders where previously they appeared in the same chapter under the heading of Mood Disorders.

EPIDEMIOLOGY

Epidemiological studies in contemporary South Africa are difficult and many yield contradicting results. This is probably the result of the enduring effects of social, political, and economic discrimination. Extreme disparities in wealth and income persist and South Africa demonstrates the second-highest level of inequality among all countries worldwide (May, 1998; Statistics SA, 2000). These disparities are generally aligned with race, and in most instances, they make the separation of racial categories from socio-economic status categories difficult. Any study of the aetiology of diseases and disorders within this setting faces the problem of complex social gradients in health, wealth, and poverty within and across diverse rural and urban communities, race, labour patterns, forms of livelihood, and population health (Myer, 2004).

ACTIVITY

Find and read the following article:

Tomlinson, M., Grimsrud, A.T., Stein, D.J., Williams, D.R., & Myer, L. (2009). The epidemiology of major depression in South Africa: Results from the South African Stress and Health study. *South African Journal of Medicine, 99*(2), 367-373.

You will notice in this article that the authors do not merely report prevalence rates, but also include demographic data such as gender, socio-economic status, etc. in their report.

In a study conducted by Tomlinson et al. (2009), a national probability sample of 4,351 South African adults was drawn. In their analysis, Tomlinson et al. (2009) made a distinction between current symptoms of depression as well as symptoms of depression 12 months prior to the study. In this sample they found an incidence of Major Depression of 9.7%, while 4.9% of the sample also showed symptoms of Major Depression 12 months prior to the study being conducted.

In a similar study, Herman et al. (2009) came to the conclusion that South Africa has a relatively high 12-month prevalence of mood disorders when compared with other countries, with only Belgium, Lebanon, Colombia, the Netherlands, France, Ukraine, Israel, New Zealand, and the USA having higher rates of mood disorders. This also holds true when comparing South Africa with other African countries. In the study by Herman et al. (2009), four times as many South Africans had lifetime mood disorders when compared to Nigerians. It is difficult to explain this phenomenon and as Herman et al. (2009) point out, reasons for differences in prevalence of mental disorders in high- and low-income countries do need further investigation before plausible explanations can be stated.

Further on in this chapter we will be exploring how mood disorders manifest differently across cultural groups, and we will also be investigating how certain socio-demographic variables either contribute to or maintain mood disorders. With this in mind, it is important to discuss the prevalence of mood disorders across various socio-demographic variables, including gender, socio-economic status, and development status.

In line with international prevalence rates (e.g. see Ebmeier, Donaghey, & Steele, 2006), South African women show higher prevalence rates of depression than men (Tomlinson et al., 2009), with higher risk associated with being separated, widowed, or divorced, especially those individuals with only an elementary school education (Herman et al., 2009).

In the 2004 Global Burden of Disease study, a distinction was made between high-income and low- and middle-income countries in terms of years lost due to a non-fatal disability

(World Health Organisation, 2004). Of the top ten disabilities, in low- and middle-income countries, unipolar depression ranked first, with alcohol abuse being fourth, Schizophrenia being ranked number six and Bipolar Mood Disorder ranked at eight. In comparison, in the high-income countries, unipolar depression also ranked first, while alcohol abuse was ranked third and drug abuse ranked number six. Bipolar Disorder did not rank in the top ten in the latter countries.

In the study by Kessler et al. (2007), no great distinction was found between developed and less-developed countries in terms of prevalence rates of mental health disorders in general; however, the only exception was that of mood disorders. This study indicated that people from less-developed countries were more at risk for developing a mood disorder than those people from more developed countries.

The reasons for these differences remain largely unclear; however, a Kenyan study (Ndetei et al., 2009) provides some insights into this. This study also found high rates of depression in Kenya, in particular that the prevalence is higher among women than men. However, they found differences in prevalence rates between rural and urban people, with the latter having higher rates of depression. They attribute this primarily to two reasons: a lack of traditional social support for women in cities and the cultural practice of polygamy. According to these authors, many of the women in polygamous relationships express resentment at having to share a husband. These findings are mentioned, not only to offer some kind of explanation for differing prevalence rates, but also to caution against categorising findings under such general headings as developed and undeveloped. Researchers need to look deeper and try to identify unique social patterns.

LIFE COURSE

In terms of the life course of this disorder, Moore and McLaughlin (2003) state that the risk of depression in children, adolescents, and the elderly is on the increase.

In the DSM-5 mood disorders in childhood are accommodated in two ways:

- Firstly, although the Bipolar and Depressive Disorders list the criteria for adults, many of these criteria make provision for symptoms manifesting differently in children.
- For example, depressed children often present with an irritable, rather than a depressed, mood, which may contribute to the difficulties in making this diagnosis. Another contributing problem, especially in adolescents, is that the disorder may go unnoticed as irritability is often ascribed to 'normal moodiness'.
- Secondly, a new disorder, Disruptive Mood Dysregulation Disorder, has been created for children in the Depressive Disorders category. This disorder was included to address the concerns about potential overdiagnosis and overtreatment of bipolar disorder in children.

Ebmeier et al. (2006) reviewed numerous international research publications and estimated that the worldwide average peak age for the risk of depression is 32 years. In comparison, in South Africa the mean age of onset is 26 years (Tomlinson et al., 2009), with a relatively low risk during childhood, followed by an increasing risk from adolescence onwards.

At the other end of life, the elderly are particularly vulnerable to depression, one of the main reasons being a lack of social support (Rodriguez, Brathwaite, & Dorsey, 2002). In contrast with depression in childhood, in the elderly it is characterised by cognitive symptoms, such as memory impairments. It is therefore often difficult to distinguish symptoms of depression from symptoms of neurocognitive disorders (see Chapter 7). Furthermore, depression is often co-morbid with physical disorders common among the elderly, such as stroke, cardiovascular diseases, Parkinson's disease, and chronic obstructive pulmonary disease.

Although aging may bring about physical and physiological changes that may contribute to the development of depression, there are also psychological and social changes that may contribute to the aetiology of this disorder. As we grow older, our once extensive social support network may show a steady decline due to the loss of friends, family, and spouses. Lopata (1993) suggests that, although an elderly person's social network may expand slightly because of grandchildren being added to the network, grandchildren often do not contribute to emotional support. Table 5.2 summarises research findings on depression in the elderly.

Table 5.2: Summary of research on depression in the elderly

Researcher	Finding
Rockwood, Stolee, & Brahim (1991)	18 – 20% of elderly in nursing homes suffer from MD.
Small (1991)	Diagnosis is difficult due to presence of medical illnesses or dementia.
Lyketsos & Olin (2002)	50% of people with Alzheimer's disease suffer from co-morbid depression.
Kessler et al. (1994)	Depression the same in the elderly, or in some instances lower, than in the general population.
Beekman et al. (2002)	Milder symptoms of depression are more common among the elderly, perhaps due to accompanying illness.
Grant, Patterson, & Yager (1988)	Depression contributes to physical disease and death.
Schultz, Drayer, & Rollman (2002)	Depression doubles the risk of death following a heart attack or stroke.

Source: Barlow & Durand, 2005.

The high incidence of depression in the elderly is maybe apt commentary on how they are treated in modern society. Wallace and O'Hara (1992) found that many elderly people became progressively more depressed over a three-year period, largely due to declining social support and increasingly poor health. It seems that as we grow older, and become frailer we become more isolated which then leads to depression and, as can be seen in Table 5.2, the more depressed we become the greater the risk of increased problems, which could ultimately lead to death.

CLINICAL PICTURE

Although Bipolar and Depressive Disorders have been discussed as mood disorders, these are two separate categories in the DSM-5, each with its own set of disorders (See Figure 5.2). The two categories do however share the same criteria for Major Depression.

SECTION I: BIPOLAR AND RELATED DISORDERS

As far as Bipolar Disorders are concerned, DSM-5 makes distinction between Bipolar I, Bipolar II and Cyclothymic Disorders. For Bipolar I disorder, patients need to meet the criteria for a fully syndromal manic episode, and possible major depressive episodes, thereby placing more emphasis on mania than depression (See Table 5.3). Bipolar II is different to Bipolar I in that there must be at least one episode of Major Depression, and that instead of a full manic episode, there is at least one episode of hypomania (See Table 5.4).

The ICD-10 does not distinguish between Bipolar I and II, but distinguishes between different types of Bipolar based on manic vs. hypomanic episodes. Another, interesting difference between the DSM-5 and ICD-10 is that the ICD-10 makes a distinction between manic episodes with or without psychotic symptoms (See Table 5.3).

You will note in text above that a distinction between mania and hypomania is made. This is because there are variations in the severity of manic episodes, which may range from mania (during which a person may become psychotic) to hypomania. A hypomanic episode, which is a subsyndromal counterpart of mania, is characterised by a distinct period of persistently elevated, expansive, or irritable mood, lasting throughout at least four days. It is also clearly different from the person's usual mood but is not as severe as mania in that the person is not psychotic, and judgement and social and work performance are not impaired. Many patients suffering from bipolar disorders become addicted to the heightened productivity and creativity that they experience during a hypomanic phase. Hypomania can be seen as a separate and unique state, or it could be an earlier and transitional state in an episode of mania, as only 50% of those patients in a hypomanic episode develop a full-blown manic episode (Goodwin & Jamison, 1990).

HELPFUL HINT
Mnemonic used to remember the symptoms of mania is DIGFAST:

- Distractibility
- Indiscretion
- Grandiosity
- Flight of ideas
- Activity increased
- Sleep (decreased need for)
- Talkativeness (pressured speech)

Table 5.3: Comparison of Bipolar Disorders between DSM-5 and ICD-10

DSM-5	ICD-10: Bipolar affective disorder
Bipolar I Disorder • Current or most recent episode manic • Current or most recent episode hypomanic • Current or most recent episode depressed • Current or most recent episode unspecified Bipolar II Disorder Cyclothymic Disorder *Specifiers for Bipolar and Related Disorders* • With anxious distress • With mixed features ‣ Manic or hypomanic episode ‣ Depressive episode • With rapid cycling • With melancholic features • With atypical features • With psychotic features • With catatonia • With seasonal pattern	Bipolar affective disorder, current episode hypomanic Bipolar affective disorder, current episode manic without psychotic symptoms Bipolar affective disorder, current episode manic with psychotic symptoms • With mood-congruent psychotic symptoms • With mood-incongruent psychotic symptoms Bipolar affective disorder, current episode mild or moderate depression • Without somatic syndrome • With somatic syndrome Bipolar affective disorder, current episode severe depression without psychotic symptoms Bipolar affective disorder, current episode severe depression with psychotic symptoms • With mood-congruent psychotic symptoms • With mood-incongruent psychotic symptoms Persistent mood [affective] disorders • Cyclothymia

Bipolar I and Bipolar II Disorders

In order to make a diagnosis of Bipolar I Disorder the person must meet the criteria for a manic episode (See Table 5.3), and that this episode may either be preceded or followed by a hypomanic (See Table 5.4) or major depressive episode (See Table 5.8) (APA, 2013). The diagnosis of Bipolar II disorders require a current or past hypomanic episode (See Table 5.3) as well as a current or past major depressive disorder (See Table 5.4).

Table 5.4: Diagnostic criteria: Manic Episode as adapted from the DSM-5

DSM-5
A. A distinct period of abnormally and persistently elevated, expansive, or irritable mood and abnormally and persistently increased goal-directed activity or energy, lasting at least one week and present most of the day, nearly every day (or any duration if hospitalisation is necessary).

B. During the period of mood disturbance and increased energy or activity, three (or more) of the following symptoms (four if the mood is only irritable) are present to a significant degree and represent a noticeable change from usual behaviour:
   (1) Inflated self-esteem or grandiosity.
   (2) Decreased need for sleep (e.g. feels rested after only three hours of sleep).
   (3) More talkative than usual or pressure to keep talking.
   (4) Flight of ideas or subjective experience that thoughts are racing.
   (5) Distractibility (i.e. attention too easily drawn to unimportant or irrelevant external stimuli), as reported or observed.
   (6) Increase in goal-directed activity (either socially, at work or school, or sexually) or psychomotor agitation (i.e. purposeless non-goal-directed activity).
   (7) Excessive involvement in activities that have a high potential for painful consequences (e.g. engaging in unrestrained buying sprees, sexual indiscretions, or foolish business investments).

C. The mood disturbance is sufficiently severe to cause marked impairment in social or occupational functioning or to necessitate hospitalisation to prevent harm to self or others, or there are psychotic features.

D. The episode is not attributable to the physiological effects of a substance (e.g. a drug of abuse, a medication, or treatment) or to another medical condition.

Note: A full manic episode that emerges during antidepressant treatment (e.g. medication, electroconvulsive therapy) but persists at a fully syndromal level beyond the physiological effect of that treatment is sufficient evidence for a manic episode and, therefore, a Bipolar I diagnosis.

Note: Criteria A – D constitute a manic episode. At least one lifetime manic episode is required for the diagnosis of Bipolar I disorder.

Source: Reprinted with permission from the Diagnostic and Statistical Manual of Mental Disorders, (DSM), Fifth Edition, American Psychiatric Association (APA), 2013 and ICD–10 Classification of Mental and Behavioural Disorders: Diagnostic Criteria for Research. World Health Organisation (WHO), Geneva, 2007.

Table 5.5: Diagnostic criteria: Hypomanic Episode as adapted from the DSM-5

DSM-5

A. A distinct period of abnormally and persistently elevated, expansive, or irritable mood and abnormally and persistently increased activity or energy, lasting at least four consecutive days and present most of the day, nearly every day.

B. During the period of mood disturbance and increased energy or activity, three (or more) of the following symptoms (four if the mood is only irritable) have persisted, represent a noticeable change from usual behaviour, and have been present to a significant degree:
   (1) Inflated self-esteem or grandiosity.
   (2) Decreased need for sleep (e.g. feels rested after only three hours of sleep).
   (3) More talkative than usual or pressure to keep talking.
   (4) Flight of ideas or subjective experience that thoughts are racing.
   (5) Distractibility (i.e. attention too easily drawn to unimportant or irrelevant external stimuli), as reported or observed.
   (6) Increase in goal-directed activity (either socially, at work or school, or sexually) or psychomotor agitation.

(7) Excessive involvement in activities that have a high potential for painful consequences (e.g. engaging in unrestrained buying sprees, sexual indiscretions, or foolish business investments).

C. The episode is associated with an unequivocal change in functioning that is uncharacteristic of the individual when not symptomatic.

D. The disturbance in mood and the change in functioning is observable by others.

E. The episode is not severe enough to cause marked impairment in social or occupational functioning or to necessitate hospitalisation. If there are psychotic features, the episode is, by definition, manic.

F. The episode is not attributable to the physiological effects of a substance (e.g. a drug of abuse, a medication, or treatment).

Note: A full hypomanic episode that emerges during antidepressant treatment (e.g. medication, electroconvulsive therapy) but persists at a fully syndromal level beyond the physiological effect of that treatment is sufficient evidence for a hypomanic episode diagnosis. However, caution is indicated so that one or two symptoms (particularly increased irritability, edginess, or agitation following antidepressant use) are not taken as sufficient for diagnosis of a hypomanic episode, nor necessarily indicative of a bipolar diathesis.

Note: Criteria A – F constitute a hypomanic episode. Hypomanic episodes are common in Bipolar I disorder but are not required for the diagnosis of Bipolar I disorder.

Source: Reprinted with permission from the Diagnostic and Statistical Manual of Mental Disorders, (DSM), Fifth Edition, American Psychiatric Association (APA), 2013 and ICD–10 Classification of Mental and Behavioural Disorders: Diagnostic Criteria for Research. World Health Organisation (WHO), Geneva, 2007.

Table 5.6: Diagnostic criteria: Depressive Episode as adapted from the DSM-5

DSM-5
A. Five (or more) of the following symptoms have been present during the same two-week period and represent a change from previous functioning; at least one of the symptoms is either (1) depressed mood or (2) loss of interest or pleasure. Note: Do not include symptoms that are clearly attributable to a medical condition. (1) Depressed mood most of the day, nearly every day, as indicated by either subjective report (e.g. feels sad, empty, or hopeless) or observation made by others (e.g. appears tearful). (Note: In children or adolescents, can be irritable mood.) (2) Markedly diminished interest in pleasure in all, or almost all, activities most of the day, nearly every day (as indicated by either subjective account or observation). (3) Significant weight loss when not dieting or weight gain (e.g. a change of more than 5% of body weight in a month), or decrease or increase in appetite nearly every day. (Note: In children, consider failure to make expected weight gain.) (4) Insomnia or hypersomnia nearly every day. (5) Psychomotor agitation or retardation nearly every day (observable by others; not merely subjective feelings of restlessness or being slowed down). (6) Fatigue or loss of energy nearly every day. (7) Feelings of worthlessness or excessive or inappropriate guilt (which may be delusional) nearly every day (not merely self-reproach or guilt about being sick). (8) Diminished ability to think or concentrate, or indecisiveness, nearly every day (either by subjective account or observed by others).

(9) Recurrent thoughts of death (not just fear of dying), recurrent suicidal ideation without a specific plan, a suicide attempt, or a specific plan for committing suicide.

B. The symptoms cause clinically significant distress or impairment in social, occupational, or other important areas of functioning.

C. The episode is not attributatble to the physiological effects of a substance or another medical condition.

Note: Criteria A – C above constitute a major depressive episode.

Note: Responses to a significant loss (e.g. bereavement, financial ruin, losses from a natural disaster, a serious medical illness or disability) may include the feelings of intense sadness, rumination about the loss, insomnia, poor appetite, and weight loss noted in Criterion A, which may resemble a depressive episode. Although such symptoms may be understandable or considered appropriate to the loss, the presence of a major depressive episode in addition to the normal response to a significant loss should be carefully considered. This decision inevitably requires the exercise of clinical judgment based on the individual's history and the cultural norms for the expression of distress in the context of loss.

Source: Reprinted with permission from the Diagnostic and Statistical Manual of Mental Disorders, (DSM), Fifth Edition, American Psychiatric Association (APA), 2013 and ICD–10 Classification of Mental and Behavioural Disorders: Diagnostic Criteria for Research. World Health Organisation (WHO), Geneva, 2007.

The typical picture of Bipolar Disorders can be described as follows:

Cognitive symptoms

When looking at the typical cognitive symptoms of mania, one needs to distinguish between thought content and thought process. In terms of the thought content, manic patients' thoughts include themes of exaggerated self-confidence and personal power (Kaplan et al., 1994). In extreme cases, these thoughts may reach delusional proportions which usually take the form of extreme personal wealth, attractiveness, or physical or mental powers (Frude, 1998), referred to as delusions of grandeur. In terms of their thought processes, an unrestrained and accelerated flow of ideas is common. Other cognitive functions, such as memory and orientation, usually remain intact; however, manic patients may find it difficult to concentrate as they are easily distracted.

Somatic symptoms

During the manic phase, one of the most common symptoms is a decreased need for sleep. Typically, a person in a manic phase may need only a few hours of sleep a night, or may go for days without sleep and still seem to be (and claim to feel) refreshed and energetic (Frude, 1998).

Behavioural symptoms

One of the obvious symptoms of mania is *overactivity*. People in a manic episode seem to have endless energy. In less severe cases (hypomania), their high levels of activity are usually aimed at accomplishing work or social goals. This increased activity often manifests itself as over-involvement in pleasurable, impulsive, and reckless activities and it often results in negative consequences. These activities include spending money, gambling, fast and dangerous driving, and sexual promiscuity (Frude, 1998). In this way, people in a manic episode put themselves and others at risk. Kaplan et al. (1994) report that approximately 75% of manic patients may become threatening or aggressive, and that some of them may attempt suicide or homicide.

One of the manifestations of accelerated thought patterns is extremely fast speech, and these patients tend to be extremely talkative. During a manic phase, speech becomes loud, fast, and difficult to interrupt.

Emotional symptoms

The characteristic mood during a manic episode is euphoria, which involves seeing the world as a wonderful place. During a euphoric phase, the person may display endless optimism and enthusiasm (Frude, 1998). One of the main problems with manic patients, however, is that they are emotionally labile (Kaplan et al., 1994), and their euphoria can quickly to turn into irritability, which may progress into hostility and anger (Halgin & Whitbourne, 2003). This is due to a low tolerance for frustration, which causes anger when they perceive that their (often delusional) aims and goals are being blocked (Davison & Neale, 2001).

Cyclothymic Disorder

This disorder could be regarded as a less severe disorder than either the Bipolar I or Bipolar II disorders. The essential feature of this disorder is a chronic, fluctuating mood disturbance which manifests in symptoms of hypomania (but not a fully syndromal hypomanic episode) and depression (but not a fully syndromal major depressive episode) (APA, 2013).

SECTION 2: DEPRESSIVE DISORDERS

The common feature of these disorders is primarily the presence of a sad, empty or irritable mood. There are a number of associated physical and cognitive symptoms, and together these symptoms impair the functioning of a person with one of these disorders (APA, 2013).

Disruptive Mood Dysregulation Disorder

In the past there has been growing concern that children may by mis- or overdiagnosed with Bipolar Disorder. This may, in part, be the result of clinicians attributing nonepisodic irritability to a manifestation of paediatric mania (APA, 2013). The problem with this is that the DSM-5 reserves the diagnosis of bipolar for episodic presentation of bipolar symptoms (APA 2013), and that the presence of only nonepisodic irritability does not meet the criteria for this disorder. In order to address this problem, a diagnostic category for children that display nonepisodic irritability, namely Disruptive Mood Dysregulation Disorder (DMDD), was created in the DSM-5, was created. This disorder is limited to children between the ages of 6 and 18 years, but typically the age of onset is before the age of 10 years (APA, 2013). The core feature of this disorder is chronic, severe and persistent irritability that manifests in two ways, i.e. frequent temper outbursts and persistent irritable or angry mood in-between temper outbursts (APA, 2013). The specific criteria for this disorder are listed in Table 5.7

Table 5.7: Diagnostic criteria for Disruptive Mood Dysregulation Disorder as adapted from the DSM-5

DSM-5
A. Severe recurrent temper outbursts manifested verbally (e.g. verbal rages) and/or behaviourally (e.g. physical aggression toward people or property) that are grossly out of proportion in intensity or duration to the situation or provocation. B. The temper outbursts are inconsistent with developmental level. C. The temper outbursts occur, on average, three or more times per week. D. The mood between temper outbursts is persistently irritable or angry most of the day, nearly every day, and is observable by others (e.g. parents, teachers, peers). E. Criteria A – D have been present for 12 or more months. Throughout that time, the individual has not had a period lasting three or more consecutive months without all of the symptoms in Criteria A – D. F. Criteria A and D are present in at least two of three settings (i.e. at home, at school, with peers) and are severe in at least one of these. G. The diagnosis should not be made for the first time before age 6 years or after age 18 years. H. By history or observation, the age of onset of Criteria A – E is before 10 years. I. There has never been a distinct period lasting more than one day during which the full symptom criteria, except duration, for a manic or hypomanic episode have been met. Note: Developmentally appropriate mood elevation, such as occurs in the context of a highly positive event or its anticipation, should not be considered as a symptom of mania or hypomania. J. The behaviours do not occur exclusively during an episode of major depressive disorder and are not better explained by another mental disorder (e.g. autism spectrum disorder, posttraumatic stress disorder, separation anxiety disorder, persistent depressive disorder [dysthymia]). Note: This diagnosis cannot coexist with oppositional defiant disorder, intermittent explosive disorder, or bipolar disorder, although it can coexist with others, including major depressive disorder, attention-deficit/hyperactivity disorder, conduct disorder, and substance use disorders. Individuals whose symptoms meet criteria for both disruptive mood dysregulation disorder and oppositional defiant disorder should only be given the diagnosis of disruptive mood dysregulation disorder. If an individual has ever experienced a manic or hypomanic episode, the diagnosis of disruptive mood dysregulation disorder should not be assigned. K. The symptoms are not attributable to the physiological effects of a substance or to another medical or neurological condition.

The fact that this disorder does not convert into a bipolar disorder later in the lifespan provides credence for the fact that DMDD and Bipolar are two distinct disorders. Further evidence to this fact is that there are clear distinctions in the genetic markers for children with DMDD and those with a bipolar disorder. In addition to this, there is a higher prevalence of DMDD in boys than girls, whereas in bipolar disorders there is more or less an equal prevalence rate (APA, 2013).

This is not an easy diagnosis as the core symptoms of this disorder can also be considered to be symptoms of other disorders such as bipolar disorders, major depressive disorder, anxiety disorder or other childhood disorders such as oppositional defiant disorder,

ADHD and autism spectrum disorders (See Chapter 13). Furthermore there is also a high comorbidity between this disorder and other disorders, and the DSM-5 states that it is rare to find children with this disorder alone (APA, 2013).

Major Depressive Disorder

Major Depressive Disorder, also called 'clinical depression', is a serious psychiatric illness that should not be confused with temporary sadness or 'the blues'. People use the term 'depression' to mean many things, such as sadness, feeling low, and unhappiness. Major Depressive Disorder, on the other hand, is a clinical syndrome that includes symptoms of depression (as a mood), as well as a variety of cognitive, physical (somatic), behavioural, emotional, and perceptual symptoms (Sweeney & Maas, 1978), as depicted in the case study of Albert.

Major Depressive Disorder should be thought of as episodic. The minimum duration of unipolar disorder is two weeks, but it can last much longer. Although depression is heterogeneous (i.e. not all people who are diagnosed with depression necessarily display the same symptoms), there are core clinical features which are stable across cultures and time (Ohaeri & Otote, 2002). These core features are either a depressed mood or the loss of interest or pleasure in nearly all activities.

There are numerous symptoms of clinical depression including cognitive, somatic, and behavioural symptoms (see Table 5.8 for DSM-5 criteria and Table 5.10 for ICD-10 criteria). These will be described in the following sections.

CASE STUDY

Albert is a 43-year-old male. He has various degrees, is an attorney by profession, and works for a large law firm. By all accounts, he is relatively successful in his work, but feels that he is stuck and has no real career prospects. He was divorced approximately five years ago and has two sons, aged 9 and 14, whom he sees on a regular basis. He has extreme feelings of guilt about how the divorce may have adversely affected his children. He has had various relationships since the divorce, but these only last for a couple of months at a time as he has difficulty committing to a relationship out of fear that it may not succeed. He has no financial, work, or relationship problems that are out of the ordinary. Recently, he has suffered from insomnia, has lost his appetite, has difficulty concentrating and generally feels tired and demotivated. As result, he went to see his doctor, thinking that the changes in his functioning were due to stress. During the clinical interview, the following facts, signs, and symptoms emerged:

- His maternal grandmother suffered from severe depression and was on occasion hospitalised for this, mainly because she was suicidal and could no longer function on her own. There may even have been a psychotic episode, but this was never confirmed.
- His maternal uncle may also have suffered from depression, but never received any treatment.
- Albert himself frequently feels down without any apparent reason.

- Typically, when he feels down he is also tired and demotivated; however, he forces himself to get out of bed and go to work during the week. During weekends, he often remains in bed for the whole of the weekend.
- Although he feels tired, he has difficulty sleeping. According to him, this is because he has difficulty 'switching his brain off', and he often just lies in bed thinking. The problem is, however, that these thoughts are mainly negative.
- He describes himself as being lazy and prone to procrastination, but on further enquiry it seems as if this may be due to both a lack of energy as well as a lack of concentration.
- There have been times that he has contemplated suicide, but out of a sense of responsibility and duty to his sons, he has never acted on these thoughts.

The doctor, having listened to Albert, made the diagnosis of Major Depression and referred him to a psychiatrist and psychologist for further treatment.

Cognitive symptoms

Depressed patients usually have a negative view of themselves, the world, and the future (Kaplan, Sadock, & Grebb, 1994). This usually manifests in extreme beliefs that they are worthless, unimportant, and ineffectual, which could be described as an extremely low self-esteem. The cognition of people with depression cannot be described in a linear way as all the components of their cognitions tend to reinforce each other in a circular way (i.e. low self-esteem intensifies a low mood, which in turn creates a negative view of the world and self, which in turn reinforces the low self-esteem). This circular reasoning often traps people in a situation which they feel they cannot escape, thereby creating a sense of helplessness and hopelessness (Beck, Brown, Berchick, Stewart, & Steer, 1990). Kaplan et al. (1994) state that, in depression, thought content often revolves around thoughts of loss, guilt, suicide, and death. According to these authors, approximately 60% of depressed patients have suicidal ideation and about 10% to 15% of depressed patients commit suicide.

Table 5.8: Diagnostic criteria for Major Depressive Episode as adapted from the ICD-10

ICD-10
• In typical depressive episodes of all three varieties (mild, moderate, and severe), the individual usually suffers from: ‣ Depressed mood. ‣ Loss of interest and enjoyment. ‣ Reduced energy leading to increased fatigability and diminished activity. ‣ Marked tiredness after only slight effort is common. • Other symptoms include: ‣ Reduced concentration and attention. ‣ Reduced self-esteem and self-confidence. ‣ Ideas of guilt and unworthiness. ‣ Bleak and pessimistic views of the future.

- Ideas or acts of self-harm or suicide.
- Disturbed sleep.
- Diminished appetite.

Source: ICD–10 Classification of Mental and Behavioural Disorders: Diagnostic Criteria for Research. World Health Organisation (WHO), Geneva, 2007.

Other cognitive symptoms of depression include thought blocking, poverty of content, impaired concentration, and forgetfulness (Kaplan et al., 1994). In severe cases of depression (i.e. Major Depression with Psychotic Features), a person may display mood-congruent delusions. We describe these as mood-congruent as the content of these delusions may include themes of guilt, sinfulness, poverty, worthlessness, failure, persecution, and terminal physical illnesses (Kaplan et al., 1994).

Somatic symptoms

Somatic symptoms are those that result in physical problems, such as fatigue, lethargy (a constant feeling of being 'slowed down'), aches and pains (e.g. headaches, lower back pain, gastro-intestinal pain, etc.), changes in appetite, significant changes in weight (either weight loss or weight gain) and sleep patterns (insomnia, early-morning awakening, and oversleeping), anhedonia (loss of pleasure in life), and a loss of libido (sexual desire). Manifestations of depression such as weight gain, sleeping too much, and a loss of interest in sex are known as vegetative states.

A typical sign of depression is an overwhelming loss of energy. This can cause a person to stay at home and avoid social interaction, and prevent a person from starting or finishing projects, maintaining previous interests, or exercising. The effects of diminished energy compound other effects of depression, and may result in work and family obligations being compromised. The pattern of a lack of energy may differ between people suffering from depression. Some people may experience extreme tiredness in the morning (e.g. due to disturbed sleeping patterns) and may then feel more energised as the day progresses; however, in other cases people may feel relatively energised in the morning and may then progressively experience extreme tiredness, and a need to sleep, as the day progresses (Frude, 1998).

Feelings of worthlessness and self-loathing, combined with a disinterest in pleasure, may cause a loss of intimacy and a decline in sexual activity. Depressed people are typically unable to talk about the reason for their reduced sexual drive with their partners, which may cause relationship difficulties. Often a lack of sexual drive reinforces feelings of worthlessness and inadequacy, which may in turn exacerbate the symptoms of depression.

Sleep may be disturbed in one of two ways, either sleeping more (hypersomnia) or less than normal (insomnia). The latter seems to be more common as approximately 80% of depressed patients complain of trouble with sleeping (Kaplan et al., 1994). Halgin and Whitbourne (2003) state that there are clear changes in EEG sleep patterns of depressed patients which are reflected in disturbances in sleep continuity. These may include intermittent awakening during the night and early-morning awakening (terminal insomnia). An inability to sleep may lead to an exacerbation of depression as patients often lie awake and ruminate about their problems.

Furthermore, a lack of sleep can lead to a loss of energy, excessive daytime sleepiness, and fatigue. Another interesting disturbance in sleep is that there is an increased duration of rapid eye movement (REM) sleep, especially during the night, and that there are more eye movements than normal during REM sleep (Halgin & Whitbourne, 2003).

A dysphoric mood and accompanying loss of pleasure in life may also impact on other areas of physical functioning, such as eating. Many depressed patients lose their appetite, which results in erratic eating habits and subsequent weight loss. On the other hand, some people have an increased appetite and subsequent weight gain, which commonly occurs in those who also tend to sleep excessively.

Behavioural symptoms

These symptoms are typically the observable manifestation of a disorder. In the case of depression we may have two, opposite, sets of behaviour, depending on the type of depression that the person is suffering from:

- ***Psychomotor retardation***, which is typically characterised by stooped posture, very little spontaneous movement, poor eye contact, impaired coordination, slow speech, and difficulties with articulation, or
- ***Psychomotor agitation***, which is usually characterised by generalised restlessness.

A behavioural symptom that is seen often is social withdrawal. This includes a marked reduction in interpersonal contact with family, friends, and colleagues. The severity of this symptom may vary from irritability with others to total social withdrawal. In addition, depressed patients often express the need to get away, or 'leave town'. In terms of verbal communication, Kaplan et al. (1994) state that depressed patients may display a decreased rate and volume of speech and often give only monosyllabic and delayed responses to questions.

Emotional symptoms

Kaplan et al. (1994) state that, although depression is the primary symptom of mood disorders, many patients deny any feelings of depression, and may not even seem to be depressed. Generally, the emotional symptoms of depression involve a dysphoric mood that exceeds ordinary feelings of disappointment and occasional sadness. This dysphoria may appear as extreme dejection or significant loss of interest in previously pleasurable activities (Halgin & Whitbourne, 2003). Other symptoms may include sadness, feelings of guilt, and worthlessness.

Perceptual symptoms

Although uncommon, hallucinations may be present in severe cases of depression. These hallucinations differ from those that one would find in other psychotic disorders, such as Schizophrenia, in that they are usually mood congruent (consistent with the depressed mood) (Kaplan et al., 1994).

Persistent Depressive Disorder (Dysthymia)

The essential feature of this disorder is a depressed mood that occurs for most of the day, for more days than not for a period of at least two years. Other symptoms of the disorder include changes in eating and sleeping patterns, low energy, low self-esteem, concentration difficulties and feelings of hopelessness. It is not uncommon for major depressive episodes to precede this disorder, nor is the occurrence of these episodes uncommon during this disorder (APA, 2013). People with this disorder are at high risk for other comorbid conditions, specifically for anxiety disorders and substance abuse (APA, 2013).

Premenstrual Dysphoric Disorder

This disorder manifests mainly in mood lability, irritability, dysphoria and anxiety symptoms. These symptoms occur repeatedly during the premenstrual cycle and typically peak at the onset of menses and remit shortly thereafter (APA, 2013). In addition to the alteration in mood, there are also other symptoms such as decreased interest in usual activities, concentration difficulties, lack of energy, increase in eating, changes in sleeping pattern and a number of physical symptoms (APA, 2013). These symptoms have an adverse effect on work and social functioning. Of note is that this does seem to be a culture-bound syndrome and that women who use oral contraceptives have a lower risk for this disorder (APA, 2013).

CROSS-CULTURAL AND AFRICAN PERSPECTIVES

CASE STUDY

Mr Carolus is 32 years old and lives in a small rural community in South Africa. He has been working as a manual labourer for the same company for 12 years. Three years before Prof Swartz met the gentleman for the first time, Mr Carolus was travelling in a bus that overturned. Some of the passengers on the bus sustained serious injuries, but he was lucky to escape with only minor injuries. He was transported to hospital along with the other injured passengers, and on arrival reported to the doctor that he had pain in his back. The doctor did not think this complaint was serious and Mr. Carolus was discharged without an X-ray being done. The timing of the accident could not have been worse for Mr Carolus as his mother had died shortly beforehand. Due to continued back pain he found it difficult to continue with manual labour and his employers assigned him to less physically demanding work. Although this did alleviate his pain for a short period of time, the pain returned and persisted. He sought medical help for this pain on numerous occasions, but the doctors could not find anything seriously wrong. At most they would prescribe mild analgesics or book him off from work for two days at a time. His complaints were also not taken seriously by his employers or co-workers and soon became the object of derision. His wife had also lost patience with his continuous complaints of back pain.

Prof Swartz spoke to him and probed for symptoms of depression. The following information was gained from this conversation:

- He slept poorly, waking up in the early hours of the morning and then being unable to fall asleep again.
- Loss of appetite and weight loss.
- Frequent spells of crying and rumination about his deceased mother.
- Constant fear about losing his job and then being unable to support his pregnant wife.
- He obsessed about his back injury during the bus accident and the fact that this was not taken seriously.
- These constant thoughts about the accident and his injury severely affected his ability to concentrate.
- He also reported that he constantly felt tired.
- He spoke in a flat, monotonous voice and showed signs of depression on his face.

An interesting twist to the tale was when Prof Swartz asked him about his mood. Mr Carolus said that he was not sad and: '... seemed rather confused when I asked him if he thought he was depressed' (p. 98). His response to this question was that he had on occasion thought there was something wrong with his 'nerves', but he knew he was not 'crazy' and generally 'it was only women' who suffered from their nerves. Prof Swartz did the ethically correct thing by referring him back to the primary health care facility in which he suggested that Mr Carolus was suffering from depression that needed treatment. Prof Swartz later heard that Mr Carolus was feeling better and that his concerns about his back had abated (but not disappeared).

Source: Adapted from Swartz, 1998, pp. 97-99.

Mr Carolus' story is not a unique one in South Africa. One of the main features is his own inability to recognise depression in himself. This, again, is not unique in South Africa or in other societies or cultures. People's conceptualisations of depression vary widely, both within and among cultures (note, for example, how Mr Carolus thinks that problems with 'nerves' are limited mainly to women). 'Because of the lack of scientific certainty,' one commentator has observed, 'the debate over depression turns on questions of language. What we call it—"disease", "disorder", "state of mind"—affects how we view, diagnose, and treat it' (Parker, 2001, p. 857). We have already in the introduction referred to the issue of language and mood disorders.

It is against this backdrop that we investigate mood disorders in Africa. As early as 1968, Prince concluded that, during the colonial period in Africa, there was a general assumption that depression was rare amongst African people. As a direct result of apartheid, this assumption seems to have been carried through to at least the mid 1990s, when diagnoses of patients seem to have been racially skewed. In a 1992 South African study of community clinics (Freeman, 1992), it was found that black patients were predominantly diagnosed with Schizophrenia (68%, as opposed to 19% of white patients) and white patients predominantly with a mood disorder (41%, as opposed to 9% of black patients). It is not surprising that people do not seek help when one takes into account the fact that the South African community seems to view the main cause of disorders such as depression and panic disorder as a 'weak character' (Hugo, Boshoff, Traut, Zungu-Dirwayi, & Stein, 2003).

German (1987) states that there seems to be unanimous consensus that mood disorders are in fact common in Africa; however, there seems to be some dispute about the nature of the symptoms. Binitie (1975) and German (1972) conclude that while there is remarkable similarity in depression symptoms between African and UK populations, it seems as if somatic symptoms are more common in African populations (Coleman, Morison, Paine, Powell, & Walvaren, 2006) and guilt and suicide more common in the European populations.

However, research done by Orley and Wing (1979) indicated that this may not necessarily be true. The answer may be found in German's (1987) statement that one should not focus on the presence or absence of individual symptoms, but rather on the extent to which some population groups *emphasise* certain symptoms as indicative of a particular state of illness. According to German (1987), it is probably true that all depressed patients experience the same amount of somatic discomfort and guilt, but that the expression of this may be over- or under-emphasised by prevailing cultural factors.

Swartz (1998) offers three reasons why there has been such a significant change in the views of professionals about depression in Africa (see Table 5.9).

Table 5.9: Reasons for changes in perceptions about depression in Africa

Reason	International	South Africa
Depressive illnesses did occur but were not noticed	Usually only people with socially disruptive behaviour come to the attention of mental health care services, and depressed people are usually overlooked (Littlewood & Lipsedge, 1997). Due to poor services in the colonial context depressed people may be reluctant to seek help (Littlewood & Lipsedge, 1997)	Swartz (1991) noticed in psychiatric hospitals that catered for black South Africans, almost all the patients who were admitted were done so because of socially inappropriate or disruptive behaviour. Parry and Swartz (1997) found that primary health care workers were not able to detect depression, this despite epidemiological studies (e.g. Gillies, 1992) indicating high rates of depression in the communities they served.
Depression taking on different forms	Littlewood and Lipsedge (1997) drew the conclusion that guilt is a less common feature in West Africa than Britain, and that hallucinations may be a core feature of depression in West Africa.	Rumble et al. (1996) drew the conclusion that apparent paranoid features may mask depression. Swartz (1998) postulates that if the aforementioned is true, many patients may in the past have been misdiagnosed with some psychotic disorder (see text before table).
Patterns of depression may be changing	Littlewood and Lipsedge (1997) point out that the risk of depression increases as one grows older, and with the increase in life expectancy in Africa, we can expect to see increases in the rates of depression.	Based on the work of Tomlinson et al. (2009), as reported earlier in this chapter, this seems to be the case for South Africa as well.

Source: Adapted from Swartz, 1998, pp. 110-115.

In an interesting study, Lester and Akande (1997) compared Xhosa, Nigerian, and American students in terms of four factors extracted from the Beck Depression Inventory:

- ***Action components:*** crying, decision-making, personal appearance, work, sleep, and tiredness
- ***Failure components:*** hopelessness, feelings of failure, disappointment with self, and suicidal ideation
- ***Guilt components:*** guilt, punishment, and irritability
- ***Physical components:*** appetite, weight, health, and sexual interest.

They found that Xhosa students had significantly higher scores on Action and Guilt components when compared to the Nigerian students. In addition, they had significantly more Guilt and Physical components as compared to their American counterparts. The Xhosa students also had significantly higher overall depression scores than the other two groups. These researchers concluded that there were clearly different depression patterns between these three groups.

Contextual factors may also be significant in depression. Ovuga, Boardman, and Wasserman (2005) found differences in prevalence rates of depression in two districts in Uganda, which they ascribed to different levels of conflict in that country. Along the same lines, Corin and Murphy (1979), caution that one must look beyond pan-cultural factors when looking at the roots of mental illness in Africa, and focus on local cultural factors. It would therefore seem as if the historically racially skewed diagnosis of mental disorder in South Africa is not due to the different prevalence of certain disorders in certain groups, but rather to misdiagnoses due to cultural insensitivity.

Where Western societies typically ascribe the causes of mood disorders to internal states (i.e. biological or psychological), non-Western societies tend to ascribe the causes to external forces, for example, social conflict, envy, witchcraft, or sorcery (Bührman, 1986; Schoeman, 1989; Swartz, 1986).

AETIOLOGY OF MOOD DISORDERS

The causal basis for mood disorders is not clear (Kaplan et al., 1994), or rather, there is no single cause for any of the mood disorders, and the exact dynamics of the interactions between all the causal variables have not been clearly identified and described. Study of the aetiology of mood disorders must be done against the following background:

- It is erroneous to try to find causal factors for the mood disorders as a whole. Both the DSM and ICD make provision for a variety of unipolar and bipolar disorders. This is due to the fact that although these disorders may share a number of common signs and symptoms, there are sufficient differences between them to warrant separate diagnostic categories. One should then, ideally, identify aetiological factors for each of these subcategories individually (Winokur, 1997). Unfortunately, due to space constraints, we cannot do this in this chapter, and only the general causes of mood disorders will be discussed.
- There is very little conclusive evidence for the causes of bipolar disorders, especially in African countries (Segal & Douki, 2005). This creates problems in terms of treatment, as treatment is often based on the known aetiology of a particular disorder.

When one studies all the literature pertaining to the causes of mood disorders, one cannot come to any other conclusion but that this disorder is a biopsychosocial one. The biopsychosocial model (as discussed in Chapter 2) proposes that biological, psychological, and social factors all play a role in causing depression. More particularly, the diathesis–stress model specifies that depression results when a pre-existing vulnerability, or diathesis, is activated by stressful life events. The pre-existing vulnerability can be either genetic (Caspi, Sugden, & Moffitt, 2003; Haeffel et al., 2008) implying an interaction between nature and nurture, or schematic, resulting from views of the world learned in childhood (Slavich, 2008). These interactive models have gained empirical support.

Biological factors

Genetics

Despite the current advances in understanding and classifying mood disorders, it is clear that these disorders still consist of a cluster of symptoms (i.e. a syndrome). This poses a challenge for understanding causes of mood disorders from a one-dimensional perspective, like genetics (Moreno et al., 2002). Family, adoption, and twin studies have consistently shown that genetics play an important role in the development of mood disorders in general (Tsuang & Faraone, 1990). However, it cannot be singled out as the most important cause of depression as it seems that those people who are at greater genetic risk for developing a mood disorder, are also more vulnerable to stressful life events (Kendler et al., 1995). Another, and more integrative, view on this is that we inherit the vulnerability for changes in certain neurotransmitters, such as serotonin (Cervilla et al., 2007) and dopamine (Elovainio, Jokela, Kivimäki, & Pulkki-Råback, 2007), which results in a mood disorder when interacting with adverse life events.

Brain structures

Many studies based on MRI scans of patients with depression have revealed a number of differences in brain structure compared to those who are not depressed. Arnone, McIntosh, Ebmeier, Munafò, and Anderson (2011) did meta-analyses of neuroimaging studies in major depression. They concluded that, compared to controls, depressed patients had increased volume of the lateral ventricles (implying increased cortical atrophy in these areas) and of the adrenal gland. These patients also have decreased volumes of the basal ganglia, thalamus, hippocampus, and frontal lobe, specifically the orbitofrontal cortex and gyrus rectus. Hyper-intensive lesions (seen as areas of high intensity on MRI scans) have been associated with patients with a late age of onset, and have led to the development of the theory of 'vascular depression' (Herrmann, Le Masurier, & Ebmeier, 2008).

Due to the fact that we mostly know which areas of the brain are responsible for which human functions, we can almost always trace the affected underlying brain structure back from the observable symptoms. For example, if we know that a person with a mood disorder often has memory problems, we can safely assume that the hippocampus is implicated in this disorder. Mayberg (2007) proposes that there may be a link between depression and neurogenesis (birth of neurons) of the hippocampus, a centre for both mood and memory. Loss of hippocampal neurons is found in some depressed individuals and correlates with impaired memory and dysthymic mood. Interestingly, stress may slow down this neurogenesis, whereas anti-depressants, which may increase serotonin levels in the brain, stimulate neurogenesis and a resulting increase in the total mass of the hippocampus, which in turn leads to normalisation of mood and memory (Duman, Heninger, Nestler, 1997; Sheline, Gado, & Kraemer, 2003). It seems as if the same also applies to the anterior cingulate, which is responsible for modulation of emotional behaviour (Drevets, Savitz, & Trimble, 2008).

According to Posner and Raichle (1994), the prefrontal cortex, thalamus, amygdala, and the anterior cingulate are joined by a neural pathway, and activity in one of these produces activity in another. These authors postulate that, in the case of depression, the firing of a circuit in which the amygdala feeds negative feelings into the consciousness, the prefrontal cortex retrieves memories that match these feelings, the anterior cingulate inflexibly maintains attention on these memories, and the thalamus provides ongoing neural activity to maintain this circuit.

Medical illness

There are some researchers who suggest that altered physical functioning could cause mood disorders, as opposed to those who argue that altered physical functioning may be the result of depression. Some research has focused on the potential roles of molecules involved in intercellular communication, namely cytokines.

Depression may also arise from treatment of a physical illness. An example of this would be treatment for chronic Hepatitis C Virus (HCV). Leutscher et al. (2010) evaluated 325 chronically HCV-infected patients undergoing antiviral therapy and they observed that depressive symptoms among patients undergoing HCV therapy are commonly overlooked and that the emergence of depression compromises the outcome of HCV therapy. Based on these findings, they strongly suggest that HCV patients be screened thoroughly for depression to assist with overall management of the patient.

Neurochemicals

The preceding sections have already alluded to the role of neurotransmitters. As science progresses and we gain a better understanding of the brain, for example, identifying new neurotransmitters, peptides, etc., hypotheses about the role of neurotransmitters in depression have changed. According to Thase and Howland (1995), the prevailing hypothesis for many years was that depression was caused by the depletion of monoamine neurotransmitters (norepinephrine, dopamine, and serotonin). This hypothesis, however, does not fully explain the cause of depression, as many other neurotransmitter systems (for example, GABA and acetylcholine) may be altered by depression (Rush, Stewart, Garver, & Waller, 1998). The neurotransmitters that are thought to play a role in depression are:

- ***Noradrenalin/norepinephrine:*** This neurotransmitter seems to work in tandem with serotonin in the pathophysiology of depression. It was found that when noradrenergic receptors are destroyed, drugs that affect serotonin lose their normal potency and vice versa; however, why this is so is still unclear (Kaplan et al., 1994).
- ***Serotonin:*** It is widely accepted that serotonin plays a primary role in the pathophysiology of mood disorders. A simple hypothesis in this regard is that too little serotonin is associated with depression, whilst high concentrations of serotonin are associated with mania. A second hypothesis, which relates to the interaction between serotonin and

norepinephrine, states that low levels of serotonin lead to higher levels of norepinephrine, which then results in depression or mania (Kaplan et al., 1994).

- ***Dopamine:*** Although dopamine was not initially thought to play a role in mood disorders, side effects of various drug treatments seem to suggest otherwise. Drugs that reduce dopamine concentrations often lead to depressive symptoms, whilst drugs that increase dopamine seem to lead to a reduction of depressive symptoms (Kaplan et al., 1994).
- ***Gamma Amino Butyric Acid (GABA):*** Although the involvement of this neurotransmitter is unclear, it seems that it may play a role as a second-messenger system in the pathophysiology of depression; thus it acts indirectly on the development of depression through its interaction with other neurotransmitters.

Winters and Neal (1985) argue that bipolar disorders have more of a biological cause than unipolar depression; however, the exact mechanisms are still unclear. The primary neurotransmitter that seems to play a role in bipolar disorders is norepinephrine. Research in this regard by Bunney, Goodwin, and Murphy (1972), Muscetolla, Potter, Pickar, and Goodwin (1984), and Goodwin and Jamison (1990), indicated that concentrations of this neurotransmitter are low during a depressed phase, and elevated during a manic phase. More recent research, however, has moved away from the norepinephrine hypothesis, mainly because the preferred pharmacological treatment of this disorder has no effect on the noradrenergic pathways, yet it provides symptom relief.

Endocrine system

There is some evidence that major depression may be caused in part by an overactive hypothalamic-pituitary-adrenal axis (HPA axis) that results in an effect similar to the neuro-endocrine response to stress. Some studies have found increased levels of the hormone cortisol and enlarged pituitary and adrenal glands, suggesting disturbances of the endocrine system may play a role not only in mood disorders, but various other disorders as well. Over-secretion of corticotrophin-releasing hormone from the hypothalamus is thought to drive this and is implicated in the cognitive and arousal symptoms (Monteleone, 2001).

It has been mentioned a number of times that the incidence of depression is higher among women than men. One possible explanation for this may be the role of oestrogen in depressive disorders:

- Increase in risk of depressive episodes after puberty, the antenatal period, and reduced rates after menopause (Cutter, Norbury, & Murphy, 2003).
- Premenstrual and post-partum periods of low oestrogen levels are also associated with increased risk (Cutter, Norbury, & Murphy, 2003).
- Sudden withdrawal of, fluctuations in, or periods of sustained low levels of oestrogen have been linked to significant mood lowering (Douma, Husband, O'Donnell, Barwin, & Woodend, 2003; Lasiuk, & Hegadoren, 2007).

Stress

Stress has been included here as a separate section, and has deliberately been slotted in between biological and psychosocial factors, as it has its foundation in both of these. It must be kept in mind that the human body and psyche function as a well-balanced system that comprises many subsystems. One of the main links between mind and body is stress, as stress not only has emotional and cognitive effects, but also results in physical and physiological changes in the body.

Stress is a complex construct, which may play an important role in various disorders (e.g. anxiety disorders, Schizophrenia, etc.). Selye (1956) pointed out that a stressor experienced for a long time depletes both the body's physical resources and the person's emotional and cognitive resources. This is because the person may feel that they cannot control the stressor, leading to feelings of helplessness and hopelessness.

Another important factor relating to stress is the predictability of a stressor. Research by Folkman (1984) indicated that people report less stress when they are able to predict the onset of a stressor. Compare, for example, your stress levels when you know that you are going to write a test versus writing an unexpected test. Unpredictability may be due to a lack of adequate information, while uncertainty may be due to a lack of effective knowledge or skills. It may also be due to a lack of self-confidence. The issues of predictability and control should, however, be viewed together with social support (see Figure 5.3).

In terms of the physical and physiological components, we need to consider both the central nervous system (i.e. hypothalamus, hippocampus, and neurotransmitters) and the endocrine system, typically referred to as the hypothalamic-pituitary-adrenal (HPA) axis. It seems the link between stress and alteration in neurotransmitters, which results in a mood disorder, could possibly be traced to this axis and the hippocampus (Brown, Harris, & Hepworth, 1994; Frank, Anderson, Reynolds, Ritenour, & Kupfer, 1994). We have already noted that ongoing chronic stress may have damaging effects on the body (Selye, 1956); however, ongoing stress may extend beyond damaging only the body; it may also alter brain functioning.

Various researchers, such as Weiss (1991), Sapolsky (1996), and McEwan (1998), have shown that stress not only alters brain function, but in extreme cases, it may even cause structural changes in the brain. Nemeroff (1998) found that depressed people typically display heightened HPA axis activity which may result in an ongoing stress response, which in turn may lead to excessive secretion of the corticotropin-releasing hormone (CRH). This leads to effects such as decreased appetite, weight loss, decreased sex drive, and hypersomnia (Sullivan, Coplan, & Gorman, 1998). In addition, post-mortem studies of depressed people found that these people tended to have a smaller hippocampus compared to people who did not suffer from depression. This finding is significant, according to Duman, Heninger, and Nestler (1997), for two reasons:

- One of the functions of the hippocampus is to inhibit the hypothalamus; therefore, a smaller hippocampus would probably be unable to inhibit the hypothalamus. Thus, depressed people are likely to show a longer stress response to an event than others.
- The hippocampus is also responsible for the production of monoamines (such as serotonin); therefore, a smaller hippocampus implies the underproduction of these essential neurotransmitters.

Although we have up to now discussed how biological factors may cause a mood disorder, we have at most described the 'mechanics' of the disorder. We have not really provided any clear answers as to the 'content' of the disorder, nor have we really examined external triggers of these disorders. In the following sections, we will be investigating both internal, psychological factors, as well as external, social factors that may lead to this disorder.

Psychosocial factors

By now it should be clear that the aetiology of mood disorders is indeed extremely complex as there are various contributing variables. Each of these may not necessarily be causal on its own, but the cause is almost always to be found in the interaction between numerous variables. To complicate matters further, Keller, Neale, and Kendler (2007) maintain that depression is a pathoplastic syndrome; that is, different adverse life events may result in different symptoms of depression (see Table 5.8). The different mood disorders may also have their own and unique causal factors; for example, life events become a more important causal factor with increasing age, but require interaction with predisposing factors, such as a family history of a mood disorder (Ohaeri & Otete, 2002).

Table 5.10: Adverse life events and depressive symptoms

	Sadness	Loss of pleasure	Appetite		Guilt	Fatigue	Suicide ideation	Loss of concen-tration	Loss of sleep
			Gain	Loss					
Loss of loved one	X	X		X					
Problem in intimate relationship	X	X		X	X				
Long-term stress	x	x		x		X			X
Depression without clear psychosocial trigger	x		X			X	X	x	

Note: X: strong feature x: weak feature

Source: Adapted from Keller, Neale, & Kendler, 2007.

We have already suggested that depressed people may have a lack of social support, making them more vulnerable to depression (Billings, Conkrite, & Moos, 1983). However, they may also lack social support as a result of their depression, which may drive other people away, as their behaviour tends to elicit negative responses from others. Depressed people's interpersonal and social skills are typically characterised by: poor interpersonal problem-solving, difficult speech patterns (e.g. slow, monotone, and monosyllabic speech), unsatisfactory eye contact, negative content in conversations, and constant seeking of reassurance (Gotlib, 1982). These factors make it difficult to relate to them or have an enjoyable conversation with them.

Another important social factor is socio-economic status, or more specifically, poverty. Stein and Gureje (2004, p. 233) state that 'it stands to reason that when life's circumstances are harsh, people will feel stressed or depressed.' However, although there may be a strong link between adverse life circumstances like poverty and mood disorders, such circumstances can never be seen as the single cause of these disorders. Tomlinson, Swartz, Cooper, and Molteno (2004) state that poverty must be understood not only as an absence of resources, but also as a complex interaction of social, interpersonal, and psychological factors that impact not only on individuals, but also on groups and the wider society.

However, despite these links between specific life events and symptoms, there is also a group of people who develop symptoms of depression in the absence of adverse life events. When one is searching for clues to the possible causes of mood disorders in general, and depression in particular, one would almost intuitively turn to adverse life events as a probable cause; however, one should always remember that:

- Different adverse life events could lead to different depressive symptoms (i.e. equifinality).
- The same adverse life events may lead to different disorders (i.e. multifinality) such as anxiety, somatoform disorders, etc., in different people.
- Not all people who are exposed to adverse life events necessarily develop symptoms of depression (or any other disorder).

For example, Fresco, Rytwinski, and Craighead (2007) found that a rigid attributional style leads to higher levels of depression in the face of negative life events. Other factors such as dispositional optimism (Hirsch, Wolford, LaLonde, Brunk, & Morris, 2007) and positive religious coping may buffer a person against the effects of negative life events (Bjorck & Thurman, 2007). It is for this reason that life events are described here as a precipitating factor, as they may, at most, trigger the onset of a mood disorder, but they are unlikely to cause such a disorder. As Table 5.8 shows, there are a number of life events, psychosocial factors, and socio-economic factors that are strongly associated with the onset of mood disorders.

Although there has been a great deal of research on the psychological factors that may cause depression, there is a lack of research on these factors as possible causes for bipolar disorders. This is mainly because there seems to be a general consensus that the causes of bipolar disorders are mainly biological (Winters & Neale, 1985). This should not be surprising as it is difficult, if not impossible, to explain bipolar disorders from a psychological perspective, as there is often no obvious link between psychosocial factors and rapid swings in mood. Furthermore, psychological forms of treatment have achieved very little success in the treatment of bipolar disorders compared to biological treatments which are more effective in controlling the symptoms. However, psychological factors are an important part of the treatment programme in terms of dealing with the sequelae (consequences) of bipolar disorder. The remainder of this section will thus focus more on the psychological causes of unipolar depression than on bipolar disorders.

Childbirth

The birth of a baby is a major life event that necessitates psychosocial adjustment not only from the mother, but also from the father and the family at large (Madu & Roos, 2006). There is such a strong link between childbirth and depression that the classification systems make provision for a separate diagnostic category, Post-Partum Depression. This disorder is categorised by sadness, dysphoria, emotional lability, insomnia, confusion, anxiety, guilt, suicide ideation, and dependency (Dennis, Janssen, & Singer, 2004). Kaplan et al. (1994) state that this disorder may be ascribed to both biological (rapid changes in hormonal levels and the physical stress of childbirth) and psychological factors (awareness of the increased responsibility of motherhood).

Rates of pre- and post-natal depression in developing countries are generally high (Rahman & Creed, 2007) and this seems also to be true in South Africa. Madu and Roos (2000) state that this disorder affects 10% to 15% (approximately 50,000) new mothers in South Africa every year, and in some areas of South Africa, the rate may be as high as 34% (Tomlinson et al., 2002). It is interesting to note that, although there are various debates about the nature and prevalence of depression cross-culturally, there do not seem to be cross-cultural variations in Post-Partum Depression. De Bruin, Swartz, Tomlinson, Cooper, and Molteno (2004) found that the symptoms of Post-Partum Depression among Xhosa and European women were similar.

In this regard, Dennis et al. (2004) found that although socio-economic status was significantly associated with depressive symptomatology, it is not a strong predictor of Post-Partum Depression. These researchers maintain that other variables, such as a previous history of depression, personality traits, stressful life events, and a lack of support, all contribute to the onset of this disorder. In the study conducted by Tomlinson et al. (2004) amongst mothers from a poor community, it was found that the main predictors of maternal depression were a lack of financial support from the father, the father having a negative attitude towards the newly born child, a lack of support or help, and the baby being unplanned or unwanted. Unfortunately, maternal depression not only affects the mother, but may also have a negative impact on the development of the infant (Patel, DeSouza, & Rodrigues, 2003; Tomlinson, Cooper, Stein, Swartz, & Molteno, 2006).

Loss and rejection

Object loss refers to the loss of a parent, or another loved one, through death or separation (Carson & Carson, 1984). One of the earliest causes for depression that was identified was the relationship between childhood object loss and adult depression (Bowlby, 1980; Freud, 1950; Rado, 1928). Akiskal (1979), in his review of evidence underlying the object loss-depression link, found no evidence that there is a direct causal link. However, it could be that early loss predisposes people to depression when they are confronted with subsequent losses.

In his comparison between clinically depressed patients and people who were not depressed, Beck (1967) found that 27% of the depressed patients had experienced a loss of a parent before the age of 16, whereas only 12% of those people who were not depressed had the same experience. Although there seems to be some evidence implying that early loss may be a causal factor, these findings are not compelling enough to suggest that it is a significant causal factor. Thus, at most, it is one of many factors that may lead to vulnerability to depression (Brown & Harris, 1978; Paykel, 1974).

According to psychoanalytic theories of depression, loss, rejection, and repressed anger are linked. Freud (1917) noticed that symptoms of grief and depression are very similar. He postulated that real, or imagined, loss of affection could elicit excessive, irrational grief which then develops into depression. He argued further that a person feels anger towards the person who has 'rejected' him or her by dying (the death of a loved one is seen, arguably in an irrational way, as rejection). This anger is regarded by the superego as unacceptable, and the result is that the anger is repressed or turned onto the person themself. These self-directed feelings of hostility then create feelings of guilt, unworthiness, and despair. Support for this explanation is mixed, with some studies (e.g. Roy, 1981) reporting that the early loss of a parent predisposes one to depression, whilst other studies (e.g. Lewinsohn & Hoberman, 1982) show no such a relationship.

Social support

Social support refers to the physical and emotional comfort we receive from the people around us. It gives us the feeling that we are important to others and that they value us. As social beings we form a complex network of relationships with others in different contexts (i.e. family, friends, work, etc.) This network plays an important role in moderating the intensity of stress. Hause (1984) has identified four types of social support:

- ***Emotional concern:*** This refers to the caring, empathy, love, and acceptance that are expressed by others.
- ***Instrumental aid:*** This refers to giving material assistance to us when we may need it, for example, money, accommodation, transport, etc.
- ***Information:*** Information includes guidance, advice, facts, clues, and other forms of information which assist us in making decisions and formulating a plan of action.
- ***Appraisal:*** Appraisal refers to the feedback that others give us that is relevant to our own self-evaluation.

Wodka and Barakat (2007) found that, when faced with adverse life events, people may be more prone to depression (and anxiety) in the absence of family support. Although having family and friends may be beneficial, research has shown that simply having people available for support is not sufficient, if these people are not actually supportive. Ross and Mirowsky (1989) concluded that the more that people talk to others as a strategy for coping with stressful situations, the more depressed they tended to become. This may sound surprising, but this suggests that social support is a more complex construct than the name implies.

A newly identified subtype of social support, inferential feedback, seems to be significant in the development of depression. Inferential feedback from friends and family members addresses the cause, meaning, and consequences of negative life events and may influence depression through its effect on depression-inducing cognitions (DeFronzo-Dobkin et al., 2007). Furthermore, too much instrumental social support has also been shown to have negative outcomes because it promotes passivity and dependence.

The combinations of control and support (Walker, 2001) are (see Figure 5.3):

- ***High control, low support:*** This combination strengthens self-efficacy and an internal locus of control.
- ***Low control, high support:*** This reinforces dependency on others and an external locus of control (i.e. low personal control).
- ***High control, high support:*** This combination fosters belief in own capabilities as well as confidence in the support from others.
- ***Low control, low support:*** In this combination, there is a perceived lack of resources, and this results in helplessness and hopelessness.
- ***Uncertain control, uncertain support:*** This combination results in anxiety and helplessness, and strengthens an external locus of control.

Figure 5.3: Interaction between control and support

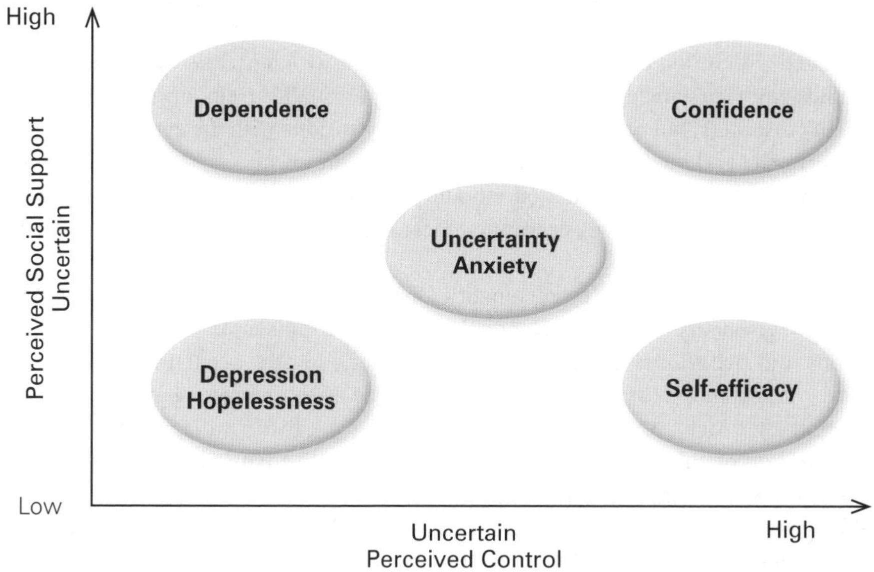

Source: Adapted from Walker, 2001.

It must be noted that Figure 5.3 mentions 'perceived support', which is different from actual support (Kanacki, Jones, & Gaibralth, 1996; Levy & Derby 1992). Perceived support is how one sees the support being received. A person's perception of their social environment may be affected by the disorder, or in many cases, is one of the causes of a disorder. As was mentioned in Chapter 1, one often needs to gather collateral information about the person, in order to ascertain to what extent their perceptions correspond with those of other people in their life. Often people report that they either have no support, or that their families and friends are overprotective, when neither of these might be the case.

A lack of social support, combined with socio-economic factors like poverty and the breakdown of kinship, is potentially a great problem in South Africa. Historically, many men from rural areas have been migrant workers who leave their families and dependants behind when seeking work in large cities. Often their wives then have to cope as single parents or, if they move to the cities with their husbands, they are far away from their own parental homes. Brown and Harris (1978) identified factors such as having nobody to confide in, as well as unemployment, as important social factors in the development of depression. If one compares the situation of many South African women to Figure 5.3, it is clear that these women have both low perceived (and real) support and very little control over their situations, greatly increasing their risk of depression.

Notwithstanding all of the problems with social support which have been raised above, it seems that support aimed at problem-solving and enhancing personal control is probably the most beneficial, and a potentially strong buffer against developing a mood disorder in the face of adverse life events.

Personality and temperament

For the purposes of this discussion, we will define a person's personality and temperament loosely as the set of his or her attitudes and beliefs as well as more enduring neurobehavioural predispositions (Hirschfeld & Shea, 1992). Typical personality traits that can be associated with mood disorders include neuroticism, avoidance, dependence, reactivity, and impulsivity (Hirschfeld & Shea, 1992). These personality traits or, in extreme cases, personality disorders, not only affect a person's ability to cope with life events, but also tend to elicit adversity and rejection (i.e. they *create* adverse life events).

Some early authors believed that one should make room for a diagnosis of a Depressive Personality Disorder. This diagnosis was first included in the DSM-II, but was removed from the DSM-III.

The DSM-IV (in Appendix B: Personality Disorders Not Otherwise Specified) defined Depressive Personality Disorder (Depressive PD) as 'a pervasive pattern of depressive cognitions and behaviours beginning by early adulthood and occurring in a variety of contexts' (American Psychiatric Association, 1994, p. 732). Depressive PD occurs before, during, and after Major Depressive Episodes, making it a distinct diagnosis not included in the definition of either Major Depressive Episode or Dysthymic Disorder. The DSM-5, however, makes no room for such a disorder.

Although this is no longer considered to be an official diagnosis, it is worthwhile reviewing the symptoms of such a disorder as it sheds some light on how personality may contribute to depression. Rather referring to a depressive personality as there seem to be people who have a generally gloomy outlook on life, themselves, the past, and the future. They are plagued by issues around developing and maintaining relationships. Recent studies have concluded that people with this type of personality are at a greater risk of developing Dysthymic Disorder than a comparable group of people with different personality types (Kwom, Kim, Chang, Park, & Yoon, 2000). These findings suggest that Depressive PD is a potential precursor to dysthymia or other depression spectrum diagnoses.

Considering personality type, Millon (2004) identified five types of depression, which he classified according to typical personality types. These are:

- ***Ill-humoured depressive:*** People with this type of depression typically show passive-aggressive personality traits. Furthermore, they tend to be hypochondriacal (see Chapter 8) and are often cantankerous, irritable, guilt-ridden, and self-condemning. They generally have a very negative view about themselves and their world.
- ***Voguish depressive:*** This type of depression is a popular and stylish mode of social disenchantment, which sees personal depression as self-glorifying, and suffering as ennobling. Typically, these people have histrionic and narcissistic personality traits. The attention from friends, family, and doctors is seen as a positive aspect of the voguish depressive's condition.
- ***Self-derogating depressive:*** Patients who fall under this subtype are self-deriding, self discrediting, see themselves as odious and dishonourable, and disparage themselves for their weaknesses and shortcomings. These patients blame themselves for not being good enough and typically display features of a Dependent PD.
- ***Morbid depressive:*** People with this type of depression experience profound dejection and gloom, are highly melancholic, and often feel drained and oppressed.

- ***Restive depressive:*** People with an Avoidant Personality Disorder are more prone to this type of depression. They are consistently unsettled, agitated, wrought in despair, and perturbed. This is the subtype most likely to commit suicide in order to avoid all the despair in life.

As can be seen from the above, it is impossible to identify a single personality trait or type as a causal factor in depression.

Behaviour

According to behaviourists, all behaviour is learnt; therefore, we could assume that all forms of abnormal behaviour are learnt as well. Behaviourists typically make use of classical conditioning and/or operant conditioning to explain the acquisition of abnormal behaviour. The main premises in these theories are that:

- Negative responses are positively reinforced.
- Positive responses are not reinforced or they are punished.

Frude (1998), based on the work of Skinner (1953), explains depressed behaviour (such as learned helplessness and hopelessness) is the result of behaviour repertoires extinguished over time. According to Skinner, behaviours that are not positively reinforced (e.g. by means of food, money, social approval, etc.), drop out of a person's behaviour repertoire.

Researchers like Ferster (1973) and Lewinsohn (1974) built on Skinner's theory by placing more emphasis on the role of self- and social reinforcement as contributors to depression. According to these theories, social reinforcement tends to lift a person's mood by making him or her feel more valued and respected. People who do not receive this kind of reinforcement tend to feel ignored and undervalued. However, the problem is that people who suffer from depression tend to withdraw themselves from others, thereby reducing their opportunities to receive social reinforcement.

According to Frude (1998), behaviour theories also offer an explanation for the maintenance of depression because depressive behaviour is often positively reinforced. Initially, the behaviourists maintained that reinforcement problems lead to the development of depression; however, they have not been able to isolate those conditions that are specific to depression (Carson & Carson, 1984). It may therefore be safer to assume that rather than causing depression, certain reinforcement patterns may affect the course of the disorder.

It is imperative that one considers a circular causal pattern (as Figure 5.4 suggests) where social factors may lead to the onset of depression but that, via a recursive feedback loop, the depression in turn impacts on social interaction (Teichman & Teichman, 1990). Coyne (1984) describes this pattern as follows: Initially a depressed person elicits sympathetic responses from others and he or she experiences a reduction of demands, which jointly reinforces the depressive behaviour. Over time, however, other people tend to become frustrated with the depressed person, which leads to an escalation of symptoms by the depressed person. This in turn leads to greater frustration in those around them, which ultimately results in rejection.

Although behaviourism offers some explanation, there has not been much support for this; also, to a certain extent, many of these explanations have been incorporated into other theories (e.g. cognitive-behavioural theories). Research has continuously indicated that internal processes, such as cognitions, perceptions, evaluations, and expectations, play a more important role in the causation of depression than merely the reinforcement, or lack of reinforcement, of behaviour.

Cognition

Cognition as an aetiological factor has been well researched and described and this section only provides a very brief summary of this research. The basic tenet of this approach is that faulty cognition is one of the main causes of depression. For this discussion, the construct 'cognition' will include perception, thought-processing, and thought content. This discussion will be an attempt to provide a more integrated view of the role of cognition, rather than referring to and explaining the different theories in detail.

Firstly, we must understand generally how depressed people perceive their world. Rotter (1966) suggested that people perceive their world in terms of their own belief in how they can affect outcomes of a situation. He stated that one either has an internal locus of control (i.e. that one perceives high personal control over the outcome of a situation) or an external locus of control (i.e. that one perceives that one has little or no control over the outcome of a situation). If people do have an external locus of control, they tend to have low self-efficacy and a low self-esteem, which in itself is not necessarily problematic, but may, in conjunction with other cognitive factors, lead to some form of pathology such as depression.

A more general theory of perception, such as that of Rotter, only gives us a vague idea of a depressed patient's cognitions. It is therefore logical that we move beyond this to a more detailed description of processing information. Abramson, Seligman, and Teasdale's (1978) Theory of Learned Helplessness postulates that people have three basic attributional structures that make up a their dominant **attributional style** (Davison & Neale, 2001):

- ***Global vs. Specific:*** This refers to whether a person thinks they are unable to deal with a certain event (specific) or whether they generally feel unable to deal with any event (global).
- ***Internal vs. External:*** People who have an internal attributional style ascribe failure to themselves, and those who have an external attributional style ascribe failure to causes out of their control.
- ***Stable vs. Unstable:*** If the person feels that the problem is stable, they expect it to be long term, as opposed to the problem being short term (i.e. unstable).

According to this theory, depressed people have a global-stable-internal attributional style; in other words, they feel that their failures are due to their own shortcomings, which will always cause problems in all situations. If this is a person's dominant attributional style, it is clear that they will, over a period of time, develop a low self-esteem and that they will feel ill-equipped to deal with life.

Beck's theory of Hopelessness (Beck, 1967) is in some regards very similar to the theory of Helplessness, as both theories attribute depression to faulty perceptions and thought-processing. According to Beck, depressed people typically display three basic negative thoughts (referred to as the negative cognitive triad), thus, they have negative views of:

- Themselves ('I am a failure.')
- The world ('All of my attempts to cope with life result in failures.')
- The future ('Because I'm a failure and I cannot cope, the future is hopeless.').

EXAMPLE

Imagine that you have just failed a Psychology test. If you are not in the grip of the negative cognitive triad, you might think that this event, while unfortunate, has to do with the lecturer, or the fact that you did not study correctly. It might not occur to you at all to doubt yourself, or to think that this event means that you are a failure and that you might as well end your studies. If your thinking process was dominated by the negative cognitive triad, however, you would very likely conclude that your failure was due to a personal failure (e.g. that you are not intelligent enough); that you will always fail Psychology tests; and that you will never be able to complete your degree. On the basis of these judgments, you will begin to feel depressed. In contrast, if you were not influenced by negative triad beliefs, you would not question your self-worth too much, and might respond to the failure by investigating your study methods, or by getting some advice from the lecturer or tutor.

All of these cognitions and perceptions, which happen quite unconsciously, form a complex interplay that may maintain a depressed person's core negative schemas. The result is often so powerful and overwhelming that the person is unable, even in the presence of strong contradictory evidence, to make a shift towards more positive thoughts.

Along the same lines Ellis (2004), like Beck, noted that depressed people tend to focus more on negative information (in the process ignoring positive information), and then overgeneralise this information to other situations. For example, they think that because some local and isolated event has turned out badly, this means that all events will turn out badly. Ellis (2004), however, goes beyond thought-processing, and maintains that faulty thought content (which he calls irrational beliefs) further perpetuates the problem. According to him, a depressed person's thoughts are often expressed in absolute statements, and there are three typical irrational beliefs that depressed people display (Ellis, 2004):

- 'I must always perform well, regardless of the conditions under which I have to work'
- Others must always treat me fairly, and with respect'
- 'My living conditions must always be perfect'.

Having read through the section on negative cognitions, one has to ask oneself what the possible origin of these negative cognitions could be. One explanation could be that people are shaped by the interactions between their behaviours, thoughts, and environment (i.e. there are processes of direct or vicarious learning). It is thought, therefore, that people learn certain cognitions through negative comments from others, adverse life conditions, traumatic experiences, failures, etc. Although these thought processes are learnt, or acquired, they need not necessarily manifest immediately. Thus they may remain latent until a new stressful life event triggers them, so that, together with a biological predisposition to depression, this ultimately results in a mood disorder such as depression.

Although these theories are logical, and one is often easily able to identify negative thoughts and thought processes in depressed people, it is debatable, firstly, as to whether these thoughts are the cause or result of depression (although there is considerable evidence indicating that they may be a cause), and secondly, whether negative thoughts, alone, are sufficient to cause depression. One must view this factor as one of many that interact with other factors to cause depression.

Integrative model

The aetiological factors that have been described in this chapter fall within many systems and subsystems. These include the broader socio-economic system (e.g. poverty, unemployment), the social system (e.g. family), and intrapersonal system (which includes different subsystems: the physiological, the neurological, perception, cognition, etc.). It is therefore important to try and integrate all of these aetiological factors in order to develop a coherent understanding of all of the findings and theories.

Figure 5.4: Interaction between different systems and subsystems in the aetiology of mood disorders

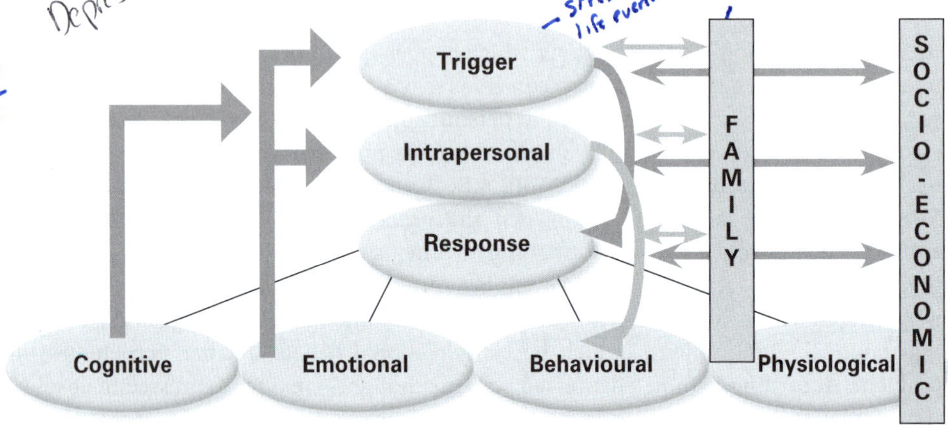

Source: © Burke, 2012.

There is strong evidence that mood disorders have a powerful genetic component, but it is important to remember that people do not inherit a specific disorder, but rather they inherit a predisposition to pathology in general. Furthermore, people inherit 'weaknesses' in certain areas (e.g. neurotransmitters) which then predisposes them to a disorder (diathesis-stress model). In the section on brain structures, it was described how there are certain overactive areas in the brain which produce and maintain negative emotions and memories. Therefore, for an integrative model, the biological predisposition would be the first ingredient.

The summary of biological causes, however, did not explain how this system is triggered. We can assume that stress, such as adverse life events may set the system in motion. Evidence that a first episode of depression is more likely to be immediately preceded by stressful life events than are recurrent ones is consistent with the hypothesis that people may become increasingly sensitised to life stress over successive episodes of depression Furthermore, the biological explanation also rests on the tendency of the person to negative emotions, as well as exposure to previous negative events (such as loss and rejection) which were stored in the long-term memory. Poverty, child abuse (physical, sexual, and emotional), as well as social isolation, are associated with increased risk of developing depressive disorders later in life. This makes sense because we learn during childhood how to become a social being.

We also develop (by means of different forms of learning) a certain perceptual style regarding others and our environment. It would seem that people who develop depression have a relatively typical inflexible and negative perception of themselves and their world (cf. Beck and Seligman). According to a biological perspective, the negative perceptual style is rigidly maintained by the anterior cingulate, which would explain why people cannot, by themselves, break this cycle of negativity.

The way in which we make meaning of ourselves and our world inevitably leads to certain behavioural responses, which in turn affects the way in which people respond to us. Depressed people may initially gain much support from others, but as was discussed earlier, their behaviour may ultimately lead to rejection by others, which in turn reinforces the way they see themselves and others (e.g. 'I am worthless', 'People don't like me', etc.).

The role of the socio-economic and social systems is twofold. On the one hand, factors such as unemployment, poverty, and childbirth may trigger a mood disorder directly or indirectly, as mentioned previously. Note that the factors mentioned are not only adverse life circumstances such as unemployment, crime, divorce, etc., but also include normal life events such as childbirth, loss of a significant other, etc. One could therefore assume that any life event which places a demand on a person which exceeds that person's ability to cope effectively with the demand is sufficient to trigger a mood disorder. This coping with the demand is obviously influenced by the way in which the person makes meaning of the event, as well as the ways in which they typically deal with life events.

The other role that the social system plays relates to the extent of, and what type of, social support a person receives. The relationship between stressful life events and social support has been a matter of some debate; the lack of social support may increase the likelihood that life stress will lead to depression, or the absence of social support may constitute a form of strain that leads more directly to depression (Vilhjalmsson, 1993). There is evidence that neighbourhood social disorder, for example, due to crime or illicit drugs, is a risk factor, and that a high neighbourhood socio-economic status, with better amenities, is a protective factor (Kim, 2008).

CONCLUSION

As far as mood disorders are concerned, it is clear that we have not reached a point of consensus on the classification of these disorders, nor do we fully understand their causes. In the future, we will have to develop a broader explanatory model that ranges from basic cellular processes to brain pathways and their links with relevant psychological constructs (Gruenberg, Goldstein, & Pincus, 2005), both pathogenic and fortigenic. The answer for future research may not lie in grouping a set of disorders together under the heading of mood disorders, but in treating each mood disorder as a separate and unique entity. After you have studied this chapter, it should be clear that the causal factors for the disorders vary from one disorder to the other. Also, individuals differ in terms of their own unique causal patterns. Thus, it may be that in some cases, disorders are predominantly biological, for example the bipolar disorders, whilst others are predominantly psychogenic. It is, however, likely in most cases that the true aetiological picture for each disorder is highly complex (on all levels) and involves many different biological, psychological, and social factors (Frude, 1998).

MULTIPLE-CHOICE QUESTIONS

CASE STUDY

Read through the following case study, and then answer the multiple-choice questions:

Ruth is a 24-year-old woman, who recently gave birth to a baby. Although her baby is healthy, Ruth has been very tearful since the birth. The nursing sisters in the ward have become worried about her, as she has become very withdrawn and tends to sleep through the day, and she shows little interest in the baby. She refuses to get out of bed, claiming that she is very tired. Her appetite is poor and, even when encouraged, she does not finish her meals. The nursing staff have also noticed that she never has any visitors and that not even the father of the baby has come to visit. Ruth has told one of the nursing sisters that she is concerned as she does not know how she will care for the baby as she lives in an informal settlement and is unemployed. According to Ruth, the father of the baby denies that it is his child, and tends to become verbally and physically abusive when she insists that it is his child. The only solution that she sees to the problem is to kill herself and the baby. When confronted about this by the doctor, she insists that a voice told her that she is bad, and needs to be punished for having a child that she cannot take care of. She is convinced that this is the voice of her mother who passed away a year ago.

1. The most appropriate diagnosis for Ruth would be a:
   a) Persistent Depressive Disorder (Dysthymic Disorder)
   b) Bipolar I Disorder
   c) Bipolar II Disorder
   d) Major Depressive Disorder

2. When considering your diagnosis, which one of the following factors influenced your diagnosis the most:
   a) the auditory hallucination (i.e. the voice that she heard)
   b) a physically abusive partner
   c) poor appetite, fatigue, and oversleeping
   d) suicidal thoughts

3. The fact that Ruth is very tearful and suicidal is an indication of a ________ mood.
   a) euphoric
   b) euthymic
   c) bipolar
   d) dysphoric

4. The voice telling Ruth that she is bad and needs to be punished, is an example of a(n):
   a) mood-congruent hallucination
   b) mood-incongruent hallucination
   c) illusion
   d) mood-congruent delusion

5. If you had to explain the cause of Ruth's disorder from a cognitive perspective, you would say that her disorder could have been caused by:
   a) low levels of serotonin
   b) high levels of monoamine oxidase
   c) negative perceptions of herself, the world, and the future
   d) a lack of social support

6. From a psychosocial perspective, the disorder may have been caused by:
   a) low social support, high perceived control
   b) high social support, low perceived control
   c) high social support, high perceived control
   d) low social support, low perceived control

PARAGRAPH AND ESSAY QUESTIONS

1. Distinguish between a Major Depressive Episode and a Manic Episode in terms of:
   a) emotional symptoms
   b) cognitive symptoms
   c) behavioural symptoms
   d) physical symptoms

2. Describe the difference between unipolar and bipolar disorders.

3. List and describe the symptoms of Major Depression.

4. Give a brief description of the biological causes of depression.

5. Describe how social factors may cause or maintain depression.

6 SCHIZOPHRENIA SPECTRUM AND OTHER PSYCHOTIC DISORDERS

Elsabe Jordaan

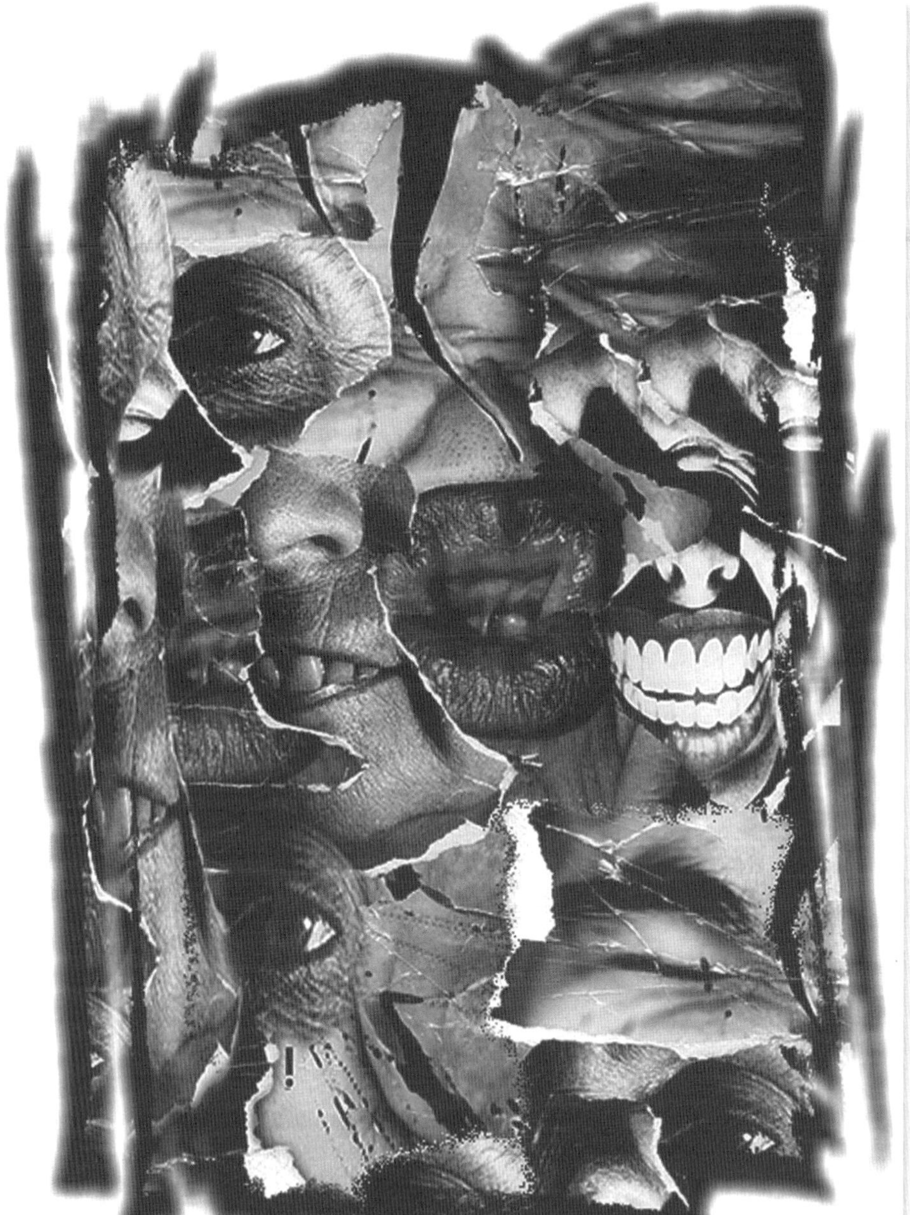

6 CHAPTER OUTLINE

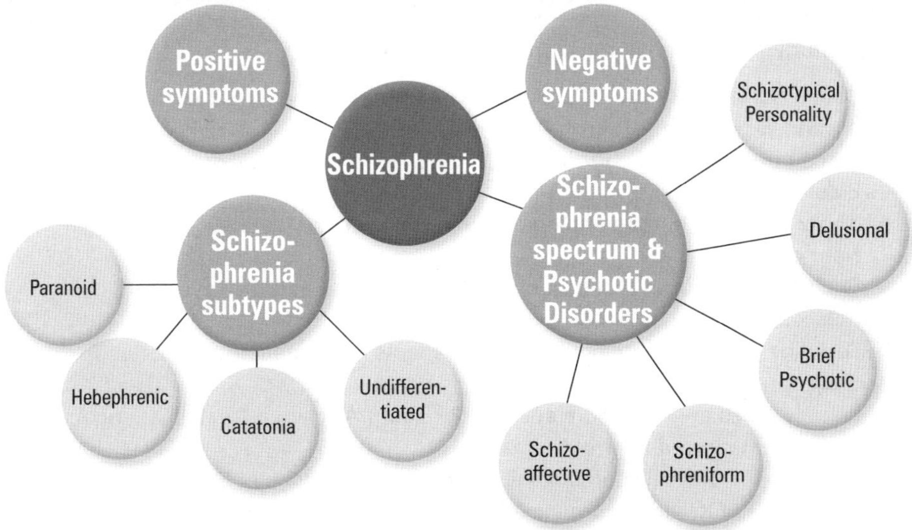

Introduction

Psychosis and the psychotic disorders

Schizophrenia
- **History of Schizophrenia**
- **Prevalence and course**

Clinical picture
- **Schizophrenia**
- **Positive symptoms**
  - Hallucinations
  - Delusions
  - Disorganised thinking (speech)
  - Disorganised or catatonic behaviour
- **Negative symptoms**
  - Flat affect
  - Avolition
  - Alogia
- **Schizophrenia subtypes (ICD-10)**
  - Paranoid Schizophrenia
  - Hebephrenic Schizophrenia
  - Undifferentiated Schizophrenia
  - Catatonia
- **Other Schizophrenia Spectrum and Psychotic Disorders**
  - Schizotypal Personality Disorder
  - Delusional Disorder
  - Brief Psychotic Disorder
  - Schizophreniform Disorder
  - Schizoaffective Disorder
- **Dangerousness and mortality risk**

Cross-cultural and African perspectives

Aetiology
- **Biological factors**
  - Genetics
  - Brain structure
  - Neurochemistry
  - Neurodevelopmental factors
- **Psychological factors**
  - Individual factors
- **Sociocultural factors**
  - The effects of social class
  - The effects of migrant status
  - Integration of aetiological factors

Controversial issues in the diagnosis and management of Schizophrenia
- **One diagnosis or many?**
  - Positive Schizophrenia versus negative Schizophrenia
  - Type I Schizophrenia versus Type II Schizophrenia
- **Normality and abnormality**
- **Labelling**
- **De-institutionalisation**

Conclusion

LEARNING OUTCOMES

After studying this chapter you should be able to:

- Define Schizophrenia and explain the difference between Schizophrenia and psychosis.
- Trace the history of Schizophrenia, including contributions of Kraepelin and Bleuler.
- Show a general understanding of Schizophrenia and distinguish Schizophrenia from other disorders.
- Distinguish between and describe the positive and negative symptoms of Schizophrenia.
- Describe the intra- and inter-personal aspects of the aetiology of Schizophrenia.
- Identify cross cultural, more specifically South African, aspects that impact on the presentation of Schizophrenia.
- Describe the clinical characteristics and major subtypes of Schizophrenia: Paranoid, Catatonic, Disorganised, Undifferentiated, and Residual.
- Describe the prevalence of Schizophrenia, including the potential genetic, neurobiological, developmental, and psychosocial contributions and risk factors.
- Describe what is known about abnormalities in neuro-cognitive and biological functioning and their relation to the symptom clusters of Schizophrenia.
- Distinguish among the different classification schemes used to describe the onset and course of Schizophrenia (e.g. process vs. reactive, poor vs. good premorbid, Type I vs. Type II) and explain why they are important.
- Describe the role of expressed emotion in the course of Schizophrenia, particularly with regard to risk of relapse.

INTRODUCTION

In the previous chapters (i.e. anxiety and mood disorders), we have dealt with disorders that could be considered to be 'milder' disorders. What is meant by this is that people suffering from those disorders, despite the severity of the disorder and irrational thoughts, are usually still able to function relatively normally. The main reason for this is that they are still 'in touch with reality'. They experience symptoms that they can, to a greater or lesser extent, recognise as abnormal. In this chapter, we will be dealing with disorders where the people suffering from these disorders lose contact with reality. In scientific language we refer to this losing of contact with reality as *psychosis*, and in this chapter we will be dealing with disorders where psychosis is the central feature.

It must be stressed that psychosis refers to a cluster of symptoms which include disruptions in mood, thoughts, perception, language, and behaviour, and which may be present in other disorders, for example, psychosis triggered by a substance and psychosis associated with a medical condition.

There are, however, DSM-5 disorders where psychosis is the primary and central set of symptoms (see Table 6.2). Due to limited space, we will be dealing mainly with Schizophrenia as it is the most common psychotic disorder. It can also be regarded as the 'classic' psychotic disorder (Kaplan, Saddock, & Grebb, 1994). Schizophrenia has been the focus of great deal of attention and research, and yet we have very little solid knowledge about many aspects of the disorder. This is despite it being a severe and persistent condition that potentially involves all areas of human psychological functioning (including behaviour, cognition, emotion, and perception) and that it usually represents an extreme deviation from normal health and functioning (Picchioni & Murray, 2008).

The impact of this syndrome on the lives of the affected individuals and their families is often disastrous; Schizophrenia usually results in lifelong impairment and disability. The individual and their families often bear direct financial and emotional costs. The costs to society are also significant, considering the loss of human potential, and the financial impact of treatment, hospitalisation, and the disability benefits that result. Schizophrenia can also be considered 'extreme' because of the absence of known causes, objective diagnostic criteria, specified course, and effective treatments for this category of disorders.

The use of the term Schizophrenia in this chapter is complicated by the classification difficulties associated with the diagnosis of Schizophrenia. Despite extensive research, no consensus exists on whether these disorders represent a single entity with symptoms arising from a common process or deficit. The DSM-5 (American Psychiatric Association, 2013) represents Schizophrenia as a defined disorder. However, Cranco and Lehman (2000) suggest that the 'Schizophrenias' can be regarded as a syndrome, considering that a set of signs and symptoms can manifest in a number of (diverse) ways. In addition, specific drugs with shared neurophysiological attributes impact on these symptoms. For the purposes of this chapter, the DSM-5 phrasing of 'Schizophrenia' (as opposed to the 'Schizophrenias', as suggested by some authors) will be used. These diagnostic issues will be revisited at the end of this chapter as part of the discussion of controversial issues related to Schizophrenia.

Due to the fact that psychosis is the central symptom, it makes sense to start with a description of what psychosis is and what it entails, before moving on to the details of the disorders that have psychosis as a central theme.

ACTIVITY

Watch the movie *A Beautiful Mind*. It is a story about a brilliant mathematician, John Nash, who was schizophrenic. The movie provides a good portrayal of what it is like for a person to live with Schizophrenia.

PSYCHOSIS AND THE PSYCHOTIC DISORDERS

The word 'psychosis' has its roots in the Greek *psyche* (mind or soul) and *-osis* (abnormal condition), therefore referring to an 'abnormal condition of the mind' (Sommer, 2011). Psychosis usually describes a break in the individual's contact with reality. This break with reality can be in the form of the experience of delusions and/or hallucinations. A delusion can be defined as a firmly held false belief or a notion that is not accepted by most members of the person's culture. Hallucinations are sensory experiences in the absence of environmental stimuli (see Table 6.1).

Table 6.1: Definition of terms

Terminology	Definition
Illusion	Misperception or misinterpretation of real external sensory stimuli.
Delusion	False belief, based on incorrect inference about external reality.
Hallucination	False sensory perception not associated with real external stimuli.

Source: Kaplan, Sadock, & Grebb, 1994.

There is a range of definitions of the concept of psychosis. Restrictive definitions may refer only to the presence of hallucinations in the absence of insight that the experiences are not 'real', while the widest definitions focus on the extent of functional impairment that a person experiences. The DSM-5 use of the term refers to the presence of specific symptoms. In Schizophrenia, Schizophreniform Disorder, Schizoaffective Disorder, and Brief Psychotic Disorder, psychosis indicates the presence of delusions, hallucinations, disorganised thinking (speech), disorganised abnormal motor behaviour (including catatonic behaviour) or negative symptoms or negative symptoms. In the case of Delusional Disorder and Shared Psychotic Disorder, psychotic refers to the presence of delusions (American Psychiatric Association, 2013).

In summary, a person experiencing psychosis may have difficulty recognising which of their sensory experiences are real, and which are not. They may also have difficulty assessing which of their thoughts are based in reality. They may struggle to organise their own thoughts, their speech, and their emotions. The person's behaviour may also be unusual and without an obvious goal. An observer may describe the psychotic person's speech, emotional expression, and behaviour as 'illogical' or 'confused'. It is highly probable that experiencing a psychotic episode will severely disrupt a person's life and they may struggle to function as they did before, at home, school, or at work. Individual experiences of psychosis may differ; despite having similar diagnoses, people may experience their symptoms differently, or experience a different combination of symptoms (American Psychiatric Association, 2000).

The notion of 'insight' is also relevant in a discussion of psychosis and the psychotic disorders. In psychology and psychiatry, 'insight' refers to a person's awareness and recognition of their own illness. The dimensions of this awareness include acknowledging the consequences of behaviour as a result of one's condition, as well as admitting to a need for treatment (Markov & Berrios, 1992).

While some disorders are typically associated with 'good insight' (e.g. phobias), Schizophrenia and the psychotic disorders are usually associated with 'poor insight' (i.e. the person has little awareness that anything is wrong with them) (Markov & Berrios, 1992).

In the initial phases of a first episode of psychosis, it may be difficult to establish with which type of psychotic disorder the person is presenting. This is because some of the criteria used to diagnose the type of psychotic disorder may not be yet known (e.g. duration and severity of symptoms). A description of the psychotic disorders enumerated in the DSM-5, follows in Table 6.2.

Figure 6.1: Schizophrenia Spectrum and other Spectrum Disorders

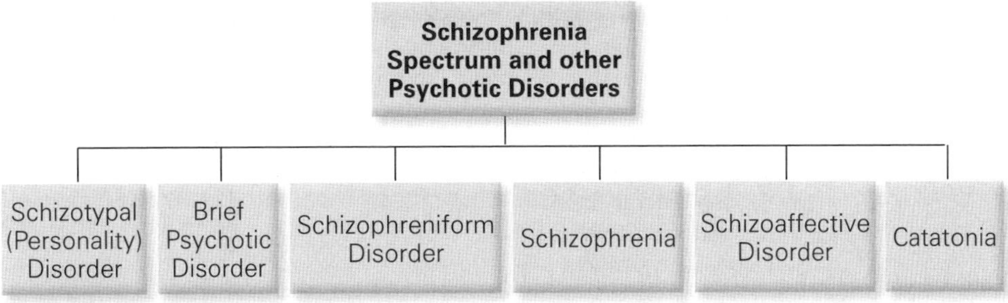

Table 6.2: Schizophrenia Spectrum and other psychotic disorders in DSM-5

Diagnosis	Diagnostic features	Duration	Subtype/ Specifiers
Schizotypal (Personality) Disorder	Listed in this category, but discussed in the Section of Personality Disorders in the DSM-5 (See Chapter 12)		
Delusional Disorder	One (or more) delusion(s)	1 month	Subtypes: Erotomanic Grandiose Jealous Persecutory Somatic Mixed Unspecified Specifier: With non-bizarre content
Brief Psychotic Disorder	One (or more) of following symptoms: • Delusions • Hallucinations • Disorganised speech • Grossly disorganised or catatonic behaviour	Change from nonpsychotic to psychotic within 2 weeks, and episode lasts for at least 1 day, but less than 1 month	Specifiers: With / without marked stressors With Postpartum onset With catatonia
Schizophreni-form Disorder	Two or more of the following: • Delusions • Hallucinations • Grossly disorganised or catatonic behaviour • Negative symptoms • No functional decline	1 – 6 months	Specifiers: With good prognostic features Without good prognostic features With catatonia

Diagnosis	Diagnostic features	Duration	Subtype/ Specifiers
Schizophrenia	Two or more of the following: • Delusions • Hallucinations • Disorganized speech • Grossly disorganised or catatonic behaviour • Negative symptoms	Minimum of 6 months; minimum of 1 month of active phase symptoms	A number of specifiers relating to course of disorder
Schizoaffective Disorder	• Uninterrupted period of illness during which there is a major mood episode concurrent with symptoms of Schizophrenia	Minimum of 2 weeks of same period of illness of hallucinations or delusions with absence of mood symptoms; mood episode present for substantial portion of active and residual periods of illness	Specifiers: Bipolar type Depressive type With catatonia A number of specifiers relating to course of disorder
Catatonia Associated with Another Mental Disorder	Three (or more) typical symptoms of catatonia (e.g. stupor, catalepsy, echolalia, echopraxia, etc.)		Indicate the name of the associated mental disorder
		No specifiers	Chronic where no intervention
		No specifiers	Variable (do not always fully remit if medical condition is treated)
		No specifiers	Variable

Source: Reprinted with permission from the Diagnostic and Statistical Manual of Mental Disorders, (DSM), Fifth Edition, American Psychiatric Association (APA), 2013.

The DSM-5 proposes to include the current category, 'Schizophrenia and Other Psychotic Disorders', in the diagnostic category 'Schizophrenia Spectrum and Other Psychotic Disorders'. The proposed changes for this category are quite extensive and of specific interest is a proposed new diagnosis, Attenuated Psychosis Syndrome, which is described as a possible diagnosis to identify increased risk for psychosis. Attenuated Psychosis Syndrome may be included in the appendix or as a disorder (American Psychiatric Association, 2012). Another interesting change is the inclusion of the Schizotypal Personality Disorder in this category. This inclusion denotes the nosological shift in DSM-5 where there is again a move to categorise disorders based on shared aetiology.

SCHIZOPHRENIA

History of Schizophrenia

The earliest descriptions of the schizophrenic disorders were made in the early 1800s. In his book *Observations on Madness and Melancholy*, John Haslam described some of the symptoms as part of what he termed 'a form of insanity' (Haslam, 1809/1976). At more or less the same time, a French physician, Phillipe Pinel was describing similar symptoms that he observed in patients across the English Channel (Pinel, 1801/1962).

In 1860, Benedict Morel, a Belgian physician, used the French term *demence precoce* (early mental deterioration) to describe a case of a bright 13-year-old boy whose functioning had declined over a period of time. This term thus refers to the age of onset of the condition, which is typically in adolescence (Berrios, Luque, & Villagrán, 2003).

By the end of the nineteenth century, a German psychiatrist, Emil Kraepelin, translated Morel's term to *dementia praecox*, again pointing out the characteristic cognitive aspects (*dementia*) and age of onset (*praecox*) of the condition. Kraepelin also described the characteristic course of the disorder, which involves deterioration over a period of time. Very importantly, he distinguished between this condition and manic (bipolar) psychosis. Kraepelin's second major contribution was the idea that various manifestations of the condition, which were earlier regarded as being distinct disorders in themselves, were variations of *dementia praecox*. The conditions that he regarded as variations of *dementia praecox* were catatonia (immobility or agitation), hebephrenia (apparent immaturity or 'silliness'), and paranoia (persecutory or grandiose delusions) (Berrios et al., 2003; Cranco & Lehman, 2000). Kraepelin distinguished hallucinations, delusions, and a decline in cognitive functioning as symptoms of the disorder. He ascribed the condition to a type of organic decline and considered the prognosis to be poor (Cranco & Lehman, 2000).

Eugen Bleuler was a Swiss psychiatrist who first coined the term Schizophrenia in 1911. This term replaced *dementia praecox*. Bleuler's definition of Schizophrenia was wider than that of Kraepelin. This was because he regarded both the age of onset and the course of the disorder as being more fluid. Bleuler differed from Kraepelin in that he believed that Schizophrenia did not always imply a course marked by deterioration. Bleuler used the term 'Schizophrenia' ('split mind') to allude to the break between thought, emotion, and behaviour that characterises the disorder (Cranco & Lehman, 2000; Daubenton & Van Rensburg, 2001). The 'splitting' referred to is a split between intellect, emotion, behaviour, and external reality, rather than 'split' or multiple personalities as in Dissociative Identity Disorder (see Chapter 8). Thus, Dissociative Identity Disorder should not be confused with Schizophrenia.

Bleuler described four fundamental or primary symptoms of Schizophrenia, resulting in his notion of mental 'splitting' that occurs in patients with Schizophrenia. He described these symptoms as affecting the 'four A's'. The four A's are autism (self-focus), associations ('loose' or unconnected ideas), affective disturbances (emotional inappropriateness), and ambivalence (lack of resolve over actions). Bleuler regarded hallucinations and delusions as secondary symptoms of the disturbance. Here he also differs from Kraepelin, who viewed delusions and hallucinations as distinguishing features (Cranco & Lehman, 2000; Daubenton & Van Rensburg, 2001).

Other notable early theorists include Martin Bleuler (son of Eugen Bleuler), who emphasised psychosis as an essential feature of these disturbances, and Adolph Meyer. Meyer regarded the schizophrenic disorders as being reactive in nature. He therefore saw Schizophrenia as a result of an interaction between a biological predisposition and an environmental stressor (Cranco & Lehman, 2000).

Internationally, a discrepancy arose in the diagnosis of the schizophrenic disorders, since practitioners in the United States tended to follow Bleuler's broader approach, while European practitioners utilised Kraepelin's view. Before the publication of the DSM-III, this resulted in almost twice as many diagnoses of Schizophrenia in the United States compared to Europe (Cranco & Lehman, 2000). The DSM-I and DSM-II utilised the four A's and Bleuler's approach. The DSM-III thus moved towards a more restrictive definition of the disorder. This trend continued in the DSM-III-R (Cranco & Lehman, 2000; Daubenton & Van Rensburg, 2001) and has also continued in the DSM-5.

One of the biggest changes in the classification of this disorder, from DSM-IV-TR to DSM-5, was the elimination of the subtypes of schizophrenia (i.e., paranoid, disorganized, catatonic, undifferentiated, and residual types). This was done because the subtypes was demonstrated to have limited diagnostic stability, low reliability, and poor validity, and did not show differences in treatment responses, nor in terms of the course of the disorders. Rather than distinguishing between different subtypes, DSM-5 adopts a more dimensional approach where the symptoms are rated in terms of severity (APA, 2013).

Prevalence and course

Schizoprenia has a similar prevalence worldwide, which appears to be in the 0.3%–0.7% range for the adult population (APA, 2013). The prevalence is greater in men throughout adulthood, but is equal towards old age (Saha, Chant, Welham, & McGrath, 2005). Some geographic and historical variations appear to exist. An example of this is that urban-born populations appear to have a higher risk than rural-born populations. Another example is that birth-cohort studies suggest a decreasing risk for younger cohorts (American Psychiatric Association, 2000).

The manifestation of Schizophrenia can be gradual or rapid. In the majority of cases, there appears to be a prodromal phase characterised by the appearance and escalation of symptoms (see Figure 6.2). The typical age of onset is in the mid 20s for males and in the late 20s for females. An early age of onset is associated with a generally poor prognosis. The onset of distinct psychotic symptoms characterises active-phase Schizophrenia. The course of the disorder appears to differ between individuals, with some presenting with relapses and remissions, while others remain chronically ill. In addition, some remain relatively stable, while others progressively decline. It appears that the negative symptoms persist and become gradually more obvious in some individuals during the course of the disorder. The phase where the intensity of the symptoms decreases and functioning improves to some extent is called the residual phase (American Psychiatric Association, 2013).

Figure 6.2 Pathway of development of a psychotic episode

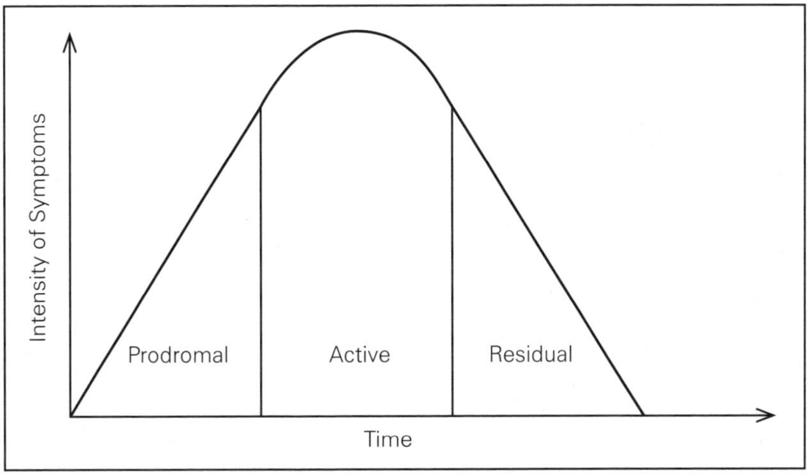

Source: © Burke, 2009.

The predictors of the course and outcome of Schizophrenia is largely unknown, and only about 20% of those diagnosed with this disorder show a favourable outcome (APA, 2013). Although psychotic symptoms may diminish with age, cognitive impairments persist (APA, 2013). Recently, the length of duration of psychosis has been increasingly emphasised as a factor that impacts the course of the disorder. Indications are that a longer duration of untreated psychosis is associated with a poorer treatment response. A shorter duration of untreated psychosis usually predicts a better response to antipsychotic medication, and consequently less severe overall psychopathology, fewer positive symptoms, fewer negative symptoms, and better functioning (Perkins, Gu, Boteva, & Lieberman, 2005).

While emphasising the need for early identification and intervention with schizophrenic patients, these findings also imply that the progressive process of decline associated with Schizophrenia could potentially be changed (Perkins et al., 2005). In order to allow for the early diagnosis of psychosis, the APA considered including a disorder, Attenuated Psychosis Syndrome, however this was not included in the main body of the text, and was only included in the section for conditions that require further study (APA, 2013).

Table 6.3: Distribution of outcome categories of chronic and acute onset

Chronic Onset	Acute Onset
Complete Remission: 0%	Complete Remission: 33%
Partial Remission: 18%	Partial Remission: 27%
No Remission: 82%	No Remission: 40%

Source: Adapted from Eggers & Bunk, 1997.

CLINICAL PICTURE

Schizophrenia

CASE STUDY

Schizophrenia

George is a 22-year-old man who is currently in a psychiatric hospital. He was in London at the time that his symptoms appeared, was hospitalised there, and as soon as his symptoms stabilised, his father fetched him and brought him back to South Africa. His background is the following:

- Parents are both Italian and they immigrated to South Africa before George was born.
- Father is a successful businessman who owns a couple of companies. No history of psychiatric illness.
- Two older sisters who have not displayed any symptoms of any psychiatric disorders.
- He grew up in a very strict Catholic home.
- Mother died of cancer when George was 12 years old.
- Learning disorders, possible Attention-Deficit/Hyperactivity Disorder (diagnosis never formally made).
- Due to a lack of academic progress, he was placed in a school for children with learning disorders but his academic performance remained below average.
- His father took him out of school when he was 16 years old and George started to work in one of his father's bakeries.
- When he turned 21, George wanted to travel to the UK and Europe and his father agreed to this.
- When he arrived in the UK, George found himself various casual jobs for extra pocket money.
- He found a place to stay in a commune where he started interacting with other people of his age. They introduced him to clubs and drugs.

After about eight months in London, George's behaviour started changing and he started to display the following symptoms:

He woke up one evening and saw a bright light and heard the voice of God. The voice told him that he was special and that he was 'the chosen one'.

Unsure of what the message meant, George started looking for more special signs. While sitting on a bench, waiting for the underground train, a woman walked past and knocked on the bench. George interpreted this as another sign from God.

George also discovered that he could communicate with world leaders via telepathy. He would often go into long conversations with them, suggesting ways and means for bringing about world peace.

He also realised that Madonna was in love with him, and they started a relationship on a spiritual plane, communicating with each other via telepathy.

George's personal hygiene deteriorated; he withdrew into his own room and became socially isolated. As a result, he lost his job and became dependent on the other people in the commune for financial assistance.

Note that:

- **Many of George's symptoms corresponded with a manic episode (e.g. he slept very little).**
- **George developed a delusion of grandeur (e.g. he was chosen by God).**
- **One of the main features was that he continuously heard the voice of God, who constantly gave him instructions.**

The other people in the commune became concerned about George and realised that something serious was wrong. They coerced him into going to a hospital, where he was finally admitted to the psychiatric ward. Here a diagnosis of Paranoid Schizophrenia was made.

Disturbances in several major areas of functioning are associated with the symptoms of Schizophrenia. These areas include thought, perception, attention, motor behaviour, affect, emotion, and life functioning. These are typically associated with gross impairment in the areas of occupational and social functioning. Although a great variety of symptoms is possible in individuals with Schizophrenia, it is rare for one person to display all of these difficulties at once. Unlike most of the diagnostic categories discussed in this text, the diagnosis of Schizophrenia does not have an essential symptom that is required in order to make the diagnosis. However, as highlighted in the case study of George, Schizophrenia is regarded in DSM-5 and ICD-10 (World Health Organisation, 2007) terms as a psychotic disorder, implying the presence of hallucinations, delusions, disorganised speech, and/or disorganised behaviour (see Table 6.4).

Table 6.4: General diagnostic criteria for Schizophrenia as adapted from the DSM-5 and ICD-10

DSM-5	ICD-10
A. Two (or more) of the following, each present for a significant portion of time during a one-month period (or less if successfully treated). At least one of these must be (1), (2), or (3): (1) Delusions. (2) Hallucinations. (3) Disorganised speech (e.g. frequent derailment or incoherence). (4) Grossly disorganized or catatonic behaviour. (5) Negative symptoms (i.e. diminished emotional expression or avolition).	• The normal requirement for a diagnosis of Schizophrenia is that a minimum of one very clear symptom (and usually two or more if less clear-cut) belonging to any one of the groups listed as (a) to (d) below, or symptoms from at least two of the groups referred to as (e) to (h), should have been clearly present for most of the time during a period of one month or more.

DSM-5	ICD-10
B. For a significant portion of time since the onset of the disturbance, level of functioning in one or more major areas, such as work, interpersonal relations, or self-care, is markedly below the level achieved prior to the event (or when the onset is in childhood or adolescence, there is failure to achieve expected level of interpersonal, academic, or occupational functioning). C. Continuous signs of the disturbance persist for at least six months. This six-month period must include at least one month of symptoms (or less if successfully treated) that meet Criterion A (i.e. active-phase symptoms) and may include periods of prodromal or residual symptoms. During these promodal or residual periods, the signs of the disturbance may be manifested by only negative symptoms or two or more symptoms listed in Criterion A present in an attenuated form (e.g. odd beliefs, unusual perceptual experiences). D. Schizoaffective disorder and depressive or bipolar disorder with psychotic features have been ruled out because either 1) no major depressive or manic episodes have occurred concurrently with the active-phase symptoms, or 2) if mood episodes have occurred during the active-phase symptoms, they have been present for a minority of the total duration of the active and residual periods of the illness. E. The disturbance is not attributable to the physiological effects of a substance (e.g. a drug of abuse, or medication) or another medical condition. F. If there is a history of autism spectrum disorder or a communication disorder of childhood onset, the additional diagnosis of schizophrenia is made only if prominent delusions or hallucinations, in addition to the other required symptoms of schizophrenia, are also present for at least one month (or less if successfully treated).	Conditions meeting such symptomatic requirements but of duration less than one month (whether treated or not) should be diagnosed in the first instance as acute Schizophrenia-like psychotic disorder and are classified as Schizophrenia if the symptoms persist for longer periods. (a) thought echo, thought insertion or withdrawal, and thought broadcasting; (b) delusions of control, influence, or passivity, clearly referred to body or limb movements or specific thoughts, actions, or sensations; delusional perception; (c) hallucinatory voices giving a running commentary on the patient's behaviour, or discussing the patient among themselves, or other types of hallucinatory voices coming from some part of the body; (d) persistent delusions of other kinds that are culturally inappropriate and completely impossible, such as religious or political identity, or superhuman powers and abilities (e.g. being able to control the weather, or being in communication with aliens from another world); (e) persistent hallucinations in any modality, when accompanied either by fleeting or half-formed delusions without clear affective content, or by persistent over-valued ideas, or when occurring every day for weeks or months on end; (f) breaks or interpolations in the train of thought, resulting in incoherence or irrelevant speech, or neologisms; (g) catatonic behaviour, such as excitement, posturing, or waxy flexibility, negativism, mutism, and stupor; (h) 'negative' symptoms such as marked apathy, paucity of speech, and blunting or incongruity of emotional responses, usually resulting in social withdrawal and lowering of social performance; it must be clear that these are not due to depression or to neuroleptic medication;

DSM-5	ICD-10
	(i) a significant and consistent change in the overall quality of some aspects of personal behaviour, manifest as loss of interest, aimlessness, idleness, a self-absorbed attitude, and social withdrawal. • The diagnosis of Schizophrenia should not be made in the presence of extensive depressive or manic symptoms or if it occurs in the presence of overt brain disease or during states of drug intoxication or withdrawal.

Source: Reprinted with permission from the Diagnostic and Statistical Manual of Mental Disorders, (DSM), Fifth Edition, American Psychiatric Association (APA), 2013 and ICD-10 Classification of Mental and Behavioural Disorders: Diagnostic Criteria for Research. World Health Organisation (WHO), Geneva, 2007.

Up to now we have referred to psychosis as the main feature of Schizophrenia; however, we need to remember that psychosis refers to a number of symptoms (or in some cases, clusters of symptoms), and that not all the symptoms of psychosis are present in all people. In fact, the different subtypes of psychotic disorders are characterised by different signs and symptoms of psychosis; that is, different disorders have different symptoms and within these, individuals show variation in their symptom presentation. One approach to these symptoms is to divide them into two broad categories: positive symptoms (active symptoms) and negative symptoms (the absence or decrease of normal functions).

Positive symptoms

The positive symptoms of Schizophrenia have an active presentation and can be seen as an excess or distortion of behaviour. These symptoms are characteristic of the active or acute phase of the disorder. The positive symptoms consist of two dimensions, which are the 'psychotic' dimension and the 'disorganisation' dimension. The psychotic dimension comprises hallucinations and delusions, while the disorganisation dimension includes disorganised behaviour and speech (American Psychiatric Association, 2000)

Hallucinations

Hallucinations are sensory events that take place in the absence of environmental stimuli. Hallucinations can therefore be regarded as distortions of perception (see Table 6.5).

Table 6.5: Summary of types of hallucinations

Sense	Hallucination	Associated with	Description
Hearing	Auditory hallucination	Most common in many psychiatric disorders such as Schizophrenia	False perception of sound most commonly, but not limited to, voices.
Vision	Visual hallucination	Most common in medical disorders	False perception of images which may be formed (e.g. people) or unformed (e.g. flashes of light)
Taste	Gustatory hallucination	Most common in medical disorders	False perception of (unpleasant) taste
Smell	Olfactory hallucination	Most common in medical conditions (e.g. epilepsy)	False perception of smell
Touch	Tactile (haptic) hallucination	Psychotic disorders such as Schizophrenia	False perception of touch or surface sensation (e.g. phantom limb after an amputation or sense of insects crawling on or under skin).
	Somatic (kinaesthetic) hallucination	Psychotic disorders	False perception of things occurring to or in the body

Source: Kaplan & Sadock, 1994, p. 307.

Although any of the senses may be affected, auditory hallucinations (hearing sounds or voices that other people cannot hear) are most common in Schizophrenia (Sartorius, Shapiro, & Jablonsky, 1974) and they commonly include the hearing of voices. The voice may be heard either inside or outside one's head and is generally considered more severe when coming from outside one's head. The voices may be male or female, recognised as the voice of someone familiar or not recognised as familiar, and may be critical or positive. The content of what the voices say is usually unpleasant and negative.

A common symptom is to hear voices conversing and/or commenting. In voices commenting, the person hears a voice making comments about his or her behaviour or thoughts, typically in the third person (such as, 'Isn't he silly?'). Sometimes the voices consist of hearing a 'running commentary' on the person's behaviour as it occurs ('She is showering.'). At other times, the voices may tell the person to do something (commonly referred to as 'command' hallucinations). These experiences can be very frightening and upsetting to the individual experiencing them. Research utilising brain imagery to observe brain activity of people experiencing auditory hallucinations implicates the speech centre of the brain, Broca's area, in the generation of auditory hallucinations, and not Wernicke's area, the area of the brain involved in language comprehension (Cleghorn et al., 1992; McGuire,

Shah, & Murray, 1993). This implies that auditory hallucinations involve listening to one's own thoughts, rather than hearing the voices of others.

Delusions

Delusions are beliefs that are firmly held contrary to reality and contrary to what most members of a society would regard as reality. Garety (1991) defines delusions as false personal beliefs that are firmly and consistently held despite logic or experiences to the contrary.

Several types of delusion were first described by a German psychiatrist, Kurt Schneider (1959). These are:

- ***Delusions of persecution:*** a belief that others are plotting against, mistreating, or even attempting to murder you; the belief that others are 'out to get you'
- ***Delusions of thought broadcasting:*** the belief that others know what you are thinking
- ***Delusions of control:*** the belief that an outside agency is attempting to influence or control you
- ***Delusions of grandeur:*** the belief that you are a powerful or famous person
- ***Delusions of reference:*** the belief that all that is happening involves or alludes to yourself
- ***Thought withdrawal:*** the belief that your thoughts are being removed from your mind by an external force.

Since the work of Schneider (1959) a number of additional delusions have been identified (see Table 6.6)

Table 6.6: Summary of delusions

Type	Subtype	Description
Nihilistic		The self, others, or the world are non-existing or ending.
Poverty		One either has no material possessions or one will be deprived of them.
Somatic		Beliefs about one's body functions (e.g. 'My brain is rotting.'). Not to be confused with somatic hallucination.
Paranoid	Persecution	One is being persecuted or victimised.
	Grandeur	Exaggerated sense of own worth, powers, or identity.
	Reference	Events or others' behaviour has a significant, negative meaning.
Self-accusation		Feelings of remorse or guilt for events for which one cannot possibly be responsible.
Control	Thought withdrawal	Belief that one's thoughts are being extracted by others.

Type	Subtype	Description
	Though insertion	Belief that thoughts are being planted into one's head by others.
	Thought broadcasting	Belief that one's thoughts are being broadcasted so that others are privy to them.
	Thought control	Other people have control over one's thoughts.
Infidelity		Extreme pathological jealousy.

Source: Adapted from Kaplan & Sadock, 1994, pp. 305-6.

Of the types of delusion discussed above, delusions of persecution are most common to Schizophrenia (Sartorius et al., 1974). Research suggests that delusions may differ in the impact they have on a person's life in that they vary in strength and disruptiveness (Brett-Jones, Garety, & Hemsley, 1987; Howard, 1992). The delusions of individuals with a diagnosis of Schizophrenia are typically of a more bizarre (highly implausible) nature than those of other diagnostic categories (Junginger, Barker, & Coe 1992).

CASE STUDY

Example of a delusion

Thandi believes that she has been admitted to a psychiatric ward because the chief psychiatrist is secretly conspiring with a political organisation that wants to know what she is thinking. In order to read her mind, 'they' inserted a device under the nail of her left big toe. This device enables 'them' to listen in on her thoughts.

Disorganised thinking (speech)

This set of symptoms was first described by Bleuler in 1911 and is also known as 'formal thought disorder'. This is regarded as characteristic of Schizophrenia. Disorganisation of speech can be defined as verbal communication in the known language of the individual which does not conform to the linguistic rules that govern the language. It is not due to intellectual, educational, or cultural disadvantage.

These unusual patterns of speech and writing result in verbal communication that holds little or no meaning for others. The listener experiences conversations with these individuals as illogical, and they may rapidly move between topics. People with Schizophrenia usually lack insight into their condition (i.e. the person is unaware of the problem themselves). Disorganised speech in Schizophrenia can take on various forms:

- ***Loosening of associations:*** This is also referred to as cognitive slippage or derailment. Loosening of associations entails the person moving between unrelated ideas in conversation. Speech may be incoherent and responses bizarre and idiosyncratic. The presence of loosening of associations is regarded as one of the most valuable diagnostic distinctions in the diagnosis of Schizophrenia.

- ***Problems with attention:*** This involves an inability to direct sustained focus to a single aspect of the environment or to organise environmental inputs (Cranco & Lehman, 2000).
- ***Neologisms:*** The speech of some people with a diagnosis of Schizophrenia may contain new words that are combinations of words in common usage.

EXAMPLE

Interviewer: *Sam, can you tell me why you were admitted to hospital?*
Sam: *I don't have time to be in hospital. The time has come for me. When time is right ... Time waits for no man!*

Note that Sam did not answer the question asked. Going off on a tangent and not answering the question is called 'tangentiality'. He also suddenly shifted between topics in the conversation, talking about unrelated areas. This is called 'loosening of associations' or 'derailment'.

Interviewer: *I believe that your mother has been to visit you?*
Sam: *Mom was here. Here today, gone tomorrow. Mom and I enjoy baking cakes together. Mom is going to take me shopping. We'll buy up a storm, and bake up a storm and shake up a storm. Our cakes are fabulicious. There was a cake sale at church. The sermon on Sunday was about the Lion and the Lamb. The Lion and the Lamb shall be together ...'*

Sam again did not answer the question. It is not clear whether he did not understand the question, struggled to focus his attention, or did not want talk about his mother. Sam's use of the word 'fabulicious' is an example of a neologism, a combination of 'fabulous' and 'delicious'.

Disorganised or catatonic behaviour

The activity levels (motor functions) of some people with a diagnosis of Schizophrenia may range from unusually high to unusually low, to the bizarre. Manifestations may include agitation, catatonia, or stereotyped movements. Agitation is shown when a person paces about rapidly, talking fast and non-stop, with arms swinging. Catatonia involves remaining in unusual physical postures for extended periods of time. Inappropriate affect, the display of emotions that are unrelated or inappropriate to those expected in a given situation, may also be present (Cranco & Lehman, 2000).

Negative symptoms

The negative symptoms of Schizophrenia refer to the absence of behaviours generally expected in a person. This term therefore refers to a deficit in usual behaviours like social interaction with others and the display of emotions. The presence of negative symptoms is generally associated with a poor prognosis. The negative symptoms of Schizophrenia include social and emotional withdrawal, blunted or flat affect, avolition (apathy), and poverty of thought and speech (alogia) (Carpenter, 1992).

Flat affect

This feature of Schizophrenia is also referred to as 'emotional blunting'. Flat affect is an absence of emotional reactions usually expected from people. This includes a lack of facial expression, poor eye-contact, a toneless voice, and an absence of emotional responses to the events in the person's environment.

Avolition

This term refers to a difficulty in starting and continuing actions. These actions include aspects of everyday life that are usually taken for granted by most people (e.g. self-care and personal hygiene). The person appears to lack the motivation or ability to engage in self-directed behaviour.

Alogia

Alogia refers to a restriction in the amount or content of speech a person produces. The term is derived from the Latin *a* (without) and *logica* (reason). People who display this symptom may be very brief and monosyllabic in their responses in conversation. Their responses may also be slow or delayed and they appear to have little interest in the conversation. Alogia is also sometimes referred to as 'poverty of speech'. This symptom is assumed to reflect a poverty of thought content, rather being merely a communication difficulty.

EXAMPLE

Interviewer: *Do you have brothers or sisters?*
Zandile: *Yes.*
Interviewer: *How many brothers or sisters do you have?*
Zandile: *Two.*

The example above illustrates the brief answers and apparent lack of interest in the conversation associated with alogia. A more usual response would be: 'Yes, I have one brother and one sister. I am the middle child. My brother lives in Durban and my sister has passed away.'

Schizophrenia subtypes (ICD-10)

Although the SM-5 no longer differentiates between sub-types of Schizophrenia, the ICD-10 does. The ICD-10 lists the subtypes of Schizophrenia as the following: Paranoid, Disorganised (DSM-5)/Hebephrenic (ICD-10), Catatonic, Undifferentiated, and Residual. These subtypes relate to the most prominent symptoms present in an individual at the time of diagnosis. The subtypes may have some implications in terms of prognosis and treatment. For instance, the Paranoid subtype is generally thought to have the best prognosis and the Disorganised subtype the worst.

However, the value of this subtype division has been questioned by various authors and appears to have limitations (McGlashan & Fenton, 1991). For example, the presentation of symptoms in an individual may change over time, or the current presentation of an individual may include symptoms associated with more than one subtype.

Paranoid Schizophrenia

This subtype appears to be the most prevalent form of Schizophrenia (Sue, Sue, & Sue, 2006). The ICD-10 describes the most salient features of this subtype as the presence of significant delusions and auditory hallucinations with relatively intact affective and cognitive functioning (see Table 6.7).

In the case of delusions, these may be multiple, but typically share a common theme. In Paranoid Schizophrenia, the content of hallucinations usually relates to the theme of the delusions (American Psychiatric Association, 2000). The case study below illustrates this.

CASE STUDY

Paranoid Schizophrenia

Mr K is a 47-year-old male who was previously a member of the South African Police Service. He went to his general practitioner telling a confused story about secret police and international agents who were after him because he had knowledge about former colleagues of his who had assumed new identities. Mr K also reported hearing the voices of those who had died in the line of police duty.

Delusions of persecution are most common, but grandiose delusions may also occur. In the case of persecutory delusions, the deluded individual is convinced that others are 'out to get them', plotting against them, talking about them, or about to disadvantage them in some way. Interpersonally, individuals with this subtype relate to others in a suspicious manner. Patients diagnosed with Paranoid Schizophrenia may also strike others as aloof, superior, or patronising in their manner. Interactions may be characterised by formality or extreme intensity. Their interpretation of the behaviour of others is often inaccurate, and typically serves to confirm the content of their delusions.

Table 6.7: Diagnostic criteria for Paranoid Schizophrenia as adapted from the ICD-10

ICD-10
• The general criteria for a diagnosis of Schizophrenia must be satisfied. The clinical picture is dominated by relatively stable, often paranoid, delusions, usually accompanied by hallucinations, particularly of the auditory variety, and perceptual disturbances. Disturbances of affect, volition, and speech, and catatonic symptoms, are not prominent. • Examples of the most common paranoid symptoms are: ‣ delusions of persecution, reference, exalted birth, special mission, bodily change, or jealousy; ‣ hallucinatory voices that threaten the patient or give commands, or auditory hallucinations without verbal form, such as whistling, humming, or laughing; ‣ hallucinations of smell or taste, or of sexual or other bodily sensations; visual hallucinations may occur but are rarely predominant.

- Thought disorder may be obvious in acute states, but if so, it does not prevent the typical delusions or hallucinations from being described clearly. Affect is usually less blunted than in other varieties of Schizophrenia, but a minor degree of incongruity is common, as are mood disturbances such as irritability, sudden anger, fearfulness, and suspicion. 'Negative' symptoms such as blunting of affect and impaired volition are often present but do not dominate the clinical picture.

Source: Reprinted with permission from the ICD-10 Classification of Mental and Behavioural Disorders: Diagnostic Criteria for Research. World Health Organisation (WHO), Geneva, 2007.

Associated features may be anxiety and anger, while persecutory content may increase the risk of suicide in these individuals. An increased risk for violence is associated with a combination between persecutory and grandiose delusions with anger (American Psychiatric Association, 2000).

Hebephrenic Schizophrenia

This subtype is characterised by a disorganisation in speech and behaviour, with flat or inappropriate affect and severe disintegration and regression to disinhibited, unorganised behaviour is associated with this subtype (Cranco & Lehman, 2000).

People with this subtype engage in aimless behaviour and they have limited goal-directed behaviour. This severely impedes the tasks of daily living (American Psychiatric Association, 2000). Thus, in terms of personal appearance, they appear neglected and uncared for. Incongruous grinning and grimacing also occur (Cranco & Lehman, 2000). Interpersonally, the behaviour of people with this subtype can be described as 'childish', 'silly', or 'bizarre'. Their emotional responses are typically flat, but with outbursts of inappropriate giggling or laughing (Cranco & Lehman, 2000).

Hallucinations and delusions, if present, are characterised by shifting themes and fragmented content. Cognitive impairment is usually found on tests of intellectual ability and on neuropsychological assessment (American Psychiatric Association, 2000).

This condition is so severe that individuals are often unable to care for themselves, which results in institutionalisation. The prognosis is poor. This subtype is associated with early and gradual onset, and a continuous course without remissions (American Psychiatric Association, 2000).

CASE STUDY

Disorganised Schizophrenia

Nivesh is a slightly built young man. His appearance is dishevelled and he is unwashed. He roams aimlessly around the hospital ward, sometimes laughing out loud for no apparent reason. At times, he stops and listens intently, presumably to voices that no one else can hear. When spoken to, Nivesh stares blankly without responding, or just giggles.

Table 6.8: Diagnostic criteria for Disorganised Schizophrenia as adapted from the ICD-10

Disorganised Schizophrenia	Hebephrenic Schizophrenia
A type of Schizophrenia in which the following criteria are met: A. All of the following are prominent: (1) disorganised speech (2) disorganised behaviour (3) flat or inappropriate affect B. The criteria are not met for Catatonic Type.	• A form of Schizophrenia in which affective changes are prominent, delusions and hallucinations fleeting and fragmentary, behaviour irresponsible and unpredictable, and mannerisms common. For a confident diagnosis of hebephrenia, a period of two or three months of continuous observation is usually necessary, in order to ensure that the characteristic behaviours are sustained. ‣ The mood is shallow and inappropriate and often accompanied by giggling or self-satisfied, self-absorbed smiling, or by a lofty manner, grimaces, mannerisms, pranks, hypochondriacal complaints, and reiterated phrases. ‣ Thought is disorganised and speech rambling and incoherent. ‣ There is a tendency to remain solitary, and behaviour seems empty of purpose and feeling. • In addition, disturbances of affect and volition, and thought disorder are usually prominent. Hallucinations and delusions may be present but are not usually prominent. • Drive and determination are lost and goals abandoned, so that the patient's behaviour becomes characteristically aimless and empty of purpose. • A superficial and manneristic preoccupation with religion, philosophy, and other abstract themes may add to the listener's difficulty in following the train of thought.

Source: Reprinted with permission from the ICD-10 Classification of Mental and Behavioural Disorders: Diagnostic Criteria for Research. World Health Organisation (WHO), Geneva, 2007.

Undifferentiated Schizophrenia

This subtype is a 'catch-all' category for individuals who clearly present with schizophrenic symptoms, but where a mixed presentation excludes them from the Paranoid, Catatonic, and Disorganised subtypes. Symptoms may include disturbances of thought and speech, hallucinations, delusions, and behavioural impairment (American Psychiatric Association, 2000).

Table 6.9: Diagnostic criteria for Undifferentiated Schizophrenia as adapted from the ICD-10

DSM-5	ICD-10
A type of Schizophrenia in which symptoms that meet Criterion A are present, but the criteria are not met for the Paranoid, Disorganised, or Catatonic Type.	• Conditions meeting the general diagnostic criteria for Schizophrenia but not conforming to any of the above subtypes, or exhibiting the features of more than one of them without a clear predominance of a particular set of diagnostic characteristics. This rubric should be used only for psychotic conditions (i.e. Residual Schizophrenia and post-Schizophrenia depression are excluded) and after an attempt has been made to classify the condition into one of the three preceding categories. • **Diagnostic guidelines:** This category should be reserved for disorders that: ‣ meet the diagnostic criteria for Schizophrenia; ‣ do not satisfy the criteria for the Paranoid, Hebephrenic, or Catatonic subtypes; ‣ do not satisfy the criteria for Residual Schizophrenia or post-Schizophrenia depression

Source: Reprinted with permission from the ICD-10 Classification of Mental and Behavioural Disorders: Diagnostic Criteria for Research. World Health Organisation (WHO), Geneva, 2007.

Catatonia

DSM-IV-TR listed Catatonic Schizophrenia as a subtype of Schizophrenia, and although DSM-5 no longer lists subtypes of Schizophrenia, it recognises that catatonia is exhibited in a wide range of disorders, e.g. neurodevelopmental, psychotic, bipolar, depressive and medical conditions APA, 2013). In order to cater for this, the DSM-5 includes a disorder called Catatonia with Another Mental Disorder. The ICD-10, in contrast to the DSM-5, lists Catatonic Schizophrenia as a subtype of Schizophrenia. Catatonia includes a wide range of psychomotor impairments. These disturbances can range from extreme activity to complete immobility. Seemingly involuntary movements, echolalia, and echopraxia may be present. Echolalia presents as the senseless and parrot-like repetition of a phrase just uttered by another person, while echopraxia involves imitating the movements of others (American Psychiatric Association, 2013).

Table 6.10: Diagnostic criteria for Catatonic Schizophrenia as adapted from the DSM-5 and ICD-10

Catatonia (DSM-5)	Catatonic Schizophrenia (ICD-10)
A. The clinical picture is dominated by three (or more) of the following symptoms: (1) Stupor (i.e. no psychomotor activity; not actively relating to environment). (2) Catalepsy (i.e. passive induction of a posture held against gravity). (3) Waxy flexibility (i.e. slight, even resistance to positioning by examiner). (4) Mutism (i.e. no, or very little, verbal response [exclude if known aphasia]). (5) Negativism (i.e. opposition or no response to instructions or external stimuli). (6) Posturing (i.e. spontaneous and active maintenance of a posture against gravity). (7) Mannerism (i.e. odd, circumstantial caricature of normal actions). (8) Stereotypy (i.e. repetitive, abnormally frequent, non-goal-directed movements). (9) Agitation, not influenced by external stimuli. (10)Grimacing. (11)Echolalia (i.e. mimicking another's speech). (12)Echopraxia (i.e. mimicking another's movements).	• The general criteria for a diagnosis of Schizophrenia must be satisfied. Transitory and isolated catatonic symptoms may occur in the context of any other subtype of Schizophrenia, but for a diagnosis of Catatonic Schizophrenia one or more of the following behaviours should dominate the clinical picture: ‣ stupor (marked decrease in reactivity to the environment and in spontaneous movements and activity) or mutism; ‣ excitement (apparently purposeless motor activity, not influenced by external stimuli); ‣ posturing (voluntary assumption and maintenance of inappropriate or bizarre postures); ‣ negativism (an apparently motiveless resistance to all instructions or attempts to be moved, or movement in the opposite direction); ‣ rigidity (maintenance of a rigid posture against efforts to be moved); ‣ waxy flexibility (maintenance of limbs and body in externally imposed positions); and ‣ other symptoms such as command automatism (automatic compliance with instructions), and perseveration of words and phrases.

Source: Reprinted with permission from the Diagnostic and Statistical Manual of Mental Disorders, (DSM), Fifth Edition, American Psychiatric Association (APA), 2013 and ICD-10 Classification of Mental and Behavioural Disorders: Diagnostic Criteria for Research. World Health Organisation (WHO), Geneva, 2007.

In the case of excessive motor activity (or 'excited catatonia'), the activity or excitement appears to be aimless and not influenced by the context. People with this subtype may talk and shout incoherently and move constantly. They sleep little, and possible risks include physical exhaustion and harm to self or others (American Psychiatric Association, 2013).

In the case of motoric immobility, the person with catatonic symptoms may adopt a strange or bizarre posture. In some instances, negativism (maintenance of a rigid posture and resistance to being moved) may be present. Catalepsy or waxy flexibility occurs when a person remains in any physical position that they are put into by someone else. While in this state, the immobile person may not eat or pay any attention to their excretory functions (American Psychiatric Association, 2013).

CASE STUDY

Catatonia

Peter is a 15-year-old boy who has been admitted to the adolescent ward of a psychiatric hospital. He is standing in the corridor with his hands above his head. He assumed this position before breakfast and is still standing like this by bedtime. He has resisted all attempts to move him or make him more comfortable. Peter has not eaten the whole day. He has also not controlled his bladder or bowel functions.

Other Schizophrenia Spectrum and Psychotic Disorders

Schizotypal Personality Disorder

Although this is a personality disorder (See Chapter 12), the DSM-5 notes it in this category as it considers it to be part of the schizophrenia spectrum disorders (APA, 2013).

Delusional Disorder

The essential feature of this disorder is the presence of one (or more) delusions that persists for at least a month (APA, 2013).

Brief Psychotic Disorder

The essential features of this disorder are that it involves the sudden onset of positive symptoms of psychosis (i.e. delusions, hallucinations or disorganized speech), or abnormal psychomotor behaviour (such as catatonia) (APA, 2013). The psychosis develops suddenly, i.e. within 2 weeks, without a prodromal phase, and a person with this disorder usually recovers fully (APA, 2013).

Schizophreniform Disorder

The symptoms of this disorder are identical to those of Schizophrenia, with the main difference between the two disorders being the duration of the two disorders (APA, 2013). This disorder follows the same pattern as that of schizophrenia, i.e. prodromal, acute and residual phases, which typically lasts for 1 – 6 months (but does not exceed 6 months) (APA, 2013).

Schizoaffective Disorder

This disorder can best be understood as an overlap between Schizophrenia and a Mood Disorder. Although this disorder requires that the person displays symptoms of schizophrenia, the symptoms of a major mood episode (depressive or bipolar) must be present for the majority of the total duration of the disorder (APA, 2013).

Dangerousness and mortality risk

As for many other aspects related to the presentation of Schizophrenia, the issue of dangerousness (risk of suicide and violence) in people diagnosed with Schizophrenia is potentially controversial and far from clear-cut.

The issue of dangerousness, particularly to others, in people with Schizophrenia is coloured by media portrayals of people with mental illness. The media often depict people with mental illness as being prone to violence, and more dangerous than the rest of the population. These portrayals are not always accurate reflections of reality, since research evidence on this issue is mixed (Lindquist & Allebeck, 1990; Steadman & Ribner, 1980).

It is difficult to predict when or how a person with a diagnosis of Schizophrenia will act in a dangerous or violent way towards to others (see Chapter 14). Individuals with a diagnosis of Schizophrenia pose a greater potential risk for violence than many other categories of disorder. Those diagnosed with the Paranoid subtype appear to pose a particular risk, since they may act rapidly and unpredictably in response to a delusion or a perceived threat. The risk is greater in those with the Paranoid subtype because they are usually able to create and execute plans of attack. This would not typically be true of people diagnosed with the Disorganised subtype, for instance, because they are unlikely to be able to organise their thoughts and behaviour sufficiently to carry out a planned attack (Cranco & Lehman, 2000).

The rates for medical illness and mortality in schizophrenic patients are significantly higher than those in the general population (Goff et al., 2005). The increased mortality rate is from both natural and unnatural causes. 28% of the increased mortality rate is associated with suicide, while accidents account for 12% of the elevation. The remainder of the mortality rate is associated with the range of conditions that cause death in the general population (Brown, 1997).

When considering suicide risk, it should be noted that up to 40% of individuals with this diagnosis attempt suicide. Approximately 10% of individuals diagnosed with Schizophrenia complete suicide within the first ten years of their diagnosis (Cranco & Lehman, 2000). Risk factors for suicide include being young, male, and having a high level of education, as well as the presence of insight. Schizophrenia-related risk factors that appear to be of importance are the number of previous suicide attempts, as well as the presence of depressive symptoms and active hallucinations and delusions (Hor & Taylor, 2010). The only consistent protective factor for suicide in Schizophrenia, is effective treatment. Prevention of suicide in patients with Schizophrenia relies on identifying those at risk and providing the best available treatment for psychosis, as well as for co-morbid depression and substance use (Hor & Taylor, 2010). The question remains whether suicide prevention interventions early in the illness could reduce this risk.

The elevated risk for medical illness associated with Schizophrenia may also be modifiable. The top six global modifiable mortality risk factors in the general population are hypertension, smoking, raised glucose levels, physical inactivity, obesity, and high blood cholesterol levels. Patients with Schizophrenia are exposed to all of these risk factors (Wildgust & Beary, 2010). The highest rates of cigarette smoking are found among schizophrenic patients in that up to 83% of these patients smoke daily (De Leon, Diaz, Rogers, Browne, & Dinsmore, 2002; Smith, Singh, Infante, Khandat, & Kloos, 2002). Increased risk in Schizophrenia patients is specifically for cardiovascular disease due to cigarette smoking, and increasingly due to diabetes and obesity. Schizophrenia patients also have higher rates of infection with HIV and infectious hepatitis. Interventions that have been applied successfully to the general population can be applied to individuals with Schizophrenia and could improve the health of Schizophrenia patients (Goff et al., 2005).

CROSS-CULTURAL AND AFRICAN PERSPECTIVES

Any discussion of cultural considerations in relation to Schizophrenia is fraught with difficulty. Cross-cultural comparisons have been criticised on the basis of reflecting diagnostic errors (see Chapter 1). For example, greater sociocultural and/or class differences between clinician and patient are more likely to result in errors in diagnosing Schizophrenia. Misdiagnosis may also be the result of racial bias and stereotyping (see Chapters 1 and 2) (Sue et al., 2006). The validity of applying diagnostic criteria developed for a white, middle-class population to other cultures has also been questioned (Adebimpe, 1981). In the United States and England, for example, proportionately more people from ethnic minority groups are diagnosed with Schizophrenia. This probably reflects misdiagnosis, rather than cultural prevalence differences (Jones & Gray, 1986; Lindsey & Paul, 1989). Differences between ethnic groupings dissolve when the groups are matched in terms of socio-economic factors and education (Carson, Butcher, & Coleman, 1988).

Cultural differences in symptomatology and in the form of disorder have been described by a variety of researchers. The content of delusions and hallucinations appears to be influenced by culture and society (Sue & Morishima, 1982), as is the type of schizophrenic disorder (Carothers, 1959). More visual hallucinations have been described in people from Mexico and Kenya, and more hallucinations of all types have been described in people from West Indian and Asian cultures (Krassoievitch, Perez-Rincon, & Suarez, 1982; Ndetei & Singh, 1983; Ndetei & Vadher, 1984). Wig (1983) describes a greater incidence of brief psychotic disorders (characterised by sudden onset, limited duration, and good prognosis), usually in reaction to an extreme psychosocial stressor, in developing countries.

Cultural differences in the clinical presentation of Schizophrenia in the South African context have been described. In the South African setting, the initial presentation is often acute (as opposed to insidious) (Daubenton & Van Rensburg, 2001). Visual hallucinations are more common in the indigenous populations of Africa, and this is also the case in the South African population (Daubenton & Van Rensburg, 2001).

In South Africa, the symptom presentation may also vary across cultures (Daubenton & Van Rensburg, 2001). The core symptoms of Schizophrenia and the presence of positive and negative symptoms appear to remain the same across South African cultural groupings (Emsley et al., 2001). However, significant differences in the clinical presentation of non-core symptoms of Schizophrenia have been found between Xhosa-speaking and English-speaking South Africans. The differences reported include higher prevalence of aggressive and disruptive behaviour in the Xhosa-speaking patients. In addition, Xhosa-speaking patients also appear to experience more symptoms of a persecutory, sexual, and fantastic nature, as well as more self-neglect and irritability.

The content of the positive symptoms also appears affected by culture in the South African context (Maslowski, Janse van Rensburg, & Mthoko, 1998). Specifically, the content of delusions is often associated with the life experience and culture of the patient. In South Africa, these themes often centre on traditional belief systems, political realities, and famous individuals. A typically South African example is that patients with Schizophrenia regularly claim to be Nelson Mandela, or to be related to him (Daubenton & Van Rensburg, 2001). These findings have been supported by the findings of a study conducted by Mosotho, Louw, and Calitz (2011) that investigated the clinical presentation of Schizophrenia among Sotho speakers. These authors found little variation in the core symptoms of Schizophrenia among Sotho speakers. However, as with the studies described above, the content of hallucinations and delusions was found to be strongly influenced by cultural aspects. The participants in this study reported frequent somatic symptoms such as headaches, palpitations, dizziness, and excessive sweating. These findings emphasise the need to change Western models such as the DSM-IV and the ICD-10 in order to account for the cultural differences found in South Africa, and in other parts of Africa (Moshoto et al., 2011).

In South Africa, the clinical presentation of Schizophrenia is often complicated by the use of substances such as cannabis (see later in this chapter), alcohol, and Mandrax, used in various combinations (Daubenton & Van Rensburg, 2001).

Schizophrenia shares a number of symptoms with some indigenous forms of 'illness' in South Africa, such as *ukuthwasa* (ancestral calling) and *amafufunyana* (spirit possession). This has led to much debate around whether to understand the presenting symptoms from within the context of the indigenous healing system (where traditional healers such as an *inyanga* or an *isangoma* would be used) or from the perspective of the biomedical model, where the individual showing the symptoms would be diagnosed with Schizophrenia. Attitudes and beliefs about Schizophrenia may differ substantially from Western assumptions in patients, family members, and mental health care workers in South Africa (Mbanga et al., 2001). Tensions exist in the interface between Western mental health care and traditional healing in the South African context (Kahn & Kelly, 2001).

The treatment of Schizophrenia with antipsychotics is further complicated by cost factors in the South African context. Newer antipsychotics have made a major impact on the treatment of Schizophrenia, but the costs of these drugs puts them beyond the reach of large sectors of the world's population. This serves to widen the gap between levels of mental health care in high-income countries like the United States and low-income countries, such as South Africa (Emsley, Oosthuizen, Joubert, Hawkridge, & Stein, 1999).

Other issues that impact on delivery of treatment to people with a diagnosis of Schizophrenia in the South African context are the chronic under-resourcing of mental health services (Lund, Kleintjes, Kakuma, Flisher, & the MHaPP Research Programme Consortium, 2010), and the consequences of de-institutionalisation policies (also see Chapter 14), specifically the rise of the revolving door phenomenon (service users who are hospitalised frequently) (Botha et al., 2010).

Relapse is considered a general problem among South Africans with this diagnosis. Relapse has many potentially negative consequences, such as hospitalisation, the development of treatment resistance, progressive structural brain damage and consequent cognitive impairment, personal distress, incarceration, and financial implications. Factors associated with relapse among South Africans with a diagnosis of Schizophrenia are a co-morbid depressed mood, poor treatment compliance due to limited insight on the part of the patient and to unpleasant medication side effects (Kazadi, Moosa, & Jeenah, 2008).

South African authors have added their voices to those questioning the view that Schizophrenia is associated with better outcomes in developing countries. The political, social, and economic challenges of life in countries in Africa, Latin America, and Asia pose psychosocial stressors that, together with limited mental health services in these regions, impact negatively on outcome for people with Schizophrenia in the developing world (Burns, 2009).

Some intriguing research findings on the aetiology of Schizophrenia are coming out of South Africa. These will be included in the discussion in the following section.

AETIOLOGY

Schizophrenia is arguably the psychological disorder that has generated the most research. In the twenty years up to 2008, Schizophrenia research has resulted in over 50,000 published studies (MacDonald & Schulz, 2009). Despite this bewildering body of work, we are far from understanding the causality of this category of disorders. Earlier in this chapter, difficulties in even attempting to define this condition were discussed. What does appear clear from the available information is that the causality of Schizophrenia is complex and characterised by multiple causes (or vulnerabilies) interacting with each other.

In the following discussion of the aetiology of Schizophrenia, possible biological factors represent a convenient starting point. Psychological and social factors will also be discussed. This section will conclude with an integrative description of the aetiology of the disorder.

Biological factors

When the biological or medical dimensions in the aetiology of Schizophrenia are considered, three aspects are typically in the forefront. These are genetics, physiological vulnerabilities, and neurochemistry.

Genetics

The hereditary component to the causality of Schizophrenia appears to be undisputed (Gottesman 1991; Ubell, 1989). Unfortunately, however, no single gene can be identified that is directly linked to the aetiology of Schizophrenia. The evidence regarding genetics indicates that multiple genes are involved. These genes give rise to an inherited vulnerability for developing the disorder (Gottesman, 1991). Possible ways to research a genetic component to the causality of Schizophrenia include family, twin, adoptee, offspring of twins, and linkage studies.

When considering family studies, research indicates that relatives of a person diagnosed with Schizophrenia are at an increased risk for the disorder, when compared to the general population. The degree of the genetic relationship influences the risk: the closer the genetic relationship with the person with Schizophrenia, the greater the risk (Gottesman, 1991). It also seems that the relatives of people with this diagnosis are also at an increased risk for other disorders, most notably Schizotypal Personality Disorder. Schizotypal Personality Disorder is sometimes regarded as a less severe variant of Schizophrenia (Kendler, Karkowski-Shuman, & Walsh 1996). The drawback of family studies is that there is no control for the influence of environment in this data.

Twin studies assume that, theoretically, the concordance rate for monozygotic (identical) twins should be 100%. If the development of Schizophrenia in an individual is solely due to genetic influences, both monozygotic twins should always develop the disorder since they share 100% of their genetic material. Similarly, the concordance rate for dizygotic (fraternal) twins should be 50%, since they share 50% of their genetic material. Research indicates that the concordance rate for identical twins is around 48%, while the concordance rate for fraternal twins appears to be about 17% (Gottesman, 1991). Thus, twin studies appear to confirm a genetic component to the causality of Schizophrenia; however, it is clear that a large part of the variance is not explained by genetics. Work by Dworkin, Lenzenweger, and Molin (1987) indicates a stronger genetic component for negative symptoms than for positive symptoms. Difficulties in interpreting twin studies include the fact that twins share a common environment from the antenatal environment to the family system. Conversely, even identical siblings can have very different social and physical childhood experiences.

Adoption studies eliminate the role of environment, as they study children who were adopted at a very young age and who were born to mothers who were diagnosed with Schizophrenia. These studies often span many years. The general conclusion that can be drawn from studies with this approach is that children of parents with a diagnosis of Schizophrenia, who were raised in families without Schizophrenia, have a higher risk for the disorder than the general population (Kety et al., 1994).

One approach that has produced some of the most compelling evidence for a genetic component in the causality of Schizophrenia is investigating the offspring of twins. This research investigates the possibility of individuals being 'carriers' of a genetic predisposition even when they do not display symptoms of the disorder themselves. Evidence from this research indicates that children of a non-symptomatic identical twin of parents with a diagnosis of Schizophrenia have the same risk for the disorder as the children of the twin with the diagnosis (17%), again suggesting a genetic component to the disorder (Gottesman, 1991).

Consensus regarding the genetic aspect of the causality of Schizophrenia (and other psychological disorders) currently appears to be that some genetic involvement can be inferred from the available information. No single gene involved in the causation of Schizophrenia (or any other psychological disorder) has been identified to date. Current thinking favours the notion of polygenetic involvement (i.e. a vulnerability to the disorder is due to a number of genes scattered throughout our chromosomes) (Gottesman, 1991).

South African research is making some notable contributions to the research into the genetic component of the aetiology of Schizophrenia. An international collaboration research project which spanned twelve years utilised a family sample of Afrikaner families afflicted with Schizophrenia in order to study rare genetic mutations that are associated with the genetics of psychiatric disorders. The Afrikaner population is a genetically relatively isolated population, characterised by close-knit family structures for which detailed medical and ancestral records are available. This facilitated the family-based genetic study and offered reliable discrimination between familial and non-familial forms of the disorder. This research served to confirm the role of new genetic mutations in non-familial cases of the disease and the presence of rare inherited structural mutations that affect many genes in familial Schizophrenia (Xu et al., 2009). This research has been described as 'offering the first clear view of the genetic landscape of Schizophrenia' (Karayiorgou & Gogos, 2011, p.2).

Brain structure

As discussed in the section on the history of the disorder, brain abnormality has been suspected as a causal factor in Schizophrenia since the earliest descriptions of the condition. Evidence indicates that abnormal neurological findings are more common in people with a diagnosis of Schizophrenia. The role of brain structure in Schizophrenia has been investigated through brain-imaging techniques and post-mortem analyses of people with Schizophrenia, as well as investigating cognitive markers through utilising neuropsychological assessment techniques.

One aspect of brain structure which has been investigated is the ventricular system. Ventricles are cavities in the brain filled with cerebrospinal fluid which cushions the brain and spinal cord. Evidence for enlarged ventricles comes from a variety of sources, including post-mortem inspection (Dwork, 1997; Heckers, 1997), CT scans, and MRI studies (Andreasen et al., 1990; Nopoulos, Flaum, & Andreasen, 1997). Enlarged ventricle size is important because it implies that brain cells have either been lost, or never developed in the first place. A relationship appears to exist between enlarged ventricle size and the negative symptoms of Schizophrenia (Crow, 1985; McGlashan & Fenton, 1992). Ventricular enlargement in people with Schizophrenia is associated with poor pre-morbid adjustment, decreased response to drug treatment, and impaired scores on neuropsychological assessment (Andreasen et al., 1992). Findings of a twin study conducted by Suddath et al. (1990) imply that ventricular enlargement in people with a diagnosis of Schizophrenia may not have a genetic origin.

Decreased activity in the frontal lobes (hypofrontality) also appears to be linked to Schizophrenia. The frontal lobes are responsible for thinking, reasoning, planning, memory, experiencing reward, and social behaviour. A relationship appears to exist between hypofrontality and the negative symptoms of Schizophrenia (Andreasen, Olsen, Dennert, & Smith, 1982).

Post-mortem studies have found prefrontal cell abnormalities and hippocampal cell abnormalities associated with Schizophrenia (Lewis et al., 2003). Medial temporal lobe structures (including the hippocampus, the superior, frontal and prefrontal cortices, and the thalamus) appear to be smaller in schizophrenic patients (Davidson & Heinrichs, 2003). Finally, a number of brain systems, including the prefrontal cortex and the temporal cortex, as well as subcortical structures, appear to experience functional abnormalities in schizophrenic patients (Van Snellenberg, Torres, & Thornton, 2006).

Neurochemistry

As with theories regarding brain abnormalities and Schizophrenia, neurochemistry as a possible causative factor has a long history and has been the subject of much research. No biochemical theory has been conclusively proven to date. Current research focus is on various neurotransmitters, including dopamine, serotonin, and norepinephrine.

One of the most enduring recent theories relating to biochemical factors in the causality of Schizophrenia is the dopamine hypothesis (Davis, Kahn, Ko, & Davidson, 1991). The dopamine hypothesis states that Schizophrenia is linked to an excess of dopamine activity at some synaptic sites (see Figure 6.3). The dopamine hypothesis is based on the fact that drugs that reduce dopamine activity in the brain reduce the symptoms of Schizophrenia. Conversely, drugs that increase the levels of dopamine in the brain have side effects that resemble the symptoms of Schizophrenia. An excess of dopamine is therefore assumed to cause some of the symptoms of Schizophrenia.

Figure 6.3: Illustration of dopaminergic pathways

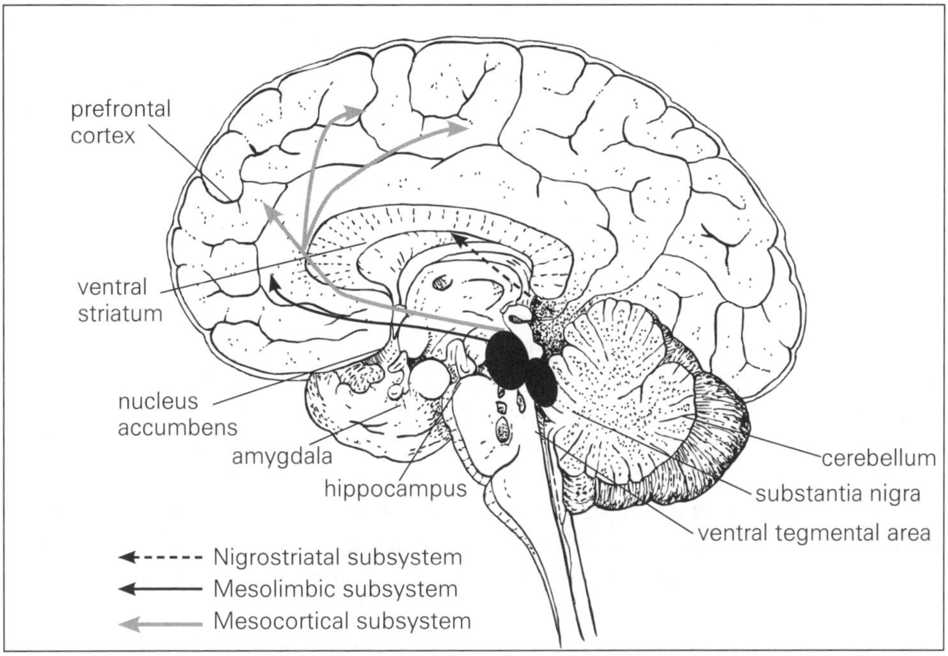

Research on the use of three different types of drugs has provided support for the dopamine hypothesis. The three types of drugs in question have the effect of either decreasing or increasing the levels of dopamine in the brain. The drugs that decrease dopamine activity are called dopamine antagonists, while drugs that increase dopamine activity are called dopamine agonists. The three types of drugs that have received the most attention in research on the dopamine hypothesis are the phenothiazines, L-dopa, and the amphetamines.

Phenothiazines are drugs that decrease dopamine activity (dopamine antagonists) in the brain by blocking the brain's use of dopamine in dopamine receptor sites in postsynaptic neurons (Davis et al., 1991). When used in the treatment of Schizophrenia, these drugs improve symptoms such as thought disorders, hallucinations, and mood symptoms.

The drug L-dopa is used in the treatment of the symptoms of Parkinson's disease such as tremors, and muscle and limb rigidity. L-dopa is converted to dopamine in the body, thereby increasing dopamine levels in the brain. In some cases, use of this drug can create Schizophrenia-like symptoms. Conversely, the phenothiazines (dopamine antagonists) can create side effects that are similar to the symptoms of Parkinson's disease (Davidson et al., 1987).

Amphetamines are stimulant drugs that elevate the brain's levels of the neurotransmitters norepinephrine and dopamine. Doses of amphetamines induce symptoms like those of acute Paranoid Schizophrenia in non-schizophrenic people (Nielsen, Lyon, & Ellison, 1983). Amphetamines also increase the severity of psychotic symptoms when administered to people with the diagnosis of Schizophrenia (Van Kammen, Docherty, & Bunney, 1982)

In summary, drugs known to decrease dopamine activity (antagonists) have the effect of decreasing Schizophrenia-like symptoms, while drugs known to elevate dopamine activity (agonists) have the effect of elevating Schizophrenia-like symptoms. It is therefore possible to conclude that the causality of Schizophrenia is linked to elevated levels of dopamine. In addition, the dopamine antagonists appear to block one specific group of dopamine receptors, the D2 receptors. The suggestion is therefore that Schizophrenia in some individuals is caused by increased dopamine activity at the D2 receptors (Davis et al., 1991).

Technological advances for the study of neural functioning and neurochemicals have focused on the receptor sites for dopamine in the brain, rather than only on dopamine levels. This research has led to the idea that an oversensitivity of the dopamine receptors, or an increased number of dopamine receptors, could be a causal factor for Schizophrenia, rather than simply an excess of dopamine (Goldsmith, Shapiro, & Joyce 1997).

Evidence contradicting the dopamine hypothesis has emerged, however. Antipsychotics in the form of dopamine antagonists are not useful in the treatment of all people with the diagnosis of Schizophrenia, neither are they effective for the treatment of all Schizophrenia symptoms. The negative symptoms, in particular, appear relatively unresponsive to these drugs (Davis et al., 1991).

In considering the effects of the various drugs on positive and negative symptoms, it is useful to study the neural pathways that utilise dopamine. The mesolymbic dopamine pathway (see Figure 6.3) appears to be involved in the positive symptoms of Schizophrenia. It also appears to be the site where the therapeutic effects of antipsychotics take place by blocking dopamine receptors. The prefrontal cortex appears to be implicated in the negative symptoms of Schizophrenia. This proposition would account for the presence of positive and negative symptoms in the same person, and account for the ineffectiveness of antipsychotics on the negative symptoms, since it is known that they have little impact on the dopamine neurons in the prefrontal cortex (Davis et al., 1991).

The dopamine hypothesis has also involved studying the relationship between serotonin and dopamine. The advent of the drug clozapine (a weak dopamine antagonist, but effective in treating Schizophrenia) has given rise to the dopamine-serotonin relationship being investigated as a causal factor for Schizophrenia symptoms. Clozapine is a serotonin antagonist in addition to being a weak dopamine antagonist, and may be involved in blocking several neurotransmitter systems at once (Kahn et al., 1993).

Our current understanding of the complex relationships between neurotransmitter systems, and the relationship between these systems and schizophrenic symptomatology, is incomplete. Advanced and complex research utilising new technologies holds the possibility of increasing our knowledge of biochemical interactions as well as our understanding of the causality of Schizophrenia and the development of new treatment options.

Neurodevelopmental factors

A number of studies have linked Schizophrenia and the influenza virus. Although the evidence is somewhat inconsistent (Westergaard, Mortensen, Pedersen, Wohlfahrt, & Melbye, 1999), studies of populations exposed to influenza epidemics indicate that individuals with antenatal exposure to the virus during the second trimester were at higher risk of developing Schizophrenia (Cannon, Barr, & Mednick, 1991; Mednick, Huttonon, & Machon, 1994). Post-mortem evidence suggests that viral infection may influence foetal brain development. Cell migration appears to be disrupted in a critical period for cortical growth during this stage of pregnancy (Akbarian et al., 1995).

Finally, other early neurological insults, most notably birth complications, may be associated with increased risk for developing Schizophrenia (Boog, 2004). Reports of an accumulation of adverse events during the pre-and perinatal periods, and the presence of behavioural and cognitive symptoms during childhood and adolescence, have given rise to a hypothesis of a neurodevelopmental aetiology for Schizophrenia. Recent interpretations of the combination of genetic and environmental factors view this interaction as potentially disrupting a normal developmental course in early life. The resultant alternative developmental paths are thought to ultimately give rise to Schizophrenia in individuals (Lewis & Levitt, 2002). South African research findings support the neurodevelopmental origin of Schizophrenia and offer possible insight into specific times of neurodevelopmental insult during antenatal development. Research conducted in the Eastern Cape by Koen, Niehaus, De Jong, Muller, & Jordaan (2006) found links between minor physical abnormalities in Schizophrenia in a Xhosa population, as compared to control groups. In addition to lending support to the neurodevelopmental view of Schizophrenia aetiology, this research also may offer a means of subtyping Schizophrenia for future genetic research.

Psychological factors

In the absence of conclusive evidence implicating an entirely biological explanation of the aetiology of Schizophrenia, psychological and environmental aspects must be considered in terms of the aetiology of Schizophrenia. This discussion of psychological factors will begin with a focus on individual factors and factors involving the family, followed by a consideration of broader social aspects.

Individual factors

Studies of high-risk children

In the 1960s, Danish researchers (Mednick & Schulsinger, 1968) followed up a group of 207 children who were identified as 'high risk' for developing Schizophrenia on the basis of their mothers having been diagnosed with the condition. A matched control group of 104 children was utilised. The children in the study were followed up for more than ten years. Several aspects were identified in this study that served as predictors for the onset of Schizophrenia. These included pregnancy and delivery complications, which were implicated in negative symptom presentations, and family instability, which was implicated in positive symptom presentations.

Predictors that were identified in similar studies in the United States and Israel were attentional dysfunction, low IQ scores, poor concentration, poor verbal ability, and poor motor abilities (Cornblatt & Erlenmeyer-Kimling, 1985; Marcus et al., 1987).

Psychological stress

Various researchers have found a high presence of stressful life events preceding the onset of the disorder (Birley & Brown, 1970; Brown, Birley, & Wing, 1972; Day et al., 1987). Similar results were found in a study that investigated the factors that predict relapse in people with a diagnosis of Schizophrenia (Ventura, Nuechterlein, Lukoff, & Hardesty, 1989). Although people with a diagnosis of Schizophrenia appeared to be impacted by the stress of their entire life situation (Forgus & DeWolfe, 1974), a number of research studies have indicated that stress associated with difficulties in close personal relationships is a precipitating factor for a Schizophrenia episode (Birley & Brown, 1970; Forgus & DeWolfe, 1974; Schwartz & Myers, 1977). South African research findings have suggested a link between exposure to trauma and the clinical presentation of first episode psychosis in South Africa. More specifically, these researchers found that previous traumatic experiences are associated with positive and affective symptoms in patients experiencing a first psychotic episode (Burns, Jhazbhay, Esterhuizen, & Emsley, 2010).

Faulty learning

A behavioural perspective that relates to the role of the family is the idea that faulty learning occurs within the family context. The faulty learning may be related to the child being conditioned into believing that the world is an unfriendly and threatening place. This happens through being exposed to early traumatic experiences, such as disruptions in parenting. Faulty learning could result from disturbed social interaction, learning from observing role models behaving in grossly inappropriate ways, and from efforts to meet inappropriate parental expectations. Such faulty learning manifests in faulty assumptions about reality, difficulties regarding a sense of self and self-worth, emotional immaturity, and a lack of effective coping skills (Carson et al., 1988).

Family influences

Various theoretical constructs have come into play in considering the role of the family in the aetiology of Schizophrenia. These include the 'schizophrenogenic' (Schizophrenia-inducing) mother, faulty communication patterns, destructive marital interactions, pseudo-mutuality and pseudo-hostility, faulty learning, and undermining of personal authenticity in the families of people diagnosed with Schizophrenia. In addition, high levels of expressed emotion were found among relatives of people with a diagnosis of Schizophrenia.

The 'schizophrenogenic mother' is a psychoanalytic concept first used by Frieda Fromm-Reichmann (1948). This term was also utilised in the early days of family therapy. This concept refers to a style of parenting which could serve to hinder childhood ego development. Behaviours and attitudes which were typically ascribed to schizophrenogenic mothers were being cold, rejecting, dominating, overprotective, and insensitive to the needs of others. This description was often linked particularly to the relationship between mother and son. This notion has been criticised on the basis that it lacks validating data and is gender biased and has fallen into disuse (Roff & Knight, 1981).

The family systems approach emerged in the 1950s and made a major impact on how the causality of Schizophrenia is viewed. The family systems view came about from research into the interaction and communication patterns of families with a member diagnosed with Schizophrenia. This research identified communication patterns that appeared to be typical of families with a family member with Schizophrenia. This typical communication pattern was called double-bind communication. This refers to communication patterns that contain 'mixed messages'.

Bateson (1959) suggested that families of people with Schizophrenia are characterised by communications that present the identified patient (diagnosed family member) with mixed messages that put them in a no-win situation. For example, a mother pays a surprise hospital visit to her son diagnosed with Schizophrenia. When he sees her, he is excited and puts his arms out to greet her. She stiffens and draws back from him. He in turn, draws back from her. She responds by asking if he is not going to greet her and whether he is not happy to see her. Together with the mixed message, there are also subtle non-verbal messages that prohibit the identified patient from either commenting on the situation or leaving the situation. Thus, double-bind communication usually takes place on both the verbal and non-verbal levels.

The double-bind theory was extremely important to the development of family systems therapy because it represented a coherent and sophisticated explanation for the link between abnormal behaviour and underlying family processes or patterns of interaction.

The family systems approach has contributed much to our understanding of the causality of Schizophrenia and other mental disorders. One major contribution is that it sees the causality as conceivably having interpersonal aspects as opposed to the intrapersonal aspects (i.e. pathology is inherent to the person, for instance, the biological view). This perspective regards the seat of pathology as being between people and not as located within the individual.

Another of the major contributions of this approach has been the notion of mutual causality or circular causality (reciprocal cause and effect). This means that patterns that are part of the cause of psychopathology are seen as vicious circles, where the interactions form a loop such that they continuously affect each other.

Other theorists who contributed to our understanding of family dynamics associated with the development and maintenance of Schizophrenia were Theodore Lidz and Lyman Wynne in the United States and R.D. Laing in the United Kingdom. Lidz described two types of problematic marital relationship patterns in families of people with a diagnosis of Schizophrenia (Lidz, Fleck, & Cornelison, 1965). These are 'marital schism' and 'marital skew'.

Marital schism occurs when constant undermining of one parent by the other takes place, with expressions that children resemble the undermined parent. Marital skew takes place when the family maintains stability by accepting the destructive and often extremely domineering behaviour of one or more of the members as normal. In both these types of families, the parents constantly compete for the children's loyalty, with the result that the children experience being torn between their parents (Lidz et al., 1965).

Wynne described families with a diagnosed schizophrenic member as having unusual and problematic emotional transactions, boundaries, and communication styles. The emotional transactions and role structure in these families were described by Wynne and his co-workers (Wynne, Ryckoff, Day, & Hirsch, 1958) as reflecting either 'pseudo-mutuality' or 'pseudo-hostility'. With pseudo-mutuality, the role structure in families of people with Schizophrenia is characterised by rigidity and conflict, while a pretence or mask of openness and mutual understanding is being maintained. This has the effect of hampering the children of the family in their attempted moves towards emotional maturity.

In the case of pseudo-hostility, there are overt expressions of conflict, with very rigid underlying coalitions between some family members. Wynne and his colleagues described the boundaries of these families as a 'rubber fence' because they allow professionals to have superficial contact with them, but resist any change to the family dynamics. The families of schizophrenics also exhibited communication deviance in that they struggled to remain focused when attempting to discuss solutions to problems (Wynne et al., 1958).

R. D. Laing, a Scottish psychiatrist who was heavily influenced by the Existentialist Movement, also emphasised the role of the family. He regarded Schizophrenia as a sane response to an insane situation. Laing used the term 'mystification' (coined by Marx) to describe the process that he observed in the parents of children diagnosed with Schizophrenia. In this process, parents denied, distorted, or relabelled their children's experiences to fit in with their own expectations. Laing argued that mystification as a result of these processes caused the development of an overtly displayed false self and a privately experienced real self. Laing (1969) believed that Schizophrenia developed when the split between these selves became too big.

The contributions of the family systems model in particular, have been criticised for methodological problems. One of these points of critique is that family interactions become the focus of study only after the diagnosis of a family member. Another related issue is a lack of use of control groups (or families) for the purposes of comparison by the family systems approach. These two issues present difficulties because conclusions are drawn about the family interactions, but whether these types of interactions will always give rise to the same types of pathology remains unclear.

Expressed emotion

Negative affective communication variables have also been the focus of research into the family dynamics associated with the development and maintenance of Schizophrenia. 'Negative affective communication' refers to the emotional tone of family interactions and attitudes. The main variable that has been distinguished is expressed emotion. Studies on these variables have mostly focused on the maintenance of Schizophrenia in families once the disorder has been diagnosed.

Expressed emotion (EE) refers to a pattern of communication which is characterised by statements expressing criticism, hostility, and over-involvement. Initial research in this area was done by Brown et al. (1972) and Brown, Bone, Dalison, and Wing (1966). This research divided families of people diagnosed with Schizophrenia into so-called 'high-EE families' and 'low-EE' families. In a nine-month follow-up of discharged patients living with their families, high relapse rates were found in the high-EE families. It appears that this aspect of the family environment also impacts on the person with a diagnosis of Schizophrenia. High-EE families also make more negative comments regarding the symptoms of Schizophrenia displayed by the patient. The negative symptoms appeared more likely to elicit negative comment, and the family members making negative comments were more likely to regard the symptoms as being within the control of the patient. In addition, unusual thoughts expressed by the patient elicited more critical comments from family members in high-EE families. In turn, an increased number of critical comments appeared to trigger a higher number of unusual thoughts in the person diagnosed with Schizophrenia. A circular (bi-directional) relationship therefore appears to exist between expressed emotion and unusual thoughts in people diagnosed with Schizophrenia and their families (Lopez, Nelson, Snyder, & Mintz, 1999; Weissman, Nuechterlein, Goldstein, & Sneider, 1998).

In terms of causality and expressed emotion, a number of issues prevent us from drawing the conclusion that high-EE is a causal factor, rather than merely a precipitating factor, in Schizophrenia. High-EE communication patterns appear to be present not only in the families of people with a diagnosis of Schizophrenia, but also in families where a member has been diagnosed with depression, Bipolar Disorder, and eating disorders (Kavanagh, 1992). Cultural differences also appear to exist in terms of high EE-communication, with Western families displaying more high-EE communication. Despite Western families apparently displaying more high-EE communication, the incidence of Schizophrenia appears to be relatively stable at about 1% across cultures (Leff et al., 1990).

Issues such as variability across cultures, high-EE not being specific to families with a member with a diagnosis of Schizophrenia, and a possible bi-directional relationship between EE and symptoms of Schizophrenia imply that, for the moment, the concept of EE may be more useful in the prevention of relapse than in understanding the aetiology of Schizophrenia.

EXAMPLE CASE

High Expressed Emotion

'I think if Mary just got some exercise, or did something constructive, she would feel much better. Just do something active ... but she won't listen to me, I am just her mother...'

Low Expressed Emotion

'I try to let Mary go at her own pace. I accept that she will take some kind of action when she feels ready.'

Cannabis use

Cannabis use appears to be an independent risk factor for Schizophrenia (Andréasson, Engström, & Rydberg, 1987). High consumers of cannabis appear to be at greater risk of developing Schizophrenia. Cannabis use also seems to be associated with poor outcome in existing Schizophrenia and may trigger psychosis not only in vulnerable individuals, but also in people who do not have a prior history of difficulties (Andréasson et al., 1987; Henquet, Murray, Linszen, & Van Os, 2005; Smit, Bolier, & Cuijpers, 2004). Cannabis use is thought to interact with genetic and environmental risk factors to cause psychotic illness (Kuepper et al., 2011). Increased public awareness of this interplay and the potential risks for developing a psychotic illness as a result of cannabis use may play a role in the prevention of Schizophrenia and psychotic illness.

To summarise, the family can be regarded as the context in which the individual's self-concept and cognitive abilities develop. Constant disqualifications of one another by members of the family, coupled with mixed messages and faulty communication, are thought to impact negatively on the developing self-concepts of the children of such a family. Similarly, these dynamics are also thought to impact on the children's development of the cognitive skills which enable them to categorise experience and communicate effectively. In this view, the person who is later diagnosed with Schizophrenia does not experience a confirmation of their personal authenticity in this family context. In this argument, the symptoms of Schizophrenia, such as identity confusion, communication problems, cognitive difficulties, and relationship problems, are related to the problematic development of cognitive skills and self-concept (Laing & Esterson, 1964; Lidz et al., 1965; Wynne et al., 1958).

Sociocultural factors

The effects of social class

Gottesman (1991) maintains that one of the most unchanging outcomes of research on Schizophrenia is that it is most prevalent among people who live in the poorest, often central, sections of large cities, who inhabit the lowest socio-economic levels, and who are employed in occupations with the lowest status. Two explanations have been put forward to make sense of this phenomenon, the sociogenic hypothesis and the social selection theory.

The sociogenic hypothesis views the stressors of a low socio-economic status as causing, or contributing to, the development of Schizophrenia. The sociogenic hypothesis regards possible sources of stress as being either environmental factors or biological factors. The environmental factors that could be associated with low socio-economic status include mistreatment and disrespect from others, lack of education, low-grade employment, and low levels of rewards and opportunities. An example of the biological factors is poor nutrition during pregnancy (Gottesman, 1991).

Social selection theory can also be described as downward drift theory. In this view, people who are in the process of developing the disorder and people with the diagnosis tend to move or drift to the poorest areas of cities due to their decreased functioning, which in turn decreases their employment opportunities and earning capabilities (Gottesman, 1991).

In attempts to clarify these issues, researchers have examined the possible downward trend in occupational status in people diagnosed with Schizophrenia (Keith, Regier, & Rae, 1991). Another research strategy has been to compare the occupational status of people diagnosed with Schizophrenia with that of their fathers. The downward drift tendency across generations was confirmed in several studies with this approach (Gottesman, 1991).

Somewhat more evidence appears to exist for the downward drift theory than for the sociogenic hypothesis. This should not be taken to imply that the social environment plays no role in the causality of Schizophrenia, however. Some evidence suggests that the stressors associated with low socio-economic status contribute to the development of Schizophrenia in some individuals (Gottesman, 1991). An explanation that includes both views is probably more accurate.

The effects of migrant status

A great deal of data is available on the incidence of Schizophrenia. One of the areas of substantial variation in incidence is migrant status (McGrath et al., 2004). A variety of studies have indicated an elevated risk for psychiatric disorder, and particularly psychotic disorders, for first generation adult immigrants. Members of ethnic minorities residing in neighbourhoods that create relative isolation have an additionally elevated risk. Most of these studies have been conducted in Europe (Menezes, Georgiades, & Boyle, 2011). Despite not all studies supporting this association, systematic reviews of the data appear to indicate that, in general, migrant groups are significantly more at risk of developing Schizophrenia than native-born populations (McGrath et al., 2004).

Some theories that have been suggested to explain this tendency emphasise psychosocial variables, such as socio-economic disadvantage, exposure to racism, and discriminatory practices, as well as factors related to family and community responses to psychiatric disorders in migrant populations (Jarvis, 1998). Other theories put forward environmental causes such as obstetric complications and perinatal infections as aetiological models (Eagles, 1991). The convergence of risk factors, such as vulnerability based on exposure to novel viruses, abnormal immunological responses, obstetric complications, and differential foetal survival have also been suggested in an attempt to explain this data (Harrison, 1990).

Integration of aetiological factors

One way in which to integrate the seemingly disjointed factors described above is to view them as predisposing, precipitating, and maintaining factors respectively. Predisposing factors imply an underlying (usually biological) vulnerability to the disorder. In the case of Schizophrenia, genetics and brain structure (including biochemical aspects) represent this biological vulnerability. Precipitating factors are the life circumstances of an individual that trigger the underlying vulnerability, thereby causing symptoms of the disorder to manifest. These factors may be either intrapersonal or interpersonal in nature. Examples of possible precipitating or triggering factors for Schizophrenia from the discussion above are psychological stress, cannabis use, faulty learning, and possibly the impact of the family system.

Once the disorder has been triggered, remission of symptoms is hindered by maintaining factors. Thus, the maintaining factors complicate and extend the course of the disorder. Factors in the discussion above that may act as maintaining factors include family dynamics and the presence of high expressed emotion in the family, cannabis use, and sociocultural factors such as social class and migrant status. Again, maintaining factors may be intra- or interpersonal aspects.

As with all the other facets of this much researched but puzzling disorder, an attempt to view the aetiology of Schizophrenia in an integrated way is far from clear cut, with some factors playing both precipitating and maintaining roles. The strong arguments for the biological basis of the disorder (and most recently, the neurodevelopmental views of the disorder) would place less emphasis on the triggering events than with other disorders, such as the mood disorders. Perhaps the metaphor of Schizophrenia as a biological time bomb is most apt. While some disorders, such as the mood disorders, can be likened to landmines, which can remain dormant for many years and that require a trigger to manifest, Schizophrenia is probably more like a time bomb ticking towards its inevitable explosion. Precipitating factors such as psychological stress and cannabis use probably serve to hasten the inevitable, while the maintaining factors, such as high expressed emotion, merely worsen the devastation left in the wake of the bomb's explosion.

CONTROVERSIAL ISSUES IN THE DIAGNOSIS AND MANAGEMENT OF SCHIZOPHRENIA

Various authors have acknowledged that Schizophrenia is probably one of the most researched, yet most confusing, of the psychological disorders (Carson, 1985). A number of controversies have been associated with the diagnosis, management, and treatment of Schizophrenia. Some of these issues will be highlighted in this section, including the question as to whether Schizophrenia represents one disorder or many, the issue of labelling and stigmatisation, the views of the anti-psychiatrists, as well as current trends towards de-institutionalisation and the impact of this on people diagnosed with Schizophrenia and their families.

One diagnosis or many?

Although the two main classification systems that are used when making a diagnosis of Schizophrenia are the DSM and ICD systems, these systems seem to be less than helpful when it comes to research and treatment of Schizophrenia. Some authors suggest that it is more appropriate to refer to this category of disorders as 'the Schizophrenias', following Bleuler's original title *Dementia Praecox or the Group of Schizophrenias* (1911/1950), thus acknowledging the complexity associated with describing and diagnosing this disorder or group of disorders (Carson, 1986).

Contributing to the difficulties related to the diagnosis of Schizophrenia, or 'the Schizophrenias', appears to be an underlying conceptual issue. If Schizophrenia is conceptualised in purely medical terms, that is, as a biological dysfunction causing a physiological disease, then a diagnosis of a single entity, 'Schizophrenia', is possible. However, there is a lack of clear diagnostic markers to aid in the diagnosis of Schizophrenia, although this can be ascribed to limitations in our current scientific knowledge (Carson, 1986).

The other alternative involves attempts to define Schizophrenia as a set of behaviours, and to allocate these behaviours to descriptive classes. This view would therefore seek to describe clusters of behaviours that would define the schizophrenic range. This approach subscribes to the notion of 'equifinality' (or multiple pathways) to the development of these behaviours. These multiple pathways involve the various subtypes and aetiological considerations associated with this group of disorders (Carson, 1986). Indeed, evidence exists for the plural view (different causal patterns and dynamics), as opposed to a unitary view of the disorder (Bellak, 1979).

From these different views, according to Tandon, Goldman, Goodson, and Greden (1990), alternative ways of studying and describing Schizophrenia have evolved. These include 'positive versus negative Schizophrenia' and 'Type 1 versus Type II Schizophrenia'.

Positive Schizophrenia versus negative Schizophrenia

We have previously referred to the positive and negative symptoms of Schizophrenia, and many authors and researchers prefer to use these symptoms to classify Schizophrenia, rather than the more traditional classification systems. Although there is some merit in this approach, it may also be too simplistic an approach to a rather complex set of disorders. The problems related to this approach include:

- It may be misleading as it seems to imply that a patient with Schizophrenia has either positive symptoms (positive Schizophrenia) or negative symptoms (negative Schizophrenia). For example, Andreasen (1982) and Andreasen et al. (1990), who can be described as the main advocates of this approach, described positive Schizophrenia and negative Schizophrenia as two distinct illnesses or at least two distinct subtypes of the same illness.
- While many studies have indicated a distinct difference between 'positive' and 'negative' patients on a number of parameters, this subtyping has not been longitudinally consistent (Kay, 1990).

- A majority of patients with Schizophrenia have been found to be have 'mixed' symptoms (Andreasen et al., 1990).
- Some research has indicated that positive and negative syndromes represent distinct dimensions and not subtypes of schizophrenic illness (Pogue-Geile & Keshavan, 1990).

Type I Schizophrenia versus Type II Schizophrenia

A further adaptation of positive and negative symptoms with regard to the classification of Schizophrenia was made by Crow (1980, 1985). He postulated two types of Schizophrenia: Type I (Reactive Schizophrenia) and Type II (Process Schizophrenia). Table 6.11 describes the differences between these two types.

Table 6.11: Summary of Type I and Type II Schizophrenia

Type I Schizophrenia	Type II Schizophrenia
• Positive symptoms • Absence of intellectual impairment • Normal brain structure • Good response to medication	• Negative symptoms • Intellectual deterioration • Enlarged cerebral ventricles • Poor response to medication

Source: Adapted from Crow, 1980, 1985.

Initially, Crow (1980) was of the opinion that Type II Schizophrenia was just a more advanced stage of Schizophrenia than Type I, but he later reformulated his theory (Crow, 1985) and described these two types as relatively independent processes. According to Crow, the two types differ in terms of their patho-physiologies, but not in terms of their aetiologies (Tandon & Greden, 1991). From the preceding discussion, one can conclude that the use of the term 'Schizophrenia' is in itself extremely complicated and that very little regarding this cluster of behaviours can be taken for granted.

'Normality' and 'abnormality'

When one tries to look at Schizophrenia in a critical way, one of the central themes is that of 'normality' versus 'abnormality'. Two main strands make up this theme. This first is that of the Anti-Psychiatry Movement (see Chapter 1), which queried whether mental illness exists at all. The second strand of the argument queries whether mental health professionals are able to distinguish between those with and those without mental illness.

A different but related question is that of labelling. Labelling theorists are interested in how psychiatric diagnoses (or labels) become self-fulfilling prophesies for those who are 'labelled'. This will be discussed in the following section.

What if 'Schizophrenia' does not exist at all? This is the view of the anti-psychiatrists (Laing, 1969; Szasz, 1961), who contest the very existence of Schizophrenia and other mental illnesses. The Anti-Psychiatry Movement holds that the act of diagnosing as well as the diagnostic categories are influenced by values, morals, and political considerations within society. Psychiatry can be seen as a form of social control. This social control is achieved by medicalising behaviour that breaks social rules. This means that any behaviour that makes other people uncomfortable, is irritating, or that questions the status quo, is approached as if it were an illness with a physical cause, needing to be diagnosed and treated (Szasz, 1970; Ussher, 1991).

The anti-psychiatrists do not agree with conventional models of psychiatric classification and diagnosis. They also disagree with the generally accepted use of an analogy between medical and mental disorders. The reason for this is that, while the characteristics of medical disorders are usually objective, the features of mental disorders are usually more a question of subjective interpretation on the part of the clinician. Szasz (1960) sees the problematic behaviours of the 'mentally ill' as 'problems of living' rather than as symptoms of underlying brain disease. While he acknowledges that the difficult behaviours of those people who would usually be described as 'mentally ill' could be strange, irritating, or even deviant, he feels that individuals should take responsibility for their actions.

In Chapter 1 (Box 1.3), reference is made to the famous Rosenhan experiment (1973). In this experiment, eight 'pseudo-patients' (research assistants) were admitted to mental hospitals after simulating symptoms of mental illness (only hallucinations: hearing voices). All were admitted, and all (but one) were discharged with diagnoses of 'Schizophrenia in remission'. In some cases, the pseudo-patients were kept in hospital for several weeks. This study therefore questions the reliability and usefulness of psychiatric diagnosis and even whether mental health professionals are able to distinguish those who are 'normal' from those who are 'abnormal'.

Labelling

A related concept is that of labelling. This refers to a tendency to view the label ascribed to a person as a description of the person as a whole, rather than merely a description of his or her behaviour. This creates expectations about how the person will act for both the labelled person and for the people around them (including clinical staff). According to Rosenhan (1973), one of the consequences of the psychiatric labels ascribed to the pseudo-patients who took part in his experiment was that ordinary behaviours exhibited by the pseudo-patients (such as taking notes or pacing up and down) were seen as signs of mental illness by psychiatric staff.

The label in this way becomes a self-fulfilling prophesy. In our use of language, the person becomes the disorder, for example, 'Margaret is a schizophrenic', as opposed to 'Margaret has a diagnosis of Schizophrenia'. This is also true for the person's own view of themselves.

De-institutionalisation

As seen above, the practice of institutionalising people with a diagnosis of Schizophrenia has been critiqued by the anti-psychiatrists as a method of social control of people who do not conform to the behaviours expected by society. The other side of the coin is then the practice of de-institutionalisation, which has had significant and controversial consequences.

In the 1980s in the United States (and in the early 2000s in South Africa), changes in legislation and policies took place that severely restricted psychiatric hospital beds. These changes also affected the possible length of stay in such facilities, as well as placing limitations on who could be committed involuntarily (Mental Health Care Act, No. 17 of 2002) (see Chapter 14). Contrast this approach to statements earlier in this chapter regarding the impact of Schizophrenia on the independent functioning of some people with this diagnosis. The aims of these policies in the United States and in South Africa were to move the mentally ill, and their care, from institutions into communities and community care structures.

In the United States, de-institutionalisation is regarded as a failure, since it resulted in a large number of people with mental illnesses (Schizophrenia, in particular) becoming homeless. An additional consideration is the unpredictable dangerousness to self (and, in some cases, to others) which characterises this population (Cranco & Lehman, 2000). The consequences of policies leading to de-institutionalisation in South Africa are not yet fully clear. However, some initial research indicates that de-institutionalising policies in South Africa are associated with 'revolving door' patients (patients who are frequently re-admitted because they remain well only for short periods of time). Early discharge was one of the contributing factors for frequent re-admissions in this research (Botha et al., 2010).

CONCLUSION

This chapter has attempted to give an overview of Schizophrenia and other disorders associated with psychosis as a cluster of disorders. Psychosis is a very serious psychiatric symptom and Schizophrenia can be regarded as the 'classic' psychotic disorder. The introduction described Schizophrenia as an 'extreme' disorder. The impact of this group of disorders and behaviours on the diagnosed individual, their family, and on the broader society is indeed extreme in terms of its emotional and financial costs.

Despite Schizophrenia being one of the most researched disorders, we still cannot make conclusive statements regarding the types of Schizophrenia, the causes of Schizophrenia, the course of Schizophrenia, possible effective treatments of Schizophrenia, and, least of all, the diagnosis of Schizophrenia itself. Even the management of people with Schizophrenia is fraught with difficulties. It appears that this cluster of behaviours, which has fascinated and puzzled mental health researchers for more than 200 years, will continue to do so for some time to come.

MULTIPLE-CHOICE QUESTIONS

1. Which of the following is *not* a typical symptom of Schizophrenia?
   a) delusions
   b) inappropriate emotions
   c) disorganised speech and behaviour
   d) refusal to maintain minimum body weight

2. Which of the following is the definition of catatonia?
   a) silly and immature behaviour
   b) *dementia praecox*
   c) immobility or agitated excitement
   d) delusions of grandeur

3. Which of the following is the definition of paranoia?
   a) silly and immature behaviour
   b) anhedonia
   c) alternating immobility and agitated excitement
   d) delusions of persecution

4. The main symptom of psychosis is:
   a) hallucinations
   b) delusions
   c) disorganised behaviour
   d) all of these

5. The most common type of hallucination experienced by schizophrenic patients is:
   a) visual
   b) auditory
   c) tactile
   d) olfactory

6. Flat affect can be described as:
   a) inability to initiate and persist in activities
   b) inability to experience pleasure
   c) lack of emotional response; blank facial expression
   d) lack of speech content and/or slowed speech response

7. Through deductive reasoning, which of the following scenarios supports the dopamine hypothesis of Schizophrenia?
   a) Antipsychotic drugs (neuroleptics) act as dopamine agonists, increasing the amount of dopamine in the brain.
   b) Antipsychotic drugs (neuroleptics) can produce symptoms similar to those of Parkinson's disease (a disorder due to insufficient dopamine).
   c) The drug L-dopa, a dopamine agonist, is used to treat symptoms of Schizophrenia in patients with Parkinson's disease.

d) Amphetamines, which activate dopamine, can lessen psychotic symptoms in people with Schizophrenia.

8. Which of the following is an independent risk factor for psychosis?
   a) a family member with a mood disorder
   b) a family with high expressed emotion (EE)
   c) cannabis use
   d) cigarette smoking

9. There seems to be evidence of neuro-anatomical causes for Schizophrenia as seen by which one of the following?
   a) All patients with Schizophrenia have smaller ventricles in their brains.
   b) In some Schizophrenia patients there is an excess amount of 'grey matter' in the cerebral cortex.
   c) The majority of Schizophrenia patients have enlarged ventricles in their brains.
   d) Many patients with Schizophrenia have increased activity in the frontal lobes of their brains.

PARAGRAPH AND ESSAY QUESTIONS

1. Describe the 'positive' and 'negative' symptoms of Schizophrenia. Explain what is meant by these terms and how they relate to prognosis and outcome.

2. Compare the major subtypes of Schizophrenia as described in the ICD-10 (Paranoid, Catatonic, Hebephrenic, Undifferentiated, and Residual) in terms of symptoms, treatment, and prognosis.

3. Discuss some of the causative factors of Schizophrenia, including genetic influences, neurotransmitter imbalances, prenatal viral exposure, and psychological stressors.

4. Define 'expressed emotion' and describe how this would impact relapse risk in a person with Schizophrenia.

5. Schizophrenia is associated with increased risk for mortality. Discuss this statement, indicating which risk factors may be modifiable.

7 NEUROCOGNITIVE DISORDERS

Basil Pillay

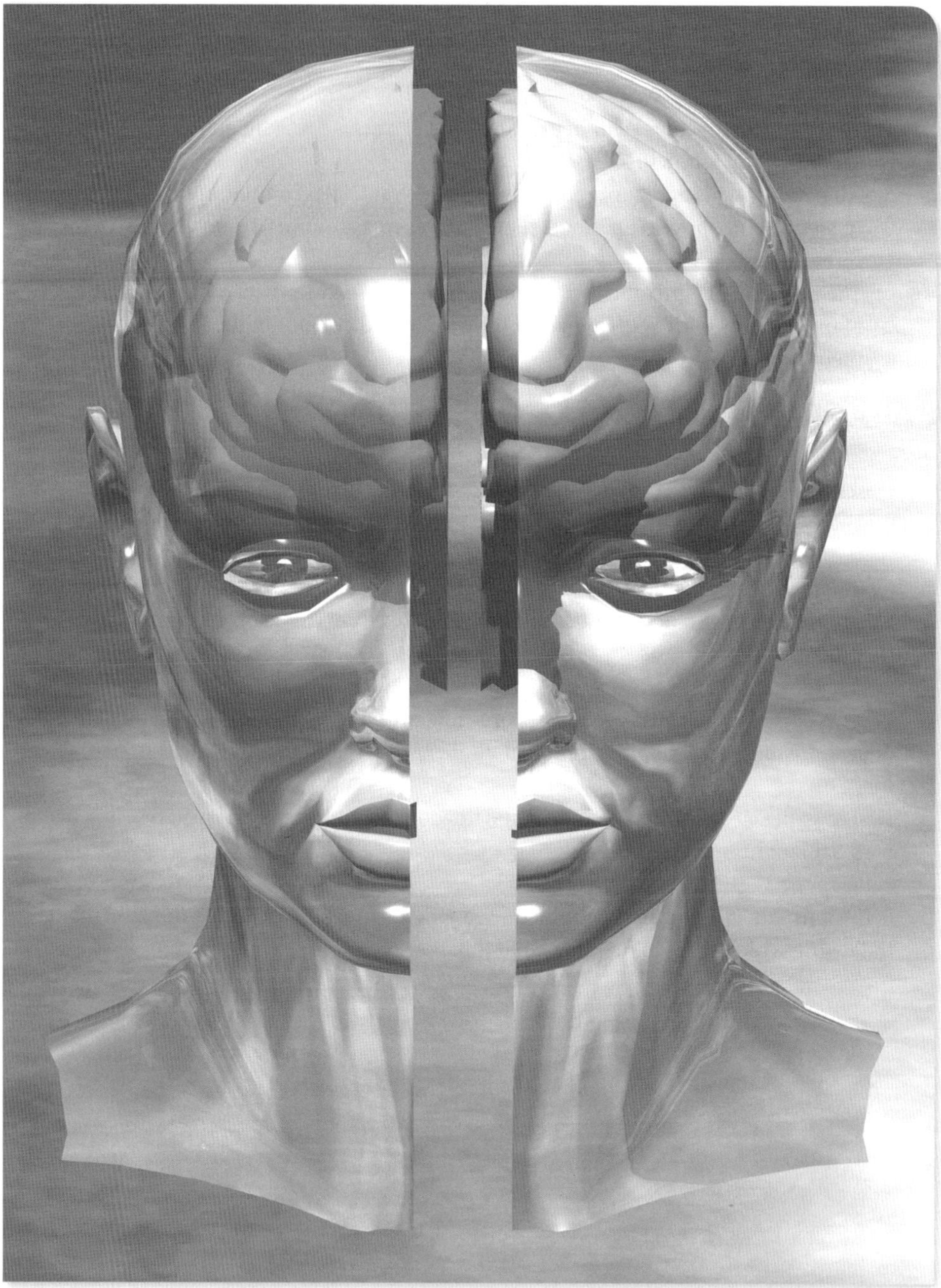

7 CHAPTER OUTLINE

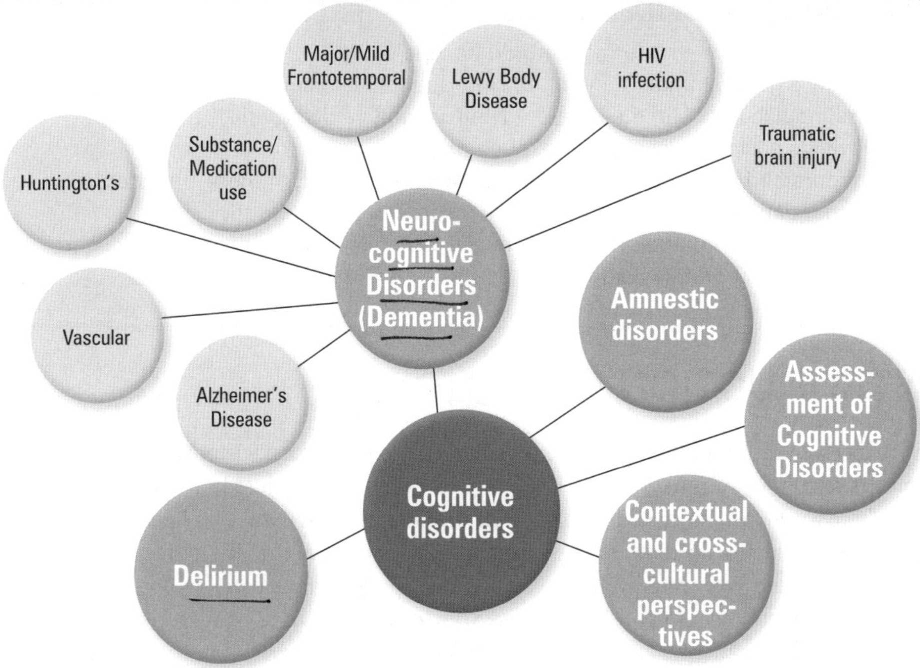

LEARNING OUTCOMES

After studying this chapter you should be able to:

- Show a general understanding of Neurocognitive disorders.
- Distinguish between the different Neurocognitive disorders.
- Provide a clinical description of each disorder.
- Understand the problems relating to the classification of these disorders.
- Understand the way Neurocognitive disorders are assessed.
- Identify cross-cultural, more specifically South African, concerns associated with Neurocognitive disorders.

INTRODUCTION

Every day we think about issues or events, solve problems, make decisions, remember things (such as telephone numbers or what we have to do), or we are just in a state of awareness (i.e. where we are, what time it is, what day or month it is). Have you ever had the experience of not being able to do these things? You may, at some time or the other, have been in a situation where you were unable to remember an important date, or not able to recall a person's name or where you had parked your car. If you have, you will know that it is usually quite embarrassing and sometimes frightening. Imagine what it would be like if this happened all the time. You would not be able to function or perform simple, routine tasks we take for granted. This is what Neurocognitive disorders are all about.

BOX 7.1: BASIC NEURO-ANATOMY

Together the brain and spinal cord form the central nervous system (CNS). The brain is divided into two hemispheres (referred to as the left and right) and is connected together by the corpus callosum. The folded or wrinkled area is referred to as cerebrum or cortex and is actually a continuous sheet folded into rises (gyri) and troughs (sulci). The cerebrum comprises four lobes: frontal, parietal, occipital, and temporal lobes. The frontal lobe is the most anterior lobe and is important for planning, organisation, abstract thought, etc. (referred to as executive functioning) as well as motor control, memory, and many other functions. The parietal lobe is

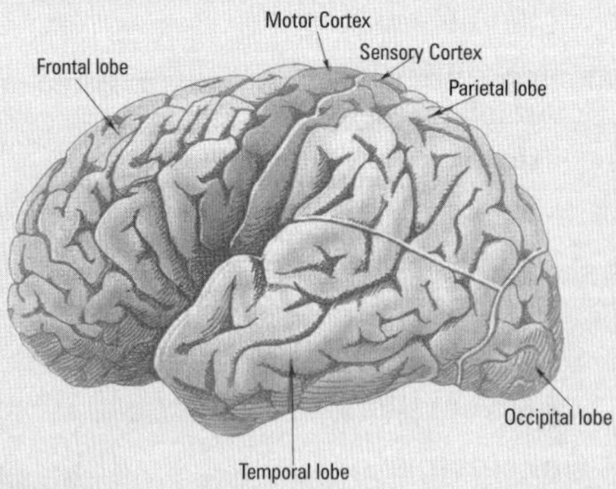

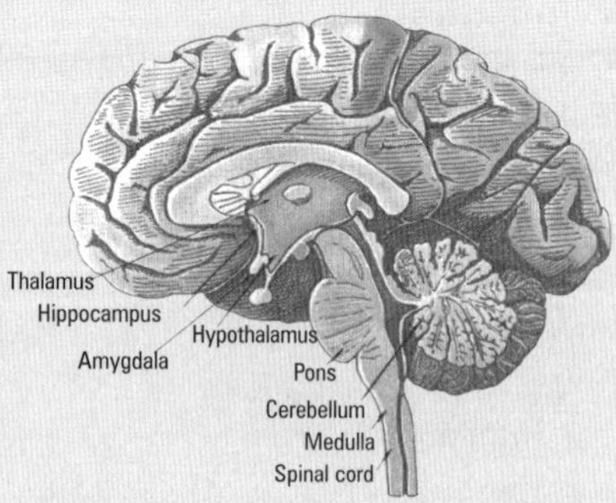

posterior (behind) to the frontal lobe and dorsal (towards the back of the brain) and is important for spatial processing, cognitive processing, motor control, memory, and other functions. The occipital lobe is most posterior and is mainly associated with visual processing. The temporal lobe is on the ventral surface (towards the bottom) of the brain and is important for auditory and visual processing, language, memory, and many other functions. Below the cortex are the subcortical areas. These structures include the hypothalamus (which supports homeostatic functions, including regulation of food intake); thalamus (important for perception and cognition), and brain stem, made up of the midbrain, pons, medulla, and cerebellum (plays an important role in motor function).

The word 'cognition' is the broad term used to refer to tasks that include memory, language, orientation, judgement, problem-solving, planning, the ability to have interpersonal relationships, and perform actions (referred to as **praxis**). When a person has significant, regular trouble in these areas of cognition, which disrupts their daily functioning, it may be due to a Neurocognitive disorder. These disruptions in cognition can be the result of many causes. These include: head injury (e.g. following a motor vehicle accident or a gunshot to the head, or from a fall); a medical condition (e.g. HIV/AIDS); or the misuse or abuse of substances (e.g. alcohol, cannabis, cocaine, etc.). Aging can also produce these cognitive problems and in some instances, like Alzheimer's disease, it can be very distressing for the sufferer and the family. In this chapter, we will focus on the common Neurocognitive disorders by explaining: how they are classified; how the disorders present themselves; the main differences between the different types of Neurocognitive disorders; their aetiology (cause); and their assessment, treatment, and management. Finally, the chapter will close with some comments on contextual and cultural issues. As you can see, Neurocognitive disorders are closely related to the brain and brain functioning. The structures of the brain and their functions are provided in Box 7.1 to help you understand some of the terminology used in this chapter (and elsewhere in this textbook) and to identify the areas to which we refer. Box 7.2 provides explanations for anatomical terms of direction used in this chapter.

BOX 7.2: ANATOMICAL TERMS OF DIRECTION

Medial	Toward the midline of the body
Lateral	Away from the midline of the body
Proximal	Toward a reference point (extremity)
Distal	Away from a reference point (extremity)
Inferior	Lower or below
Superior	Upper or above
Anterior	Toward the front
Ventral	Anterior
Posterior	Toward the back
Dorsal	Posterior

THE CLASSIFICATION OF NEUROCOGNITIVE DISORDERS

Neurocognitive disorders can be organised into two (DSM-5) or three (ICO-10) broad areas. The DM-5 distinguishes between Delirium and Major or Mild Neurocognitive Disorders, and the ICD-10 between delirium, dementia, and amnestic disorders. Within each group, there are further subgroups which are organised according to their aetiology. Table 7.1 lists the *Diagnostic and Statistical Manual of Mental Disorders* (DSM-5) (American Psychiatric Association, 2000) and the *International Classification of Disorders* (ICD-10) (World Health Organisation, 1993) classifications of cognitive disorders.

Table 7.1: Classification of Neurocognitive disorders as adapted from the DSM-5 and ICD-10

DSM-5	ICD-10
Delirium	
• Delirium Due to a General Medical Condition • Substance-Induced Delirium • Delirium Due to Multiple Aetiologies • Delirium Not Otherwise Specified	• Delirium not induced by alcohol and other psychoactive substances • Delirium, not superimposed on dementia, so described • Delirium, superimposed on dementia, so described • Other delirium • Delirium, unspecified
• Major and Mild Neurocognitive Disorders (NCD)	• Dementia
• Major or Mild Neurocognitive Disorder Due to Alzheimer's Disease • Major or Minor Frontotemporal Neurocognitive • Major or Mild Neurocognitive Disorder with Lewy Bodies • Major or Mild Vascular Neurocognitive Disorder • Major or Mild Neurocognitive Disorder Due to: ▸ Traumatic Brain Injury ▸ HIV Infection ▸ Prion Disease ▸ Parkinson's ▸ Huntington's Disease ▸ Another Medical ▸ Multiple Aetiologies ▸ Unspecified Neurocognitive Disorder	• Dementia in Alzheimer's disease • Dementia in Alzheimer's disease with early onset • Dementia in Alzheimer's disease with late onset • Dementia in Alzheimer's disease, atypical or mixed type • Dementia in Alzheimer's disease, unspecified • Vascular dementia • Vascular dementia of acute onset • Multi-infarct dementia • Subcortical vascular dementia • Mixed cortical and subcortical vascular dementia • Other vascular dementia • Vascular dementia, unspecified • Dementia in other diseases classified elsewhere • Dementia in Pick's disease • Dementia in Creutzfeldt-Jakob disease • Dementia in Huntington's disease • Dementia in Parkinson's disease • Dementia in human immunodeficiency virus (HIV) disease

DSM-5	ICD-10
	• Dementia in other specified diseases classified elsewhere • Unspecified dementia • Amnestic Disorders • Organic amnestic syndrome, not induced by alcohol and other psychoactive substances
Other mental disorders due to brain damage and dysfunction and to physical disease	
	• Organic hallucinosis • Organic catatonic disorder • Organic delusional (schizophrenia-like) disorder • Organic mood (affective) disorder • Organic anxiety disorder • Organic dissociative disorder • Organic emotionally labile (asthenic) disorder • Mild cognitive disorder • Other specified mental disorders due to brain damage and dysfunction and to physical disease • Unspecified mental disorders due to brain damage and dysfunction and to physical disease
Personality and behavioural disorders due to brain disease, damage, and dysfunction	
	• Organic personality disorder • Post-encephalitic syndrome • Post-concussional syndrome • Other organic personality and behavioural disorders due to brain disease, damage, and dysfunction
Other Cognitive Disorders	
• Unspecified Neurocognitive Disorder	• Unspecified organic or symptomatic mental disorder

Source: Reprinted with permission from the Diagnostic and Statistical Manual of Mental Disorders, (DSM), Fifth Edition, American Psychiatric Association (APA), 2013 and ICD–10 Classification of Mental and Behavioural Disorders: Diagnostic Criteria for Research. World Health Organisation (WHO), Geneva, 2007.

HISTORY OF NEUROCOGNITIVE DISORDERS

In the DSM-111 and previous editions of the DSM these disorders were referred to as 'organic mental disorders' or organic brain disorders because they are linked to an identifiable pathology such as a brain tumour or a cerebral disease. In the DSM-5, the term 'organic mental disorder' was replaced with Cognitive Disorders because the previous term incorrectly implies that disorders *not* in this group of disorders (i.e. the so-called 'nonorganic' or functional mental disorders, like depression) do not have a biological basis. You will notice from Table 7.1 above that the ICD-10 still retains the use of the word 'organic'.

The DSM-5, however, went a step further and renamed this category 'neurocognitive disorders' which clearly indicates these 'cognitive disorders' have a clearly delineated neurological aetiology.

DELIRIUM

Clinical picture

Delirium is usually seen as a temporary state of mental confusion with fluctuating consciousness. It usually occurs rather suddenly and is characterised by mental confusion, the inability to pay attention, and the inability to think clearly. This condition is generally reversible. In addition, it is accompanied by anxiety, disorientation, and incoherent speech. Delirium is an abnormal mental state and not a disease. It is sometimes also referred to as an 'acute confusional state' or 'acute brain syndrome'. The main feature of the disorder is the impairment in consciousness. By consciousness, we mean awareness that can vary from being fully alert to being comatose (unconscious) – see Figure 7.1 for a graphical representation of how the levels of consciousness are rated. In order to diagnose dementia, there are specific features that must be present. See Table 7.2 for the DSM-5 and ICD-10 criteria for delirium.

Figure 7.1: Levels of consciousness

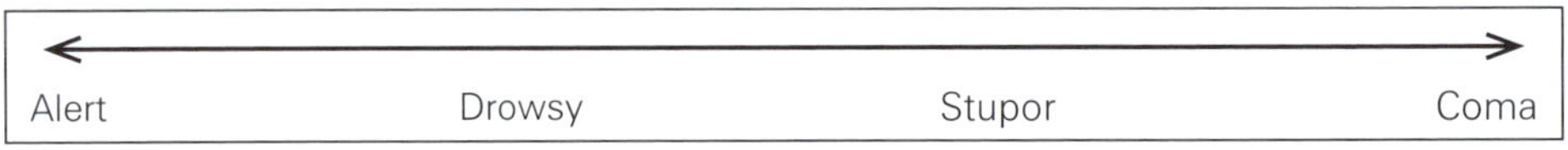

The cognitive changes in delirium include memory impairment, disorientation, language disturbance, and perceptual disturbance. In addition, emotional disturbances commonly occur. There may be anxiety, fear, depression, irritability, anger, euphoria (excitement or elation), and apathy, all of which can occur rapidly and with unpredictable shifts from one emotional state to another.

Epidemiology

According to the DSM-5 (2000), delirium is likely to occur in about 0.4% of the adult general population between the ages of 18 and 55 years, and in about 1.1% of those 55 years and older. In medical inpatients, it is more common and ranges from 10% to 31%, increasing significantly in the elderly. The incidence of new delirium per admission ranges from 3% to 29% and occurrence rate per admission varies between 11% and 42%.

Aetiology

Delirium is further classified according to its aetiology. For example, if the aetiology of the delirium is a consequence of a general medical condition (i.e. a seizure or renal failure), then Delirium Due to a General Medical Condition is diagnosed. If it is a consequence of a drug misuse or abuse, then Substance Intoxication Delirium or Substance Withdrawal Delirium is diagnosed. The category Delirium Due to Multiple Aetiologies is used when there may be several causes for the delirium, or Delirium Not Otherwise Specified is considered when the aetiology is not established or not known. There are several common causes of delirium (see Table 7.3).

Table 7.2: Diagnostic criteria for delirium as adapted from the DSM-5 and ICD-10

DSM-5	ICD-10
A. The disturbance in attention (i.e. reduced ability to direct, focus, sustain, and shift attention) and awareness (reduced orientation to the environment). B. The disturbance develops over a shirt period of time (usually hours to a few days), represents a change from baseline attention and awareness, and tends to fluctuate in severity during the course of a day. C. An additional disturbance in cognition (e.g. memory deficit, disorientation, language, visuospatial ability, or perception). D. The disturbances in Criteria A and C are not better explained by another preexisting, established, or evolving neurocognitive disorder and do not occur in the context of a severely reduced level of arousal, such as coma. E. There is evidence from the history, physical examination, or laboratory findings that the disturbance is a direct physiological consequence of another medical condition, substance intoxication or withdrawal (i.e. due to a drug of abuse or to a medication), or exposure to a toxin, or is due to multiple aetiologies.	For a definite diagnosis, symptoms, mild or severe, should be present in each one of the following areas: • Impairment of consciousness and attention (on a continuum from clouding to coma; reduced ability to direct, focus, sustain, and shift attention); • Global disturbance of cognition (perceptual distortions, illusions, and hallucinations – most often visual; impairment of abstract thinking and comprehension, with or without transient delusions, but typically with some degree of incoherence; impairment of immediate recall and of recent memory but with relatively intact remote memory; disorientation for time as well as, in more severe cases, for place and person); • Psychomotor disturbances (hypo- or hyperactivity and unpredictable shifts from one to the other; increased reaction time; increased or decreased flow of speech; enhanced startle reaction); • Disturbance of the sleep–wake cycle (insomnia or, in severe cases, total sleep loss or reversal of the sleep–wake cycle; daytime drowsiness; nocturnal worsening of symptoms; disturbing dreams or nightmares, which may continue as hallucinations after awakening); • Emotional disturbances, e.g. depression, anxiety or fear, irritability, euphoria, apathy, or wondering perplexity. The onset is usually rapid, the course is diurnally fluctuating, and the total duration of the condition less than six months.

Source: Reprinted with permission from the Diagnostic and Statistical Manual of Mental Disorders, (DSM), Fifth Edition, American Psychiatric Association (APA), 2013 and ICD–10 Classification of Mental and Behavioural Disorders: Diagnostic Criteria for Research. World Health Organisation (WHO), Geneva, 2007.

Table 7.3: Some common causes of delirium

Central nervous system	Epilepsies and seizures, migraine, head trauma, brain tumour, stroke
Metabolic disorder	Diabetes
Systemic illness	Infection (malaria, sepsis, viral, syphilis), dehydration, nutritional deficiency, burns, heat stroke
Medical conditions	Cardiac failure or surgery, leukaemia, renal failure, hepatitis, etc.
Medications	Pain medication, antibiotics, antivirals, antifungals, steroids, cardiac medication
Over-the-counter (OTC) medications	Herbal remedies and nutritional supplements
Drugs of abuse	Intoxication and withdrawal from drugs such as alcohol, cannabis (dagga), MDMA (Ecstasy), Crystal meth (Tik), cocaine, heroin, etc.
Toxins	Intoxication and withdrawal from aluminium, pesticides, etc.

Source: Adapted from Sadock & Sadock, 2007.

Treatment and management of delirium

The symptoms of delirium usually develop suddenly (e.g. after a head injury) or they can develop over hours to days. Delirium is dangerous and is sometimes fatal, especially in the elderly. Since delirium is often associated with an underlying physical cause, recovery is to be expected if it is treated appropriately. Recovery from the delirium may occur in a few hours to days, or symptoms may persist for weeks to months, this being common in the elderly or those with co-existing dementia. The management of delirium involves identifying and correcting the underlying problem and symptomatically managing any behavioural or psychiatric symptoms. If the underlying aetiological factor is promptly treated, recovery is usually quick and likely to be complete. Recovery is also related to pre-morbid cognitive and physical abilities. If a person had good cognitive and physical functioning before the illness, they have better recovery from delirium. Those with previous episodes of delirium may be at increased risk for recurrent symptoms.

Although most individuals recover fully, delirium may progress to stupor, coma, seizures, or death, especially when the underlying cause is untreated. However, in the elderly, full recovery is less likely. Even when there is recovery in the elderly, there are often persistent cognitive deficits. In the medically ill, delirium is associated with more medical complications and higher mortality.

So-called 'environmental interventions' are generally recommended for patients with delirium. These interventions are designed to reduce or eliminate environmental factors that exacerbate delirium. They include providing an optimal level of environmental stimulation, reducing sensory impairments, and making environments more familiar.

In addition, cognitive-emotional support provides patients with reorientation and reassurance. In particular, information concerning delirium may reduce fear or discouragement. Doctors may also use certain drugs (e.g. antipsychotic drugs) to control agitation in the patient.

NEUROCOGNITIVE DISORDERS (DEMENTIA)

The DSM-IV-TR referred to these disorders as Dementia, and ICD-10 still uses this description. Although the DSM-5 now refers to these disorders as Neurocognitive Disorders (NCD), the term dementia is still retained to certain extent (APA, 2013). The APA (2013) states that the term dementia is a customary description of degenerative disorders for older adults, however, the term NCD is more inclusive as it includes NCD that affect younger people as well (APA, 2013). The APA (2013) views these disorders as unique when compared to the other DSM-5 categories as the underlying pathology and aetiology can be easily determined. The primary diagnosis would be Major or Mild NCD, followed by an aetiological subtypes (e.g. Alzheimer's disease, Parkinson's disease, HIV infection, etc.) (See Table 7.1).

To understand the clinical picture of these disorders, it is necessary to note which neurocognitive domains are affected. The DSM-5 describes these as follows (APA, 2013):

- *Complex attention*: Sustained, divided and selective attention as well as processing speed.
- *Executive functioning*: Planning, decision making, working memory error detection and correction, inhibition and mental flexibility.
- *Learning and memory*: All memory registers (e.g. short-term, semantic, autobiographical) and implicit learning.
- *Language*: Expressive and receptive language.
- *Perceptual-motor:* This includes visual perception, visuo-constructional abilities, perceptual-motor, praxis and gnosis.
- *Social cognition:* Recognition of emotions and theory of mind.

Clinical picture

In order to accommodate both the DSM-5 and ICD-10 descriptions of these disorders, we will refer to them as NCD (Dementia) in the rest of this chapter. In NCD (Dementia) there is the gradual loss of mental abilities or cognitive skills such as thinking, remembering, and reasoning, which results in a person not being able to do simple, everyday activities, such as getting dressed or eating. They may lose their ability to solve problems, experience difficulty controlling their emotions, and undergo a personality change. They may sometimes become agitated or hallucinate (i.e. see or hear things that are not there). Memory loss is a common symptom of NCD (Dementia). However, many different diseases can cause dementia (Sadock & Sadock, 2007). Table 7.4 lists the DSM-5 for NCD and ICD-10 criteria for dementia. Note that the DSM-5 makes a distinction between Major and Mild NCD, but that this distinction is based on severity, rather than type, of symptoms. Table 7.4 only reports the symptoms of Major NCD, but Minor NCD can be deduced from this as a less severe condition.

Table 7.4: Diagnostic criteria for dementia as adapted from the DSM-5 and ICD-10

Disorders (DSM-5)	Dementia (ICD-10)
A. Evidence of significant cognitive decline from a previous level of performance in one or more cognitive domains (complex attention, executive function, learning and memory, language, perceptual-motor, or social cognition) based on: (1) Concern of the individual, a knowledgeable informant, or the clinician that there has been a significant decline in cognitive function; and (2) A substantial impairment in cognitive performance, preferably documented by standardized neuropsychological testing or, in its absence, another quantified clinical assessment. B. The cognitive deficits interfere with independence in everyday activities (i.e. at a minimum, requiring assistance with complex instrumental activities of daily living such as paying bills or managing medications). C. The cognitive deficits do not occur exclusively in the context of a delirium. D. The cognitive deficits are not better explained by another mental disorder (e.g. major depressive disorder, schizophrenia).	The primary requirement for diagnosis is evidence of the following: • There is a decline in both memory and thinking which is sufficient to impair personal activities of daily living, as described above. • The impairment of memory typically affects the registration, storage, and retrieval of new information, but previously learned and familiar material may also be lost, particularly in the later stages. • Dementia is more than dysamnesia; there is also impairment of thinking and of reasoning capacity, and a reduction in the flow of ideas. • The processing of incoming information is impaired, in that the individual finds it increasingly difficult to attend to more than one stimulus at a time, such as taking part in a conversation with several persons, and to shift the focus of attention from one topic to another. The above symptoms and impairments should have been evident for at least six months for a confident clinical diagnosis of dementia to be made.

Source: Reprinted with permission from the Diagnostic and Statistical Manual of Mental Disorders, (DSM), Fifth Edition, American Psychiatric Association (APA), 2013 and ICD–10 Classification of Mental and Behavioural Disorders: Diagnostic Criteria for Research. World Health Organisation (WHO), Geneva, 2007.

NCD (Dementia) is an extremely common condition among the elderly. However, it must not be confused with normal decline in cognitive functioning that occurs with aging. The diagnosis of NCD is made when there is greater memory and other cognitive impairment than would be expected due to normal aging and when the symptoms cause considerable impairment in the person's everyday functioning (Sadock & Sadock, 2007).

As described before, there are several areas of cognitive disturbance that may occur. One of the critical ones is memory impairment, which is understood to be a prominent early symptom and is required to make the diagnosis of NCD (Dementia). The person is not able to learn new things or forgets previously learned information. As a result, the person will lose or forget things, such as wallets, keys, or the food cooking on the stove, or they may become lost in unfamiliar surroundings. In the advanced stages of the disorder, the person may actually forget their occupation, schooling, birthday, family members, and sometimes even their name.

Another area of potential deterioration is that of language function (aphasia). The person may have difficulty naming people and objects. Speech may become vague, long-winded, and repetitive with excessive use of non-specific words such as 'thing' and 'it'. In the advanced stages of dementia, the person may even be mute or have a deteriorated speech pattern characterised by echolalia (i.e. echoing what is heard) or palilalia (i.e. repeating sounds or words over and over).

A further area of potential deterioration is the failure to recognise or identify objects despite there being intact sensory function (agnosia). The person may not be able to recognise familiar objects, such as a table or a pen. As the dementia progresses, the person may be unable to recognise family members or even their own reflection in the mirror.

Common in NCD (Dementia) are problems with the ability to plan, organise, sequence, and abstract (referred to as executive functioning), which is associated with frontal lobe functioning. Patients with this disorder may also become spatially disorientated, have difficulty with spatial tasks, and have poor judgment and insight. They may not be aware of their memory loss or other cognitive deterioration and may do things that are not in keeping with their actual abilities, for example, driving a car erratically, or making huge purchases or sales. They may demonstrate disinhibited behaviour. This may include tactless, rude, or even offensive actions that don't follow the usual social rules about what to say or where to do something. This includes things like making inappropriate jokes, neglecting personal hygiene, or being inappropriately familiar with strangers. Sometimes people with NCD (Dementia) may become violent and harm others. Depression and suicidal behaviour commonly occur in dementia. Some individuals may also have motor disturbances, resulting in an unsteady gait, which may contribute to falls that result in injuries with serious consequences and complications (Sadock & Sadock, 2007).

ACTIVITY

Watch the movie *The Notebook*, based on the novel by Nicholas Sparks. It is a moving story that has an older man (James Garner) regularly reading a love story from a notebook to his aging companion (Gena Rowlands) who is suffering from Alzheimer's disease – the most common NCD (Dementia) that affects the elderly. The movie provides a good portrayal of what it is like for a person suffering from a NCD (Dementia), and their family.

Epidemiology

The prevalence of NCD (Dementia) depends on age and the extent of the cognitive impairment. There is a rise in prevalence as a result of the growing aging population. Major NCD (Dementia) is present in about 1–2% of the general population that is older than 65 years, and 30% of the general population older than 85 years (APA, 2013). Prevalence of Minor NCD varies from 2–10% at age 65 and 5–25% by age 85 (APA, 2013).

Very few studies on prevalence of NCD (Dementia) have been carried out in Africa. A series of studies from Ibadan, Nigeria, have produced consistently low rates for NCD (Dementia), especially for Alzheimer's disease (Hall et al., 1994). More recent studies reveal rather higher rates, but still lower than surveys carried out elsewhere (Ineichen, 2000). There are several possible reasons for these findings, including differential survival rates, the hiding of cases by relatives because of stigma, reluctance to seek medical assistance as it is considered inappropriate, poor access to medical care, the feeling that the old person has come to the end of their useful life, and defective case-finding techniques (Ineichen, 2000). The statistics on prevalence of NCD (Dementia) in developing societies are incomplete but the estimate of people suffering with NCD (Dementia) in developing countries is 6.8% (Brodrick, 2002). The prevalence of different causes of NCD (Dementia) (e.g. infections, nutritional deficiencies, traumatic brain injury, endocrine conditions, cerebrovascular diseases, seizure disorders, brain tumours, substance abuse, etc.) varies substantially across cultural groups.

Aetiology

The NCD (Dementias) are subcategorised according to presumed aetiology (see Table 7.1). For the purposes of this book, only some of the aetiological subtypes will be discussed.

NCD (Dementia) due to Alzheimer's Disease

Alzheimer's disease is the most common cause of NCD (Dementia), occurring in 50% or more of all cases. Factors that are considered major risks are family history of Alzheimer's disease, genetic factors (e.g. links to chromosomes 1, 14, and 21, multiple E4 genes, and amyloid deposits), and head injury. While there are variations or subtypes of Alzheimer's disease, generally speaking the onset is subtle, in that there are initial symptoms of memory impairment and gradual, general deterioration in cognitive abilities (Sadock & Sadock, 2007). The pathology is associated with the parietal and temporal regions of the brain.

NCD (Dementia) due to Vascular Disease

Cerebrovascular disease, which affects blood vessels in the brain, is considered to be the second-most common cause of NCD (Dementia). Mainly small and medium-size vessels may undergo infarction, which is death or damage as a result of obstruction to the local blood supply. This results in multiple lesions, involving changes to structures in the brain. These infarctions may be due to injury or disease in the brain. NCD (Dementia) associated with cerebrovascular disease usually has an abrupt onset and fluctuating course. The risk factors associated with this NCD (Dementia) are hypertension, diabetes, advanced age, stroke, alcoholism, and other cardiovascular risk factors such as smoking and obesity. This disorder tends to be more common in men. Compared to Alzheimer's disease, patients with Vascular NCD (Dementia) are more like to have depression, affective changes, disturbance of gait, and confusion, which is often more noticeable in the evenings (Sadock & Sadock, 2007).

Parkinson's disease is a disorder that affects nerve cells in the part of the brain controlling muscle movement. It is a disease of the basal ganglia and belongs to a group of conditions called motor system disorders, which are the result of the loss of dopamine-producing brain cells. The sufferer typically demonstrates slow movement. This NCD (Dementia) is commonly associated with depression.

NCD (Dementia) due to Huntington's disease

Huntington's disease results from genetically influenced degeneration of brain cells in subcortical areas of the brain (brain stem, thalamus, basal ganglia, or tracts connecting these areas to the frontal lobe). Huntington's disease is passed genetically from parent to child. Each child of a Huntington's disease parent has a 50–50 chance of inheriting the Huntington's disease gene. If a child does not inherit the gene, they will not develop the disease and cannot pass it on to subsequent generations. A person who inherits the gene will sooner or later develop the disease. The NCD (Dementia) associated with this disease is characterised by more motor abnormalities (slow or uncontrolled motor movement) and fewer language abnormalities. This degeneration also causes loss of intellectual abilities and emotional disturbance. The person with this disease has difficulty with complex tasks.

Figure 7.2: MRI image – demonstrates bilateral atrophy of the head of the caudate nuclei and compensatory ventricular dilatation of the frontal horns bilaterally suggestive of Huntington's disease

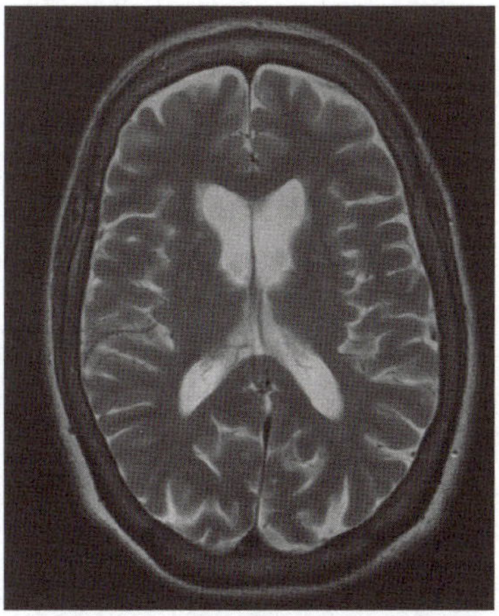

Major or Mild Frontotemporal NCD (Dementia)

In the DSM-IV-TR this disorder was referred to as Dementia due to Pick's disease, but this has changed in DSM-5 to reflect the neuroanatomical area that is affected, rather than the underlying aetiology. This disorder is characterised by atrophy or shrinking of the frontal and temporal regions of the brains (see Figure 7.3). In the early stages of this disorder, there is some executive dysfunction however personality and behavioural changes are prominent with cognitive functions remaining intact.

Figure 7.3: CT scan of Pick's disease

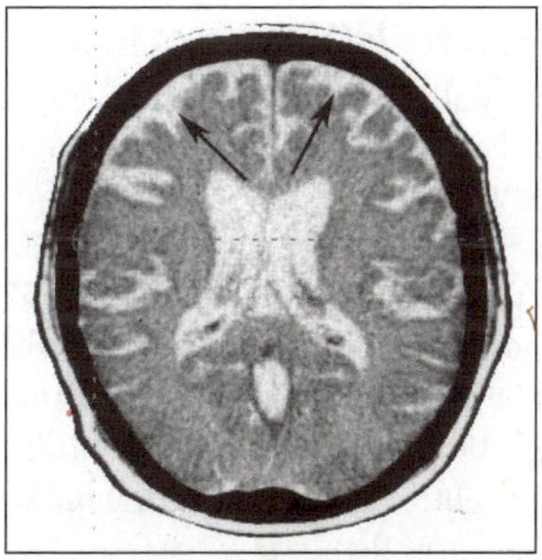

Source: http://petscans.info/PETfdgPicks.jpg&imgrefurl/

NCD (Dementia) due to Lewy body disease

Lewy body disease is a NCD (Dementia) associated with Lewy inclusion bodies found in the cerebral cortex (see Figure 7.4). Lewy bodies are round deposits which contain damaged nerve cells. It is believed that they are formed as the cells try to protect themselves from attack. This disorder presents in a similar way to Alzheimer's but is more rapid and characterised by greater deficits in attention, psychomotor speed, and verbal fluency. Other features are hallucinations, Parkinsonian-type and other motor features, and extrapyramidal signs (abnormal involuntary movements, alterations in muscle tone, and postural disturbances).

Figure 7.4: Microscopic image of a Lewy body

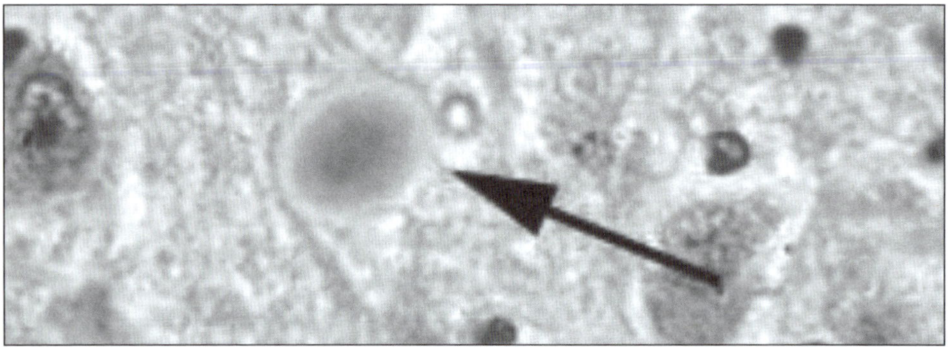

Source: http://www.nlm.nih.gov/medlineplus/images/lewybody.jpg

NCD (Dementia) due to Prion disease

This disorder includes NCDs due to a group of subacute spongiform encephalopathies (e.g. Creutzfeldt-Jakob disease, which is more commonly known as 'mad cow disease') (APA, 2013) is. The disorder has an insidious onset with rapid progression of impairment (from minor to major impairments within six months) (APA, 2013). Motor symptoms, such as ataxia, abnormal movements are prominent in this disorder.

NCD (Dementia) due to HIV infection

HIV/AIDS contributes substantially to the burden of disease in developing countries and in sub-Saharan Africa in particular. There are an estimated 25 million individuals living with HIV across Africa (UNAIDS/WHO, 2006). NCD (Dementia) that is associated with direct HIV infection of the central nervous system is typically characterised by forgetfulness, slowness, poor concentration, and difficulties with problem-solving. Behavioural manifestations most commonly include apathy and social withdrawal. Occasionally, these may be accompanied by delirium, delusions, or hallucinations. NCD (Dementia) in association with HIV infection may also result from accompanying central nervous system tumours (e.g. primary central nervous system lymphoma) and from opportunistic infections (e.g. tuberculosis and syphilis).

Figure 7.5: HIV particles adhering to a CD4 lymphocyte

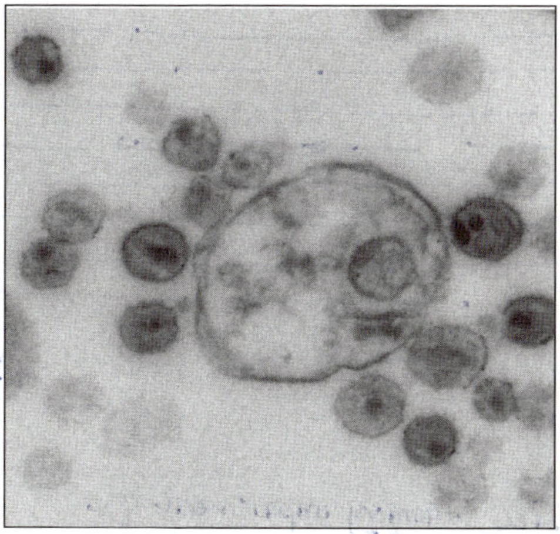

Source: Courtesy of Optics and and Imaging Centre Nelson R Mandela School of Medicine, University of KwaZulu-Natal.

NCD (Dementia) due to traumatic brain injury

The prevalence of head trauma is extremely high in South Africa given the high rate of motor vehicle accidents (MVAs) and high level of violence. The extrapolated prevalence of traumatic brain injury for South Africa and other countries is presented in Table 7.5. Head injury-related NCD (Dementia) is characterised by emotional lability, dysarthria (speech impairment), and impulsivity.

Table 7.5: Traumatic brain injury in southern Africa (extrapolated statistics)

Country	Prevalence	Population
Angola	21 957	10 978 552
Botswana	3 278	1 639 231
South Africa	88 896	44 448 470
Swaziland	2 338	1 169 241
Zambia	22 051	11 025 690
Zimbabwe	7 343	12 671 860

Source: http://www.wrongdiagnosis.com/t/traumatic_brain_injury/stats-country.htm

NCD (Dementia) due to substance/medication use

This disorder results from the abuse of drugs or medication, or from toxin exposure. Such substances include alcohol, inhalants, sedatives, hypnotics, or anxiolytics (medication for the treatment of anxious states).

Treatment and management of NCD (Dementia)

As with delirium, treating the underlying cause of NCD (Dementia) is necessary although the condition most often is not reversible. However, by understanding the aetiology of the NCD (Dementia), it may be possible to arrest or reverse the process. In some cases, especially in NCD (Dementia) due to Vascular disease, preventative measures may be possible. Preventative measures may include changes in diet and exercise, as well as blood-pressure monitoring. Changes in cognitive function significantly affect sufferers who can benefit immensely from supportive and educational psychotherapy. In addition, assistance in dealing with loss and grief is also important for both the individual and their family.

AMNESTIC DISORDERS (ICD-10)

Historically, the DSM-IV-TR made provision for a group of disorders known as amnestic disorders. Although the DSM-5 no longer has this category, the ICD-10 does.

Clinical picture

An amnestic disorder is characterised by memory impairment in the absence of other significant accompanying cognitive impairments. The syndrome is characterised by the inability to learn new information (anterograde amnesia), and the inability to recall knowledge stored from before the onset of the disorder (retrograde amnesia). Short-term and recent memory is usually affected. Patients often cannot remember what they had for breakfast or the name of their doctor. The onset can be sudden (e.g. when the cause is trauma, cerebrovascular events, or toxic substances) or gradual (e.g. cerebral tumours). Amnestic disorders are also subcategorised according to presumed aetiology: Amnestic Disorder Due to a General Medical Condition (such as head injury), Substance-Induced Persisting Amnestic Disorder (induced by, for example, excessive alcohol consumption or carbon monoxide poisoning), or Amnestic Disorder Not Otherwise Specified (Sadock & Sadock, 2007). The criteria for amnestic disorders are specified in Table 7.6.

Table 7.6: Diagnostic criteria for amnestic disorders as adapted from the ICD-10

Amnestic Disorders
The primary requirements for this diagnosis are: • Memory impairment as shown in impairment of recent memory (learning of new material); disturbances of time sense (rearrangements of chronological sequence, telescoping of repeated events into one, etc.). • Absence of defect in immediate recall, of impairment of consciousness, and of generalised cognitive impairment. • History or objective evidence of chronic (and particularly high-dose) use of alcohol or drugs. • Personality changes, often with apparent apathy and loss of initiative, and a tendency towards self-neglect may also be present, but should not be regarded as necessary conditions for diagnosis. • Although confabulation may be marked, it should not be regarded as a necessary prerequisite for diagnosis.

Source: Reprinted with permission from the ICD–10 Classification of Mental and Behavioural Disorders: Diagnostic Criteria for Research. World Health Organisation (WHO), Geneva, 2007.

Epidemiology

There are no adequate studies on the incidence and prevalence of amnestic disorders. They are most commonly found in association with excessive use of alcohol and traumatic head injury. We would imagine the prevalence to be significantly high in South Africa given the high levels of head injury due to motor vehicle accidents and other violence (e.g. armed assaults, grievous bodily harm, and domestic violence). This violence is often complicated or exacerbated by irresponsible use of alcohol.

Aetiology

The main brain areas that are implicated in the amnestic disorders are the temporal lobes, midline nuclei of the thalamus, hippocampus, mamillary bodies, and the amygdala. The left hemisphere is more implicated than the right.

Some symptoms associated with the frontal lobes are usually seen in amnestic disorders. These symptoms include confabulation (fabrication of detailed, plausible experiences and events to cover gaps in memory) and apathy. There are several possible causes for amnestic disorders.

These include (Sadock & Sadock, 2007):

- Systemic conditions (such as thiamine or Vitamin B_1 deficiency)
- Hypoglycaemia (low blood sugar)
- Brain-related conditions like hypoxia (low oxygen)
- Seizures and epilepsies
- Surgical procedures to the brain
- Infections (e.g. herpes simplex encephalitis)
- Tumours
- Cerebrovascular diseases
- Substance-related conditions (related to e.g. alcohol, neurotoxins, sedatives, and many over-the-counter drugs).

Some of these causes are discussed in more detail below:

- ***Cerebrovascular diseases:*** These usually affect the hippocampus and involve the posterior cerebral and basilar arteries and their branches. Infarctions rarely involve only the hippocampus but, more commonly, also affect the occipital and parietal lobes.
- ***Multiple sclerosis:*** Memory disorder is the most common cognitive complaint in patients with multiple sclerosis.
- ***Korsakoff's syndrome:*** This is an amnestic syndrome caused by thiamine deficiency and is commonly associated with chronic alcohol abuse. The neglect of proper eating by chronic alcohol abusers is the cause for the thiamine deficiency. Individuals with Korsakoff's also demonstrate personality changes and a lack of initiative, spontaneity, and general interests. Confabulation, apathy, and passivity are also common.
- ***Alcoholic blackouts:*** Individuals with severe alcohol abuse may present with memory loss of the events that occurred while they were intoxicated.
- ***Head injury:*** Amnesia is a common symptom in head injury. Usually the amnesia is retrograde and includes the actual traumatic event.

- ***Transient Global Amnesia:*** This syndrome is characterised by the abrupt loss of the ability to recall recent events or to remember new information. It is associated with mild confusion, lack of insight, and the inability to perform previously learned complex tasks. The condition usually last for 24 hours.

Treatment and management of amnestic disorders

As in all of the cognitive disorders, the primary approach to treatment of the amnestic disorders is to treat the underlying cause. Thus, the initial treatment is directed to the underlying pathological process.

If the underlying cause is primary, systemic, or cerebral, the treatment may include the use of thiamine, antiretroviral medication, or aspirin. Sometimes drugs which seem to improve memory in patients with Alzheimer's disease may be used. However, despite the variety of pharmaco-therapeutic trials that have been undertaken, no drug treatments have been proved effective in amnestic disorder (Sadock & Sadock, 2007).

For mild cases of amnesia, rehabilitation may involve teaching memory techniques and employing the use of memory tools, such as calendars, lists, notes, timers, and association techniques. These memory exercises and retraining can be very useful. Helpful prompting of the date, time, and location is also known to reduce anxiety.

Patients with amnestic disorder also experience considerable difficulty in their social and occupational functioning. To help such patients, emotional and social support may be necessary. They may also require supervised living conditions to ensure that appropriate feeding and care occurs. Many patients do slowly recover over time and sometimes they may even recover memories that were formed before the onset of the amnestic disorder. It is useful, particularly after the remission of the amnestic episode, to provide psychotherapy or counselling in order to help the individual adjust to their period of illness and to aid their recovery.

ASSESSMENT OF NEUROCOGNITIVE DISORDERS

The assessment usually begins with a review of the clinical notes of doctors or information recorded in the hospital or clinic files. This is followed by clinical interviews, observation, and basic screening tests.

Several simple screening tests and/or rapid assessments are undertaken by the clinician. The most common is the Mini Mental Status Examination (MMSE), which is a quick way to evaluate cognitive function. The test has a set of questions and tasks that assess orientation, memory, attention, concentration, calculation, language, and consciousness (see Table 7.7). The MMSE has been traditionally used to screen for cognitive impairment in a variety of dementia illnesses, including HIV-associated dementia.

Table 7.7: Mini Mental Status Examination

Task	Instructions
Date orientation	'Tell me the date?'
Place orientation	'Where are you?'
Register three objects	Name three objects slowly and clearly. Ask the patient to repeat them.
Serial sevens	Ask the patient to count backwards from 100 by 7. Stop after five answers. (Or ask them to spell 'world' backwards.)
Recall three objects	Ask the patient to recall the objects mentioned above.
Naming	Point to your watch and ask the patient 'What is this?' Repeat with a pencil.
Repeating a phrase	Ask the patient to say 'no ifs, ands, or buts'.
Verbal commands	Give the patient a plain piece of paper and say 'Take this paper in your right hand, fold it in half, and put it on the floor.'
Written commands	Show the patient a piece of paper with 'CLOSE YOUR EYES' printed on it.
Writing	Ask the patient to write a sentence.
Drawing	Ask the patient to copy a pair of intersecting pentagons on a piece of paper.

Source: Adapted from Folstein, Folstein, & McHugh, 1975.

Probably the most widely used test to quantify the level of consciousness is the Glasgow Coma Scale (GCS). It is simple and correlates well with outcome following severe brain injury. Scores are given for eye-opening response (e.g. whether the patient does not open their eyes, or opens their eyes spontaneously, or opens their eyes to a painful stimuli or to light), verbal response (e.g. whether the patient makes no sounds, makes incomprehensible sounds, utters inappropriate words, or responds normally to questions), and motor response (e.g. whether the patient makes no movement, responds to painful stimuli by withdrawing, or obeys a command to perform a motor activity). Performance on the GCS total score is used to establish the level of consciousness.

Another simple and commonly used test is the Clock Drawing Test (CDT). The CDT is used to assess cognitive functioning in psychiatric and neurological settings. The patient is asked to draw the face of a clock with all the numbers on it. The patient is then asked to draw the hands pointing to ten past eleven. The drawing is scored for accuracy of the representation of the clock face, the layout of numbers, and the position of the hands. Total cut-off scores are used to indicate whether the drawing is suggestive of dementia. The test is used as a clinical screening task for visuo-spatial and constructional disabilities and can be useful as a dementia screening device (Spreen & Strauss, 1991). For examples of the deterioration on the CDT see Figures 7.6 and 7.7.

Figure 7.6: Examples of stimulus-bound and conceptual errors on the Clock Drawing Test

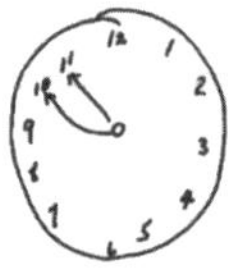

(a) 'Pure' stimulus-bound response.

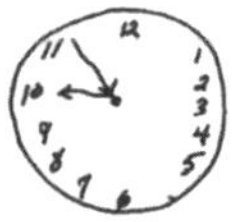

(b) SB(B): stimulus-bound and conceptual error.

(c) 'Closing-in' in the copy condition.

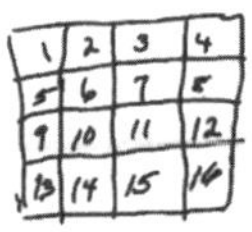

(d) Misrepresentation of the clock (and a spatial error).

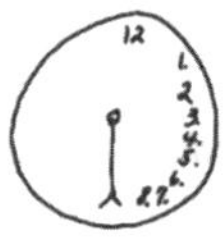

(e) Misrepresentation of the clock (and a spatial error).

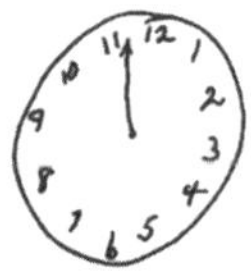

(f) Misrepresentation of the time on the clock.

Source: © Rouleau et al., 1996. Reprinted from: Brain and Cognition, 32(1), Rouleau, I., Salmon, D. P., Butters, N. Longitudinal analysis of clock drawing in Alzheimer's disease patients, pp. 17-34 © 1996, with permission from Elsevier.

Figure 7.7: Examples of spatial and/or planning deficits in the layout of numbers and perseverative errors on the Clock Drawing Test

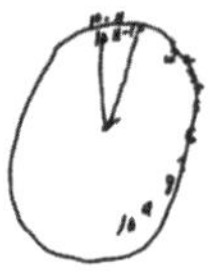

(a) Neglect of the left hemispace (and a conceptual error).

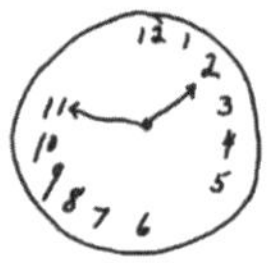

(b) Planning deficit.

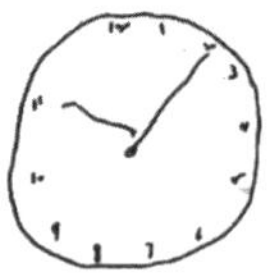

(c) Nonspecific spatial errors in the layout of numbers.

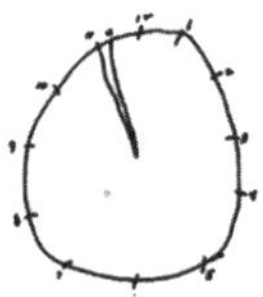

(d) Numbers written outside the clockface.

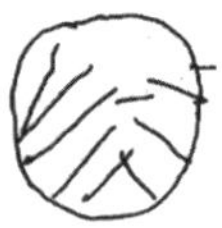

(e) Perseveration of hands.

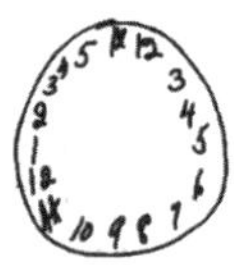

(f) Perseveration of numbers.

Source: © Rouleau et al., 1996. Reprinted from: Brain and Cognition, 32(1), Rouleau, I., Salmon, D. P., Butters, N. Longitudinal analysis of clock drawing in Alzheimer's disease patients, pp. 17-34 © 1996, with permission from Elsevier.

There are several dementia scales that are used to rate the patient's functioning on various criteria. Some of these scales are rated by the attending practitioner or family/caregivers so that the clinician is not dependent on the report of the ill patient. Commonly used scales are the International HIV Dementia Scale (HDS), Deterioration Cognitive Observee (DECO), or the Clinical Dementia Scale (CDS). The HDS was developed as a bedside evaluation test to differentiate patients with HIV-associated dementia from those who are cognitively normal. A South African study found that the HDS correlates positively with the MMSE and identified more participants demonstrating cognitive impairment than the MMSE (Ganasen, Finchama, Smit, Seedat, & Stein, 2007). In another South African study, the DECO scores were also found to correlate well with MMSE scores and clinicians' ratings (Lenger, De Villiers, & Louw, 1996). See Table 7.8 for an example of a few items from the DECO (Ritchie & Fuhrer, 1992; 1994).

Table 7.8: Instructions and sample of DECO items

We would like you to tell us how your relative was a year ago. The following questions ask about a number of everyday situations. We would like you to tell us whether in these situations he/she is doing about the same, not as well, or much worse, than a year ago. Put a cross in the square to show your reply.

	Better or about the same	Not as well	Much worse
Does he/she remember as well as before which day and which month it is?			
When he/she goes out of the house, does he/she know the way as well as before?			
Have there been changes in his/her ability to remember his/ her own address or telephone number?			

Source: Ritchie & Fuhrer, 1994.

There are more sophisticated neuropsychological assessments which are normally done after the initial screening tests indicate a cognitive disorder. Such neuropsychological assessments are usually administered and conducted by experienced psychologists and those specialising in neuropsychology. These neuropsychological tests may be administered individually or as a complete battery. See Chapter 1 for a more detailed discussion of these tests.

Other useful and also necessary assessments are the neuro-imaging techniques such as X-rays, Magnetic Resonance Imaging (MRI), Functional Magnetic Resonance Imaging (fMRI), and Positron Emission Tomography (PET) scans, as well as other laboratory tests. These are extremely helpful in the diagnosis of cognitive disorders but are extremely expensive and not always readily available.

CONTEXTUAL AND CROSS-CULTURAL PERSPECTIVES

Individual and group beliefs and attitudes influence health behaviour. Therefore, all disorders and illness behaviours are strongly influenced by cultural and contextual factors. Further, cultural and social beliefs, and environment, also influence the way health care facilities are used (Pillay, 1996). Although Western medicine plays a dominant role in the mass control of disease, traditional or folk medicine continues to play an important role in the health care of communities. People possess unique attitudes, values, and beliefs about health and illness which integrally influence their health behaviour. When working in multicultural settings, it is important to be aware of the cultural and language differences that can influence a diagnosis of cognitive disorders.

In addition to culture and social background, educational background and environmental factors must be taken into consideration when one evaluates an individual's mental capacity or disorders (Jinabhai et al., 2004; Ngcobo & Pillay, 2008; Pillay, 2000). In South Africa, past inequalities in education, and the consequent lack of facilities and resources, significantly impact on the evaluation and understanding of individuals with cognitive disorders.

Some of the symptoms associated with cognitive disorders, such as disorientation, changes in consciousness, forgetfulness, amnesia, seizures, dissociation, delusions, or changes in behaviour and personality, may be accounted for differently by different indigenous world views. For example, according to traditional African views, some of these symptoms may be explained as:

- *Ukuthwasa*, the calling to be a traditional healer whose role is to help in the caring and healing process of the whole person, addressing the condition, and also restoring balance by addressing the alleged causes of the illness.
- *Ukufa kwabantu*, which broadly means 'the illnesses of the people' and is not recognised by the patient as an illness or disease per se, but as a disturbance caused by breaking a taboo or displeasing an ancestor, or due to a spell that has been cast on the patient. These include:
    - *Indiki*, *ufufunyane*, or *izizwe* (spirit possession)
    - *Umnyama* (pollution or contamination)
    - *Ubuthakathi* (bewitchment or sorcery)
    - *Ukuphonsa* (curses or spells)
    - *Umkhondo/umeqo/idliso* (some form of poisoning).

BOX 7.3

Ubuthakathi is the 'direct' use of traditional herbs or ointments or medicines which can be either sprinkled over someone else's food or yard or applied anywhere in order to come into physical contact with the person. It always has evil intentions.

Ukuphonsa is 'indirect'. Literally translated as 'throwing', it implies distance. It can be done even when there is no way of actually coming into contact with the medicine that is used. It may have good intentions, e.g. to gain the love of someone.

All cultures and religious groups have traditional explanations for 'abnormal behaviour'. In Islam, magic, sorcery, and witchcraft all fall under the term *sihr*. Belief in demonic possessions and the existence of *jinn* also form part of the culture of Islam.

According to Hussain and Cochrane (2002), jinn are a separate 'race' that can appear in different forms and can cause harm by possessing a human. Jinn can also cause physical illness, anger, or sadness. They can be used by sorcerers to wreck marriages, cause mental illness, and inflict constant pain in the body or even epilepsy (Abdussalam-Bali, 2004; Hussain & Cochrane, 2004; Karim, Saeed, Rana, Mubbashar, & Jenkins, 2004). Jinn possession also manifests with bizarre, multiple behaviours, and odd movements. Similar explanations about spirit possession are common in other Eastern religions, as well as among some Christian groups.

It seems that Western patients rely mainly on answers from technological medicine whereas more traditional cultures or religious groups seek divination from a healer, who can restore the equilibrium of their lives. About 80% to 90% of people from developing societies rely on traditional healing for health care. The DSM-5 uses the term 'Culture-Bound Syndrome' for many of these conditions; this refers to 'recurrent, locality-specific patterns of aberrant behaviour and troubling experience that may or may not be linked to a particular DSM-5 diagnostic category'.

Meyer, Moore, and Viljoen (2002) argue that it is essential to consider a patient's cultural context when they present in a health care setting. Ignoring (or being ignorant of) a patient's cultural context and their belief system risks misdiagnosis, the application of inappropriate therapeutic techniques, and great distress and pain for the patient.

Further, most neuropsychological and psychological assessments were developed in Western contexts but are widely used in South Africa, and other developing countries, where the contexts are very different. In addition, level of education significantly contributes to the variations in the scores on these tests (Brodrick, 2002; Lenger, de Villiers, & Louw, 1996) and cultural differences in cognitive and perceptual information-processing are known to influence performance even on the non-verbal tests. Individuals from some backgrounds may not be familiar with the information used in certain tests of general knowledge (e.g. names of presidents, geographical knowledge), memory (e.g. date of birth in cultures that do not routinely celebrate birthdays), or orientation (e.g. sense of place and location may be conceptualised differently in some cultures). Thus, in some populations (such as immigrants), attributing low scores to pathological processes rather than to other factors can result in diagnostic error and/or over-diagnosis of significant morbidity, as well as over-prescribed treatment (Klimidis & Tokgoz, 2008).

CONCLUSION

Increasing longevity as a result of better health, diets, and living conditions, as well as changes in lifestyle, contribute to the steady increase of the prevalence of cognitive disorders. Depending on the classification system being used, cognitive disorders may be divided into three main groups: delirium, dementia, and amnestic disorders. In each category, the aetiology of the disorder influences the onset, course, treatment, and outcome of the disorder. Symptoms of different cognitive disorders also occur in other medical conditions. This, as well as the influence of beliefs, and cultural and contextual factors, makes diagnosis and treatment of these disorders complicated and difficult.

MULTIPLE-CHOICE QUESTIONS

1. The three categories of cognitive disorders in the ICD-10 are:
   a) delirium, dementia, and amnestic disorders
   b) delirium, dementia, and Alzheimer's
   c) Alzheimer's, delirium, and amnestic disorders
   d) Alzheimer's, organic, and amnestic disorders

2. The symptoms of delirium tend to develop:
   a) very slowly, over the course of several years
   b) very quickly, over the course of a few hours to a few days
   c) moderately slowly, over the course of several months
   d) either very quickly or very slowly, depending on the cause

3. The gradual deterioration of brain functioning that affects judgement, memory, language, and other cognitive processes, is called:
   a) Major or Mild Neurocognitive disorders (dementia)
   b) delirium
   c) amnestic disorder
   d) mental retardation

4. Neurocognitive disorders that are caused by HIV appears to be due to:
   a) infection by the HI virus
   b) side effects of antiretroviral treatment
   c) opportunistic infections that occur in HIV patients
   d) imbalances in the neurotransmitters

5. Compared to most disorders, Huntington's disease is very unusual because it is:
   a) the result of one gene
   b) influenced by many genes

c) always a cause of dementia
d) associated with subcortical impairment

6. The main impairment in amnestic disorders is an inability to:
   a) transfer information from the short-term memory into long-term memory
   b) remember significant events from the distant past
   c) perform basic arithmetic
   d) remember one's own name

PARAGRAPH AND ESSAY QUESTIONS

1. Define 'Neurocognitive disorders'.

2. Name the three main types of Neurocognitive disorders as described in the DSM-5.

3. Name the maintpps of Neurocognitive disorders as described in the ICD-10 and describe how each of these disorders are subclassified?

4. Provide a description of the main domains of Neurocognitive functions?

5. Write an essay on the clinical picture, epidemiology, aetiology and treatment of Major or Minor Neurocognitive disorders.

6. Distinguish between delirium and NCD (Dementia).

7. With reference to the ICD-10, how are amnestic disorders different from delirium and dementia?

8. Describe the aetiological subtypes of NCD.

9. Briefly explain Korsakoff's Syndrome.

10. What are the common assessments used in establishing a Neurocognitive disorder?

11. Write a brief essay on the assessment of Neurocognitive disorders.

12. Neurocognitive disorders (like all mental disorders and illness behaviours) are strongly influenced by cultural and contextual factors. Explain.

8 DISSOCIATIVE AND SOMATIC SYMPTOM AND RELATED DISORDERS

Larise du Plessis and Conrad Visser

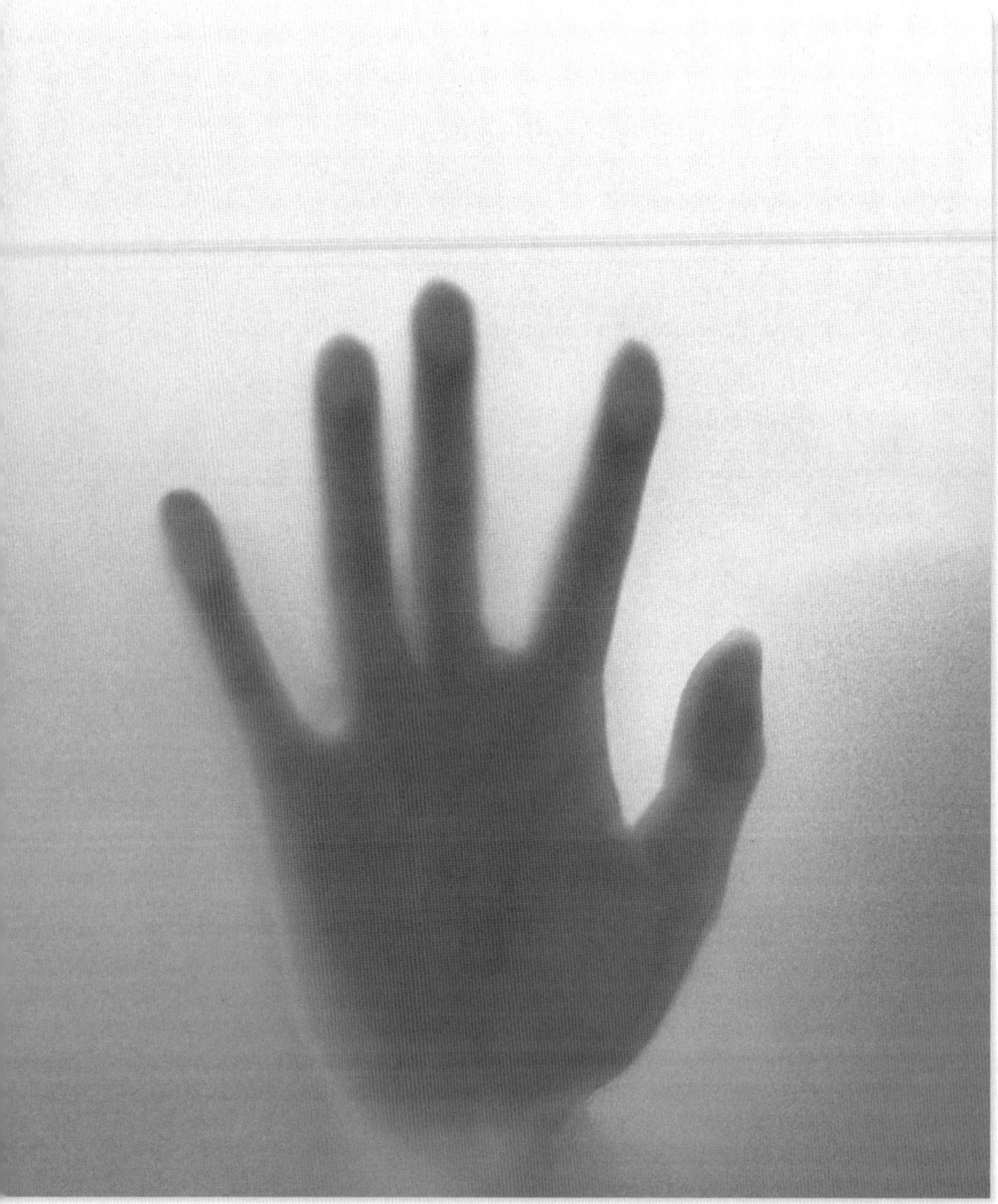

8 CHAPTER OUTLINE

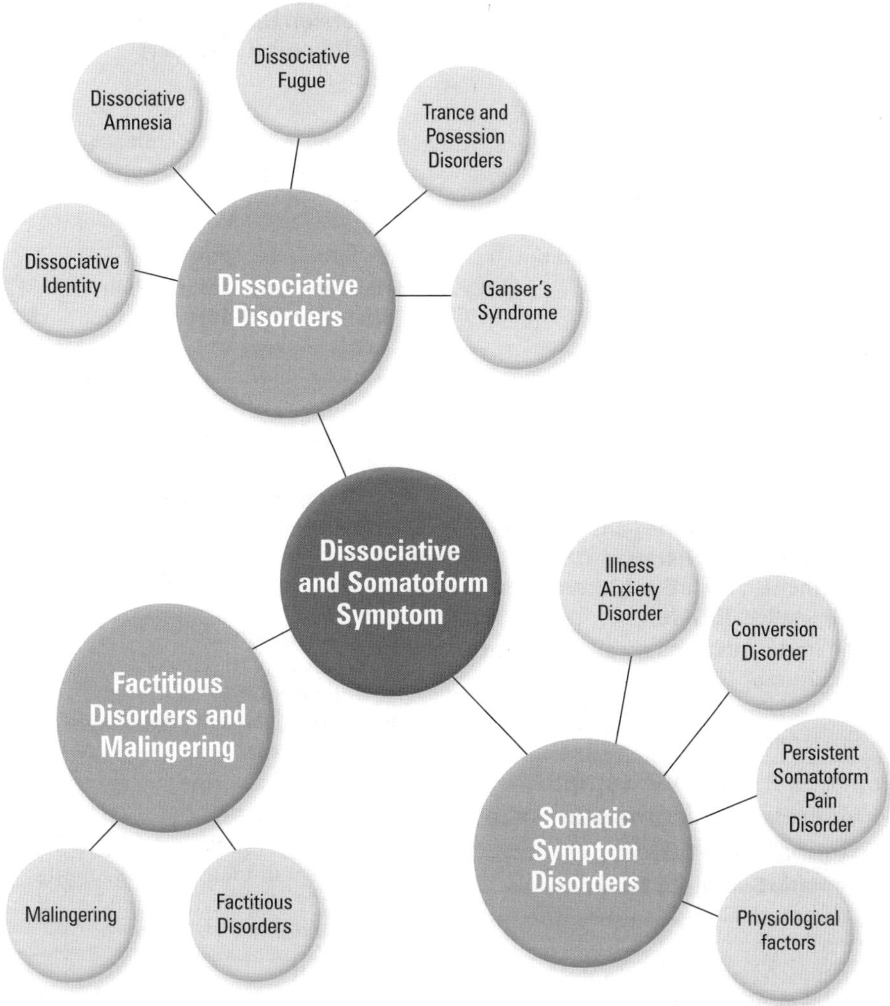

LEARNING OUTCOMES

After studying this chapter you should be able to:

- Describe the concepts of dissociation and somatising.
- Discuss the association between early adversity, trauma, dissociation, and somatising.
- Provide an overview of the psychological processes of compartmentalisation and detachment.
- Provide an overview of current nosological approaches to dissociative and somatoform disorders.
- Describe the aetiology, pathogenesis, epidemiology, clinical features, and differential diagnoses of dissociative and somatic symptom and related disorders, as classified by the DSM-5.
- Describe conditions other than the dissociative disorders which are characterised by prominent dissociation.
- Describe culture-specific conditions with strong dissociative phenomena.
- Discuss *amafufunyana* and *ukuthwasa* in relation to dissociation.
- Describe Ganser's Syndrome.
- Discuss Psychological factors affecting other medical conditions.
- Describe the factitious disorders.
- Define malingering and give an approach to the detection of deceit in clinical practice.

INTRODUCTION

The DSM-5, as was the case with the previous editions of the DSM, has two separate categories for these disorders; however, for the purposes of this book, we have elected to combine the dissociative disorders (Section 1) and somatoform disorders (Section 2) together in one chapter. Our decision to preserve this format is based on the obvious neuroscientific and clinical similarities exhibited by the two categories.

Attempts at systematic classification of dissociative and somatising conditions began in the nineteenth century. Ever since, conceptualisations and classifications have undergone repeated revisions. In the first edition, we considered the limitations of the existing DSM and ICD approaches to the disorders and speculated about future reconceptualisation and categorical realignment of disorder constructs. Speculation was fuelled by the prevailing unwieldiness of some of the constructs, on the one hand, and useful insights gained from advances in neuroscience over the past two decades, on the other. In their continuing effort to make disorder constructs more practicable, the authors of the fifth edition of the *Diagnostic and Statistical Manual of Mental Disorders* (DSM-5) have proposed a set of refinements to the alignment, terminology, and diagnostic criteria of dissociative and somatoform conditions (see Figure 8.1).

Since much categorical overlap exists between disorders characterised by dissociation and somatising, we decided to discuss representative conditions without dogmatically assigning each to one or the other diagnostic category. We also provide a comparative overview of related conditions from around the world as well as South African culture-specific syndromes. We also include the factitious disorders and malingering in the chapter, as they may present with bodily symptoms and are regulars on differentials lists.

Figure 8.1: Summary of Dissociative Disorders and Somatic Symptom and Related Disorders in DSM-5

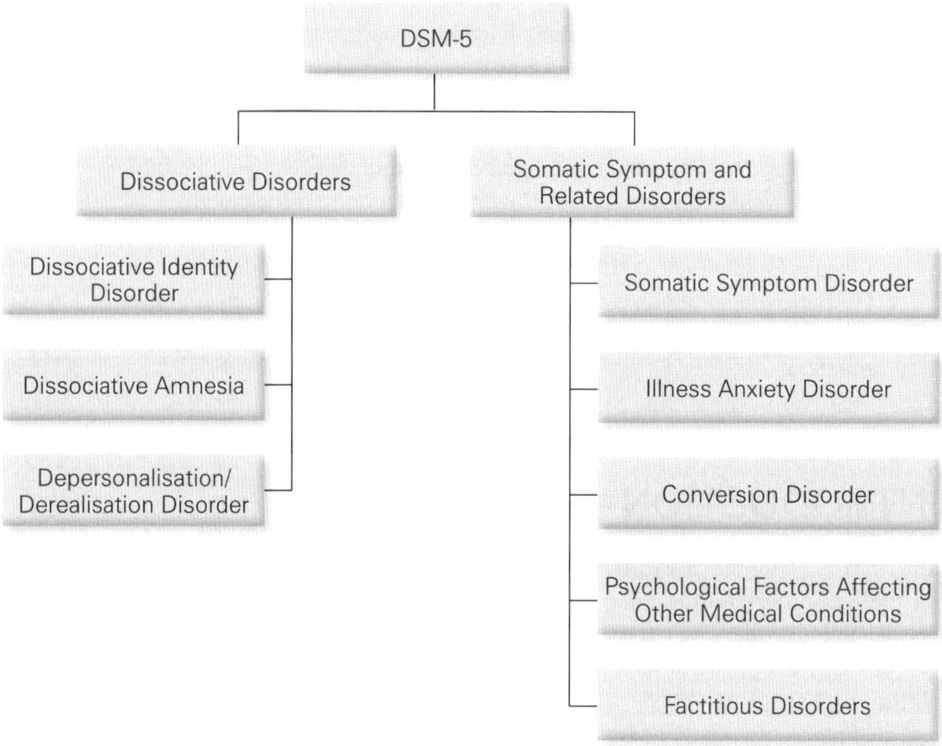

DISSOCIATION, SOMATISING, AND STRESS

What is dissociation?

As a phenomenon, dissociation is common. We have all experienced it in one form or another. In the course of normal human experience, when faced with a major threat, we can feel detached from ourselves, as if we look upon our own actions from the outside, experience the world as unreal, or have little or no recall of a trauma. Normal dissociation is not limited to stressful situations; it also occurs when bored, engaged in monotonous activities, and when meditating, tired or sleepy. But, dissociation can also mean pathology where we recognise a surprisingly wide range of conditions. Table 8.1 summarises states and conditions causing dissociation.

What causes dissociation?

Cardeña's (1994) overview of dissociation provides a simple model and practical point of departure to understanding how dissociation relates to threat. He viewed dissociation as comprising three distinct features:

- Suspended integration of mental modules (mental systems or information streams)
- Altered state of consciousness
- A defence mechanism.

Recent insights into the neural mechanisms at play in dissociation highlight these very features. Mindful of this, its expression in animals and the fact that dissociation is not limited to stressful situations, we propose to restate Cardeña's model to broaden its conceptualisation: Dissociation is a genetically endowed trait, adapted as a defence to threat that suspends the integration of mental systems and alters consciousness. As a defence mechanism, it partners 'fight' and 'flight'. It operates throughout the animal kingdom and, by virtue of the survival advantage it confers, is preserved across generations. Cardeňa further conceptualised dissociation to involve two distinct psychological processes: compartmentalisation and detachment. Each process possesses its own distinct nearal circuitry.

Table 8.1: Conditions and situations associated with dissociation

Mental disorders
Dissociative disorders Panic Attack (partially mediated by metabolic effects of hyperventilation) Acute Stress Disorder and Posttraumatic Stress Disorder Borderline Personality Disorder Somatoform disorders Schizophrenia and other psychotic states Somnambulism ('sleepwalking') Dementia and delirium
Substance-related states
Alcohol Cannabis (dagga) Sedative-hypnotics (e.g. benzodiazepines like diazepam; older antihistamines like cyclizine) Hallucinogens (e.g. lysergic acid diethylamide – LSD; phencyclidine and ketamine) Opiates (morphine-like) Steroids Antipsychotic agents Lithium Anticholinergic agents

Neurological and general medical conditions
Hypoxia (insufficient oxygen-supply to brain)
Metabolic disturbances (e.g. alkalosis, hypoglycaemia, hyponatraemia, hypocalcaemia)
Organ failure (kidney and liver)
Hypertensive encephalopathy
Cerebral infections (e.g. herpes simplex encephalitis, falciparum malaria)
Cerebral neoplasms (e.g. astrocytoma, glioblastoma multiforme, metastases)
Postconcussion
Stroke (especially if involves brain stem, basal forebrain, thalamic and medial attentional structures)
Transient Global Amnesia
Wernicke-Korsakoff Syndrome (Vitamin B1 – Thiamine – deficiency)
Epilepsies (e.g. temporal lobe epilepsy)
Migraine
Post-operative states (unique combination of stress response and fluid, electrolyte, and metabolic changes)

Compartmentalisation

Corresponding to the suspension of mental integration, compartmentalisation is the inability to control processes and take actions through acts of volition. Put differently, compartmentalisation is the inability to bring information usually accessible to consciousness (and thereby susceptible to conscious influence) into conscious awareness. Compartmentalised processes continue to function in spite of their disconnection from conscious awareness and other mental processes. Compartmentalisation can manifest as amnesia and other deficits like blindness, loss of tactile sensation, and paralysis.

Anatomically and functionally, the brain's cortex is arranged hierarchically. Primary cortical regions are devoted to single operations and are subordinate to higher-order or association cortical regions. Compartmentalisation relies on this top-down regulation of subordinate cortical regions responsible for sensory or motor processing by the higher-order cortices. If the motor system is involved, paralysis results, without any demonstrable pathology of the apparatus of movement. If it involves modality-specific sensory systems, the patient becomes blind, deaf, or loses the sense of touch. The 'lesion' responsible for this dissociation is not anatomical, but functional. With paralysis, it is as if the primary motor cortex, responsible for transmitting the final command for the contraction of a muscle group, had been 'taken off-line', its activity suspended by higher-order motor cortex like the prefrontal cortex. Evidence for this exists in functional brain imaging. Figures 8.2 and 8.3 illustrate compartmentalisation.

This apparently bizarre situation is one expression of the fear response and confers survival advantage on animals possessing the trait. In the animal kingdom, paralysis is a common defensive behaviour. We have all heard of an animal rolling over and 'playing dead'. In neuroscientific parlance, 'playing dead' is called 'freezing', or 'tonic immobility'. The immobile prey survives a possible death as it escapes detection by its predator. The sensory equivalent can result in anaesthesia and analgesia, with diminished tactile sensation and dampened experience of pain. Freezing and anaesthesia partner fight and flight as behavioural phenomena characteristic of the fear response. A behaviour not unlike tonic immobility probably became entrenched in Neolithic man, conceivably increasing the odds on surviving battle.

Figure 8.2: This diagram depicts the hierarchical arrangement of motor integration and information flow in the brain. Sensory and other information is fed to higher-order motor cortices (prefrontal cortex and cingulate gyrus), represented by Process AA. Process A indicates hierarchical flow of information from highest to lowest order motor cortex (viz. prefrontal to primary) whence the final instruction is passed onto the appropriate muscles to contract. Process B indicates the modulating influence of higher-order cortex over subordinate cortex – an example of top-down regulation.

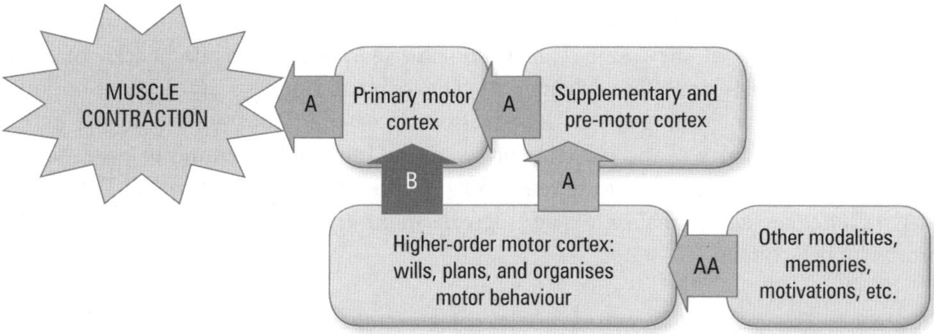

Source: © Visser, 2009.

Figure 8.3: Depicts the same process as Figure 8.2. High-order association cortex inhibits the primary motor cortex via Process B, interrupting information passage for further motor-processing. The result of this compartmentalisation is a failure to 'will' or release the motor behaviour - despite an intact neural network, functional paralysis ensues. The higher-order association cortex has suspended activity of the primary motor cortex, in effect 'taking it off line'. Modality-specific sensory losses would follow a similar plan, but recruit different cortical areas.

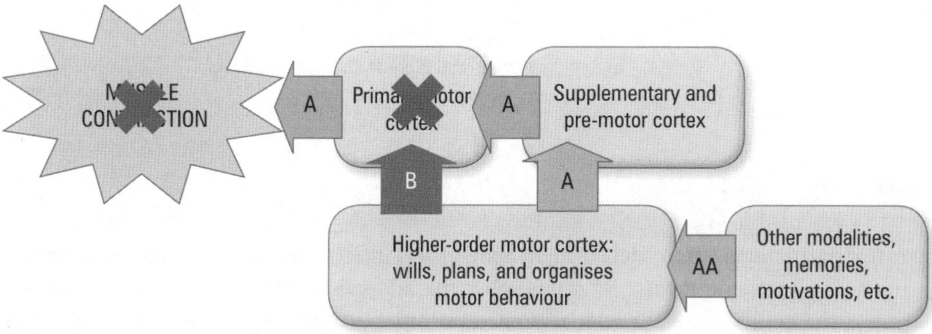

Source: © Visser, 2009.

Detachment

Detachment corresponds to an altered state of consciousness. Subjectively, it involves the experience of alienation of the self or the world outside. Emotional experiences are numbed, or blunted, and the person may experience depersonalisation or derealisation. The altered state of consciousness interferes with encoding of traumatic information, disturbing the memory trace of the event. The person also fails to integrate the emotional with the contextual aspects of the experience.

As memory is state dependent, these weakly integrated traces can be brought into conscious experience when the person is faced with a new stressful event in the future. As a result, aspects of the trauma can be re-experienced, like the 'flashbacks' of Post-traumatic Stress Disorder (see Chapter 4). Detachment can also snuff out emotional experience when, for example, the right prefrontal cortex inhibits activity in the limbic system. Likewise, parts of the parietal cortex can be inhibited, resulting in disturbances in the internal representation of the self and its relation to the external world. The person then experiences depersonalisation and derealisation. Figures 8.4 and 8.5 illustrate the process of detachment.

Figure 8.4: This diagram illustrates the flow of information when experiencing an event. Process A indicates incoming sensory information. Process AA represents passage of integrated sensory experience to prefrontal executive cortex. The limbic system mediates the emotional experience of the event and is reliant on integrated sensory information. Process B sets sensitivity of limbic information-processing.

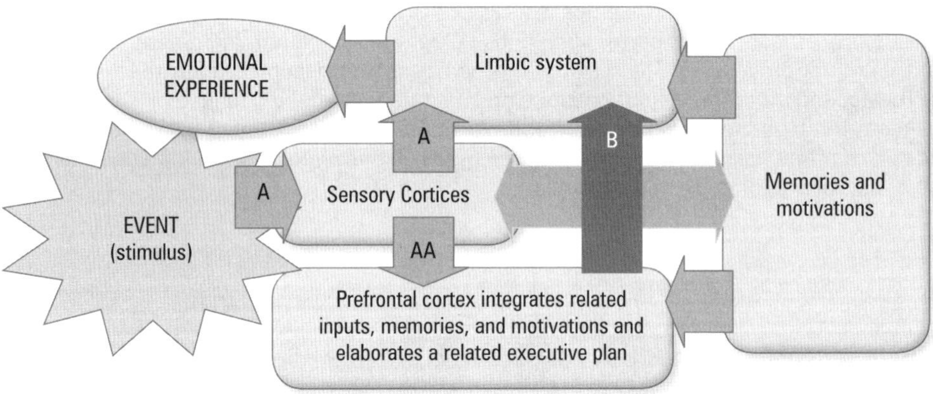

Source: © Visser, 2009.

Like compartmentalisation, detachment may also confer survival advantage on a person in the face of extreme threat. By attenuating the adverse emotional aspects of the stress response, the brain's finite attentional capacity is rationed and can remain focussed on the primary task at hand, thereby averting threat.

Figure 8.5: This diagram illustrates the same neural system as Figure 8.4. Process B depicts detachment of the limbic system by the prefrontal cortex inhibiting it. Inhibition of the limbic system gives rise to numbing of emotional experience related to the traumatic event. Depersonalisation follows a similar path, but involves different areas of cortex, e.g. parietal cortex (inferior lobule).

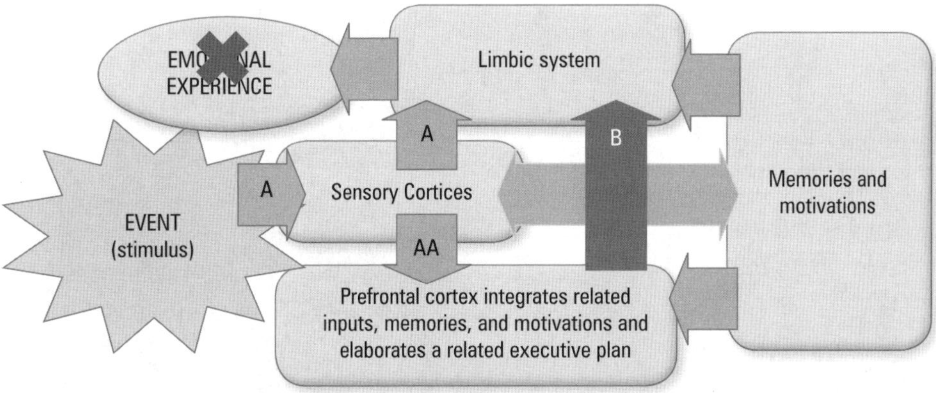

Source: © Visser, 2009.

Early adversity and future pathology

So, how can a once-adaptive system become the seat of such disabling pathology? The answer lies in early adversity. When exposed to severe threat, like physical and sexual abuse, or severely inconsistent attachment, a child may respond defensively through compartmentalisation or detachment. If repeatedly traumatised, the dissociative response is strengthened in a use-dependent way through conditioning and becomes established as the preferential response to threat. In other words, the more a neural process – in this case, dissociation – is used, the more efficient it becomes and the more easily it is engaged. Later, when faced with a significant psychosocial threat, dissociation is engaged as the preferential response and produces symptoms like blindness, paralysis, amnesia, attentional narrowing, disturbed personal identity, and alienation. Somatising phenomena may also include sensory disturbances of various kinds that point towards dissociation: pain, sensory loss, dizziness, and abdominal discomfort are examples that come to mind. Figure 8.6 summarises the genesis of dissociative pathology.

Figure 8.6: A likely pathogenetic explanation for pathological dissociation is given in this diagram. In vulnerable individuals, early adversity leads to dissociation as expression of the fear response. Given the salience of the traumatic event, the patient becomes conditioned to respond preferentially with dissociative phenomena if faced with significant psychosocial stressors. As a result, future trauma unleashes dissociative phenomena and sets the scene for the emergence of dissociative and somatoform disorders, as well as related conditions like Acute Stress Disorder.

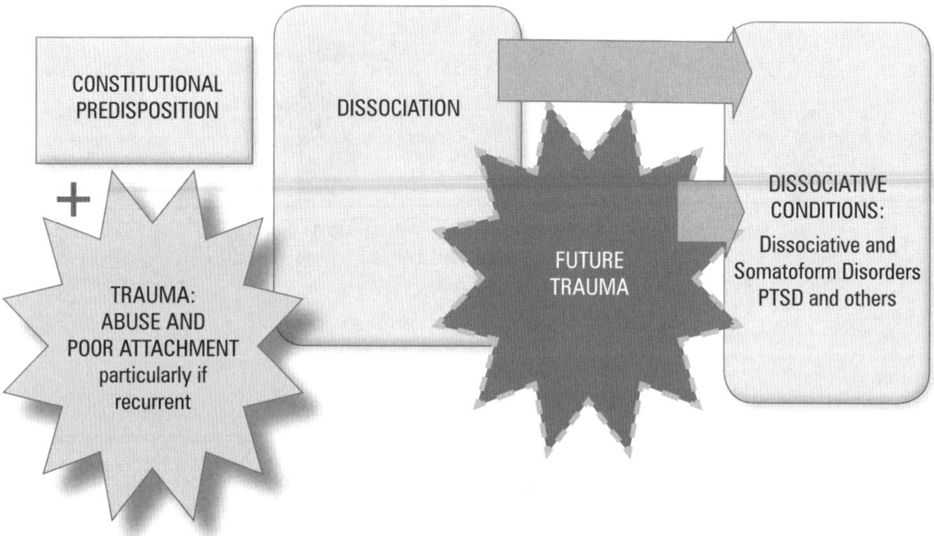

Source: © Visser, 2009.

SECTION 1: DISSOCIATIVE DISORDERS AND THEIR COMPARATIVE NOSOLOGY

According to the DSM-5, dissociative disorders are typically characterised by "... a disruption of and/or discontinuity in the normal integration of consciousness, memory, identity, emotion, perception, body representation, motor control and behavior" (American Psychiatric Association, 2013, p. 291). What follows are descriptions of the individual conditions included under the category of dissociative disorders. The DSM-5 recognises three dissociative disorders: Dissociative Amnesia (with Dissociative Fugue as a specifier), Dissociative Identity Disorder, and Depersonalisation/Derealisation Disorder (American Psychiatric Association, 2013).

Table 8.2: Comparative nosology of dissociative disorders

DSM-5	ICD-10
Dissociative Amnesia	Dissociative Amnesia Dissociative Fugue
Depersonalisation/ Derealisation Disorder	Depersonalisation/ Derealisation Disorder*
Dissociative Identity Disorder	Multiple Personality Disorder Dissociative Trance & possessions
Other Specified Dissociative Disorders Unspecified Dissociative Disorders	Dissociative (Conversion) Disorder, Unspecified
	Dissociative Stupor** Dissociative Motor Disorders** Dissociative Convulsions** Dissociative Anaesthesia and Sensory Loss** Mixed Dissociative (Conversion) Disorders**
	* Listed under Other Neurotic Disorders ** Conforms to DSM-5 Conversion Disorder and Functional Neurological Disorder where they are considered Somatoform/Somatic Symptom Disorders

Now in its tenth edition, the *International Statistical Classification of Diseases and Related Health Problems*, or ICD-10 (World Health Organisation, 2007), takes a somewhat different view on dissociative conditions by considering conversion as a dissociative condition. ICD-10 lists: Dissociative Amnesia, Dissociative Fugue, Dissociative Stupor, Dissociative Trance and Possession Disorders, Dissociative Motor Disorders, Dissociative Convulsions, Dissociative Anaesthesia and Sensory Loss, Mixed Dissociative (Conversion) Disorders, and Other Dissociative (Conversion) Disorders. Diagnosis of dissociative disorders using the ICD-10 approach requires the fulfilment of the general criteria for dissociative disorders as well as those for the specific disorders. This requirement does not apply to Depersonalisation/Derealisation Disorder. Table 8.3 lists ICD-10 general criteria for dissociative disorders.

The Dissociative Motor Disorders, Convulsions, Anaesthesia, and Mixed Disorders are equivalent to DSM-5's Conversion Disorder. Not listed as a Dissociative (Conversion) Disorder but instead under Other Neurotic Disorders is Depersonalisation/ Derealisation Disorder. Table 8.2 tabulates the comparative nosologies of Dissociative Disorders. The shaded rectangles indicate homology between the different classifications and the ellipses the central dissociative element.

HELPFUL HINT
Common features of dissociative disorders

- Constitutional predisposition
- History of childhood trauma
- Symptoms emerge following psychosocial stressor
- Symptoms include amnesia, identity disturbance, and alterations in sensory experience.

Table 8.3: General criteria for dissociative disorders (ICD-10)

G1. There must be no evidence of a physical disorder that can explain the characteristic symptoms of this disorder (although physical disorders may be present that give rise to other symptoms).
G2. There are convincing associations in time between the onset of symptoms of the disorder and stressful events, problems, or needs.

Source: Reprinted with permission from the ICD–10 Classification of Mental and Behavioural Disorders: Diagnostic Criteria for Research. World Health Organisation (WHO), Geneva, 2007.

Dissociative Identity Disorder

Even in the United States, Dissociative Identity Disorder is highly controversial. Across the globe, its validity as a clinical or pathological entity is doubted. Conceptually, Dissociative Identity Disorder represents a chronic dissociative disorder characterised by the existence of two or more distinct identities or personalities. It typically follows childhood sexual or physical abuse and is considered the most serious of the dissociative disorders.

Because of its apparent rarity outside the United States, it is sometimes considered an example of an American culture-bound syndrome. Golub (1995) showed that more than 60 per cent of cases worldwide emanated from the United States. It has even been suggested that the condition is non-existent in Great Britain, Russia, India, and South East Asia. Even in the United States, the condition is rarely diagnosed in Hispanic or Asian Americans (Escobar, 2004). In Turkey, an incidence between 1.1% and 1.7% was found in the general, non-psychiatric, population (Akyüz, 1999). Studies in Iran, Germany, Australia, Sweden, and the Netherlands have yielded a wide incidence range (2 to 17%) among psychiatric patients (Hales, 2008).

Before the nineteenth century, Dissociative Identity Disorder was probably considered as a possession state. Benjamin Rush, the father of American psychiatry and signatory of the American Declaration of Independence, described a syndrome not unlike Dissociative Identity Disorder in the early 1800s. Charcot and Janet did likewise in France; Freud and Bleuler also recognised it and described its symptoms. It was not until the seventies and eighties, following the universal attraction of the films *Sybil* and *The Three Faces of Eve,* that the condition, then called Multiple Personality Disorder, entered pop culture. Incorporation of the condition into the DSM-III in 1980 cemented the condition's status. In late 2011, debate erupted across the globe about claims that Sybil was indeed a hoax. Perhaps it is sobering to consider that, with our ever-deepening understanding of the pathogenic mechanisms underlying the dissociative disorders in general, the set of phenomena now known as Dissociative Identity Disorder possesses neuro-scientific validity.

Epidemiology

A full understanding of the incidence and prevalence of Dissociative Identity Disorder has not been achieved and estimates range widely. The overwhelming majority of cases are female with onset commonly in adolescence, with a mean age of onset of thirty. There appears to be an inherited basis to the condition – first-degree relatives of probands diagnosed with Dissociative Identity Disorder have a greater risk of developing the condition than the population at large.

Aetiology and pathogenesis

As a dissociative condition, Dissociative Identity Disorder shares its pathogenic mechanism with other dissociative conditions. It is recognised that nearly 100% of cases involve a traumatic event during childhood – usually physical or sexual abuse, the latter often incestuous. Lack of emotional support surrounding the trauma and poor attachment add to the risk. Other traumatic events, like the death of loved one, may also prove sufficient as risk factors.

Table 8.4: Diagnostic criteria for Dissociative Identity Disorder as adapted from the DSM-5 and for Multiple Personality Disorder as adapted from ICD-10

DSM-5 Dissociative Identity Disorder	ICD-10 Multiple Personality Disorder*
A. Disruption of identity characterised by two or more distinct personality states, which may be described in some cultures as an experience of possession. The disruption in identity involves marked discontinuity in sense of self and sense of agency, accompanied by related alterations in affect, behaviour, consciousness, memory, perception, cognition, and/or sensory motor-functioning. These signs and symptoms may be observed by others or reported by the individual.	In this residual code, the general criteria (G1 AND G2) for dissociative (conversion) disorders must be met. A. Two or more distinct personalities exist within the individual only one being evident at a time.

B. Recurrent gaps in the recall of everyday events, important personal information, and/or traumatic events that are inconsistent with ordinary forgetting. C. The symptoms cause clinically significant distress or impairment in social, occupational, or other important areas of functioning. D. The disturbance is not a normal part of a broadly accepted cultural or religious practice. **Note:** In children, the symptoms are not better explained by imaginary playmates or other fantasy play. E. The symptoms are not attributable to the physiological effects of a substance (e.g. blackouts or chaotic behaviour during alcohol intoxication) or another medical condition (e.g. complex partial seizures).	B. Each personality has its own memories, preferences, and behaviour patterns, and at some time (and recurrently) takes full control of the individual's behaviour. C. There is inability to recall important .personal information which is too extensive to be explained by ordinary forgetfulness. *Other Dissociative (Conversion) Disorder

Source: Reprinted with permission from the Diagnostic and Statistical Manual of Mental Disorders (DSM), Fifth Edition, American Psychiatric Association (APA), 2013 and ICD-10 Classification of Mental and Behavioural Disorders: Diagnostic Criteria for Research. World Health Organisation (WHO), Geneva, 2007.

Diagnosis, clinical presentation, and course

DSM-5 diagnostic criteria for Dissociative Identity Disorder require the presence of at least two or more distinct personalities or an experience of possession (APA, 2013), and the absence of a general medical condition, like certain epilepsies and the exclusion of effects of psychotropic substances. Table 8.4 lists the DSM-5 criteria for Dissociative Identity Disorder and the ICD-10 diagnostic criteria for Multiple Personality Disorder.

The average number of personalities ranges from five to ten but only two or three are usually evident at diagnosis. Transitions between personalities can occur gradually, but more frequently occur rapidly and quite dramatically. Whilst possessing one personality, the patient is amnesic of the others. Occasionally, one personality retains awareness of another's qualities. Classically, each alter has a well-developed set of attributes.

Patients may appear coy or seductive, look depressed or anxious, but mental state examination is usually normal. It is rare for a switch between alters to occur during a clinical encounter. Sometimes patients report hallucinations. Conversion symptoms may also be present, typically non-epileptic seizures. Different alters may exhibit different conversion or other somatic symptoms.

In children, the condition may look more trance-like. During adolescence, Dissociative Identity Disorder can take two forms. In the first, symptoms are similar to those of Borderline Personality Disorder or a rapid-cycling bipolar condition, with unstable moods, impulsivity, risk-taking, and self-injury. In the second form, adolescent patients are socially withdrawn and reason in a childlike manner. Although rare, adolescent males can display prominent antisocial behaviour.

Dissociative Identity Disorder can emerge as early as three years of age. The earlier the onset, the worse the prognosis is likely to be. Severity is determined by early age of onset, chronicity, the number of alters, and the coexistence of other mental conditions. Mood, anxiety, and substance use disorders are commonly diagnosed as co-morbid conditions, as is Borderline Personality Disorder. Prognosis is typically guarded and recovery incomplete.

Differential diagnosis

Dissociative Amnesia is an obvious differential diagnosis of Dissociative Identity Disorder. However, in Dissociative Amnesia the adoption of different identities does not occur and tends to run an acute course, while Dissociative Identity Disorder is chronic. In Schizophrenia and other psychotic disorders, patients may adopt a new identity as expression of a delusional state. But Schizophrenia's typical affective incongruence and silliness, and the presence of delusions and formal thought disorder, make for ready differentiation. In both rapid-cycling bipolar conditions and Borderline Personality Disorder, the absence of distinct personalities distinguishes them from Dissociative Identity Disorder.

Complex partial epilepsy may be confused for Dissociative Identity Disorder, but is associated with typical phenomena suggesting epilepsy. Factitious disorders and malingering should always be considered. However, atypical presentations and, in the case of malingering, the identification of an obvious external motivation for the behaviour, steers diagnosis away from Dissociative Identity Disorder.

Dissociative Amnesia

Amnesia, or the inability to recall, is common to almost all dissociative disorders and is prominent in Dissociative Amnesia and Dissociative Identity Disorder. However, when amnesia is the predominant mode of presentation, a diagnosis of Dissociative Amnesia is most appropriate.

Dissociative Amnesia shows the following characteristics:

- The amnesia involves episodic memory, with loss of autobiographical recollection of events and important personal information.
- The amnesia is not the result of failure to encode, store, or retrieve information as occurs in Wernicke-Korsakoff Syndrome, stroke, or other lesions involving the medial memory structures. As a consequence, it is possible to recover lost memories, and deficits are usually reversible.
- Commonly, the amnesia involves a discrete period and does not involve vagueness or poor retrieval. Instead, a full range of information is simply not accessible. Uncommonly, people are unable to recall any personal information and they are then said to experience generalised amnesia. Systematised, or selective, amnesia concerns the failure to recall certain, but not all, events during a relatively short period.
- The amnesia is predominantly retrograde. Retrograde amnesia refers to amnesia for past events, or events before an index event (like trauma). Anterograde amnesia refers to the inability to form new memories following an index event and is the most pronounced aspect of amnesia of physical origin like concussion (see Chapter 7). In Dissociative Amnesia, new information can still be learnt and anterograde amnesia, except for a very brief period following the index trauma, is unusual.
- The amnesia involves events of a stressful or traumatic nature like incidents of child abuse. Other events, like the death of a spouse, can also trigger Dissociative Amnesia.
- It is not uncommon to experience amnesia for many events.

- Patients with Dissociative Amnesia appear normal in other respects: memory for general information is intact as are non-declarative memory (including procedural memory for tasks like riding a bike or changing gears) and other cognitive functions.
- The amnesia is too expansive for ordinary forgetfulness to have been the cause.
- Occasionally, if associated with minor head trauma, the trauma is too slight to have physiological consequences on memory function matching what is observed.
- Although uncommon, travel away from familiar surroundings can occur in Dissociative Amnesia. Currently, travel is the defining feature of Fugue. However, in a move away from previous DSM's, where this Dissociative Fugue was considered to be a distinct disorder, DSM-5 has included Fugue as a specifier, rather than a distinct disorder in Dissociative Amnesia.

HELPFUL HINT

Clues to Dissociative Amnesia

- Blackouts or time losses of discrete duration
- Reports of behaviour patient cannot account for
- Appearance of unexplained possessions
- Unexplained changes in relationships
- Wandering away
- Unexplained changes in abilities, tastes, knowledge
- Incomplete recall of life events
- Episodes of mistaken identity.

Source: Adapted from Hales, 2008.

Epidemiology

Dissociative Amnesia is considered the most common of the dissociative disorders, but as is common with dissociative disorders in general, epidemiological data are limited. Dissociative Amnesia appears to be more common in women than men and in young, rather than older adults. Its incidence rises during war and social unrest and seems to correlate with natural and human-made disasters (e.g. the 9/11 attacks in the US). A direct relationship appears to exist between the severity of trauma and the incidence of amnesia.

Aetiology and pathogenesis

In keeping with the general model for dissociation, faced with significant trauma, patients with Dissociative Amnesia fail to integrate the emotional aspects of experience with its context and story. Constitutional predisposition is a likely added risk factor.

Table 8.5: Diagnostic criteria for Dissociative Amnesia as adapted from the DSM-5 and ICD-10

DSM-5	ICD-10
A. An inability to recall important autobiographical information, usually of a traumatic or stressful nature, that is inconsistent with ordinary forgetting. **Note:** Dissociative amnesia most often consists of localised or selective amnesia for a specific event or events; or generalised amnesia for identity and life history.	A. The general criteria for dissociative disorder must be met. B. There must be amnesia, either partial or complete, for recent events or problems that were or still are traumatic or stressful.

B. The symptoms cause clinically significant distress or impairment in social, occupational, or other important areas of functioning. C. The disturbance is not attributable to the physiological effects of a substance (e.g. alcohol or another drug of abuse, a medication) or a neurological or other medical condition (e.g. partial complex seizures, transient global amnesia, sequelae of a closed head injury/traumatic brain injury, or other neurological condition). D. The disturbance is not better explained by dissociative identity disorder, posttraumatic stress disorder, acute stress disorder, somatic symptom disorder, or major or mild neurocognitive disorder.	C. The amnesia is too extensive and persistent to be explained by ordinary forgetfulness (although its depth and extent may vary from one assessment to the next) or by intentional simulation.

Source: Reprinted with permission from the Diagnostic and Statistical Manual of Mental Disorders (DSM), Fifth Edition, American Psychiatric Association (APA), 2013 and ICD–10 Classification of Mental and Behavioural Disorders: Diagnostic Criteria for Research. World Health Organisation (WHO), Geneva, 2007.

Diagnosis, clinical features, and course

Table 8.5 lists comparative diagnostic criteria for Dissociative Amnesia. Most cases have their onset following an emotionally stressful event (see the case study of Thandiwe). Onset is usually abrupt, but this is not a diagnostic requirement. Most patients are aware of the memory loss; some appear upset about it, others indifferent. Infrequently, patients may wander away from familiar surroundings. Rarely, patients may also assume new identities. The extent and depth of amnesia may vary across clinical encounters. Other cognitive functions are unaffected. Patients are usually alert before and after the onset of amnesia, but clouding of consciousness can be apparent surrounding the trauma. Anxiety and depression commonly co-occur with the amnesia and stressful event. The end of an amnesic episode is usually abrupt and complete.

Differential diagnosis

Conditions listed in Table 8.2 must be considered when making a diagnosis of Dissociative Amnesia. Aiding differentiation, the cognitive deficits of dementia and delirium (see Chapter 7) are readily apparent and extend well beyond memory. Loss of personal information in dementia usually indicates advanced disease when obvious other signs of dementia are manifest. Post-concussion amnesia involves both retrograde and anterograde elements. The retrograde component is typically short and always shorter than the anterograde amnesia (see Figure 8.7). History and physical evidence of head trauma further support a diagnosis of post-concussion amnesia.

Figure 8.6: The temporal pattern of amnesia as a result of acute derangement of brain function, like concussion or a seizure consists of an anterograde and a retrograde component. The graph depicts time on the horizontal axis and density of memory loss on the dependent, vertical axis. The time of insult is indicated by the thick black arrow. Amnesia for antecedent events constitutes the retrograde amnesia; the period of amnesia following the insult constitutes the anterograde amnesia. The gradual return of memory following a brain insult outstrips the period of memory loss predating it.

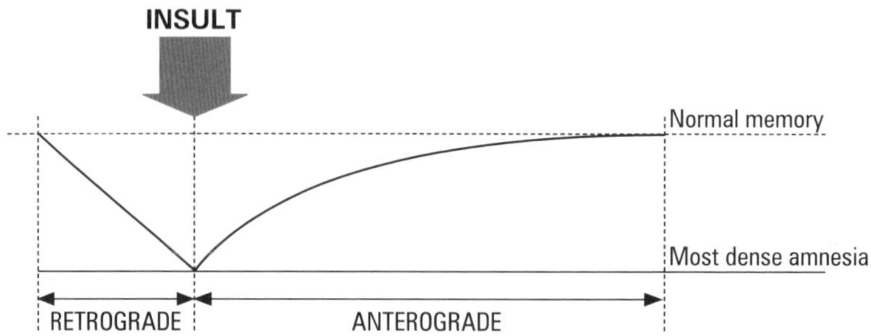

Source: © Visser, 2009.

CASE STUDY

Thandiwe (18 years old) had recently moved to a well-known South African university town to commence studies in journalism. One night during orientation week, she was found sitting outside the university's administration block by a patrolling police officer. She was crying and looked anxious. Concerned, the officer took her to the nearby provincial hospital where she was able to give her name, age, and a few other personal particulars but she could remember none of the events of that day. With gentle persuasion from the casualty officer, she eventually related how she could recall a 'dream-like' image of 'two dark figures'. Following the recommendations of the casualty officer, she admitted herself to the local mental hospital the next morning. She continued to be amnesic for recent events, but was able to recount her life story. She was also able to learn new information and easily adapted to the hospital milieu. Although aware of her amnesia, she seemed detached and indifferent to it.

Thandiwe's family history was as follows: She grew up in an abusive home. Her father, a wealthy businessman in Cape Town, was well known as a 'sex addict' and often cheated on Thandiwe's mother. He often arranged lavish receptions at their home where people 'partied hard'. Once, Thandiwe was drawn into a sexual orgy involving her father, two unknown women, and her brother. Her father eventually committed suicide when investigated for molesting the daughter of his personal assistant.

Thandiwe related how her move from Cape Town to study at university had been particularly stressful. She found some comfort with her new boyfriend and appeared to have become heavily dependent on him. Despite his apparent support, she felt increasingly anxious, inadequate, and fearful. She experienced ever-more-frequent headaches and insomnia. A res-mate of hers later indicated that on the day she was found roaming the streets, she had walked in on her boyfriend 'making out' with another girl. She apparently ran out of the residence, screaming. A friend found her a short while later, sitting outside, looking dazed and saying nothing. The friend suggested that they seek help from the university counselling centre, but Thandiwe objected and walked off. Thandiwe has never used drugs, and a casualty drug-screen was clear. She has no medical history.

Within days of admission, she made a complete recovery and was able to relate events leading to the amnesic episode. After discharge, she was referred for psychotherapy.

Epilepsy commonly interrupts recall. A seizure can result in precipitous memory impairment. Whilst epileptic patients are prone to increased seizure activity during periods of emotional stress, seizures are typically associated with other predictable and stereotypic phenomena. These include convulsive movements, incontinence, tongue-biting, aimless stereotypes (repetitive behaviours like plucking at clothes, fumbling with an object, smacking of the lips, and fluttering of eyelids), unresponsiveness, and a glazed look during a non-convulsive seizure. A history of epileptic aura characterised by emotional changes, memory aberrations like déjà vu, and aberrant sensory experiences like smelling burning rubber is often noted as well (see Appendix A).

Although sleepwalking, or somnambulism, may resemble a dissociative state, it occurs during sleep and usually at night. In contrast to the sleepwalker's glazed look and lack of responsiveness, patients with Dissociative Amnesia appear normal to casual observers and do not let on that anything is amiss.

Acute and Posttraumatic Stress Disorders are characterised by dissociative symptoms and memory disturbances. Hyperarousal, psychic numbing, phobic avoidance, and depression are also more prominent. Factitious disorders and malingering must be considered if the presentation is atypical. Where gain is suspected, like escaping trial, malingering must be a prime consideration.

Dissociative Fugue (ICD-10)

As mentioned before, in DSM-5 Fugue is considered to be only a specifier for Dissociative Amnesia, and not a distinct disorder; however, it is listed as a distinct disorder in ICD-10. Although rare, Dissociative Fugue is an apt reminder of the adaptive origins of dissociative conditions. Fight and flight are the archetypical defensive behaviours among animals. 'Fugue', derived from the Latin *fugare* meaning 'to flee', refers to the 'flight' behaviour characteristic of the fear response; travel from a person's customary home or place of work indeed defines Dissociative Fugue. Amnesia of important aspects of personal identity is another prerequisite. Although patients classically adopt a new identity during a fugue episode, this is not common.

Epidemiology

Dissociative Fugue is believed to be rare and is encountered during periods of high stress, such as war, civil unrest, natural disasters, and following intense interpersonal conflict.

Aetiology and pathogenesis

Like Dissociative Amnesia, the pathogenesis of Dissociative Fugue conforms to the general model for dissociation. Patients with mood disorders and certain personality disorders, notably Borderline, Histrionic, and Schizoid Personality Disorder, are at greater risk of responding with fugue-like behaviour following trauma. Marital, financial and occupational stress, violence, and war experiences serve as the trigger in most instances. Other risks include the presence of depression, previous suicide attempts, substance abuse, and brain injury.

Diagnosis, clinical presentation, and course

In the aftermath of a traumatic life event, the patient with Dissociative Fugue wanders away from home, work, or their usual social environment, often for days on end. During an episode, sufferers have complete amnesia of personal information and past experiences and are characteristically unaware that something is amiss with their ability to recall information. During the fugue, the patient functions otherwise normally and can even secure employment and earn a living. Like Dissociative Amnesia, very little attracts the attention of the casual observer to its existence. Once resolved, patients can recall events preceding the fugue but are amnesic for events during it. A fugue is usually short lived, lasting mere hours to a few days, with spontaneous recovery occurring as abruptly as its onset. Rarely, fugues may last months and involve distant travel. Recurrence is rare. Table 8.6 lists the ICD-10 diagnostic for Dissociative Fugue.

Differential diagnosis

Wandering is not an unusual behavioural manifestation of psychopathology. It is not unusual to read a newspaper headline about a patient who had strayed from a hospital ward and gone missing. Such wanderings usually involve acute psychosis, mania, delirium, or dementia. While the travel in Dissociative Fugue is purposeful and organised in its execution, the wanderings of a demented or delirious patient are aimless. Other cognitive impairments are usually obvious in dementia and delirium (see Chapter 7).

Wandering may be encountered in complex partial epilepsy. Dissociative Amnesia occasionally involves travel. In Dissociative Identity Disorder, the new identities or 'alters' are more completely established than the new identity in Dissociative Fugue and switching between identities dominates the clinical picture.

Table 8.6: Diagnostic criteria for Dissociative Fugue as adapted from the ICD-10

ICD-10
A. The general criteria for dissociative disorder must be met. B. The individual undertakes an unexpected yet organised journey away from home or from the ordinary places of work and social activities, during which self-care is largely maintained. C. There is amnesia, either partial or complete, for the journey which also meets criterion C for Dissociative Amnesia.

Source: Reprinted with permission from the ICD–10 Classification of Mental and Behavioural Disorders: Diagnostic Criteria for Research. World Health Organisation (WHO), Geneva, 2007.

Depersonalisation/Derealisation Disorder

Depersonalisation is conceptualised by DSM-5 as a persistent or recurrent alteration in the perception of self, resulting in the suspension of a person's sense of their own personal reality (APA, 2013). Experientially, depersonalisation states include feelings of estrangement from the self, being like a machine, dead, in a dream, or being detached from the body. In derealisation, individuals or objects are experienced as unreal, dreamlike, or visually distorted. The person experiences a sense of unreality or detachment with respect to their surroundings. Patients maintain intact reality-testing and experience depersonalisation/derealisation with full awareness of its abnormality.

Symptoms of Depersonalisation/Derealisation are usually transient. They often occur at the same time as anxiety states. Depersonalisation/Derealisation are common in panic attacks. Whereas depersonalisation is a feeling that the body or self is altered and not real, derealisation involves the perception that the external world is not real. The experiences of depersonalisation and derealisation are collectively referred to as alienation. Although these experiences are not recognised as separate diagnostic entities by DSM-5, the distinction is useful inasmuch as it provides for a better account of a patient's personal experience.

ICD-10 considers Depersonalisation/Derealisation Disorder not as a dissociative (conversion) disorder but under the rubric of Other Neurotic Disorders where it finds itself in the motley company of Neurasthenia, the Asian culture-specific syndromes of *latah, koro* and *dhat*, Psychaesthenia, psychaesthenic neurosis, psychogenic syncope (fainting) and occupational neurosis (e.g. writer's cramp).

Epidemiology

Depersonalisation/derealisation are common and occur from time to time in up to 70% of otherwise healthy individuals. The sexes are equally affected. Depersonalisation/derealisation are particularly common during adolescence. There are limited data on the occurrence of pathological depersonalisation/derealisation. A recent community-based study in the United States found a prevalence of Depersonalisation Disorder of 0.8% (Johnson, 2006). Surveys in the United Kingdom and Canada have revealed one-month prevalence rates between 1.2 and 1.7% (Hales, 2008) Onset is usually between the ages of 15 and 30, but can occur as young as 10. The prevalence of depersonalisation/derealisation in the psychiatric population is substantially higher, occurring most notably with Posttraumatic Stress Disorder, Major Depressive Disorder, Panic Disorder, Schizophrenia and substance-use disorders.

Aetiology and pathogenesis

The general pathological mechanism involved in depersonalisation/derealisation involves dissociative detachment. Detachment is the subjective experience of an altered state of consciousness characterised by alienation of the self or the external world. Detachment arises during periods of stress and represents an adaptive response whereby the expression of anxiety mediated by the limbic system is inhibited in a top-down fashion by the prefrontal cortex. As a result, anxiety is kept in check, freeing the brain to devote processing capacity to averting extreme threat. Depersonalisation/derealisation can be likened to a soldier persevering with combat despite sustaining otherwise debilitating wounds. The soldier remains focussed and performance is not curtailed by pain that would normally cause incapacitation. Table 8.7 lists common conditions and substances typically associated with the emergence of depersonalisation/derealisation.

Diagnosis, clinical features, and course

The DSM-5 diagnostic criteria for Depersonalisation/Derealisation Disorder are provided in Table 8.8. ICD-10 lists Depersonalisation/Derealisation Disorder as a Non-psychotic Neurotic Disorder (F48.1). Patients with depersonalisation/derealisation do not cease to have bodily experiences and remain aware of the external world. However, the quality of experience is changed. Alienation results in body parts taking on a foreign feel. Commonly, body parts, particularly the extremities, are experienced as changing shape or size.

Table 8.7: Causes of Depersonalisation/Derealisation

CAUSES OF DEPERSONALISATION/DEREALISATION			
Mental	**Substances of abuse**	**Medical**	**Other**
Panic attack Generalised Anxiety Disorder Phobias Obsessive-Compulsive Disorder Posttraumatic Stress Disorder Acute Stress Disorder Major Depressive Episodes Mania Schizophrenia Somatoform disorders Conversion Disorder Other dissociative disorders	lcohol intoxication & withdrawal Cannabis Opioids Hallucinogens Stimulants Solvents **Medicinal substances** Anticholinergic agents AAntihistaminergic agent Barbiturates Benzodiazepines Beta-blockers	Botulism Cardiac arrhythmias Cerebral infections Cerebral ischaemia Cerebral neoplasm Cerebral trauma Epilepsies Huntington's disease Hypocalcaemia Hypoglycaemia Hyponatraemia Hypoxia Hypothyroidism Lupus erythematosus Migraine Multiple sclerosis Myocardial ischaemia	Boredom Electrical stimulation Emotional trauma Exhaustion Sensory deprivation

Borderline Personality Disorder Histrionic Personality Disorder Schizoid Personality Disorder Schizotypal Personality Disorder Dementia Delirium	Digoxin Neuroleptic agents Opiate analgesics Scopolamine	Spinocerebellar degeneration Hemi-depersonalisation Right (non-dominant) parietal cortical lesions	

Table 8.8: Diagnostic criteria for Depersonalisation/Derealisation Disorder as adapted from the DSM-5 and ICD-10

DSM-5	ICD 10
A. The presence of persistent or recurrent experiences of depersonalisation, derealisation, or both: (1) Depersonalisation: Experiences of unreality, detachment, or being an outside observer with respect to one's thoughts, feelings, sensations, body, or actions (e.g. perceptual alterations, distorted sense of time, unreal or absent self, emotional and/or physical numbing). (2) Derealisation: Experiences of unreality or detachment with respect to surroundings (e.g. individuals or objects are experienced as unreal, dreamlike, foggy, lifeless, or visually distorted). B. During the depersonalisation or derealisation experiences, reality testing remains intact. C. The symptoms cause clinically significant distress or impairment in social, occupational, or other important areas of functioning. D. The disturbance is not attributable to the physiological effects of a substance (e.g. a drug of abuse, medication) or another medical condition (e.g. seizures). E. The disturbance is not better explained by another mental disorder, such as schizophrenia, panic disorder, major depressive disorder, acute stress disorder, posttraumatic stress disorder, or another dissociative disorder.	For a definite diagnosis, there must be either or both of A and B, plus C and D: A. Depersonalisation symptoms, i.e. the individual feels that his or her own feelings and/or experiences are detached, distant, not his or her own, lost, etc.; B. Derealisation symptoms, i.e. objects, people, and/or surroundings seem unreal, distant, artificial, colourless, lifeless, etc.; C. An acceptance that this is a subjective and spontaneous change, not imposed by outside forces or other people (i.e. insight); D. A clear sensorium and absence of toxic confusional state or epilepsy.

Source: Reprinted with permission from the Diagnostic and Statistical Manual of Mental Disorders (DSM), Fifth Edition, American Psychiatric Association (APA), 2013 and ICD–10 Classification of Mental and Behavioural Disorders: Diagnostic Criteria for Research. World Health Organisation (WHO), Geneva, 2007.

Occasionally, patients may experience a sense of removal from their own body, as if the conscious self has been evacuated from the confines of the physical body. Autoscopy is one example of this, where patients feel as if they are viewing themselves from the outside, often from above and a short distance away. These out-of-body or extracorporeal experiences are often encountered in accounts of near-death experiences and in the paranormal literature.

With reduplication phenomena, patients have the experience of being duplicated and present in two different places at once. For example, patients may confirm their presence in the consulting room whilst, at the same time, believe that they are at home. The patient may be at pains to convince the doctor of the reality of the experience. Reduplication is also experienced in active psychosis, dementia, delirium, seizures, migraine, and focal lesions involving the parietal cortex.

Derealisation often partners depersonalisation. However, during childhood or adolescence, it is not uncommon for derealisation to occur in isolation, divorced from any depersonalisation. Frequently, anxiety, even panic, accompanies depersonalisation, underscoring their commonality as stress responses. During an episode, a patient may appear preoccupied and dysphoric. Reality-testing remains intact. When depersonalisation is experienced frequently, patients start ruminating about their experiences and phobic avoidance towards situations that may cue depersonalisation may ensue. Often, depersonalisation symptoms make a sudden first appearance, accompanied by intense anxiety and hyperventilation.

In more than half of cases, Depersonalisation/Derealisation Disorder tends to be a chronic condition. For most patients, symptom intensity remains fairly constant and symptoms cluster in episodes separated by periods of remission. Like other dissociative conditions, depersonalisation/derealisation tend to occur during periods of increased psychosocial stress. However, relaxation, boredom, and use of medicinal substances can also precipitate spells of depersonalisation/derealisation.

Differential diagnosis

As Table 8.7 demonstrates, causes of depersonalisation/derealisation are many and varied. Depersonalisation/derealisation may occur in Major Depressive Episodes, Schizophrenia, and other experiences of psychotic alienation, but a meticulous history and mental state examination should provide enough information to make the diagnostic distinction. Enquiry must be made into the use of psychoactive substances – even the unsuspecting use of medicinal agents like colic remedies known to produce depersonalisation/derealisation phenomena.

The occurrence of isolated depersonalisation/derealisation in the absence of other psychopathology should warn of the possibility of serious physical pathology like cerebral neoplasm or central nervous system infection and warrants thorough neurological examination, including brain-imaging.

Classically, epilepsy is considered the archetypal physical or non-psychiatric cause of depersonalisation/derealisation. The abrupt onset of a seizure and its predictable accompaniments like convulsive movements, stereotypies, disturbed consciousness, and amnesia assist with accurate differentiation.

Depersonalisation/derealisation can occur during a migrainous aura. In migraine, the aura comprises primarily sensory disturbances that announce the imminent onset of headache. The migrainous aura is differentiated from Depersonalisation/Derealisation Disorder by the presence of severe, classically one-sided and pulsatile (throbbing) headache, photosensitivity, hyperacusis (heightened sensitivity to sound), nausea, and vomiting. Migraine-equivalents, where aural phenomena occur in the absence of the typical headache, are cause for serious diagnostic challenge.

Trance and Possession Disorders (ICD-10)

Dissociative Trance Disorder was categorised in DSM-IV-TR as a separate and distinct disorder; however, this is no longer considered to be such in the DSM-5 and has been subsumed in Dissociative Identity Disorder and is also described in Other Specified Dissociative Disorders in the DSM-5. Despite this, we still provide a separate discussion of Trance and Possession Disorders, not only for the peculiar and puzzling nature of its symptoms, but also the universality of the phenomenon, as well as that it is described in the ICD-10 as a distinct disorder.

Observing trance and possession states and the rituals of many cultures yields remarkable similarities. Shamans are common in Latin America, South East Asia, Japan, the Pacific Islands, India, the Middle East, and sub-Saharan Africa. Typically, a medium or shaman may preside over a séance-like event. When the shaman enters a dissociative state, an entity from another realm or spirit world takes over conscious awareness and influences behaviour.

The commonest features of trance states are amnesia, emotional disturbance, and loss of personal identity (Spiegel, 1997), features that bear resemblance to Dissociative Identity Disorder. Altered states of consciousness, stereotyped motor behaviour, short duration, fatigue in the aftermath, normal behaviour between trances, onset before age 25, limited education, low socio-economic status, and having witnessed a trance previously have all been found in relation to this condition (Kua, 1986).

Table 8.9 provides the ICD-10 criteria of Trance and Possession Disorders. Dissociative Trance Disorder must be coded as a Dissociative Disorder Not Otherwise Specified in the DSM-5.

HELPFUL HINT

Trance and Possession Disorders

- Trance and possessed states are common
- Encountered in all peoples of the world
- Onset often before age 25
- Often follows psychosocial trauma
- Amnesia is characteristic
- Loss of personal identity is common
- Marked emotional disturbance
- Dissociative Identity Disorder probably related
- Can be normal or pathological
- Travel, wandering from familiar surroundings
- Assumption of new identity.

Source: Adapted from Hales, 2008

Table 8.9: Diagnositic criteria for Trance and Possession Disorders as adapted from ICD-10

TRANCE AND POSSESSION DISORDERS – ICD-10 diagnostic criteria
The general criteria for dissociative disorder must be met. A. Either of the following must be present: (1) *Trance*. There is temporary alteration of the state of consciousness, shown by any two of: (a) loss of the usual sense of personal identity; (b) narrowing of awareness of immediate surroundings, or unusually narrow and selective focusing on environmental stimuli; (c) limitation of movements, postures, and speech to repetition of a small repertoire. (2). *Possession disorder.* The individual is convinced that he or she has been taken over by a spirit, power, deity, or other person. B. Both (1) and (2) of criterion B must be unwanted and troublesome, occurring outside or being a prolongation of, similar states in religious or other culturally accepted situations. C. *Most commonly used exclusion clause:* The disorder does not occur at the same time as Schizophrenia or related disorders, or mood (affective) disorders with hallucinations or delusions.

Source: Reprinted with permission from the ICD–10 Classification of Mental and Behavioural Disorders: Diagnostic Criteria for Research. World Health Organisation (WHO), Geneva, 2007.

Worldwide, predictable psychosocial stressors have been identified as precipitants of trance states. In South Africa, Szabo (2005) identified Major Depressive Episodes and bereavement as triggers. Catholic exorcisms, directed at driving out a demon that possesses the sufferer, are also considered dissociative states (Ferracuti, 1996).

Ganser's Syndrome (Unspecified Dissociative Disorder: DSM-5; Other Dissociative (Conversion) Disorder: ICD-10)

This curious condition, also known as the 'Syndrome of Approximate Answers' or 'Twilight Hysteria' was first described by Sigbert Joseph Maria Ganser (1853–1931) in 1898. In a paper entitled *Concerning an Unusual Hysterical Confusional State (Über einen eigenartigen hysterischen Dämmerzustand)*, Ganser described his observations of a behavioural syndrome found among young men freshly admitted to a Dresden prison. The pre-eminent feature of the condition is paralogia, or the giving of approximate answers.

The paralogic phenomenon, known by the German *vorbeireden* is illustrated by the following examples. When asked to do a simple calculation like '3 + 1', the patient may answer '5'; asked to name a pencil, the patient responds with 'pen'. Believed to be common, such so-called 'Ganserian' phenomena occur on a continuum of severity. Unusual psychosocial stress and neurological factors have been implicated in its causation. Its pathogenesis is likely dissociative in nature. However, patients often have antisocial or histrionic premorbid personalities and the condition is frequently encountered in prisoners facing trial, fuelling the sceptics' argument against its existence (Allen, Postel, & Berrios, 2000; Sadock & Sadock, 2000).

It is appealing to speculate about a possible pathogenic mechanism. A constitutionally vulnerable young male, of low intellect and a background of social adversity, is faced with a severe threat, like incarceration. Dissociation of some kind likely ensues with attentional impairment, disorientation, amnesia, hallucinations, conversion, somatising, and paralogia. The argument for Ganser's Syndrome being a form of transient, even Schizophrenic, psychosis or a delirium remains unsettled. In the DSM-IV-TR, Ganser's Syndrome was considered a Dissociative Disorder Not Otherwise Specified and, in ICD-10, it is listed under Other Dissociative (Conversion) Disorder along with Multiple Personality Disorder.

BOX 8.1: FEATURES OF GANSER'S SYNDROME

1. Sense of space and time is disorganised.
2. The patient tends to 'suspend' information at his or her disposal and gives 'I don't know'-answers.
3. Clouding of consciousness.
4. Despite intact understanding of a question, the patient displays a psychogenic inability to answer.
5. Answers are true to the semantic sphere of the question. Ganser referred to this phenomenon as vorbeireden (to talk past the point) and exemplified it thus: When at a railway station, '... a railway employee gave you a ticket at random rather than the ticket you asked for; the point being that he did not give you a bucket of water or a cup of tea.'
6. The patient may hallucinate and re-enact, in a hallucinatory manner, certain traumatic experiences.
7. General or partial analgesia that can migrate across the body.
8. Even innocuous questions like 'What is your name?' may cause difficulty and trigger vorbeireden.
9. Symptoms appear all at once and leave in a staggered manner, leaving a 'mode of being' similar to the personality before onset of the twilight state.
10. Later, when told about the behaviour, the patient expresses surprise.

Source: Allen, Postel, & Berrios, 2000.

Related conditions across different cultures

In Latin America, a common condition is *ataque de nervios,* a dissociative-like state characterised by a dramatic display of negative emotions and somatic symptoms in the wake of a psychosocial stressor. Co-existence of *ataque de nervios* with major depression and anxiety disorders correlates with a history of childhood abuse.

In China, the diagnosis of *yi-ping*, meaning hysteria, typically affects women with histories of interpersonal conflict, illness, or following the death of a loved one. The symptoms of *yi-ping* appear not unlike the general schema for dissociative disorders: memory disturbance, loss of personal identity, lessened awareness of surroundings, and excessive emotionality.

It is not difficult to align the so-called 'running syndromes' with Dissociative Amnesia, Fugue, or Trance Disorders. *Amok* is the prototypical 'running syndrome' and is found in Malay men. It produced the expression 'to run amok'. A man so affected enters a trance-like state and, imbued with a mysterious energy, runs or takes flight, a behaviour he can sustain for long hours on end. In its wake he remembers very little, if anything; experiences fatigue and could commit suicide. *Amok* is attributed to interpersonal conflict, personal abuse, intolerable embarrassment, slight, shame, and loss of honour. Running *amok* is seen as a way to seek revenge and restitution for a perceived insult to a man's dignity. The person running *amok* is not regarded as possessing responsibility for his actions as he is believed to be spirit-possessed. The amnesia is also regarded as prejudicial to sufferers when called to account.

Another much debated condition from the Malaysian peninsula and Indonesian archipelago is *latah*. *Latah* can be normal or pathological and is characterised by exaggerated startle responses. Sufferers habitually jump violently when startled, something they find most unpleasant. Trance-like states with automatic obedience may occur. The sufferer may feel compelled against his will to imitate the speech and behaviour of others (echolalia and echopraxia) (Eisenberg, 1959; Ropper, 2001; Tanner, 2001; World Health Organisation, 1992). Coprolalia, or the compulsive-like, irresistible utterances of profanities, is not uncommon. Behaviours continue even if the sufferer realises that his tormentors, believed to be controlling him, want to ridicule and degrade him. *Myriachit* is an identical condition found in the Arctic regions of Siberia. *Latah* is listed under Other Neurotic Disorders in ICD-10.

Pibloktoq is a typical running syndrome recognised by the Inuit peoples of the Arctic. (*Pibloktoq*, itself a transliteration, is variously spelt *pibloktok* and *pivloktoq* and sometimes erroneously referred to as 'Arctic Psychosis'). *Pibloktoq* is characterised by prodromal listlessness, fatigue, dysphoria, and mental 'confusion'. A 'seizure' of disruptive behaviour ensues during which sufferers strip off their clothing and embark on a spell of frenzied running and rolling in the snow. Echolalia and echopraxia emerge, along with destructive behaviours directed at objects, not people. Episodes are brief, often lasting mere minutes, and followed by loss of consciousness. Afterwards, the person has no recollection of the episode. Interpersonal stress is a likely precipitant.

From the tropics and Arctic, we move to New England and Canada where Jumper Disease of Maine, a condition much in the vein of *latah*, is found. Jumper Disease of Maine is also known as 'Jumping Frenchmen of Maine', 'Jumpers', 'Shakers' and 'Barkers'. The 'Jumpers' were members of an isolated, socially backward Francophone community in the Goosey Lake area of Northern Maine. They were descendants of a deviant Methodist sect which settled in New England four hundred years ago. 'Jumpers' are so called for their fierce startle response, with violent jumping and twisting. When startled, they also display echolalia and echopraxia. As a religious service reaches rapture, 'Jumpers' would jump and roll around in ecstasy, crawl about on all fours whilst making barking noises and emitting incoherent utterances understood by fellow worshippers as speaking in tongues (Eisenberg, 1958; Ropper, 2001). Speaking in tongues or glossolalia is considered normal and even desirable in certain Pentecostal churches. In the early nineties, genetic linkage analyses demonstrated that point mutations in the gene coding for the glycine receptor are present in patients with hyperekplexia, or excessive startle as found in Jumpers. Glycine is an amino acid neurotransmitter and modulates neural stimulation (Ropper, 2001; Shiang, 1993).

Whereas the neural mechanism of dissociation is universal, its appearance depends on the prevailing cultural context. Among Africans and East Asians, where communalism is more prominent, the dissociation readily manifests with possession of the patient by an external agency – a demon, a deity, or another person. In the West, particularly North America, where individual and personal experience are primary, dissociation in the form of Dissociative Identity Disorder manifests with competing versions of the self.

Amafufunyana and *ukuthwasa*

Among South Africa's black population, the occurrence of demon possession and the role of shamans or mediums are well known (Heap, 1991). *Amafufunyana* is found among the Xhosa-, Zulu- and Tswana-speaking peoples of southern Africa. Translated, *amafufunyana* means 'evil spirits'. *Ukuthwasa* refers to a person 'arising', upon his or her calling, to become a diviner or traditional healer. Whilst it is apparent that *amafufunyana* and *ukuthwasa* overlap with Schizophrenia (Niehaus, 2004), they also conform to the construct of Dissociative Trance Disorder with Possession.

Traditional beliefs about the causation of *amafufunyana* understand it to be a manifestation of ancestral anger, causing angry spirits to enter the mind of an affected person. Bewitchment is a frequent explanatory theme, or cause. Other causes are failure to observe a traditional ritual, stepping over a dangerous track, evil spirits, poisoning with soil and ants from the grave, and a variety of witch-familiars like the river snake, *impundulu* (evil lightning bird) or *tokoloshe* (dwarf-like creature with baboon-like facial features). The Xhosa people in the Cape Peninsula believe 'nerves', relationship problems, drug or alcohol abuse, and the Lord's Will to cause *amafufunyana*. But, the most widely held belief among the Xhosa about its causation is that it is multifactorial, with spiritual, social, interpersonal, and other influences (Ensink, 1996; Kruger, 2007).

The earliest warning of impending *amafufunyana* is social withdrawal. Listlessness, poor appetite, grunting, falling down, and overt aggression may follow. Vocalisations may emerge, believed to be the *amafufunyana* or evil spirits speaking through the person once they have seized control of his or her mind. The vocalisations can be in a foreign language or sound like those of an entirely different person, even of the opposite gender. Communication disturbances are present with incoherence and neologisms that can take the guise of formal thought disorder. During the acute phase, the person may also thrash around wildly and walk on all fours. Outlandish movements, not unlike convulsions, may occur. After effects include an inability to recall events during the affliction and feeling dazed and tired. Cataloguing the phenomenology of *amafufunyana* highlights conspicuous similarities between it and syndromes like *amok*, *pibloktoq* and the exaggerated startle, or hyperekplexia, of *latah* and Jumper Disease of Maine.

Ukuthwasa concerns a calling from ancestors for a person to undergo diviner or *thwasa* training and usually follows on misfortune befalling the person. Clinical manifestations of *ukuthwasa* are varied including anxiety, labile moods, loss of appetite, 'confused' feelings, and auditory and visual hallucinations. Somatic complaints, most typically involving the joints, emerge. The affected person can become restless and wander, sometimes disappearing from home. Personal hygiene is neglected and social isolation sets in. Sexual desire may be heightened or lost, with infertility supervening. Antisocial behaviour, violence, and aggression have been noted in *ukuthwasa* (Buhrman, 1984; Ensink, 1999). The prominence of dreams in *ukuthwasa* is noteworthy with water the near-universal theme. Dreams often involve an attraction for rivers and other bodies of water, as well as the urge to be submerged. Other common themes concern forests and animals.

Symptoms do not remit until the call for training is accepted. If not heeded, 'madness' and death may follow. If *thwasa* training is not completed, the original *ukuthwasa* may be transformed into *ukuphambana*, a Xhosa word for unspecified insanity (Ensink, 1996). Interestingly, in their survey of Xhosa-speakers in the Cape Peninsula, Ensink, and Robertson (1999) found that most respondents viewed alcohol or drug abuse as the principal cause of *ukuphambana*.

The bewildering variety of symptoms associated with *ukuthwasa* allows for its placement within several diagnostic categories. The interpretation of spiritual influence, or being under the spell of an external agency, aligns it with Dissociative Trance Disorder with Possession or Dissociative Identity Disorder as proposed in DSM-5. However, when hallucinations and social withdrawal are present, Schizophrenia or other psychotic states must be considered. *Amafufunyana* and *ukuthwasa* affect adults and children alike (Ensink, 1996). It appears that the majority of patients with *amafufunyana* had experienced an earlier episode of *amafufunyana*, whilst few reported previous *ukuthwasa*. A family history of Schizophrenia or another psychiatric disorder was more common for those with *ukuthwasa* than *amafufunyana*.

Epidemic Hysteria

It is not unheard of for a collection of people, usually participating in a single activity, to exhibit dissociative-like behaviour and report experiences of dissociation, somatising, or anxiety. Epidemic Hysteria is strictly defined as a constellation of symptoms suggestive of bodily illness, but without identifiable cause, that occurs between two or more people who share beliefs in those symptoms (Philen, Kilbourne, McKinley, & Parrish, 1989). Rather than viewing the phenomenon as a group of people each with an individual dissociative disorder, Boss (1997) suggests that Epidemic Hysteria should be viewed as a social phenomenon involving otherwise healthy people.

Two characteristic patterns of Epidemic Hysteria are recognised. In the first, the anxiety variant, abdominal pain, headache, dizziness, fainting, nausea, and hyperventilation are the most common symptoms. In the second type, or motor variant, frenetic dancing, convulsions, laughing, and loud utterances are noted (Boss, 1997). Characteristically, girls are more affected than older women, boys, or men. It is also recognised among young performers, at schools, and religious gatherings (Small, 1991; Wittstock, 1991).

Symptom propagation is believed to occur through social networks, mediated, at least in part, by sight and sound. Observing a friend become sick is a good predictor of the development of symptoms (Small, 1991), but multiple psychological and physical mechanisms most likely contribute to outbreaks. The case vignette, concerning a widely-reported event at a school in Mthatha, is illustrative.

CASE STUDY

For over a week in late May 1999, a group of girls attending St. John's College, a church school with over a thousand pupils in Mthatha (formerly Umtata) in the Eastern Cape Province of South Africa, started behaving strangely: they screamed, foamed at the mouth, fainted, and jerked. Newspaper reports spoke of an 'outbreak of hysteria'. No boys were affected. Whilst initially sceptical, fearing the looming June examinations had precipitated a large-scale hoax, the principal was eventually obliged to appeal to the church to intervene.

The Anglican Archdeacon called upon was frustrated at his first attempts at exorcism and noted that 'the spirit was moving from one girl to another' where they had been gathered in one classroom. Subsequently, he set about doing individual exorcisms. Shortly thereafter, thirty-two girls were admitted to the provincial hospital. Twenty-five were effectively sedated and discharged home; four were observed in casualty; two admitted to the internal medicine unit for suspected but unspecified 'illness' and one was referred to the psychiatric unit. A hospital spokesman described the girls as being in a 'very hysterical state'. The school was closed for a week following the exorcism.

Although newspapers reported this phenomenon as possession by evil spirits, they also reflected the public's ambivalence regarding the supernatural. An alternative context soon emerged, one that was sociological and secular. It highlighted the tense relationship between religion and mental health in a context of rapid social change and the transition from traditional society to the often confusing urbanised, competitive Western culture.

Source: Parle, 2003.

Soccer crowds, audiences at pop concerts, and protestors can all display so-called 'mass hysteria'. Public protest can transform into collective rampage with wanton destruction and looting. In another manifestation of group behaviour, more than 900 followers of the charismatic Reverend Jim Jones committed suicide in November 1978 at the People's Temple Agricultural project, referred to as Jonestown, in Guyana. Reminiscent of Jonestown was the behaviour of the Branch Davidians, followers of David Koresh, in 1993 in Waco, Texas, and the North Korean Sun Myung Moon Cult. Stage hypnotists draw capacity audiences who witness or keenly participate in group hypnosis, another manifestation of group dissociation.

Although influenced by many external factors, crowd behaviour at soccer stadium disasters, like Hillsborough in the United Kingdom in 1989, and the Orkney and Ellis Park tragedies in South Africa in 1991 and 2001 respectively, may have been partially influenced by dissociative-like group behaviour.

SECTION 2: SOMATIC SYMPTOM AND RELATED DISORDERS AND THEIR COMPARATIVE NOSOLOGY

Somatising lies at the heart of these disorders. It refers to a tendency to experience bodily, or somatic, distress in the face of psychological stress. While intuitively logical, robust evidence for a causal link between stress and somatising is still lacking. In the DSM-5 (American Psychiatric Association, 2013), the diagnosis is made on the basis of positive symptoms and signs (i.e. distressing somatic symptoms along with abnormal thoughts, emotions and behaviours in response to these symptoms), rather than the absence of medical reasons for these symptoms.

Seven types of somatoform disorder are recognised in DSM-5. These are: Somatic Symptom Disorder, Illness Anxiety Disorder, Conversion Disorder (Functional Neurological Symptom Disorder), Psychological Factors Affecting Other Medical Conditions, Factitious Disorder, Other Specified Somatic Symptom and Related Disorder and Unspecified Somatic Symptom and Related Disorder (APA, 2013).

ICD-10 takes a distinctly different tack. The most noteworthy differences are the absence of Conversion Disorder, considered a Dissociative Disorder, and Body Dysmorphic Disorder – subsumed under Hypochondriacal Disorder. Listed disorders are: Somatisation Disorder, Undifferentiated Somatoform Disorder, Hypochondriacal Disorder, Somatoform Autonomic Dysfunction, Persistent Somatoform Pain Disorder, Other Somatoform Disorders, and Somatoform Disorder, Unspecified.

Table 8.10: Comparative nosology of somatoform disorders

DSM-5	ICD-10
Somatic Symptom Disorder *Specifier: with pain as predominant symptom*	Somatisation Disorder Undifferentiated Somatoform Disorder Persistent Somatoform Pain Disorder
Illness Anxiety Disorder	Hypochondriacal Disorder
Conversion Disorder (Functional Neurological Disorder)	
Factitious Disorder??	
Other Specified Somatic Symptom and Related Disorder Unspecified Somatic Symptom and Related Disorder	Somatoform Autonomic Dysfunction Other Somatoform Disorders Somatoform Disorder, Unspecified
Psychological Factors affecting Medical Condition	

Table 8.10 lists disorders of the different nosologies. Dotted rectangles group together homologous symptoms or symptoms of a like nature; central lighter-coloured rectangles indicate DSM-5 equivalents. The central darker rectangle illustrates how DSM-5 Complex Somatic Symptom Disorder incorporates discrete DSM-IV-TR and ICD-10 conditions, including Pain Disorder and Hypochondriasis. Note how DSM-5 treats Hypochondriasis as two separate disorders.

Somatic Symptom Disorder (Somatisation Disorder: ICD-10)

Not altogether unlike Conversion Disorder, Somatic Symptom Disorder has also been known for millennia and considered a form of hysteria. In the seventeenth century, Thomas Sydenham recognised that 'antecedent sorrows' or psychosocial stressors were involved in the pathogenesis of the condition. In France, in the mid-1800s, Paul Briquet recognised the involvement of multiple organ systems and noted the condition's chronicity. To this day, Somatisation Disorder is alternatively known as Briquet's Syndrome. In the 1950s, Purtell resurrected Briquet's Syndrome and interest grew with Feighner's comprehensive list of diagnostic criteria for it. Feighner's criteria are considered the gold standard against which to measure Somatisation Disorder. However, they are complex and unwieldy, deterring doctors from adopting them for everyday practice. Dauntingly, Feighner identified 59 criteria spread across ten groups. Positive diagnosis required the presence of 25 criteria, representing nine of the ten groups.

The term 'Somatisation Disorder' was introduced for the first time in the DSM-III in 1980. Although simpler than Feighner's, the DSM criteria were also complex and daunting. Despite attempts at truncating and simplifying criteria, most psychiatrists continue to find the criteria difficult to use and dodge diagnosis as a result (Hales, 2008). This operational difficulty of diagnosis harms its recognition in primary care, where it usually makes its presence felt. In DSM-5, this disorder is labelled Somatic Symptom Disorder and the criteria have been simplified compared to the previous DSM-IV-TR.

Epidemiology

Somatic Symptom Disorder is believed common in primary health care and general medical practice, affecting as many as 10% of patients and, because of the difficulties with diagnostic criteria as discussed above, is probably under diagnosed. The condition predominantly affects females with an incidence five-fold that for males. The higher than expected incidence in men of Greek and Puerto Rican extraction implicates cultural factors modifying the sex ratio (American Psychiatric Association, 2000). Somatic Symptom Disorder mainly affects people of low socio-economic standing and limited education. By definition, the onset has to be before age 30; most commonly, onset is in adolescence.

Aetiology and pathogenesis

Not unlike Conversion Disorder, psychoanalytic theories about the causation of Somatic Symptom Disorder suggest that symptoms are substitutes for repressed unacceptable impulses of a sexual or violent nature. As a social communication, it is seen to produce secondary gain through avoiding work and garnering sympathy and support. Parental teaching may also play a role. The presence of significant psychosocial trauma, particularly in childhood, appears important to its development. Functional neuro-imaging studies have implicated the frontal and non-dominant parietal lobes in the neural dysfunctions of Somatic Symptom Disorder. Decreased blood flow has been demonstrated in the cerebellum, frontal and temporo-parietal regions, as well as reduced metabolism and size of subcortical structures, notably the caudate nucleus. Distractibility, poor habituation to repetitive stimuli, and circumstantial associations are neuropsychological abnormalities shown in the disorder. Evoked potential studies have shown abnormal sensory-processing.

An appealing but unproven theory holds that cytokines play a role in the expression of symptoms in Somatic Symptom Disorder. Cytokines are signalling molecules that mediate communication between different cells involved in the immune response. Serum concentrations of cytokines, particularly Interleukins 1, 2, and 6, as well as Tumour Necrosis Factor α, are raised during infections, notably the influenza-A virus. Cytokines are believed responsible for the constitutional symptoms of lethargy, depression, poor sleep, and lack of appetite characteristic of systemic infection and certain cancers. Although supporting data are lacking, abnormal cytokine production may account for some of the symptoms of Somatic Symptom Disorder. Cytokine abnormalities are also associated with major depression and Schizophrenia (see Chapters 5 and 6).

Data suggest that Somatic Symptom Disorder is at least partly genetically determined. For example, it occurs in up to 20% of first-degree female relatives of Somatic Symptom Disorder probands. Interestingly, both substance abuse and Antisocial Personality Disorder are over-represented in families of female Somatic Symptom Disorder probands (Cloninger & Yutzy, 1993). In contrast, relatives of male probands cluster with anxiety disorders. We could argue that males and females manifest with Somatic Symptom Disorder of different aetiology or pathogenesis (Hales, 2008). A 29% concordance for Somatic Symptom Disorder in monozygotic twins, as well as suggestive evidence from adoption studies, lends further credence to a genetic basis for the condition.

Diagnosis, clinical presentation, and course

In summary, the defining feature of Somatic Symptom Disorder is the occurrence of multiple bodily symptoms emanating from multiple organ systems. Symptoms include pseudo-neurological ones. The condition is further characterised by cognitive distortions about the symptoms, anxiety about them, and dysphoria. Early psychosocial adversity (mostly in childhood) is reported by patients and time of onset is related to trauma. The specific presence of histrionic or borderline personality traits, conversion and dissociative phenomena, sexual difficulties, menstrual irregularities, and strained relationships assist with recognition (Hales, 2008). Tables 8.11 lists DSM-5 and ICD-10 diagnostic criteria for this disorder. Somatic complaints can be grouped according the structure provided by criterion B of the DSM-5 or ICD-10 diagnostic criteria. Examples of specific symptoms are provided in the diagnostic criteria of the ICD-10.

Although similar in content, the approach adopted by ICD-10 differs from that of DSM-5 in a number of important ways. The DSM-5 approach is primarily concerned with examples of somatic symptoms associated with significant distress and impairment. The ICD dwells more on the process of the condition, as well as peculiarities of its course and natural behaviour. For example, attention is drawn to the chronicity of the disorder and the variable nature of symptoms.

The quality of psychological distress and related behaviours are also described in ICD-10 and include: preoccupation, anxiety, and resultant increased utilisation of resources (e.g. 'repeated consultations') and use of alternative resources including traditional healers where logistical constraints prevail. The ineffectiveness of reassurance by professionals (and others) is emphasised. Somatic symptoms listed in ICD-10 differ qualitatively from those in DSM-5, including, for example, 'bad taste' and 'excessively coated tongue'. ICD-10 does not list pseudo-neurological symptoms, thus emphasising the distinction between Conversion and Somatisation Disorders. Dissociative symptoms are also not specified.

Somatic Symptom Disorder: Rules of thumb

- Affects predominantly females
- Psychologically unsophisticated, lower socio-economic standing and education
- History of childhood trauma
- Symptoms related to psychosocial trauma
- Poly-symptomatic, multiple organ systems
- Chronic course.

Whilst still untested in large clinical settings, the leaner approach of DSM-5 appears practical. DSM-5 recognises that Somatic Symptom Disorder, Illness Anxiety Disorder, and Undifferentiated Somatoform Disorder share the following characteristics: multiple somatic symptoms or health concerns referable to different organ systems, the presence of related cognitive distortions, chronicity, dysfunction, and reduced quality of life. In previous editions of the DSM, Pain Disorder was described as a separate disorder, but in DSM-5 pain is included as a specifier for Somatic Symptom Disorder.

DSM-5 also addresses the major criticisms of the previous Somatoform Disorder (DSM-IV-TR), namely over-reliance on counting physical symptoms to reach diagnostic threshold and lack of any substantial psychological criteria. DSM-5 Somatic Symptom Disorder emphasises symptoms that are singularly psychological: cognitive distortions, high health-related anxiety, disproportionate and persistent concerns about the seriousness of symptoms, and excessive time and energy devoted to the symptoms and health concerns.

On examination, it becomes apparent that patients often present their complaints in an exaggerated manner, peppered with colourful descriptions. Accounts of their multiple bodily complaints can be vague and ineffectual. The historical description of their symptom careers is often faulty and patients sometimes fail to distinguish between current, recent, and past symptoms in their convoluted stories.

Table 8.11: Diagnostic criteria for Somatic Symptom Disorder as adapted from the DSM-5 and the ICD-10

DSM-5 Somatic Symptom Disorder	ICD-10 Somatisation Disorder
A. One or more somatic symptoms that are distressing or result in significant disruption of daily life.	A. There must be a history of at least two years of complaints of multiple and variable physical symptoms that cannot be explained by any detectable physical disorders. (Any physical disorders that are known to be present do not explain the severity, extent, variety, and persistence of the physical complaints, or the associated social disability.)

<table>
<tr><th>DSM-5
Somatic Symptom Disorder</th><th>ICD-10
Somatisation Disorder</th></tr>
<tr><td>B. Excessive thoughts, feelings, or behaviours related to the somatic symptoms or associated health concerns as manifested by at least one of the following:
(1) Disproportionate and persistent thoughts about the seriousness of one's symptoms.
(2) Persistently high level of anxiety about health or symptoms.
(3) Excessive time and energy devoted to these symptoms or health concerns.
C. Although any one somatic symptom may not be continuously present, the state of being symptomatic is persistent (typically more than 6 months).</td><td>If some symptoms clearly due to autonomic arousal are present, they are not a major feature of the disorder in that they are not particularly persistent or distressing.
B. Preoccupation with the symptoms causes persistent distress and leads the patient to seek repeated (three or more) consultations or sets of investigations with either primary care or specialist doctors. In the absence of medical services within the financial or physical reach of the patient, there must be persistent self-medication or multiple consultations with local healers.
C. There is persistent refusal to accept medical reassurance that there is no adequate physical cause for the physical symptoms. (Short-term acceptance of such reassurance, i.e. for a few weeks during or immediately after investigations, does not exclude this diagnosis.)
D. There must be a total of six or more symptoms from the following list, with symptoms occurring in at least two separate groups:
Gastrointestinal symptoms
(1) abdominal pain;
(2) nausea;
(3) feeling bloated or full of gas;
(4) bad taste in mouth, or excessively coated tongue;
(5) complaints of vomiting or regurgitation of food;
(6) complaints of frequent and loose bowel motions or discharge of fluids from the anus;
Cardiovascular symptoms
(7) breathlessness without exertion;
(8) chest pains;
Genito-urinary symptoms
(9) dysuria or complaints of frequency of micturition
(10) unpleasant sensations in or around the genitals;
(11) complaints of unusual or copious vaginal discharge;
Skin and pain symptoms
(12) blotchiness or discolouration of the skin;
(13) pain in the limbs, extremities, or joints;
(14) unpleasant numbness or tingling sensations.
E. Most commonly used exclusion clause: Symptoms do not occur only during any of the schizophrenic or related disorders, any of the mood (affective) disorders, or panic disorder.</td></tr>
</table>

Source: Reprinted with permission from the Diagnostic and Statistical Manual of Mental Disorders (DSM), Fifth Edition, American Psychiatric Association (APA), 2013 and the ICD–10 Classification of Mental and Behavioural Disorders: Diagnostic Criteria for Research. World Health Organisation (WHO), Geneva, 2007.

Patients recount frequent visits to doctors, clinic sisters, and casualty departments. Interpersonal conflict, chronic distress, anxiety, and depression are not uncommon. Acts of deliberate self-harm and threats of suicide are also not unusual. Female patients may dress in a seductive manner or appear demure in consultation – an observation not unfamiliar in Borderline or Histrionic Personality Disorder (see Chapter 12). Patients also tend to be self-absorbed, display an external locus of control, seek praise, behave dependently, and manipulate interpersonal situations.

The nature and occurrence rates of symptoms vary across different cultures. Burning sensations in extremities, the feeling of worms crawling in the head and formication (ants crawling under the skin) are pseudo-neurological phenomena more common in Africa and South Asia than North America. In parts of the world where concern about semen loss is rife, symptoms referable to the genitalia are more common (American Psychiatric Association, 2000). In India, this syndrome is known as *dhat*. A whitish discharge in urine is interpreted by patients as semen loss. Both men and women are afflicted as females are also thought to secrete semen. A similar condition, known as *shen-k-uei,* is found in Taiwan (World Health Organisation, 1992).

Somatic Symptom Disorder is a chronic, disabling condition. Increases in symptom severity coincide with periods of heightened psychosocial stress. Symptoms come in spurts, lasting around six to nine months. Relatively symptom-free periods last around six months; it is rare for a patient to be symptom free for more than a year. Common co-morbid psychiatric conditions are Major Depressive Disorder, personality disorders, substance-related disorders, Generalised Anxiety Disorder and phobias. The most serious complication of Somatic Symptom Disorder is iatrogenic ('iatrogenic' literally means 'caused by the doctor' – *iatros* is doctor in Greek) and involves the risks of invasive diagnostic procedures, medication side effects, and repeated surgery.

Differential diagnosis

It stands to reason that the differential diagnoses of Somatic Symptom Disorder include general medical and neurological illness. Conditions with non-specific, transient, and fluctuating clinical manifestations present as the most likely candidates. As for Conversion Disorder, multiple sclerosis and myasthenia gravis are primary considerations. Systemic lupus erythematosus, acute intermittent porphyria, and porphyria variegata (also known as South African porphyria, most commonly encountered among certain Afrikaans families), hyperthyroidism, hyperparathyroidism, and haemochromatosis, or haemosiderosis (excessive deposition of iron in tissues) must be considered. Hyperparathyroidism, a surprisingly common condition among the elderly, causes sustained high concentrations of serum calcium, or hypercalcaemia, the consequences of which are manifold and affect many organ systems.

Features suggestive of Somatic Symptom Disorder rather than physical disease

- Association with psychosocial stressor
- Involvement of multiple organ systems
- Absence of characteristic findings on examination and laboratory investigations
- Absence of structural abnormalities.

Whereas syphilis was known as the 'great mimicker' in the pre-antibiotic era, acquired immune deficiency syndrome (AIDS) is its modern-day counterpart. Given its variable manifestations, AIDS warrants inclusion on the list of differential diagnoses. In older patients, particularly over the age of 40, the onset of multiple bodily symptoms must alert the doctor, or psychologist, to the possible presence of a medical condition. Obvious psychiatric differentials for Somatic Symptom Disorder are Illness Anxiety Disorder, Conversion Disorder, and Pain Disorder. Other psychiatric conditions presenting with unexplained physical symptoms notably include Schizophrenia, where psychotic bodily experiences and beliefs, like kinaesthetic (bodily) hallucinations, are surprisingly common. Somatic complaints, even psychotic ones, occur in Major Depressive Disorder. Panic Attacks are also defined by many bodily sensations.

Illness Anxiety Disorder (DSM-5)/Hypochondriacal Disorder (ICD-10)

Also known since the Hippocratic era and heavily entrenched in the minds and vernacular of the lay public, Hypochondriasis (as it was previously known in the DSM-IV-TR), in its current conceptualisation, concerns the morbid preoccupation with a disease conviction which involves the fear of contracting, or the belief of having, a serious disease. Exaggerated awareness and frankly inaccurate interpretation of bodily symptoms and functions give rise to the erroneous beliefs and fears. The ancient Greeks attributed the syndrome to visceral disturbances in the 'hypochondrium' (*hypo* refers to below, *chondrium* to cartilage), or the area of abdomen below the cartilaginous border of the ribcage. In the nineteenth century, Hypochondriasis referred specifically to unexplained conditions limited to the anatomical hypochondrium.

Illness Anxiety Disorder/Hypochondriacal Disorder has virtually always been subservient to another mental disorder, like an anxiety disorder or major depression. Since its induction into the modern nosologies, its validity as a separate condition has been questioned. The location of this disorder within the Somatic Symptom/Somatoform Disorders has also been the topic of debate.

Symptoms of this disorder often occur in depressive and anxiety disorders. In addition, it is not unusual for it to exist co-morbidly with these conditions. This observation has led to it being conceptualised as a symptom dimension, rather than diagnostic category. Symptom dimensions recognise the occurrence of clusters of symptoms across different disorders, but do not regard the clusters as diagnostic entities in their own right. For example, fever is a typical symptom dimension in general medicine: we recognise its occurrence in many conditions but do not talk of 'fever disorder'.

Epidemiology

In a general medical population, the six-month prevalence of this disorder ranges between 4% and 6%, although a wide range has been found by various studies (Escobar, 1998). Information from Africa about its prevalence and other epidemiological characteristics is negligible. In contrast with Conversion and Somatic Symptom Disorders, the sexes are equally affected. Age of onset is typically in the twenties, although the condition can start at any age. Social class, education, and marital status appear not to affect its expression.

Aetiology and pathogenesis

Extensions of psychoanalytic theory explain this disorder as disturbed object relations, displacement of repressed hostilities to the body in order to better communicate anger – albeit indirectly – and an interplay between masochism, guilt, conflicted dependency, and the need for suffering and receiving love. Defences against low self-esteem, inadequacy, and conditioned reinforcement of the sick role have also been considered causative. The most compelling evidence points toward it as a variant expression of other mental conditions, notably anxiety disorders and depression. It seems these conditions establish a hyper-vigilant state which is biased towards the detection of harm, including probable noxious signals originating from the person's own body. It is like an overly-sensitive smoke detector, raising the alarm for evacuation on detecting the smoke of a single cigarette wafting in from an office balcony. If this hypothesis holds sway, disturbances in the neural substrate of fear are implicated in the condition's pathogenesis.

Illness Anxiety/ Hypochondriasis: Rules of thumb

- Preoccupation with having a disease
- Absence of demonstrable pathology
- Anxious disposition
- Reassurance not helpful
- Symptoms correlate with psychosocial stress.

Table 8.12: Diagnostic criteria for Illness Anxiety Disorder (DSM-5) and Hypochondriacal Disorder (ICD-10)

DSM-5 Illness Anxiety Disorder	ICD-10 Hypochondriacal Disorder
A. Preoccupation with having or acquiring a serious illness. B. Somatic symptoms are not present or, if present, are only mild in intensity. If another medical condition is present or there is a high risk for developing a medical condition (e.g. strong family history is present), the preoccupation is clearly excessive or disproportionate. C. There is a high level of anxiety about health, and the individual is easily alarmed about personal health status. D. The individual performs excessive health-related behaviours (e.g. repeatedly checks his or her body for signs of illness) or exhibits maladaptive avoidance (e.g. avoids doctor appointments and hospitals). E. Illness preoccupation has been present for at least 6 months, but the specific illness that is feared may change over that period of time.	A. Either of the following must be present: (1) a persistent belief, of at least 5 months' duration, of the presence of a maximum of two serious physical diseases (of which at least one must be specifically named by the patient) (2) a persistent preoccupation with a presumed deformity or disfigurement (Body Dysmorphic Disorder) B. Preoccupation with the belief and the symptoms causes persistent distress or interference with personal functioning in daily living and leads the patient to seek medical treatment or investigations (or equivalent help from local healers). C. There is persistent refusal to accept medical reassurance that there is no physical cause for the symptoms or physical abnormality. (Short-term acceptance of such reassurance, i.e. for a few weeks during or immediately after investigations, does not exclude this diagnosis.)

DSM-5 Illness Anxiety Disorder	ICD-10 Hypochondriacal Disorder
F. The illness-related preoccupation is not better explained by another mental disorder, such as somatic symptom disorder, panic disorder, generalised anxiety disorder, body dysmorphic disorder, obsessive-compulsive disorder, or delusional disorder, somatic type.	D. Most commonly used exclusion clause: The symptoms do not occur only during any of the schizophrenic and related disorders or any of the mood (affective) disorders.

Source: Reprinted with permission from the Diagnostic and Statistical Manual of Mental Disorders (DSM), Fifth Edition, American Psychiatric Association (APA), 2013 and the ICD–10 Classification of Mental and Behavioural Disorders: Diagnostic Criteria for Research. World Health Organisation (WHO), Geneva, 2007.

Diagnosis, clinical presentation, and course

Table 8.12 lists the DSM-5 diagnostic criteria for Illness Anxiety Disorder and the ICD-10 criteria for Hypochondriacal Disorder.The most notable difference between the DSM-5 and ICD-10 diagnostic approaches is the latter's integration of Body Dysmorphic Disorder with Hypochondriacal Disorder (Criterion A (2)). In contrast, DSM-5 explicitly excludes Body Dysmorphic Disorder in Criterion F, and has included Body Dysmorphic Disorder in the Obsessive-Compulsive Disorders. ICD-10 also specifies Schizophrenia as a primary differential diagnosis.

The heterogeneity of patients with a DSM-5 diagnosis of Illness Anxiety is widely recognised. Around one-quarter of patients with this disorder display 'classical' illness anxiety, or fear of having a serious medical condition, but do not report somatic symptoms. The rest display a mix of illness anxiety and somatic symptoms.

This disorder commonly coexists with a depressive or anxiety disorder. Illness concerns fluctuate and typically intensify during periods of increased psychosocial stress, most notably the death of a loved one or serious illness affecting a person important to the patient. The disorder follows an episodic course with symptomatic episodes lasting months to years. Periods of remission are of similar duration. Significant long-term improvement is expected in one-third of cases. Predictors of good prognosis are: high socio-economic status, sudden onset of symptoms following a distinct stressor, the absence of significant personality pathology, no serious medical illness, and treatment-responsive anxiety or depression.

Differential diagnosis

As health concerns are about bodily disease, this disorder must be differentiated from general medical conditions. Like Somatic Symptom Disorder, medical conditions with ill-defined, transient, and fluctuating phenomena present as primary candidates for differential diagnosis. Examples of these include multiple sclerosis, systemic lupus erythematosus, and occult neoplasms (present but undetected cancers) are good examples in this regard. The distinction between Illness Anxiety Disorder and Somatic Symptom Disorder depends on the focus of the patient's concern: in the former, the concern is the presence or risk of developing a specific *disease;* in the latter, the patient complains of identified symptoms, not disease entities. Illness

Anxiety Disorder patients mostly list none or fewer symptoms than do patients with Somatic Symptom Disorder. The latter also involves multiple bodily systems.

Conversion Disorder can be distinguished from Illness Anxiety Disorder by the preponderance of female patients and the sudden and dramatic onset of pseudo-neurological symptoms. *La belle indifférence* also points toward Conversion Disorder. Body Dysmorphic Disorder – considered a variant of Hypochondriasis by the ICD – involves preoccupation with an anatomical abnormality, not illness anxiety. If illness concerns are of delusional intensity, psychotic disorders must be considered. Anxiety and depressive disorders often coexist with Illness Anxiety Disorder and hypochondriacal complaints are not infrequent in these conditions.

Conversion Disorder (Functional Neurological Disorder)

Although neuroscientific evidence for a dissociative neural mechanism in its expression is suggested (Spitzer, 2006), a precise understanding of the pathogenesis of Conversion Disorder continues to elude us. Once considered a dissociative disorder by the DSM, Conversion Disorder was reclassified as a Somatoform Disorder in DSM-III (1980) and remains so till today. For DSM-5, it retains its location under the category Somatic Symptom Disorder (APA, 2013). This recognises its primary presentation as somatic whilst avoiding inferences about a pathogenic mechanism. In contrast, ICD-10 continues to consider Conversion Disorder as a group of dissociative disturbances.

History

Conversion has been recognised since antiquity. The concept of 'hysteria' was first introduced by Egyptian physicians around 1900 BCE who regarded the emergence of symptoms to be a consequence of a 'wandering uterus'. Hysteria is derived from the ancient Greek word *'hyster'*, meaning 'uterus'. The term is attributed to the ancient Greek physician Hippocrates and included in the *Corpus Hippocraticum*. During the explosion of medical and psychological knowledge in the nineteenth century, a consideration of hysteria was revived, laying the foundations for its modern understanding. In his *Personnalité Hystérique,* Briquet proposed that the disorder resulted from brain dysfunction following stressful environmental events acting on the 'affective part of the brain'.

Reynolds reasoned that symptoms resulted from a patient forming some notion, or 'idea' about the patient's body. Jean Martin Charcot evoked and manipulated signs of hysteria through hypnosis. He also proposed that the disorder arose in individuals predisposed by heredity and once exposed to a traumatic event, a 'functional' or 'dynamic' brain lesion resulted. Pierre Janet, who introduced the concept of dissociation, viewed hysteria as a disturbance in selective attention (Black, 2004; Ford, 1985). Sigmund Freud first introduced the term 'conversion' to medicine. In psychoanalysis, conflict exists between instinctual impulses, like aggression or sexuality, and the prohibition of their expression. Conversion refers to the repression of unconscious intrapsychic conflict and the consequent conversion of the associated anxiety into a physical, or somatic, symptom. As a consequence, the patient avoids conscious confrontation of unacceptable, intolerable impulses. The resolution of intrapsychic conflict is considered the primary gain. But, in communicating a need for special treatment through the expression of the conversion symptom, the patient may derive additional benefits from others, bringing about the so-called secondary gain that can be seen as a way of non-verbally manipulating others and the environment (Ford, 1985; Sadock & Sadock, 2000). Despite the logical appeal provided by the psychoanalytic understanding of conversion, clinical experience has failed to show convincingly that any gain is derived.

Over the ensuing decades, other aetiological theories emerged, including theories relating to social, communication, and behavioural aspects. The ascent of neuroscience in the late twentieth century saw a resurgence of interest in the biological mechanisms at play in Conversion Disorder. Clinical experience, neuropsychological evidence, and advances in neuro-imaging and neuro-physiological techniques have yielded insightful and practical pathogenic theories of conversion and Conversion Disorder.

Epidemiology

Conversion symptoms of severity insufficient to warrant medical attention occur in as many as one-third of all people. Among psychiatric patients, the incidence of conversion symptoms is between 5% and 15%. Females outnumber males by up to five to one. In men, conversion symptoms mainly relate to occupational accidents, military service, being on trial, and serving a prison sentence. Onset can be at any age, but is most common in adolescence. Conversion Disorder is most common in the youngest child in a family; in lower socio-economic classes; subaverage intelligence; educational underachievement; rural domicile; and exposure to war and combat (Ford, 1985).

Conversion Disorder is universal but the type of symptoms depends on sociocultural contexts. In Nigeria and India, the most common pseudo-neurological complaints are feelings of heat, peppery and crawling sensations, numbness, burning hands, and a hot peppery sensation in the head. 'Brain fag', a condition originally described in Nigerian university students and believed not uncommon in South Africa, presents with the aforementioned symptoms. Pseudo-neurological symptoms are also common in *ataque de nervios* and include heat rising to the head, numbness of extremities, and pseudo-seizures (Escobar, 2004).

Aetiology and pathogenesis

To facilitate understanding of its pathogenesis, we need to explore the important clinical manifestations of Conversion Disorder. Conversion involves the emergence of a single symptom, or set of symptoms, referable to the nervous system. This mode of presentation is called 'monosymptomatic' and 'pseudo-neurological' and can affect any aspect of neurological function, including abnormal movements, paralysis, gait disturbances, non-seizural convulsions, mutism, urinary retention, hallucinations, pain, blindness, deafness, analgesia, and disequilibrium symptoms like giddiness and a sense of lurching.

On neurological examination, inconsistencies abound: simultaneous contraction of opposing agonist-antagonist muscle groups; fluctuating weakness; sensory losses that do not follow anatomical boundaries; and dramatic and implausible movement and gait disturbances. *La belle indifférence* (the flippant lack of concern for the apparently serious neurological handicap shown by the patient) reminds of lesions involving the non-dominant parietal cortex. When a stroke affects the non-dominant parietal cortex, the patient tends to neglect, or deny the existence of, the opposite part of the body; this is called hemi-neglect.

The patient may also seem unaffected by the affliction and carry on as if there is nothing wrong at all, a phenomenon called anosognosia meaning 'failure to recognise disease'. Because the left side of the body is represented mainly in the right hemisphere of the brain, the preponderance of left-sided symptoms in Conversion Disorder further implicates non-dominant hemispheric involvement because, in most people, the non-dominant hemisphere is located on the right. Alexithymia and anxiety are also common in Conversion Disorder.

Slater (1965) found that more than 50% of patients with a current diagnosis of Conversion Disorder proceed to develop a recognisable neurological condition within ten years of original diagnosis. Although this claim has become controversial, the presence of Conversion Disorder does not rule out concurrent or future neurological disease. Likewise, actual neurological disease does not exclude Conversion Disorder (Black, 2004). Ludwig (1972) posited that sensory information feeding into the cortex is inhibited by other cortical regions thereby barring somatic information from consciousness. Findings suggesting bi-frontal and right parietal dysfunctions (as suggested by *la belle indifférence* and the preponderance of left-sided symptoms) supported this notion (Flor-Henry, 1965, cited in Black, 2004). In addition, subtle verbal imprecision, impaired vigilance and memory, affective incongruence, and disordered processing of endogenous somatic percepts (internal sensory and experiential representations of the body) are also demonstrable and support left-dominant impairments. Impaired inter-hemispheric communication further compounds the picture (Black, 2004; Sadock & Sadock, 2000).

Conversion Disorder: Rules of thumb

- Affects females more than males
- Psychologically unsophisticated
- History of childhood trauma
- Symptoms associated with psychosocial stressor
- Mono-symptomatic and pseudo-neurological
- Symptoms: sensory, motor, seizure, and mixed
- Usually brief course
- Coexistence of other neurological illness common.

Functional neuro-imaging findings provide more support for the neurological basis of Conversion Disorder. For example, activation of the anterior cingulate gyrus and association motor cortices (areas concerned with the initiation and planning of movements), and inactivity of the primary motor strip (the area of cortex that transmits the final signal for muscle contraction), have been demonstrated in conversion paralysis (refer to Figure 8.3). Right inferior parietal dysfunction is also demonstrable on functional imaging. Unlike the primary sensory cortices (the first cortical port of call for incoming sensory information), the body is not conformally mapped onto the inferior parietal cortex. In this instance, conformal mapping means that bodily features are represented in the cortex in a manner that their relationships and relative sizes are maintained. It is analogous to a map drawn of Africa faithfully showing South Africa at the tip of the continent embracing a much smaller land-locked Lesotho and that the much larger Congo, with which it shares no border, lies to its north. In higher-order cortices, conformity is not maintained and the bodily representation is distorted. As a consequence, dysfunction in a higher-order sensory cortex, like the inferior parietal cortex, may explain the disregard for anatomical constraints so characteristic of sensory conversion symptoms.

Since the nineteenth century, most observers have noted the universality of early trauma as a predictor of Conversion Disorder. The earlier the trauma and the longer its duration, the more severe conversion symptoms are likely to be. Incestuous experiences appear to confer additional risk. Although specific details of abuse may be questionable, patients probably experienced significant problems with attachment, impaired object relations, and a dysfunctional family system (Krahn, 2008).

Conversion Disorder appears to be the result of dynamic restructuring of neural networks leading to the disconnection of volition, sensory experience, and movement. In the absence of an identifiable anatomical lesion, the disconnection is considered 'functional' and emerges as a result of dissociative compartmentalisation related to early adverse experience. Whilst primary perception and motor control are intact, integration of sensory percepts and motor planning is not. As a result, when disruption occurs at the level of preconscious motor planning, paralysis ensues; when modality-specific attention is disrupted, sensory losses like blindness and anaesthesia follow (Black, 2004; Krahn, 2008; Mailis-Gagnon & Israelson, 2003; Sierra, 1998; Spence, 2000). Disturbances of right fronto-parietal networks may cause disturbances in self recognition and the sense of 'selfhood' (Black, 2004; Sierra, 1998). The well-documented occurrence of 'negative affectivity' most likely relates to non-dominant frontal disturbances (Black, 2004). Our current understanding of conversion as an evolutionary adaptation underlies its existence as a brain response type.

Diagnosis, clinical presentation, and course

Tables 8.13 and 8.14 provide diagnostic criteria for Conversion Disorder of DSM-5 and ICD-10 respectively. Conversion symptoms fall into four broad categories: sensory, motor, seizure, and mixed. Conventionally, diagnosis has been one of exclusion, but the nature of conversion symptoms alone can alert the doctor to their presence. Conversion symptoms do not observe neurological constraints and demonstrate, to a greater or lesser degree, incongruence and internal inconsistencies. The DSM-5 emphasises this and recommends using them as positive indicators of conversion. Finely-honed observation and command of neuro-anatomy are invaluable allies in the unmasking of conversion symptoms. Examples of incongruent and inconsistent symptoms are provided in the discussion on individual symptom categories.

A history of physical or sexual abuse is sometimes reported. A psychological trauma that precedes onset of the index conversion symptom is usually identifiable, although it remains unclear whether this is a prerequisite for symptom development. Over and above the conversion symptom, history and mental state examination will often reveal a person of low intellect who is psychologically unsophisticated. Patients may come across as depressed or anxious. Alexithymia, or the inability of a patient to 'read' his or her own mood, is common during the conversion episode and as an enduring trait in patients prone to conversion (Grabe, 2000). About 50% of patients display *la belle indifférence.* Cognitive deficits are not clinically conspicuous, although very slight verbal expressive difficulties may be noted. Insight is often poor. Personality styles commonly associated with Conversion Disorder are passive-aggressive, dependent, antisocial, and histrionic. Conversion patients are at heightened risk of suicide and self-harm (Black, 2004; Ford, 1985; Krahn, 2008; Sadock & Sadock, 2000).

Sensory symptoms

Anaesthesia (loss of sensation) and paraesthesia (abnormal sensations like 'pins and needles') are common in Conversion Disorder and tend to involve the extremities. Anaesthesia often follows a 'glove and stocking' distribution uncharacteristic of peripheral neuropathy, spinal cord or brain pathology. Likewise, hemi-anaesthesia (loss of sensation over one half of body) strictly observing the patient's midline with perfect demarcation of anaesthetic skin and normal skin suggests Conversion Disorder or feigning. All sensory modalities fall prey to Conversion Disorder, including the organs of special sensation: blindness, tunnel vision, monocular diplopia (double vision in one eye only), deafness, and loss of smell and taste. Careful neurological examination usually uncovers normal sense organs and intact pathways; for example, pupils respond appropriately to light and 'blind' patients can negotiate obstacles without help.

Motor symptoms

Weakness, paralysis, abnormal movements, and gait disturbances are all encountered. In a paralysed limb, muscle tone and reflexes remain normal. Wasting is usually absent, except in cases of chronic conversion paralysis where disuse atrophy sets in. Fasciculations – small ripple-like contractions in a muscle indicative of loss of innervation to the muscle – are absent. Hoover's sign may be observed, where the heel of an ostensibly paralysed limb presses down onto the doctor's hand when the patient is asked to raise the other leg. Conversion paralysis involving one side of the body is contradicted by a patient's failure to turn his or her head to that side when instructed. Movement disturbances are often grotesque and involve the extremities, trunk, head, and face. Swaying, rhythmical tremors, tic-like and choreiform (dance-like) movements occur. Bobbing of the head on the trunk is a strong indicator of Conversion Disorder. Abnormal movements typically worsen when attention is drawn to them. Astasia-abasia – an outrageous gait with a general wildness uncharacteristic of true ataxia is typical of Conversion Disorder. Patients with astasia-abasia rarely fall, and when they do, rarely hurt themselves. As with sensory disturbances, weakness and other motor abnormalities tend to fluctuate from examination to examination.

Pseudo-seizures

Pseudo-seizures are convulsive events resembling true seizures. To complicate matters, nearly one-third of patients with pseudo-seizures have confirmed epilepsy. Certain pseudo-seizures may have their origins in the expression of a complex learnt response to stress that recruits the same or similar neural networks to those usually active during a true seizure. Predating the onset of pseudo-seizures, an epileptic patient might have responded to a psychological trauma with a true seizure. Conforming to a dissociative mechanism, this 'seizure response' becomes the preferential response to future trauma. When challenged again by similar trauma, neural networks behave as is usual during a seizure. This produces the observable phenomena without demonstrable seizural electrical activity.

Clinically then, the patient shows behaviour indistinguishable from a true seizure, but without the occurrence of an electrophysiological storm. Indicators for the occurrence of pseudo-seizures include the absence of injuries during falls, no tongue-biting, absence of urinary incontinence, intact light and gag reflexes, and no rapid increase in serum prolactin concentration. Prolactin is a hormone released by the pituitary and promotes lactation; a seizure stimulates sudden release of prolactin into the blood stream. A most useful aid in diagnosing pseudo-seizures is constant video EEG telemetry.

Other symptoms

Communication disturbances, usually of an expressive kind, range from mutism to bizarre and changeable disturbances of articulation. Aphonia, or the inability to produce the necessary voice on which words are grafted through articulation, is also encountered. Conversion aphonia is distinguished from true aphonia (e.g. damage to the recurrent laryngeal nerve or resection of the larynx) by the retained ability to vocalise whilst coughing or sneezing. Globus hystericus, or 'lump in the throat', common in states of anxiety and experienced by normal people, is likely to be a mixed sensory and motor conversion phenomenon.

Obviously non-physiological and fanciful symptoms tend to occur in least educated patients. Conversion patients' proneness to suggestion adds to the difficulty in securing reliable symptoms (American Psychiatric Association, 2000). False memories, particularly of childhood physical and sexual abuse, are now considered conversion phenomena (Krahn, 2008) but are not accommodated by DSM-5 or ICD-10 schemata. The concept is also at odds with the DSM's declared stance on limiting phenomena encountered in somatoform disorders, the category to which Conversion Disorder belongs in the DSM-5, to the bodily aspects. That said, conversion hallucinations, or pseudo-hallucinations, differ from psychotic hallucinations, hallucinations found in delirium, and those associated with Posttraumatic Stress Disorder, Acute Stress Disorder, and Dissociative Trance Disorder. Pseudo-hallucinations may take on a useful, supportive quality, like a distressed girl hearing the voice of her boyfriend comforting her. They may also contain magical and childlike imagery. Insight into their 'unreality' is mostly retained (Hales, 2008).

Conversion Disorder Symptoms

- **Mono-symptomatic and pseudo-neurological**
- **Symptoms do not adhere to neurological constraints and are incongruent and internally inconsistent**
- **Sensory: blindness, tunnel vision, hearing loss, loss of sensation over skin (e.g. glove-and-stocking)**
- **Motor: paralysis, abnormal movements, gait disturbance (astasia-abasia)**
- **Pseudo-seizures**
- **Common: weakness, blindness, sensory loss, and mutism**
- **Extravagant symptoms correlate with psychological naivety.**

Course

In 90% to 100% of cases, conversion symptoms resolve within a few days. One in four patients experiences recurrence of conversion during periods of psychosocial stress. Good pre-morbid psychosocial adjustment, sudden onset of symptoms following a clearly identifiable stressor, no co-morbid psychiatric or medical conditions, and the absence of civil or criminal litigation improve prognosis. The longer conversion symptoms remain present, the worse the outcome. The delayed emergence of a neurological condition always remains likely, necessitating meticulous examination and rigorous surveillance.

Table 8.13: Diagnostic criteria for Conversion Disorder as adapted from the DSM-5

DSM-5 Conversion Disorder (Functional Neurological Symptom Disorder)
A. One or more symptoms of altered voluntary motor or sensory function. B. Clinical findings provide evidence of incompatibility between the symptom and recognised neurological or medical conditions. C. The symptom or deficit is not better explained by another medical or mental disorder. D. The symptom or deficit causes clinically significant distress or impairment in social, occupational, or other important areas of functioning or warrants medical evaluation.
Specify symptom type: **(F44.4) With weakness or paralysis** **(F44.4) With abnormal movement** (e.g. tremor, dystonic movement, myoclonus, gait disorder) **(F44.4) With swallowing symptoms** **(F44.4) With speech symptom** (e.g. dysphonia, slurred speech) **(F44.5) With attacks or seizures** **(F44.6) With anaesthesia or sensory loss** **(F44.6) With special sensory symptom** (e.g. visual, olfactory, or hearing disturbance) **(F44.7) With mixed symptoms**

Source: Reprinted with permission from the Diagnostic and Statistical Manual of Mental Disorders (DSM), Fifth Edition, American Psychiatric Association (APA), 2013.

Differential diagnosis

It stands to reason that neurological conditions involving sensory and motor symptoms, as well as seizures, are differential diagnoses. The range of candidate pathologies is wide, including cerebrovascular disease, cerebral neoplasia, infection, neuro-degenerative conditions, epilepsies, and dementias. Other conditions include myasthenia gravis (progressive muscle weakness, worsened by fatigue, caused by auto-immune destruction of the junction of motor nerves onto muscles) and other myopathies (muscle diseases).

Multiple sclerosis (an auto-immune inflammation and destruction of white matter in the central nervous system degrading nerve conduction) can mimic sensory and motor conversion symptoms. Affective disturbances often accompany both multiple sclerosis and Conversion Disorder. A related condition, optic neuritis (inflammation of the retina and optic nerve) causing visual loss can be misdiagnosed as Conversion Disorder. Other conditions with confusing symptoms include Guillain-Barre Syndrome, a condition involving the spinal cord and causing progressively ascending paralysis involving more and more of the body.

Table 8.14: Diagnostic criteria for Dissociative Equivalents of Conversion Disorder as adapted from the ICD-10

DISSOCIATIVE MOTOR DISORDERS
A. The general criteria for dissociative disorder must be met. B. Either of the following must be present: (1) Complete or partial loss of the ability to perform movements that are normally under voluntary control (including speech). (2) Various or variable degrees of incoordination or ataxia, or inability to stand unaided.
DISSOCIATIVE CONVULSIONS
A. The general criteria for dissociative disorder must be met. B. The individual exhibits sudden and unexpected spasmodic movements, closely resembling any of the varieties of epileptic seizure, but not followed by loss of consciousness. C. The symptoms in criterion B are not accompanied by tongue-biting, serious bruising or laceration due to falling, or urinary incontinence.
DISSOCIATIVE ANAESTHESIA AND SENSORY LOSS
A. The general criteria for dissociative disorder must be met. B. Either of the following must be present: (1) Partial or complete loss of any or all of the normal cutaneous sensations over part or all of the body (specify: touch, pinprick, vibration, heat, cold). (2) Partial or complete loss of vision, hearing, or smell (specify).
MIXED DISSOCIATIVE (CONVERSION) DISORDERS

Schizophrenia, depression and anxiety conditions can also be associated with strange bodily phenomena. Somatic Symptom Disorder can have pseudo-neurological symptoms. The presence of other somatic symptoms and their chronicity sway diagnosis in the direction of Somatic Symptom Disorder. Hypochondriasis concerns a preoccupation with disease and patients do not focus on specific symptoms. Malingering and factitious disorders remain the greatest diagnostic challenge when faced with a patient presenting with atypical or implausible symptoms.

CASE STUDY

Claudia Z lives in a small coastal town in the Eastern Cape. She is a 27-year-old single mother of two toddlers, one of whom is mentally retarded. Since her father's death three years ago, she has been responsible for supporting her ailing mother, working as a packer at a small supermarket in town. A few weeks before the collapse, she met a police officer on secondment from Port Elizabeth. A romantic relationship developed but was soon spoiled by mistrust, resentment, and physical violence. One Monday, Claudia collapsed at work and was taken to the local hospital.

She was found to be fully conscious and able to give an adequate account of herself and recent events. She described a sudden and complete loss of sensation in her lower limbs and could no longer move. Her general examination was unremarkable. She was unable to lift her legs off the bed, let alone stand. Muscle tone and deep tendon reflexes were normal and Hoover's sign present. She also demonstrated a dense sensory loss affecting both lower limbs, but not conforming to any known neurological distribution. She was transferred to Port Elizabeth where detailed special investigations failed to uncover any focal neurological lesions. A psychiatrist who consulted her whilst in Port Elizabeth commented that she appeared childlike and displayed a glib disregard for her apparently grave neurological condition. During her stay in hospital, she received regular visits by the hospital clinical psychologist who provided supportive therapy. Exactly a week after the sudden onset of paralysis and sensory loss, Claudia stood up and discharged herself from hospital.

Persistent Somatoform Pain Disorder (ICD-10)

The International Association for the Study of Pain (Merskey & Bogduk, 1986, p. 209) defines pain as 'an unpleasant sensory and emotional experience associated with actual or potential tissue damage, or described in terms of such damage'. This definition stresses the subjective nature of pain. Chronic pain is defined as 'pain that persists beyond the normal time of healing' (Merskey & Bogduk, 1986, p. 209).

Acute pain is a cardinal adaptive response to tissue damage, initiated by nociception (stimulation of nerves conducting pain) and accompanied by behaviours that limit tissue damage. Chronic pain, on the other hand, involves layers of pain experience, suffering, and pain behaviour, and is a dysfunctional remnant of a once-adaptive behaviour. Pain behaviour encompasses a patient's efforts to avoid factors that may precipitate or aggravate pain where behavioural restrictions adversely affect all experience. The maintenance of pain is mediated through several mechanisms located in the peripheral and central nervous systems. In addition, emotional and motivational aspects exert their influence through conditioning. Although pain experienced in Pain Disorder may have had a definite nociceptive origin, psychological factors are foremost in its persistence.

The validity of Pain Disorder has been questioned since its first incarnations as Somatoform Pain Disorder in DSM-III-R (American Psychiatric Association, 1987). During the preparations for the DSM-IV, much consideration was given to the omission of Pain Disorder from the somatoform disorders. Favouring exclusion was recognition that pain without nociceptive origin is unusual and that separating the psychological and physical aspects of chronic pain is nearly impossible. This complication was acknowledged by the DSM-IV Work Group and reflected in the eventual DSM-IV diagnostic criteria. ICD-10 continues to lack an equivalent disorder. The Persistent Somatoform Pain Disorder of ICD-10 is more restrictive in its definition and is limited to chronic pain without any demonstrable nociceptive origin. DSM-5 includes pain as a specifier of Somatic Symptom Disorder. DSM-5 Somatic Symptom Disorder emphasises the psychological aspects of the disturbance with reference to cognitive distortions and emotional impacts, and supports 'pain behaviour' as a manifestation of chronic pain.

Epidemiology

Pain is the commonest complaint in all of medicine. The general practitioner will attest to this with frequent encounters with patients complaining of lower back pain, joint pains, and headaches. In the developed world, estimates of the occurrence of chronic pain range between 25% and 30% of the general population. Thousands of people are given disability benefits each year because of chronic pain. In the Netherlands, it is estimated that 10,000 new cases of chronic pain are added annually, with substantial burden on the fiscus (Verhaak, Kerssens, Dekker, Sorbi, & Bensing, 1998). Persistent Somatoform Pain Disorder is diagnosed twice as commonly in women as in men. Onset is usually in the fourth or fifth decade of life. Demographically, Persistent Somatoform Pain Disorder is associated with lower educational achievement and lower socio-economic standing.

Aetiology and pathogenesis

A review of the complex neurobiology of pain is beyond the bounds of an undergraduate psychology textbook. Chronic pain has multifactorial origins, but a constitutional predisposition is likely. First-degree relatives of Persistent Somatoform Pain Disorder probands are at increased risk of developing it. Developmental risks include childhood adversity like parental separation, alcohol abuse in the home, quarrelling parents, and lack of physical affection towards the child. An association between chronic pain and depressive conditions has long been reported, yet its neural mechanism remains elusive. The conscious experience of pain is modulated by the cerebral cortex through descending inhibitory pathways using serotonin as neurotransmitter.

Endorphins also modulate the expression and experience of pain. Endorphins are opioid-like molecules that occur naturally in the central nervous system. A primary lesion in one of these modulatory systems could result in true Persistent Somatoform Pain Disorder, as opposed to a disorder characterised by chronic pain co-occurring with another mental condition like depression or emerging on the back of actual tissue damage and nociceptive pain.

Kindling is the systematic amplification of a nerve's responsiveness following repeated low-grade or sub-threshold stimulation of post-synaptic nerve. Kindling, through long-term potentiation and other forms of neural plasticity, is considered an essential mechanism in the formation of memory. In the development of chronic pain, kindling may be active in neural networks that relay pain-

Chronic physical pain

- **Pain fluctuates**
- **Patients can be distracted from pain experience**
- **Analgesics provide relief**
- **Examples:**
  - **Neuropathies (e.g. diabetic)**
  - **Neuralgia (e.g. trigeminal, post-herpetic)**
  - **Neuroma (e.g. arising from severed nerve)**
  - **Cancer (especially pancreatic carcinoma)**
  - **Arthritis (e.g. rheumatoid, osteoarthritis)**
  - **Peripheral vascular disease.**

related information between the cortex and limbic system (Rome, 2000). In the spinal cord and peripheral nervous system, commandeering of non-nociceptive nerves to mediate pain (e.g. nerves that characteristically conduct fine touch now come to relay pain), sensitisation (increased responsivity), and amplification (increased nerve signal intensity) are further mechanisms that can maintain pain in the absence of tissue damage (Dworkin & Wilson, 1993; Shipton, 2008).

Psychodynamic theories of chronic pain relate to patients symbolically expressing intrapsychic conflicts by means of the body. Others may regard emotional suffering as weakness, thus displacing the problem to the body. Pain can also function as a mechanism for obtaining love and nurturance as well as averting responsibilities. These secondary gains reinforce pain and maintain the pain-related behaviour. Intractable pain has also been conceptualised as a means to manipulate others and to gain the upper hand in tense interpersonal situations, like a strained marriage.

CASE STUDY

Frans, 42, is a machine operator at a bottling plant outside Pretoria. He is divorced and has two teenage children living with his ex-wife. His general practitioner referred him to the specialist psychiatric clinic of a local teaching hospital for evaluation and further management. Five years ago, Frans injured his neck when he was knocked over by a forklift. He sustained what appeared to be a minor sprain to his neck muscles with no fracture or dislocation. Due process for lodging an injury-on-duty claim was followed. But, after a protracted dispute and escalating tension between Frans and his employer, his claim for compensation was rejected. In the ensuing months, Frans found it increasingly hard to work. He was always in pain and struggled to move his neck. Eventually, he went on an extended sick leave. For the past six months, Frans has been on unpaid leave of absence and has struggled to make ends meet.

When examined by the attendant clinical psychologist, Frans came across as miserable. He struggled to describe his feelings and repeatedly brought the conversation back to his intractable pain, his suffering, and inability to enjoy life the way he used to before the injury. He stopped playing club rugby after the accident, gave up fly-fishing, no longer tinkers in the garage, and has even stopped visiting friends. Never free of pain, he has resorted to a daily intake of over-the-counter analgesics, often taking excessive amounts causing unpleasant side effects and occasional withdrawal symptoms. His alcohol intake has also escalated. Recently, he was convicted for driving under the influence of alcohol. The embarrassment of the conviction and the relentless pain made him contemplate suicide for the first time. He implored the psychologist to do his best, for he claimed that were it not for the pain, his life would be 'back on track'.

Diagnosis, clinical presentation, and course

The ICD-10 diagnostic criteria for Persistent Somatoform Pain Disorder are provided in Table 8.15. ICD-10 criteria for Persistent Somatoform Pain Disorder draw attention to the all-consuming nature of the disorder, where pain-related behaviours have superseded adaptive functioning and ruined experience. DSM-5 considers pain as a somatic symptom, regardless of origin. When pain is the focus of presentation and the patient's psychic life is fashioned around it, it becomes a disorder in its own right. In stark contrast, chronic nociceptive pain, without negative modification by psychological factors, is not a mental disorder, for example, chronic cancer pain, post-herpetic neuralgia (pain following reactivation of chickenpox), and peripheral vascular disease in an otherwise well-adjusted individual with good pre-morbid psychosocial adaptation.

Persistent Somatoform Pain Disorder: Rules of thumb

- Pain is focus of presentation
- Feelings, motivations, and behaviours become subordinate to pain experience
- Pain behaviour is demonstrated with cognitive distortions and depression
- Chronic course.

In Persistent Somatoform Pain Disorder, all kinds of pain can be present: low back pain, facial pain, headache, or pelvic pain. Any pathological process can be responsible for the initiation of pain - trauma, surgery, or degeneration. The pain experience is all-consuming and colours every aspect of the patient's world. Patients can become utterly preoccupied with the pain and blame all their miseries and misfortunes on it. If not for the pain, an idealised life is imagined. Patients may deny any other causes of distress.

On history and examination, evidence of depression is present in nearly all patients. Typical depressive phenomena are anhedonia, lack of energy, decreased libido, insomnia, weight loss, psychomotor retardation, and irritability.

Persistent Somatoform Pain Disorder is often complicated by substance abuse, commonly painkillers and alcohol. Common co-morbid conditions are Major Depressive Disorder – present in 25-50% of cases – and Dysthymic Disorder. Persistent Somatoform Pain Disorder usually runs a chronic, unremitting, and disabling course. Antecedent personality pathology, marked passivity, substance abuse, and a long pain history predict a guarded outcome. Litigation and potential compensation predict a poorer prognosis.

Differential diagnosis

The following characteristics of nociceptive pain help to differentiate it from Persistent Somatoform Pain Disorder: physical pain fluctuates and is sensitive to emotions and contextual factors; distraction is usually possible and analgesics provide relief. Persistent Somatoform Pain Disorder may be difficult to distinguish from Somatic Symptom Disorder, but in the latter, multiple systems are involved and non-pain symptoms are present. Illness Anxiety/Hypochondriasis is characterised by a preoccupation about being ill, as opposed to the presence of pain. Conversion Disorder is typically short-lived and symptoms are limited to a single pseudo-neurological set. Pain, by definition, is also not considered a manifestation of Conversion Disorder.

Factitious disorders provide a diagnostic challenge. Also challenging, malingering typically occurs in a context where external motivations, like avoiding prosecution or obtaining compensation, are identifiable. However, diagnosis is made difficult because Persistent Somatoform Pain Disorder patients may well be motivated to malinger given the prospect of financial reward through disability compensation or the payment of damages.

Table 8.15: Diagnostic criteria for Persistent Somatoform Pain Disorder as adapted from ICD-10

ICD-10 Persistent Somatoform Pain Disorder
A. There is persistent severe and distressing pain (for at least 6 months, and continuously on most days), in any part of the body, which cannot be explained adequately by evidence of a physiological process or a physical disorder and which is consistently the main focus of the patient's attention.
B. *Most commonly used exclusion clause:* This disorder does not occur in the presence of Schizophrenia or related disorders, or only during any of the mood (affective) disorders, Somatisation Disorder, Undifferentiated Somatoform Disorder, or Hypochondriacal Disorder.

Source: Reprinted with permission from the ICD–10 Classification of Mental and Behavioural Disorders: Diagnostic Criteria for Research. World Health Organisation (WHO), Geneva, 2007.

Psychological factors affecting other medical conditions

This diagnostic category is included in this chapter for the sake of completeness. Where psychological factors are adjudged to adversely affect the expression of established physical illness, this diagnosis is justified. Psychological factors are considered ways of responding to stress, interpersonal style, maladaptive coping, denial, and non-compliance. By contrast, a psychological reaction to a physical condition is best considered an Adjustment Disorder. Obviously, physical illness can precipitate any psychiatric disorder.

FACTITIOUS DISORDERS AND MALINGERING

The factitious disorders and malingering are considered to be illness-endorsing behaviours and involve the volitional and untruthful presentation of phenomena suggestive of illness or impairment. A good understanding of their clinical nature is also an invaluable aid to the process of diagnosis. Illness-endorsing behaviours show a professed belief in something that is untrue, where efforts are directed at endorsing the truth of a claimed illness. Any symptom, or combination of symptoms, whether physical or psychological, can be presented. Factitious disorders and malingering are disorders involved in such illness-endorsing deception.

Deceit involves a subject about which the person chooses to deceive, the deceptive distortion introduced into the subject, and a behaviour that communicates this untruth to the target of deceit. For example, in an effort to avoid being punished by his schoolmistress for not handing in his homework, a boy fabricates a story that his dog has eaten it. Here, the homework constitutes the subject of deceit, the alleged behaviour of his dog the distortion, and the boy's relaying of events the behaviour. In illness-endorsing behaviours, the subject of deceit concerns a chosen illness and the distortion lies in the manifestations of the chosen illness as displayed by the person carrying out the deception. The behaviour involves this person's attempts at convincing the examiner, or target of deceit, of the reality of the illness.

In malingering, the ruse involves the intentional endorsing of a false illness to avert threat or receive unfair advantage. An accused person may pretend to be psychotic so as to avoid trial. Another may feign chronic pain to obtain disability benefits. In malingering, the motivation is external and the malingerer is aware of it. In factitious disorders, the motivation is internal, or intrapsychic, and the patient unaware of it. In both malingering and factitious disorders, the deception is volitional and occurs with full awareness. The behavioural aspect of deceit concerns the quality of perpetration or how the deception is 'pulled off'.

The success of deceit rests on two pillars: familiarity with the subject of deceit and a style of communication that avoids raising suspicion. Deceitful communication succeeds if it appears natural and targets an unsuspecting audience. Deceitful communication is a skill honed through practice. Anxiety is its greatest foe. Suspicion is more often raised by the nature of the communication than by factual errors about the subject of deceit. While factual knowledge is a necessity to test the truth of any claim, recognising the presence of deceit also rests on keen observation and familiarity with human nature. In both factitious disorders and malingering, the untruthfulness of a claim exists on a continuum: deceitful symptoms may involve exaggeration of current ones, displacement of symptoms from one site or system to another, mislabelling innocuous experiences as symptoms, reporting past symptoms, and outright fabrication (Du Plessis, 2003).

Factitious Disorders

DSM-5 departs from the previous approaches to factitious disorder by relocating them to the Somatic Symptom Disorder category. This move highlights the importance of differentiating factitious disorders from other disorders characterised by somatic symptoms. DSM-5 also draws attention to the objective identification of deceit, or recognition of a 'pattern of falsification'.

According to DSM-5, factitious disorders involve the intentional production or feigning of physical or psychological symptoms in order to assume the sick role. Not only do patients deceive in their reporting of symptoms, they misrepresent their medical histories, and often their lives. The ICD-10 takes a similar approach.

DSM-5 identifies two factitious disorders, the first being Factitious Disorder imposed on Self. Table 8.16 provides the DSM-5 diagnostic criteria for Factitious Disorder Imposed on Self. Factitious Disorder Imposed on Another, also called Münchhausen by Proxy, is a disturbing situation where a caregiver, usually a mother, intentionally produces or feigns signs and symptoms in a person entrusted to their care, usually a child.

Aetiology, pathogenesis, and epidemiology

The aetiology is unknown. Men are more often affected than women. It is believed that many factitious patients suffered childhood abuse, poor attachment and perceived their parents as rejecting. Frequent contact with doctors and nurses and repeated hospitalisation may have been seen as a source of care and nurturance and an escape from harsh familial environments. This care and nurturance received may have served as reward, in turn reinforcing the illness-endorsing behaviour. Yet such patients appear to provoke repeated rejection, at first by a parent, then later by doctors and other caregivers. Rejection is thus re-enacted with masochistic regularity. Patients who present with predominantly psychological features have often had first-hand experience in living with, or taking care of a relative with a mental disorder. Patients often have above-average medical or psychological knowledge, gained from relatives or their own training and employment as laboratory technicians or nurses. Statistical data on factitious disorders are limited.

Diagnosis, clinical presentation, and course

Patients with factitious disorders challenge the doctor-patient relationship in that the patient enters the relationship from a position of intentional deceit and decimation of trust. Sparked by this apparent betrayal, and fuelled by our primitive punitive streak, the temptation to strike back must be resisted with all the power we are able to muster. Confrontation, exposure at all costs, and blaming attitudes are not helpful and may even precipitate severe personality disintegration, impulsive acts of self-harm, and frank psychosis.

Factitious Disorder Imposed on Others is popularly known as Münchhausen Syndrome, after the extravagant Karl Friederich Hieronymus Freiherr von Münchhausen (1720–1797) from Bodenwerder, now in Germany. A retired German cavalry officer and raconteur, he was renowned for his lavishly exaggerated tales of conquest and travel. He claimed, for instance, to have extracted himself from a swamp by his own hair and to have ridden a bisected horse into battle. Like the Baron, patients can present with pseudologia phantastica (pathological or compulsive lying), which is an elaborate, often fancifully embellished account of a person's exploits, where limited factual material is seamlessly mixed with outright fantasy. The patient also appears to believe his or her patently fallacious stories.

Münchhausen patients can present with a bewildering array of signs and symptoms and become remarkably adept at manipulating laboratory tests and clinical techniques. Their symptoms can cover the entire spectrum of internal medicine, surgery, and other disciplines. In time, patients become experts at symptomatology. Combined with oft-rehearsed performances to an assortment of medical specialists, some patients can turn even the doubters among these professionals into believers, strengthening and perpetuating the patient's dependency on health care. Patients submit themselves to repeated dangerous diagnostic procedures. The so-called washboard or gridiron abdomen is well known in surgical wards and speaks of repeated abdominal surgery. Co-morbid conditions like Borderline Personality Disorder and depression are common. Factitious psychotic symptoms are more likely with Borderline patients and those with a close relative who is mentally ill. Such patients have a prognosis worse than Bipolar I or Schizoaffective Disorder (Sadock & Sadock, 2000). Factitious Disorder runs a chronic, mostly unremitting course. Morbidity is presumed high because of exposure to multiple diagnostic and therapeutic interventions.

In spite of the deceitful nature of their presentations, patients with Factitious Disorder are distressed and dysfunctional. Often, Factitious Disorder is an even stronger reason for intervention than the fallacious presenting condition. Factitious Disorder also does not provide patients with immunity from other illnesses.

Table 8.16: Diagnostic criteria for Factitious Disorder Imposed on Self as adapted from DSM-5

DSM-5 Factitious Disorder as Imposed on Self
A. Falsification of physical or psychological signs or symptoms, or induction of injury or disease, associated with identified deception. B. The individual presents himself or herself to others as ill, impaired, or injured. C. The deceptive behaviour is evident even in the absence of obvious external rewards. D. The behaviour is not better explained by another mental disorder, such as delusional disorder or another psychotic disorder.

Differential diagnosis

As Factitious Disorder is almost always a diagnosis of exclusion, the differential diagnosis involves any conceivable condition. Psychiatric differential diagnoses include Somatic Symptom Disorder, Illness Anxiety Disorder/Hypochondriacal Disorder, Persistent Somatoform Pain Disorder, Borderline, Antisocial, and Histrionic Personality Disorder, Schizophrenia, and malingering. Ganser's Syndrome must be considered because of similarities in response style (e.g. *vorbeireden* or talking past the point).

CASE STUDY

Pule, a single man of thirty, presented to a well-known Johannesburg surgeon. Pule has a confirmed Bachelor's degree in biochemistry and had been employed as a laboratory technician at a private pathology laboratory until his retrenchment a year earlier. In the interim, he has worked as a waiter in Melville. He informed the surgeon that, for the past year, he had been experiencing repeated spells of light-headedness and fainting after meals. Pule produced a pile of reports from special investigations suggesting that he had experienced periods of sustained hypoglycaemia (low blood sugar). The surgeon immediately entertained the possibility of insulinoma – an insulin-secreting tumour of the pancreas. As an earlier dedicated arteriogram of the pancreas had failed to demonstrate a tumour, the surgeon organised admission for a repeat arteriogram and other investigations.

While examining Pule, the surgeon noticed that he must have undergone many laparotomies (major abdominal surgery) and remarked about his 'grid-iron abdomen'.

Pule admitted to this, listing appendectomy, cholecystectomy, and several exploratory laparotomies. Curiously, Pule could not provide any documentary evidence of the previous operations and was hesitant to divulge names of previous doctors and details of admissions. Pule described how, as a youngster, he had been sickly and often in hospital for 'months at a time'. He claimed to have spent weeks in ICU, requiring cardiopulmonary resuscitation on four occasions. Pule further related how, after graduating, he had worked for Medicin sans Frontiers in the Congo and Darfur, was involved in an exchange programme with a Libyan university, taught English in Taiwan, travelled across Tibet, met the Dalai Lama, played as a jazz saxophonist in Cape Town, worked as a clerk at the South African embassy in Guatemala, and spent three years in exile in the former East Germany.

Pule's very full life and improbable experiences left the surgeon uneasy and suspicious. In the first two days in hospital, Pule experienced three episodes of severe hypoglycaemia, culminating on one occasion in a grand mal seizure. For reasons she could not explain, an experienced nurse on the eve of retirement became suspicious of his presentation. When Pule had another hypoglycaemic attack, she decided to inspect the drawer of his bedside table. Perhaps not unsurprisingly, she discovered several half-empty blister packs of metformin, an oral treatment for diabetes and the most likely explanation for Pule's hypoglycaemic spells. With the surgeon's support, she approached Pule, gently enquiring about the tablets. Enraged, he accused both of them of criminal negligence and threatened litigation. But, minutes later, Pule fled the hospital never to be seen again.

Malingering

Malingering is not a mental disorder. Cunnien (1997) frames malingering as a conscious and deliberate behaviour that constitutes a form of pretence, fabrication, or feigning in the presence of an objectively identifiable goal. Rogers (1988) offers a similar understanding, but added that malingering can coexist with true illness. Turner (2000) emphasised that malingering per se, is neither symptom nor illness, but behaviour. Unrelated to Münchhausen's by Proxy, Malingering by Proxy involves the reporting of untruthful symptoms in another and is motivated by an identifiable external incentive, like securing a child support grant (Hales, 2008). Extended Malingering involves the co-opting of others to endorse the index malingerer's deceitful claims. Dysfunctional Malingering Syndrome involves continuation of hapless attempts at malingering despite the malingerer's realisation of its lack of success.

Table 8.17: Definition of Malingering as adapted from DSM-5

DSM-5 Malingering
The essential feature of malingering is the intentional production of grossly exaggerated physical or psychological symptoms, motivated by external incentives such as avoiding military duty, avoiding work, obtaining financial compensation, evading criminal prosecution, or obtaining drugs. Under some circumstances, malingering may represent adaptive behaviour – for example, feigning illness while a captive of the enemy during wartime. Malingering should be strongly suspected if any combination of the following is noted: 1. Medico-legal context (e.g. the person is referred by an attorney to the clinician for examination) 2. Marked discrepancy between the person's claimed stress or disability and the objective findings 3. Lack of cooperation during the diagnostic evaluation and in complying with the prescribed treatment 4. The presence of Antisocial Personality Disorder.

Source: Reprinted with permission from the Diagnostic and Statistical Manual of Mental Disorders (DSM), Fifth Edition, American Psychiatric Association (APA), 2013.

Epidemiology, clinical presentation, and assessment

Malingering is surprisingly common. In a general psychiatric population, Rogers (1993) found its incidence among people undergoing evaluation in personal damages suits at close on 50% and 21% in those undergoing assessment in criminal matters. In South Africa, the occurrence of malingering is not well studied. The clinical picture of malingering is rightly confusing and differential diagnoses embrace all of medicine and psychology. Its proper detection requires an alertness to inconsistency and a healthy dose of scepticism, all without sacrificing compassion. Exposing malingering is both satisfying and annoying, but it is humbling for professionals to realise their vulnerability to being deceived. The literature is replete with psychological tests tailored for the assessment of malingering. By virtue of their design and the predictable manner in which test takers respond, most psychometric and neuropsychological tests are de facto malingering screening devices. Most clinicians rely on their pattern-recognition ability to unmask malingering and do not employ systematic protocols; however, novice practitioners lack this experience.

Aware of the novice's needs and potential benefits of a systematic model, one of the authors of this chapter (Du Plessis, 2003) developed the 'Expert Model' for the clinical detection of malingering (see Tables 8.18, 8.19, and 8.20). The Expert Model is synthesised from clinical approaches taken by experts in forensic psychiatry. As it is generic and systematic, the Expert Model can assist the practitioner in any branch of clinical medicine.

Expert Model for the detection of malingering

The Expert Model follows a three-step approach:

- Suspicion – formation of the initial malingering hypothesis.

- Iterative hypothesis testing – the deductive stage.
- Clinical confirmation.

Table 8.18: 'Expert Model': Step-wise approach

STEP 1 – SUSPICION
1. Raised by context. 2. Raised by Symptomatology and/or Assessment Behaviour Dimension. 3. Psychological testing, laboratory investigations, and information from third parties.
STEP 2 – ITERATIVE HYPOTHESIS TESTING
1. Reviewing the domain or domains in which suspicion originally raised. 2. Examining other domains (Symptomatology and Assessment Behaviour) for supportive evidence. 3. Strengthened by formal psychological testing, laboratory investigations, information from third parties.
STEP 3 – CLINICAL CONFIRMATION
1. Presentation is implausible or impossible. 2. Sufficient iterations, rigorous cross-referencing to amass sufficient evidence. 3. Confession. 4. Direct observation of production of symptoms. 5. Escape from assessment not accounted for by another reason.

Table 8.19: 'Expert Model': Symtomatology dimension – domains and examples

SYMPTOMATOLOGY DIMENSION
Explanatory notes
• Requires expert knowledge and appraisal of symptoms. • Can be least labour and resource intensive, relying mainly on the clinical interaction, nursing, and incidental interactions. • Special investigations can add valuable information when least expected. Behaviour during test-taking or when undergoing laboratory procedures is often revealing (e.g. no anxiety in MRI tunnel in person claiming claustrophobia). • The dimension has four domains: Atypicality, Incongruence, Fluctuation-Variability, and Longitudinal.
Domains with examples
Atypicality Domain Psychopathological phenomena are mostly stereotypical and reflect pathological functioning in neural systems. Memory impairments conform to impairments in attentional, learning, and memory systems and have predictable features, viz. anterograde and retrograde components. Likewise, disturbances in language, praxis, and gnosis have typical manifestations. Psychotic phenomena are surprisingly stereotypical in presentation.

Incongruence Domain
It is most unusual for a disease or disorder to be characterised by a single phenomenon: 'orphan' symptoms draw immediate attention to their improbability. Symptoms typically keep predictable company and occur in predictable clusters, referred to as syndromes. Malingering is often characterised by the occurrence of orphan symptoms or arbitrary clustering of symptoms not conforming to any known, or likely, pathophysiological process.

Fluctuation-Variability Domain
Disease processes run a course that is mostly predictable. For example, diurnal fluctuations characterise mood disturbances: depression is typically worse in the mornings, or afternoons, but not stable. Sleep disturbances display typical patterns. By virtue of their neurobiological origins, typical psychotic hallucinations are worse when alone or at night; hallucinating whilst having a conversation is most unusual. This is the first point of departure of this assessment domain: the clinician must appraise whether expected changes across time and contexts are observed. Secondly, the malingerer may be unable to maintain the deceit over time. He or she may also present differently across contexts: whilst being interviewed by the psychiatrist, the malingerer may display a certain set of symptoms and behaviours, yet, when in the dining hall, observed by nurses, his or her guard may be down and symptoms disappear. 'Fluctuation' refers to unusual, unexpected, and atypical changes in presentation over time, and 'variability' to changes across contexts.

Longitudinal Domain
Whereas the aforementioned domains rely heavily on clinical interaction, nursing observation, observation during psychological testing, and other activities, the Longitudinal Domain taps into the malingerer's behaviour and mental state outside the assessment context. Reports by relatives, friends, colleagues, police officials, prosecutors, correctional service members, teachers, and previous doctors and psychologists may be invaluable in shedding light on a person's behaviour, mental state, and adaptation before the assessment. Pathological conditions have natural histories and conditions often take months to resolve. In certain conditions, signs and symptoms of disturbance are always present: viz. Mental Retardation, Dementia, and Schizophrenia. A person's history should support the current presentation. Discrepancies between psychiatric history, reported mental state, and adaptive functioning with assessment findings raise suspicion.

As a form of deceit, malingering is detectable along two dimensions: errors of fact and errors of communication. Errors of fact involve the subject of deceit (e.g. illness, like psychosis) and the distortion introduced by the malingerer (factors adjudged by the malingerer to create the guise of psychosis, like fake delusions). Errors of fact concern symptomatology and are amenable to clinical assessment, provided the assessor is sufficiently au fait with the field's symptomatology. Special investigations, neuropsychological measures, and information from third parties may assist in detecting false symptoms.

Errors of communication concern the manner in which the malingerer communicates the deception and are also amenable to clinical appraisal. Both error dimensions are composed of domains designed to assist the doctor or psychologist with the detection of malingering. In the Expert Model, errors of fact are appraised in the 'Symptomatology Dimension' (so named because the subject of deceit and deceitful distortion concern symptoms). The communicative behaviour always plays out in an assessment context and is thus represented by the 'Assessment Behaviour Dimension'. Table 8.18 summarises the three steps employed by the Expert Model in the detection of malingering. Tables 8.19 and 8.20 explain and list examples of 'Symptomatology' and 'Assessment Behaviour'.

Table 8.20: 'Expert Model': Assessment Behaviour Dimension

ASSESSMENT BEHAVIOUR DIMENSION
Explanatory notes
• This dimension of assessment does not rely on expert knowledge of a specific discipline, but on keen observation. • Least labour and resource intensive, relying mainly on the clinical interaction, nursing reports, other incidental interactions. • Consists of eight domains: Interactional Style, Response Style, Paralingual, Affective Display, Motoric Behaviour, Autonomic Phenomena, Temporo-contextual Inconsistency and General Deceitfulness. • Assessment behaviour is in operation across all contexts where the subject of an elaborate assessment process interprets the contexts as scrutiny. The more naturalistic a setting, like when mixing with patients in the courtyard of a ward or during dinner time, the less likely the person will react with overt assessment behaviour. But, we should be mindful that assessment is stressful and many sincere people, normal or mentally ill, react to assessment with awkward affectedness.
Domains and examples
Interactional Style • Unduly familiar, obsequious or unduly formal. • Bland and insincere. • Lack of cooperation: unwilling to answer, contrariness, sarcasm. **Response Style** • Directing focus of conversation: either towards, or away from a topic. • Unexpected shifts: from specifics to generalities, or vice versa. • Requests for clarifications or repetitions: 'pardon', 'I did not get that', 'can you repeat that?'. • Qualifiers/modifiers: 'but', 'however', 'ordinarily', 'essentially', 'specifically'. • Expanded contractions: 'cannot', 'did not', 'were not', 'will not 'instead of 'can't', 'weren't', 'won't'. • Covert denials of lying: 'frankly', 'obviously', 'to tell the truth', 'honestly, believe me'.... • Bamboozlers: Q: 'Have you phoned the client?' A: 'I have not managed to get through to her.' Q: 'Isn't this room a bit damp?' A: 'The owner used to use it as a studio.' • Communication errors, changes of thought in mid-cadence, unexpected grammatical errors. • Stilted language. **Paralingual** Pause fillers: 'Uh', 'err', 'ah', 'eissh'. • Pregnant pauses. • Prosodic changes: increased pitch, speaking with a clenched jaw ('lying through his teeth'), slower pace, response delays. • Stuttering and throat clearing.

Affective Display Domain

- Forced, unnatural smiling: linear smile, absence of canthic creases.
- Smiling, laughing, and giggling: increased frequency, often incongruent and insincere.
- Affective responses following utterance: affect always precedes awareness and utterance.
- Unexpected affective responses.

Motoric Behaviour

- General agitation: psychomotor restlessness, hand-wringing, handling objects, lower limbs restless.
- Posture: more leaning and postural shifts.
- Gestures: less finger pointing, fewer hand gestures but more pronounced shoulder shrugs.
- Emergence of movement disorders.
- Ward-off: hand obscuring face, hand-to-face movements, facial grooming, touching nose, crossing arms, closing hands, interlocking fingers.

Autonomic

- Breathing: sighs, deep or shallow breathing, 'discordant breathing'.
- Decreased saliva: dry mouth sound, drinking, swallowing, throat clearing.
- Tremor: wavering phonation, manipulating objects, may tend to hide hands.
- Sweaty palms.

Temporo-contextual Inconsistency

- Marked inconsistencies in behaviour, interaction, and performance across different contexts, e.g. no interaction during consultation with psychiatrist but engages freely with nurses and others on ward, playing darts and serving at meal times.

General Deceitfulness

Doctors and psychologists are trained to relieve suffering, rehabilitate, and restore dignity. We tend to trust our patients. Forensic evaluations fight against the grain of what the healing professions are about. Entering a consultation with the presumption that the patient is malingering is cynical and dark. However, naively believing everything a patient reports is playing with fire. Striking that delicate balance is what the art of medicine and psychology is about.

CONCLUSION

At first glance, the dissociative and somatoform disorders appear inordinately complex with an unsettled classification and often unwieldy, if not quirky, diagnostic criteria. Management is frequently difficult and a strained therapist-patient relationship not uncommon. The fact that a compact unitary biopsychosocial explanatory model eludes us further compounds things. Despite these difficulties, we can get to grips with these conditions. What follows is a distillation of what we do know about dissociative and somatising conditions and attempts to draw attention to their defining and differentiating features. To keep things clear, matters of classificatory contention are not considered in the summary.

Pathogenesis

Dissociative and somatoform disorders mostly follow a similar pathogenic process:

- Early adversity or trauma: child abuse, trauma, serious illness, and poor attachment.
- Constitutional predisposition exists.

- Dissociation is expressed as a defensive response to trauma and partners fight and flight.
- Detachment and compartmentalisation are neural information processes at play.
- Dissociative compartmentalisation and detachment operate to produce predictable disturbances in:
    - Memory
    - Sensory experience
    - Motor behaviour
    - Representation of the self and the external world.

Symptom expression

- Emergence, exacerbation, or maintenance of symptoms follows, or is related to exposure to trauma or adversity.
- Symptoms consist of a variable mix of dissociative phenomena and somatising.
- A mix of mental and bodily symptoms is the norm.
- Somatic symptoms can occur in almost any bodily system or affect almost any function.
- Negative affects and limited capacity to describe experienced feelings are common co-occurrences.
- Somatic symptoms do not yield to medical explanation.
- Course is often chronic.

Using the psychopathological mode of presentation and the course of the condition as parameters, the following table provides a useful guide to recognise and differentiate conditions:

Table 8.21: Primary mode of presentation and course of dissociative and somatoform disorders

Category	Disorder	Subtype/ Specifier	Primary mode of presentation	Course
Dissociative Disorder	Dissociative Identity Disorder		Disturbed personal identity	Recurrent, chronic
	Dissociative Amnesia		Amnesia	Transient, brief
		Fugue	Amnesia, travel, disturbed personal identity	Transient, days to months
	Depersonalisation/ Derealisation Disorder		Alienation from self	Recurrent, brief

Category	Disorder	Subtype/ Specifier	Primary mode of presentation	Course
Somatic Symptom and Related Disorders	Somatic Symptom Disorder		Multiple symptoms in different organ systems	Chronic
		Pain	Pain overwhelms all experience and behaviour	Chronic
	Illness Anxiety Disorder/ Hypochondriasis		Preoccupation with disease, not specific symptoms	Chronic
	Conversion Disorder		Sensory, motor disturbance, pseudo-seizures	Transient, can be chronic

Dissociation and somatising as symptom dimensions

- Dissociation is not limited to the dissociative disorder construct. It occurs across a wide spectrum of psychiatric and medical conditions:
  - Acute Stress Disorder
  - Posttraumatic Stress Disorder
  - Panic attack
  - Other anxiety disorders
  - Schizophrenia and other psychotic disorders
  - Depressive disorders
  - Borderline Personality Disorder.
- Somatising and somatic phenomena also occur across a wide spectrum of mental conditions:
  - Depressive disorders
  - Schizophrenia and other psychotic disorders
  - Panic attack
  - Generalised Anxiety Disorder and other anxiety disorders.
- In these instances, dissociation and somatising occur as fairly predictable symptom clusters, or dimensions but do not define the conditions.
- In Posttraumatic Stress Disorder, Obsessive-Compulsive Disorder and Borderline Personality Disorder, prominence of dissociative symptoms predicts a poorer long-term outcome.
- Both dimensions are not infrequent in a variety of conditions usually considered as 'culture-bound syndromes' in the current classificatory systems (e.g. running syndromes, spirit possessions, etc.).

Psychosomatic conditions

- Phenomenology appears not unlike dissociative and somatoform disorders.
- A primary bodily locus of disease is recognised. Expression of the condition is influenced by psychological factors.
  - Differentiation from dissociative and somatoform disorders is often difficult.

Malingering and factitious disorders

- Presentation is deceitful.
- Symptoms are deliberately feigned or exaggerated.
- Presentation can involve mental and bodily symptoms.
- May resemble dissociative and somatoform disorders.
- Malingering:
  - Recognition of external motivation essential for Malingering.
  - Malingering is not a disorder, but can coexist with true mental or bodily illness.
  - Patients with confirmed psychiatric of medical conditions can also malinger.
- Factitious disorders:
  - Risks are not unlike those for dissociative and somatoform disorders.
  - Morbidity in factitious disorders can be severe.
  - Course is mostly chronic and patients may abscond from therapy.

Disease burden

- Symptoms are real.
- Distress and dysfunction are real and can be severe.
- Somatoform and factitious conditions often present a greater burden of disease than the conditions suggested by their primary presentation.
- Psychiatric co-morbidity and medical complications are common and add to disease burden.
- Presentations can tax the doctor/psychologist-patient relationship and add to a sense of therapeutic nihilism.

Final word

- Symptoms, distress, and dysfunction of dissociative and somatoform disorders are real.
- Diagnosis and management require a rigorous and empathic approach.
- Diagnosis is often one of exclusion.
- Treatment is mostly a long-term undertaking.
- Treatments are modestly successful.
- Factitious disorders are likewise real, with real distress and dysfunction.
- Although a blatant act of deceit, Malingering can co-exist with true illness.

MULTIPLE-CHOICE QUESTIONS

1. Dissociation:
   a) is a phenomenon only encountered in mental disorders
   b) involves severance of connection between one's sense of identity, feelings, thinking, and behaviour
   c) comprises the psychological processes of containerisation and detachment
   d) cannot occur during bereavement

2. Somatising:
   a) is dominated by fear and perplexity
   b) involves mental anguish sublimated into meditation-like dissociation
   c) is encountered in a broad spectrum of mental disorders
   d) is an uncommon finding in patients with depression and anxiety disorders

3. Dissociative disorders:
   a) are characterised by recurrent episodes of brief psychosis
   b) may involve disturbances in memory, personal identity, and perception
   c) are very rare in developed Western societies
   d) are noted for their insidious onset without identifiable stressors

4. Indicate the true statement:
   a) As it is a mental condition, Persistent Somatoform Pain Disorder is not associated with morbidity.
   b) Hypochondriasis is defined as the occurrence of many symptoms, referable to different organs.
   c) Somatic Symptom Disorder is typically brief in duration.
   d) Conversion Disorder may occur in epileptic patients.

5. Indicate the true statement:
   a) In factitious disorders, the patient does not deliberately feign or exaggerate symptoms.
   b) Munchausen's by Proxy Disorder concerns the fabrication of symptoms in the presence of a clear, identifiable external motivation.
   c) Malingering is not a mental disorder.
   d) As there is no true pathology, patients with factitious disorders experience no distress.

PARAGRAPH AND ESSAY QUESTIONS

1. Describe dissociation with reference to the fear response and the processes of compartmentalisation and detachment. Mention how symptoms correlate with the two constructs.

2. Give an account of *amafufunyana*, *ukuthwasa*, and selected culture-specific syndromes from the rest of the world with reference to dissociation and somatising.

3. Describe the aetiology, epidemiology, clinical presentation, and differential diagnosis of: Dissociative Amnesia, Conversion Disorder, and Illness Anxiety Disorder/ Hypochondriasis.

4. Compare and contrast malingering and factitious disorders.

9 SEXUAL DYSFUNCTIONS, DYSPHORIA AND PARAPHILIC DISORDERS

Juan A. Nel & T. Melanie Lake

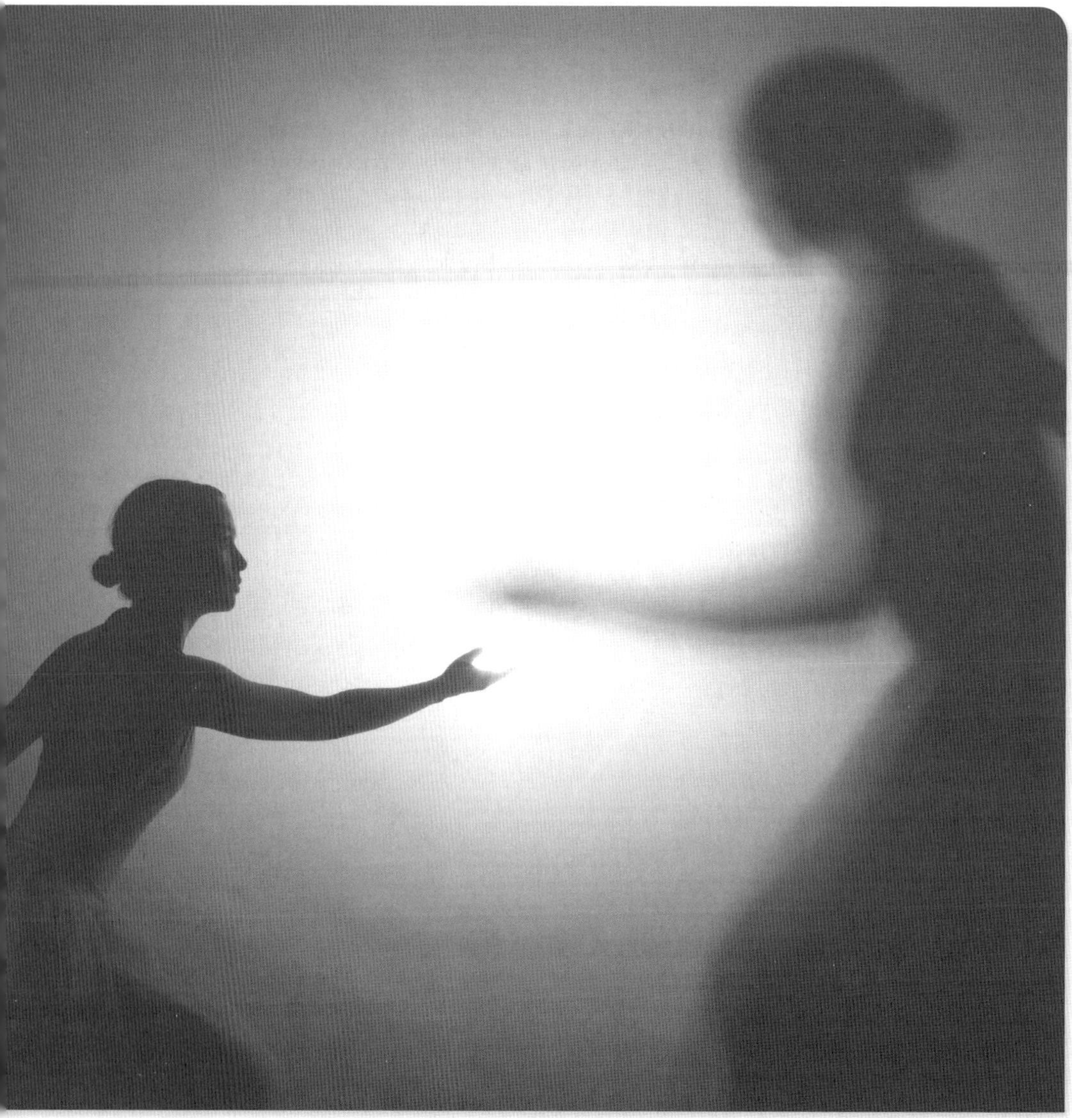

9 CHAPTER OUTLINE

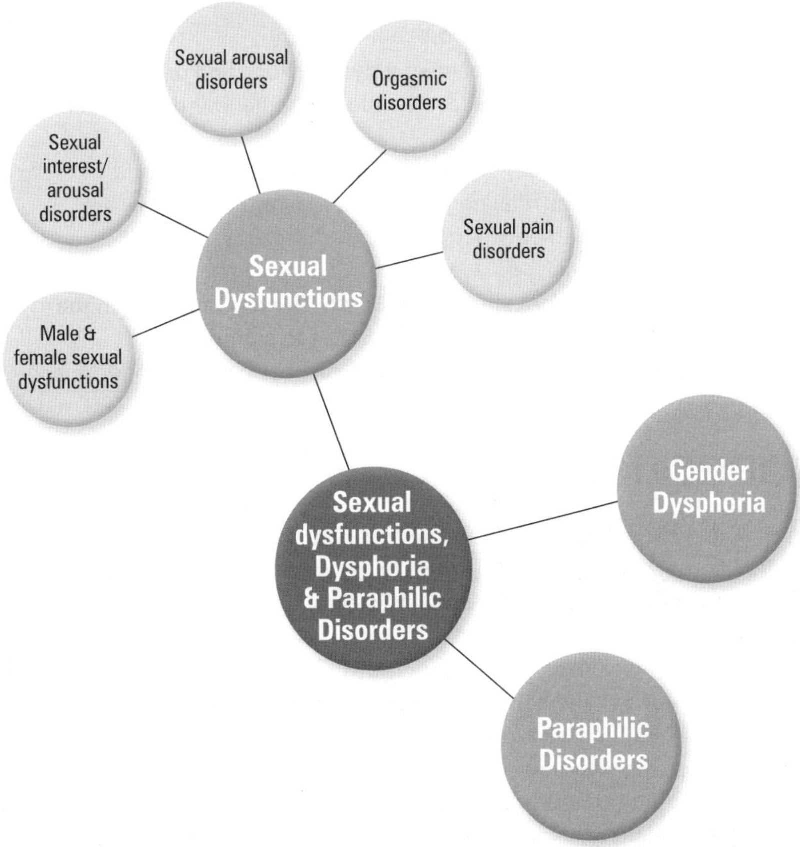

LEARNING OUTCOMES

After studying this chapter you should be able to:

- Show a general understanding of sexual dysfunctions and gender dysphoria, and be able to distinguish sexual dysfunctions and gender dysphoria from other disorders.
- Describe the history of sexual dysfunctions and gender dysphoria.
- Understand the problems relating to the nosology of these disorders.
- Describe, and distinguish between, sexual dysfunctions, paraphilias, and Gender Identity Disorder.
- Identify cross-cultural, more specifically South African, variations in the presentation of sexual dysfunctions and gender dysphoria.
- Formulate an aetiological model of sexual dysfunctions and gender dysphoria.

INTRODUCTION

This chapter deals with the fascinating, and yet for many people intensely personal, aspects of human functioning: sexuality and gender. More specifically, we will be exploring the diagnostic criteria and aetiology of three major categories of disorders classified under the sexual dysfunctions and gender dysphoria. These are the sexual dysfunctions, paraphilic, and gender disorders. As you progress through this chapter, it will become clear that the distinction between 'normal' and 'abnormal' sexual and gender behaviour is not too clear. This is a very important point that needs special emphasis here. To contextualise this discussion, we return to our earlier definitions of abnormality as behaviours that are statistically rare (atypical), cause intense personal distress and impairment in global functioning or psychological dysfunction (breakdown in cognitive, emotional, or behavioural functioning), and/or are culturally inappropriate or not expected (see Chapter 1).

The very definition of some sexual and gender behaviours as disordered or abnormal is contentious. Sexuality remains a sensitive and emotive issue in most societies, including South Africa, and for many it is still a taboo subject. However, the importance of people's sexual selves, as well as healthy sexual functioning and expression, is undisputed. In many somewhat conservative modern homes, even discussions on healthy sexual functioning may be out of the question. One can imagine the extra layers of embarrassment and secrecy that might accompany the experience of sexual dysfunction or diversity.

From the study of both physical and psychological human functioning, we know that sexuality is a powerful driving force (Pigg & Adams, 2005). At the same time, it is typically regulated by a host of social conventions. Societal norms and values tend to prescribe, and often prohibit, the sexual behaviours from which we may choose. This can result in a conflict of interests between individual freedom and the pressure to conform to the expectations of the masses. Moreover, sexual standards and acceptable practices can change (and certainly have changed) according to the particular society or culture, religion, language group, and/or historical context that people find themselves in.

Something as biologically determined as being male or female is likely to be accompanied by different sets of sexual expectations or privileges. Thus, the abnormality criterion of 'culturally inappropriate or not expected' may exert a lot of influence when it comes to the sexual dysfunctions and gender dysphoria. An important criticism levelled at this criterion is that it is inappropriate, because social norms and values are merely constructions; they do not exist in any absolute sense outside this context (that is, people merely agree to agree on them) and social constructions run the risk of being reified (made into 'real' objects or accepted as 'truth'). See the case study below as an example.

Use of the term 'pathology' in reference to diverse sexual behaviours is problematic (Hekma, 2009; Pan-American Health Organisation [PAHO] & World Health Organisation [WHO], 2000). Long-standing controversies regarding terminology relate to whether to refer to these sexual behaviours as 'variations', 'preferences', 'deviations', or 'diseases' (Seligman & Rosenhan, 1998). It is important to bear in mind that while the medical community is interested in the consequences of unusual sexual practices for health, many psychologists consider paraphilias to be compulsive behaviours. However, many people who practice diverse sexual behaviours do not feel that they fall into either of these categories. For these individuals, there are only two non-negotiable issues when it comes to human sexual behaviour: that coercion of others (especially children and adolescents) into sexual activities is never permissible, and that people must not be led by their sexual urges into regrettable, dangerous, detrimental, or mutilating practices (Love, 1995). It is important to note that the psychiatric fraternity is increasingly acknowledging the substantial shifts that have occurred in how sexual diversity is perceived. This can, amongst others, be seen in the proposed changes to diagnostic criteria applied to paraphilias in the DSM-5.

CASE STUDY

DISORDERED OR JUST DIFFERENT?

- A young male psychology student who has been living quite happily with his mild PVC (polyvinyl acetate, a common plastic) clothing fetish, a paraphilia, for the last few years may experience no personal distress. If his family does not know of his choice while a few close friends accept it and his girlfriend loves it, he may encounter no problems in social functioning. If he is doing well in his studies and looking forward to his working years, we might not find impairment in his academic and/or occupational contexts either. His PVC fetish may very well be less frequently encountered in the general population than the more common sexual arousal patterns, but this criterion alone is not enough to consider him disordered. The only problem that this young man experiences might be the prejudice of the less well informed in society, who would consider him a pervert, or even dangerous, if they were to find out.

Sexual dysfunctions and gender dysphoria remain a contentious issue because sexual and gender functioning is both a sensitive and a powerful topic. Other historical and current hot debates in the area include:

- Sexual minority groups, such as bisexual people, who may suffer the broader societal expectation that heterosexuality is the only 'normal' way, or even pressure from people with a same-sex sexual orientation to 'make up their minds'.
- Women's liberation groups that have issues with psychological theories, such as Freudian psychoanalysis, which holds that certain types of sexual functioning in women (vaginal orgasm) are 'mature' whereas others (clitoral orgasm) are 'immature'.
- Transsexual (obsolete term for gender identity disorder) activists who have come to mistrust psychologists as health-care providers while needing them, for instance, for assessments and motivations for sex reassignment surgery.
- Men and women who have had difficulties accepting the historically male constructions of sexual norms or roles (such as that only the man should initiate sex).

When those who get to judge the sexual diversity, sexual orientation, or gender expressions of others are in positions of power (such as psychologists, politicians, and religious leaders), the effects of their disapproval can be devastating in terms of the associated neglect, de-prioritisation, marginalisation, exclusion, discrimination, and victimisation.

Gender is also a highly politicised concept. In recent years, feminist scholars have successfully challenged the status quo and contributed to a body of knowledge that suggests that any consideration of human sexuality is incomplete unless it takes 'masculinity' and 'femininity' to be cultural concepts (PAHO & WHO, 2000). In the context of this chapter, the difference between biological sex (male and female) as fixed and gender (including gender roles) as flexible is of paramount importance.

In human beings, there are two distinct biological sexes, male and female. Men possess male gonads and various other male anatomical features whereas women possess female gonads and other recognisable female anatomical features. The vast majority of people will be easily distinguishable as either one or the other.

However, this is not the case with the very small percentage of individuals who are intersex (hermaphrodites), who are born with either both male and female gonads or with ambiguous genitals. It has been said that the prevalence of intersex in South Africa is amongst the highest in the world. Extrapolating from international figures, which estimate that between one in 500 and one in a 1,000 is affected to a significant degree, at the very least 45,000 to 90,000 South Africans are intersexed to a significant degree (Gross, n.d.). Medical practitioners observing anatomical sexual ambiguity after birth have often treated the situation as an emergency, immediately performing surgery. Depending on the mix of characteristics, such babies have often been 'assigned' to one or other sex and given medical and psychosocial treatments considered supportive of that gender. Much criticism has been levelled at the medical practice of 'deciding' such an important part of an individual's identity in such cases (Barlow & Durand, 2011; Samelius & Wägberg, 2005). Increasingly, surgery is only considered as a last resort and implications for a specific psychological gender identity are borne in mind.

The complexity of human sexual functioning can be seen in the reality that biological or anatomical sex does not necessarily relate in a direct sense to one's sexual orientation, or to one's gender identity, for that matter. Also, 'sexuality is not reducible to a body part or a drive; it must be understood as integral to an entire matrix of social, economic, cultural, and relational forces; it is constructed rather than given' (Petchesky, 2008, p. 12). Sexuality, like gender, is complex and multidimensional. In practice, this implies that what people do sexually (their behaviour) may differ from both their sexual orientation and desire (i.e. object choice or fantasy) and also their sexual identity. Their sexual identity, in fact, may or may not correspond with their behaviour or their desire. As Petchesky (2008) emphasises, all three of these aspects are again distinct from gender behaviour, gender orientation, and gender identity.

A recent comparison of studies involving large samples of adults across the United Kingdom, France, and the United States suggests that the overwhelming majority of people have engaged in only heterosexual (sexual relationships with members of the opposite sex) behaviour. In addition, while 75% of American men have engaged in oral sex, only one-fifth report having engaged in anal sex (Barlow & Durand, 2011). Roughly 1% of men studied had engaged exclusively in homosexual (sexual relationships with members of the same sex) behaviours, and this figure rises to 2%–4% of men who had engaged in sexual relationships with members of both the same and the opposite sex, or bisexual behaviours. If same-sex attraction is taken into consideration in addition to behaviour, almost 9% of women and 10% of men reported same-sex attraction and behaviour.

Earlier reviews of prevalence studies (Gonsiorek & Weinrich, 1991, in Eliason, 1996) concluded, however, that the rate of same-sex sexuality in the United States is between 4% and 17% (depending on whether bisexuals are included and how same-sex sexuality is defined). It is important to note that same-sex sexual orientation (most often called gay or lesbian) and bisexual orientation are seen as sexual variations nowadays rather than as problems, and are generally not considered to be indications for treatment. Nonetheless, the majority of people engage in heterosexual, vaginal intercourse within a relationship with one partner.

Due to some of the issues of contention given above, sexuality has been an under-researched area. Therefore, both nationally and internationally, reliable and valid data on the common and less common sexual practices is lacking. It does, however, seem that sexual practices and what constitutes sexual satisfaction is increasingly similar globally (Barlow & Durand, 2011). Nonetheless, the body of scientific knowledge on sexuality is growing and various aspects can be defined as follows (Samelius & Wägberg, 2005). Sexology is the study of sexuality and is a rather small, but growing, field. Internationally, research on sexuality issues is mainly the domain of the humanities and social sciences, most notably within the disciplines of history, literature, ethnology, sociology, and social anthropology (Pigg & Adams, 2005). Interestingly, psychology is not at the forefront of related research. Clinical sexology is that subdiscipline of sexology that focuses on the prevention and treatment of sexual problems pertaining to sexual dysfunctions, compulsive sexual behaviours, gender dysphoria, and syndromes following sexual victimisation (PAHO & WHO, 2000). Sexual health concerns and problems refer to life situations related to sexuality that impact on wellness and quality of life. For this reason, they require interventions by individual health practitioners, often medical doctors and psychologists, and/or society in the form of raising awareness. These concerns and problems include, amongst others, the sexual dysfunctions, sexual violence, and the HIV/AIDS pandemic (PAHO & WHO, 2000).

Although there are gender differences in sexual behaviour, the sexes are drawing closer in terms of their sexual attitudes and behaviours (Kimmel, 2000). The previous societal 'double standard' (found, for instance, in the outdated idea that viewed promiscuous men in a positive light and promiscuous women in a negative light) has all but disappeared in Western societies. This outdated idea had the effect of socialising a number of women to develop conservative, embarrassed, self-conscious, or behaviour-inhibiting 'sexual self-schemas' whereas many other women developed schemas including passion, romance, and openness to sexual experience (Andersen & Cyranowski, 1994; Barlow & Durand, 2011). On the other hand, men were found not to develop negative core beliefs about sex (Andersen, Cyranowski, & Espindle, 1999).

There are a number of gender differences in sexual behaviour. For example, a much higher percentage of males than females report masturbating (Kimmel, 2000). This is the largest gender difference in sexual behaviour, and may be because masturbation is more anatomically convenient for men or more socially permissible, although women have been encouraged to self-explore sexually for years. Males also express more permissive attitudes and behaviours toward casual and premarital sex than do females. Females report having had fewer sexual partners than males and a lower frequency of intercourse. Women tend to desire more intimacy and demonstrations of love during sex, while men tend to emphasise arousal (Nel, 1999). College students and young adults engage in alarmingly high rates of sexual risk behaviour (Sarason & Sarason, 1993). The number of partners and types of sexual activity practised by college women has remained fairly constant since 1975, although the use of condoms has increased (Nel, 1999). Barlow and Durand (2011) report than more than 23% of American men have had 20 and more sexual partners.

Sexual activity can, and does, continue into old age for many. Sexual behaviour can continue past the age of 80 for some. Barlow and Durand (2011) report that 50% of men and 36% of women aged 75 to 79 are sexually active. The decreases in sexual activity that are found in some aging people may be related to more general decreases in mobility and overall health. Various diseases of old age, and the treatments given for them, may have vasocongestive response effects and arousal-reducing effects that interfere with sexual behaviour. Aging males may have a difficult time achieving or maintaining an erection and aging women may experience a reduction in vaginal lubrication. Overall, high levels of both physical and mental health, and good relationship quality, have been found to be the best predictors of sexual well-being (Laumann, et al., 2006).

There are four categories of sexual dysfunctions with, in most instances, differences between how they manifest in males and females. These are sexual desire disorders, sexual arousal disorders, orgasmic disorders, and sexual pain disorders. There are eight major paraphilias described in the DSM-IV-TR and numerous less common ones that have been the topic of specific studies and dedicated research (Money, 1984, 1988). The sexual dysfunctions and gender dysphoria are perhaps the most contested of all the behaviours considered abnormal. The reasons mentioned above cover some of the material inherent in these controversies. The increased advocacy by social movements for recognition of, respect for, and the protection of the rights of sexual minorities has been added to this arena. Interestingly, as will be highlighted in the following sections, many of the contestations have been incorporated in the proposed revisions to be included in DSM-5. What is also significant is that while the so-called sexual disorders and gender dysphoria are currently inclusive of the sexual dysfunctions, Gender Identity Disorder and the paraphilias, the DSM-5 is considering separating each of these into stand-alone categories (American Psychiatric Association, 2012).

HISTORY OF SEXUAL DYSFUNCTIONS AND GENDER DYSPHORIA

> *In the 1960s you were sick if you liked being a homosexual; now you are sick if you do not like being a homosexual.*
>
> — MacDonald, 1976, in Steffens & Eschmann, 2001, p. 7.

The distinction between sex and gender in the English language was only emphasised in the 1950s and 1960s by British and American psychiatrists and other medical professionals working with intersex and transsexual people (Esplen & Jolly, 2006).

Not so long ago, same-sex sexual orientation was seen as psychopathology within the biomedical model and treated as a mental disorder. Same-sex sexuality was declassified as a disorder by the American Psychiatric Association in 1973 (Shidlo & Schroeder, 2002). In 1975, the American Psychological Association passed a resolution supporting this action (American Psychological Association, 1998) and encouraging professionals to work against the prevailing idea that same-sex sexuality was 'perverse' (Goldfried, 2001). The American National Association of Social Workers brought out its first policy statement related to same-sex sexuality shortly thereafter, in 1977. This statement emphasised that the Association's position of non-discrimination and equal status for all, regardless of sexual orientation, best served the mental health and welfare interests not only of affected individuals, but also of society as a whole (Tully, 2000). However, the 'expert' opinion of same-sex sexuality as undesirable, along with research aimed at 'converting' same-sex sexual behaviour to that of the mainstream, persisted until the late 1970s (Sandfort & De Keizer, 2001).

From the early 1970s, the term 'homosexual' was increasingly rejected as pathologising and replaced with the term 'gay' by same-sex minorities and affirmative health-care practitioners alike. Gonsiorek (1988) reported that 'ego-dystonic homosexuality', an incomprehensible diagnosis, unpopular with many mental health professionals who did not agree with it, was excluded from the revision of the DSM-III in 1987. While the American Psychiatric Association's DSM classification system declassified homosexuality as pathology in 1973, the World Health Organisation (WHO) followed suit only in 1990 with the *International Classification of Diseases* (ICD) delisting homosexuality in 1999 (Ministerial Advisory Committee on Gay and Lesbian Health [MACGLH], 2002). Now 'officially' seen as a sexual variation rather than a problem, same-sex sexual orientation, itself, is not a condition to be treated. See Table 9.1 for a brief overview of the history of sexual dysfunctions and gender dysphoria.

Table 9.1: Summary of history of sexual dysfunctions and gender dysphoria

Dates	Theorist	Description
1856–1939	**Sigmund Freud**	The father of psychoanalysis, Freud developed theories regarding the effect of sexual development on behaviour in a period when others steered away from sexuality-related research or discussions.
1859–1939	**Havelock Ellis**	Ellis introduced sexual information and outlooks that were revolutionary and polemic (Godow, 1982). Made up, primarily, of a series of six research volumes from the years 1896 to 1910 on *Studies in the Psychology of Sex*, these findings convinced Ellis that the norm in human sexuality was variability, both across and within cultures. He found so much variability in human sexual expression that a definitive appraisal of what was 'normal' was extremely difficult to make. Ellis introduced a number of highly progressive ideas for his time, including the contention that heterosexuality and homosexuality are not absolutes, but instead manifested in terms of varying degrees on a continuum. Ellis propagated a tolerant attitude towards individual sexual choices.
1868–1935	**Magnus Hirschfeld**	Informed by his travels in Africa, Hirschfeld was convinced that puritanical European society had inflicted unnecessary sexual mores on people in the process of colonisation. He also first discovered that hormones influenced sexual behaviour and that irregularities in development 'caused' sexual deviance (Tully, 2000).
1872–1922	**Iwan Bloch**	Author of among others, *Psychopathia Sexualis*, Bloch suggested that sexual problems could not be understood based exclusively on theology, medicine, law, or anthropology. He considered biological observation and cultural research as the two fundamental pillars of sexual investigation, which required a restricted, independent rigorous science.
1948	**Alfred Kinsey and associates**	Released findings from 16,000 interviews in the book *Sexual Behaviour in the Human Male* (Kinsey, Pomeroy, & Martin, 1948). A few years later, the book *Sexual Behaviour in the Human Female* (Kinsey, Pomeroy, Martin, & Gebhart, 1953) followed. These pioneering works offered findings that surprised many people, most notably the report that roughly 10% of people engaged in same-sex sexual relationships. This data has since been presumed to be inaccurate due to the less sophisticated sampling procedures of his day and the contradictory findings of many recent studies (Barlow & Durand, 2009).

Dates	Theorist	Description
1952		Christene Jorgensen had the first successful sex reassignment surgery in Denmark (Tully, 2000).
1966	**William H. Masters and Virginia E. Johnson**	Conducted research in couple's sex therapy and published their pioneering work in the book *Human Sexual Response*. This was based on 13 years of experience in treating infertility problems in their St Louis laboratory during the 1950s and 1960s. They identified four distinct stages during sexual activity: arousal (or excitement), plateau, orgasm, and resolution (Masters & Johnson, 1976).
1979	**Harry Benjamin**	The Harry Benjamin International Gender Dysphoria Association releases the first version of the standards of care, specifying the minimum requirements for proper care and protection of both the person with Gender Identity Disorder and the professionals who provide treatment.
1921–2006	**John Money**	First formulated and defined the concepts of gender role and gender identity. Amongst others, his clinical contributions include sex reassignment treatments in transsexualism and extensive work with the paraphilias (Money, 1984, 1988).
1987	**DSM-III**	'Ego-dystonic homosexuality' excluded from revised DSM-III
1998		First oral treatments of male sexual dysfunction become available.

Scientific interest in sexual dysfunctions and their treatment has soared since 1998, when oral treatments for male sexual dysfunction first became available (Brotto & Klein, 2007). The availability of effective and safe medications not only to improve, but also to modify, the sexual functioning of individuals has similarly brought about renewed interest in the prevalence and consequences of compulsive sexual behaviour (PAHO & WHO, 2000) (also see Chapter 10). For example, use of anti-androgen medication, for example Androcur, is associated with the hypothesis that the higher prevalence of paraphilias in males is due to increased androgens (South African Sexual Health Association [SASHA], n.d.). Another example is the use of selective serotonin re-uptake inhibitors (SSRIs) and other antidepressants to treat premature ejaculation and compulsive forms of sexual behaviours (PAHO & WHO, 2000).

CLINICAL PICTURE

In previous editions of the DSM, sexual dysfunctions, gender identity disorder and paraphilias were all categorised under Sexual and Gender Identity Disorders. The DSM-5 splits these disorders into three distinct categories, i.e. Sexual Dysfunctions, Gender Dysphoria and Paraphilic Disorders (See Figure 9.1). For the purposes of this book, these disorders will all be discussed in one chapter, under different sections.

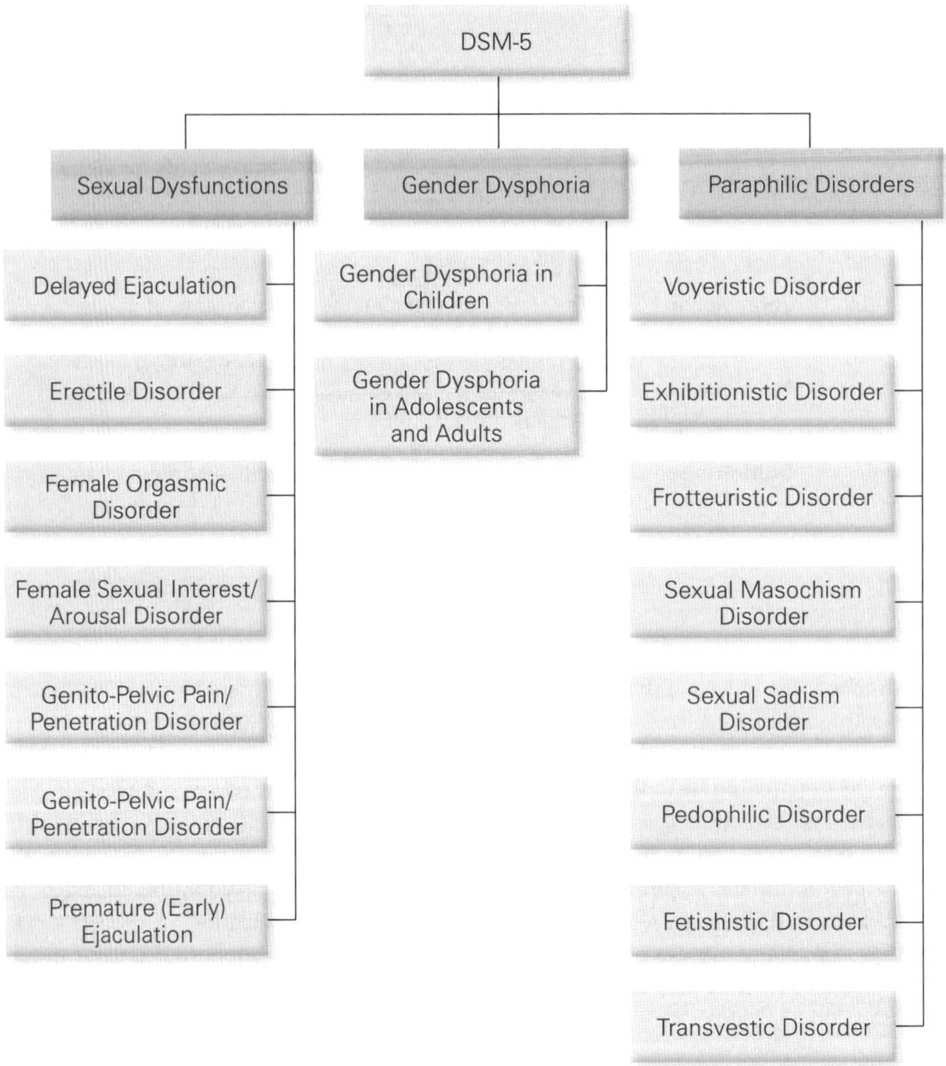

SECTION 1: SEXUAL DYSFUNCTIONS

Reflecting its development from a medical rather than social model, the DSM classification of sexual dysfunction does not include what have been termed 'sexual difficulties' (McConaghy, 2005). Such difficulties may relate to the emotional tone of sexual relations, an inability to relax, too little foreplay before intercourse, disinterest, partners choosing an inconvenient time, being 'turned off', and being attracted to people other than an intimate partner (McConaghy, 2005).

If we accept that it may be very difficult to ask the question of what constitutes 'normal' sexual behaviour, we may need to rephrase our question. The question, 'What makes sexual behaviour that differs somewhat from the norm a disorder?' makes more sense and acknowledges many of the issues raised above. It would probably be the question asked by a mental health practitioner sensitive to these issues. It is important to note that anyone may experience aspects of these difficulties occasionally, which may fall within so-called 'normal' parameters. Experiencing occasional problems with one's sexual functioning is extremely common (Nolen-Hoeksema, 2008). These difficulties are diagnosed as dysfunctional only when they are enduring, cause the person significant emotional distress, and interfere with intimate relationships.

In light of this point, sexual dysfunctions are understood to exist when an individual persistently finds it difficult to function adequately while having sex. This set of disorders involves people having trouble engaging in sexual relationships with others and enjoying a sexual act to the point of sexual satisfaction. In order to examine what adequate sexual functioning might be, we must name and understand the phases of the human sexual response. As indicated above, sex researchers Masters and Johnson (1976) identified four distinct phases during sexual activity: arousal (or excitement, which refers to a subjective sense of sexual pleasure and physiological signs of arousal), plateau (the brief period before orgasm), orgasm (in males, feelings of the inevitability of ejaculation followed by ejaculation, and in females, involuntary contractions of the walls of a section of the vagina), and resolution (the decrease in arousal after orgasm has occurred, especially in men).

A fifth stage, the 'desire phase' (when sexual urges occur in response to sexual cues or fantasies), that precedes the arousal phase, was suggested by Kaplan (1979) and has been the topic of research and psychotherapeutic interventions ever since (Talmadge & Talmadge, 1986; Verhaege, 1998). This has important implications for the study of sexual dysfunctions as one disorder category refers specifically to inadequate desire-phase functioning.

'Sexual dysfunction' refers to some inadequacy in functioning at one of the phases of desire, arousal, and/or orgasm. Strictly speaking, no sexual dysfunction can occur during the phases of plateau or resolution. An inability to feel sexual desire, to become sufficiently aroused to have sex, or to achieve orgasm would be considered sexual dysfunctions. These are typically sexual problems related to the sexual response cycle or to pain. The stages of sexuality (desire, arousal, and orgasm) are each associated with specific dysfunctions. Impairment may be experienced in only one of the three areas of sexuality, or in two or in all three.

The DSM-5 specifies four categories of sexual dysfunction (see Table 9.2).

Table 9.2: Sexual dysfunctions in males and females, according to DSM-5

Sexual dysfunction	Males	Females
Sexual arousal desire disorders	Male Hypoactive Sexual Desire Disorder Sexual Aversion Disorder Erectile Disorder	Female Sexual Interest Arousal Disorder
Orgasmic disorders	Delayed Ejaculation Premature (Early) Ejaculation	Female Orgasmic Disorder
Sexual pain disorders		Genito-Pelvic Pain/Penetration Disorder

Source: Reprinted with permission from the Diagnostic and Statistical Manual of Mental Disorders (DSM), Fifth Edition, American Psychiatric Association (APA), 2013

Diagnoses also indicate specifiers, including: lifelong (i.e. the person has always had the problem) versus acquired (i.e. new in onset); generalised (i.e. experienced in all situations and with all partners) versus situational (i.e. the difficulty is experienced in selected situations or with certain partners); and whether the problem is due to psychological factors or to biological and psychological factors combined (Seligman & Rosenhan, 1998).

There are numerous biological factors that can cause and maintain various sexual dysfunctions. These include vascular and hormonal abnormalities, undiagnosed diabetes, and the use and/or abuse of certain drugs. For this reason, a thorough psychological assessment, with the intention of diagnosing and treating a sexual dysfunction, should be preceded by a physiological examination by a medical doctor or specialist. The purpose of this is to exclude any physiological factors before a psychologist conducts the assessment to look for psychological factors that may be playing a role in the sexual dysfunction. General medical conditions and other physiological problems may be the primary cause of the problem, as well as being much easier to treat than psychological problems. Many medical drugs are available nowadays that promise effective treatments.

The psychological factors that may cause and maintain various sexual dysfunctions include certain psychological disorders (depression or Schizophrenia) and maladaptive attitudes and cognitions. Closely related are the sociocultural factors such as relationship problems, traumatic experiences, and cultural taboos against sex (such as from one's cultural upbringing or society). These aetiological factors will be discussed in more depth later in the chapter. Aetiology is important to identity as this is likely to guide treatment options available to a patient. However, when making clinical judgements about the presence of a sexual dysfunction, clinicians should always give recognition to an individual's ethnic, cultural, religious, and social background in so far as they may influence sexual desire, expectations, and attitudes about performance (American Psychiatric Association, 2000).

Male and female sexual dysfunctions

Males may experience a dysfunction in terms of lack of desire for sex or they may experience sexual aversion, the inability to attain and/or maintain an erection, the inability to control or delay ejaculation (premature ejaculation), or the inability to ejaculate at all. Females may experience a dysfunctional level of desire for sex or they may experience sexual aversion, an inability to become sexually aroused, an inability to become aroused enough to achieve orgasm, or an inability to tolerate vaginal penetration. Below we will work through both the male and female versions of the disorders of sexual desire, arousal, orgasm, and sexual pain. Female and male sexual dysfunctions can have a major impact on quality of life and interpersonal relationships. They are multicausal and multidimensional problems, combining biological, psychological, and interpersonal determinants.

The lack of sexual desire and impaired physical excitement, in what would typically be considered arousing situations, is known as sexual unresponsiveness (previously called 'frigidity'). Unresponsiveness and difficulty reaching orgasm are the most common sexual dysfunctions in women. The most common sexual dysfunctions in men are ejaculating too quickly, and impaired excitement, known as erectile dysfunction (previously called 'impotence') (Brotto & Klein, 2007).

The Masters and Johnson four-stage Human Sexual Response Cycle, which informs the classification system of sexual dysfunctions, has been criticised with regard to its lack of generalisability for women (Brotto & Klein, 2007). This model may describe male sexual functioning well but that of women less so. It has also been suggested that sexual difficulties in women have been over-diagnosed and medicalised and that the designation 'dysfunction' is unhelpful (Brotto & Klein, 2007).

This criticism is what informs many of the changes currently underway in the classification and diagnosis of sexual dysfunctions in women, in particular. It is purported that the current standard for diagnosing a sexual dysfunction often results in inflated estimates of the proportion of women meeting criteria for sexual dysfunction. Going forward, the presence of more symptoms in women's sexual functioning, the reporting of distress, as well as revised duration and severity criteria, will help to ensure that short-term, and possibly even adaptive, changes in sexual functioning are not labeled as a dysfunction (American Psychiatric Association, 2012). Nonetheless, in terms of the DSM-5, both men and women may experience the full scope of sexual disorders, and, as indicated, people of heterosexual, bisexual, and same-sex sexual orientations are also all prone to these problems. Difficulties with and/or the inability to become aroused or reach orgasm are as common in same-sex as in heterosexual relationships (Barlow & Durand, 2011).

Sexual interest/arousal disorders

As is indicated in Table 9.2, three conditions are placed under the category of sexual interest and arousal disorders, namely, Female Sexual Interest Arousal Disorder, Erectile Disorder and Male Hypoactive Sexual Desire Disorder.

Female Sexual Interest/Arousal Disorder and Male Hypoactive Sexual Desire Disorder

A man or woman with this disorder has a level of interest in sexual activities that is so low as to be considered abnormal. The person typically does not imagine sexual activity or fantasise, does not wish for more sexual activity, and does not seek out actual sexual relationships. This may be the case even during times of being in a romantic relationship with a potential sexual partner or someone with whom they used to have sex.

Hypoactive sexual desire is difficult to define in absolute terms (such as how often one wants to have sex in one month) given the lack of reliable population norms. However, the definition emphasises the persistent lack or deficiency of well-accepted 'markers' of desire, such as sexual thoughts or fantasies, as well as absent or deficient receptivity to sexual initiation by a partner. The definition also requires that the man or woman be significantly distressed by this deficiency in desire and/or experience significant interpersonal (romantic relationship) difficulties due to it.

Table 9.3: Diagnostic criteria for Hypoactive Sexual Desire Disorders as adapted from the DSM-5 and the ICD-10

DSM-5 Female Sexual Interest/Arousal Disorder	DSM-5 Male Hypoactive Sexual Desire Disorder	ICD-10
A. Lack of, or significantly reduced, sexual interest/arousal, as manifested by at least three of the following: (1) Absent/reduced interest in sexual activity. (2) Absent/reduced sexual/erotic thoughts or fantasies. (3)No/reduced initiation of sexual activity, and typically unreceptive to a partner's attempts to initiate. (4) Absent/reduced sexual excitement/pleasure during sexual activity in almost all or all (approximately 75–100%) sexual encounters (in identified situational contexts or, if generalized, in all contexts). (5) Absent/reduced sexual interest/arousal in response to any internal or external sexual/erotic cues (e.g. written, verbal, visual). (6) Absent/reduced genital or nongenital sensations during sexual activity in almost all or all (approximately 75–100%) sexual encounters (in identified situational contexts or, if generalized, in all contexts). B. The symptoms in Criterion A have persisted for a minimum duration of approximately six months.	A. Persistently or recurrently deficient (or absent) sexual/erotic thoughts or fantasies and desire for sexual activity. The judgment of deficiency is made by the clinician, taking into account factors that affect sexual functioning, such as age and general and sociocultural contexts of the individual's life. B. The symptoms in Criterion A have persisted for a minimum duration of approximately six months. C. The symptoms in Criterion A cause clinically significant distress in the individual. D. The sexual dysfunction is not better explained by a nonsexual mental disorder or as a consequence of severe relationship distress or other significant stressors and is not attributable to the effects of a substance/medication or another medical condition	• The subject is unable to participate in a sexual relationship as they would wish. • The dysfunction occurs frequently, but may be absent on some occasions. • The dysfunction has been present for at least six months. • The dysfunction is not entirely attributable to any of the other mental and behavioural disorders in ICD-10, physical disorders (such as endocrine disorder) or drug treatment. • There is a lack or loss of sexual desire, manifest by diminution of seeking out sexual cues; thinking about sex with associated feelings of desire or appetite; or sexual fantasies.

C. The symptoms in Criterion A cause clinically significant distress in the individual. D. The sexual dysfunction is not better explained by a nonsexual mental disorder or as a consequence of severe relationship distress (e.g. partner violence) or other significant stressors and is not attributable to the effects of a substance/medication or another medical condition.		• There is a lack of interest in initiating sexual activity either with partner or as solitary masturbation, at a frequency clearly lower than expected, taking into account age and context, or at a frequency very clearly reduced from previous much higher levels.

Source: Reprinted with permission from the Diagnostic and Statistical Manual of Mental Disorders (DSM), Fifth Edition, American Psychiatric Association (APA), 2013 and ICD-10 Classification of Mental and Behavioural Disorders: Diagnostic Criteria for Research, World Health Organisation (WHO), Geneva, 2007.

This diagnosis is subtyped as: lifelong or acquired, generalised or situational, and of an aetiological origin that is predominately psychological (psychogenic) or a combination of psychological and physical factors (mixed), or unknown. Sexual desire disorders that are exclusively physical (organic) in origin would not be considered to be psychological disorders. A full diagnosis must first exclude the possibility of organic origin and be based on the best available evidence from the medical history, laboratory tests, and physical examinations done on the patient.

A number of factors are well known to have an impact on men's and women's general sexual desire, also sometimes called libido (one's sex drive). (In the original Freudian terminology, the libido referred to an instinctual pressure for gratification of sexual desires.) So-called 'positive factors' tend to increase levels of sexual desire whereas negative factors tend to decrease these levels. Table 9.4 highlights some of the physiological, psychological, and socio-cultural factors on both sides.

Table 9.4: Factors that affect libido

Positive factors	Negative factors
• Good health • Effective stimulation • Good body image • High self-esteem • Privacy • Security • Trust • Affection • Good relationship(s) • Good communication	• Disease • Stress • Fatigue • Lactation in women • Alcohol and other substances (use and abuse) • Medical drugs (e.g. antidepressants) • Dyspareunia (genital pain with intercourse) • Depression or other psychological difficulties • Anxiety or anger • Inhibitions • Traumatic experience(s)

Source: Adapted from SASHA, n.d.

The New Definitions Committee (Basson et al., 2003, in Brotto & Klein, 2007) provides new definitions and diagnostic criteria for female sexual dysfunctions, including sexual desire disorders in women. For diagnosis with Female Sexual Interst Arousal Disorder, a woman must present with: the persistent or recurrent deficiency (or absence) of sexual thoughts, fantasies, and/or desire for, or receptivity to, sexual activity, which causes personal distress. This move may help to counter the pathologising of women who merely experience lower sexual desire than their partners do or than some expected 'norm'. Some women report experiencing low sexual drive but may not be distressed by this and not be motivated to change it.

The two important elements in the new definition are the persistent lack of desire and resulting personal distress. Thus, the definition would not apply to the woman who lacks desire only in some circumstances (for example, during periods of marital conflict) or at certain times (for example, before or during menstruation) (Basson et al., 2003, in Brotto & Klein, 2007). Similarly, even if sexual desire was persistently lower than that of the partner or women of comparable age and socio-economic status, the definition would not apply in the absence of personal distress in response to the situation.

As far as the arousal component of this disorder is concerned women with this disorder would experience recurrent or persistent inability to achieve or maintain the necessary physical responses (lubrication and swelling) of sexual excitement while engaging in sexual behaviours. Moreover, the disorder must cause the woman to experience a significant level of emotional distress and/or interpersonal (intimate relationship) problems. Female Sexual Arousal Disorder is associated most strongly with difficulty becoming aroused during penile sexual intercourse. The woman's desire for sexual activities may be strong but she typically finds her body becoming unresponsive during the sexual act (see Table 9.3).

Female Sexual Arousal Disorder may be lifelong or acquired and may be generalised across sexual activities or situational (depending upon the partner, and/or circumstances). Prevalence rates are harder to estimate for women with Female Sexual Arousal Disorder because they may be less likely than men to seek treatment for this condition.

In conclusion, it ought to be noted that Female Sexual Arousal Disorder will in all probability be incorporated with Hypoactive Sexual Desire Disorder in a new term, Sexual Interest/Arousal Disorder in Women (SIAD). This proposed change is informed by empirical findings suggesting that desire and (at least subjective) arousal overlap substantially in the experiences of women. Also, it is purported that in some women desire precedes arousal, while in other women it follows. Yet another reason for the proposed new term relates to variations in how women define desire, ranging from a focus on sexual behavior as an indicator of desire, to spontaneous sexual thoughts and fantasies, with others emphasising the responsive nature of women's desire (American Psychiatric Association, 2012).

Sexual Aversion Disorder (ICD-10)

As opposed to a person with Hypoactive Sexual Desire Disorder described above, a person (man or woman) with Sexual Aversion Disorder may be interested in sex and even enjoy sexual fantasising. He or she is also quite likely to enjoy and practise masturbation to the point of orgasm. However, the individual is repulsed by the notion of engaging in the actual sex act (or parts thereof) with another person. The most important difference between these first two disorders is that individuals with Hypoactive Sexual Desire Disorder seem to have no interest in sexual activity, whereas individuals with Sexual Aversion Disorder associate sexual thoughts and activities with fear, panic, and/or disgust.

Sexual Aversion Disorder, then, is characterised by the active dislike and avoidance of genital contact with a would-be sexual partner. This dislike and avoidance must also cause the individual emotional distress and/or interpersonal (romantic relationship) problems. Some people may experience a generalised dislike and avoidance of all sexually intimate behaviours, whereas others dislike and avoid only specific facets of sexual activity between people (such as vaginal penetration).

CASE STUDY

MALE HYPOACTIVE SEXUAL DESIRE DISORDER

A 45-year-old male business executive presents at a clinic with the problem of fatigue for the past four months and, related to that, he has noticed that his desire for intimacy and sexual intercourse has decreased.

On further inquiry, it is ascertained that he holds a senior position at work and that he is always under pressure to meet deadlines. Because of this, he continuously feels anxious and angry, and he feels depressed if he does not meet some of his deadlines. He does take alcohol, but does not think that he has a drinking problem.

DISCUSSION

This client presents with low sexual desire. His main problem, however, is fatigue, resulting from his heavy schedule at work. Typically, the psychologist or doctor always has to ask about sexual function because, if not asked, most clients or patients will not volunteer such information. Many may believe that such a problem will either get better with time or that the psychologist or doctor will be uncomfortable discussing it.

In this particular client, we find that there are a few factors that put him at risk of developing erectile dysfunction (to be discussed below) as well, and these are the following:

- Anxiety
- Anger
- Alcohol
- Aging.

In others, there may also be the following risk factors:

- Drugs
- Deliberate control
- Dissociation (past negative experiences)
- Depression.

Note: These are popularly known as the '4As' and the '4Ds'.

Table 9.5: Diagnostic criteria for Sexual Aversion Disorder as adapted from the ICD-10

ICD-10
• The subject is unable to participate in a sexual relationship as they would wish. • The dysfunction occurs frequently, but may be absent on some occasions. • The dysfunction has been present for at least six months. • The dysfunction is not entirely attributable to any of the other mental and behavioural disorders in ICD-10, physical disorders (such as endocrine disorder), or drug treatment. • Sexual aversion: ‣ The prospect of sexual interaction with a partner produces sufficient aversion, fear, or anxiety that sexual activity is avoided, or, if it occurs, is associated with strong negative feelings and an inability to experience any pleasure. ‣ The dysfunction is not due to performance anxiety (reaction to previous failure of sexual response). • Lack of sexual enjoyment: ‣ Genital response (orgasm and/or ejaculation) all occur during sexual stimulation, but are not accompanied by pleasurable sensations or feelings of pleasant excitement. ‣ There is an absence of manifest and persistent fear or anxiety during sexual activity.

Source: Reprinted with permission from the ICD-10 Classification of Mental and Behavioural Disorders: Diagnostic Criteria for Research, World Health Organisation (WHO), Geneva, 2007.

This diagnosis is subtyped as: lifelong or acquired, generalised or situational, and of an aetiological origin that is predominately psychological (psychogenic) or a combination of psychological and physical factors (mixed), or unknown. The New Definitions Committee (Basson et al., 2003, in Brotto & Klein, 2007) provides new definitions and diagnostic criteria for Sexual Aversion Disorder in women. These are: the persistent or recurrent phobic aversion to, and avoidance of, sexual contact with a sexual partner, which causes personal distress.

Sexual arousal disorders

Sexual arousal disorders occur in both females and males, as Female Sexual Interest Arousal Disorder (as discussed in the previous section), Male Hypoactive Sexual Desire Disorder and Erectile Disorder respectively.

Erectile Disorder

A man with Erectile Disorder (or erectile dysfunction – ED) would experience the recurrent, partial or complete inability to achieve or maintain an erection while engaging in sexual behaviours. This must also cause the man emotional distress and/or interpersonal (intimate relationship) problems. The man may still retain an active interest in sexual behaviours, and even engage in them with a flaccid penis but with less intense pleasure than would be experienced with an erection. The inability to achieve or maintain an erection sufficient for satisfactory sexual 'performance' has historically or colloquially been called 'impotence', but the term 'erectile dysfunction' is preferable.

Male Erectile Disorder is said to have either an organic or psychogenic origin (McConaghy, 2005). Organic origin would refer to an onset not related to life events, with previously normal functioning and the man's libido intact. Here, the aetiology is most likely to be post-operative, vascular, neuropathic, or metabolic in nature, or due to drugs, dyspareunia, aging, or physical trauma. Psychogenic origin would refer to a man with fully turgid morning erections and/or erections with masturbation, and otherwise intact neurological, circulatory, and endocrine systems as well as genitalia. The aetiology here is most likely life events or other psychosocial factors.

Table 9.6: Diagnostic criteria for Erectile Disorder as adapted from the DSM-5 and ICD-10

DSM IV-TR	ICD-10
A. At least one of the three following symptoms must be experienced in almost all or all (approximately 75 – 100%) occasions of sexual activity (in identified situational contexts or, if generalized, in all contexts): (1) Marked difficultly in obtaining an erection during sexual activity. (2) Marked difficultly in maintaining an erection until the completion of sexual activity. (3) Marked decrease in erectile rigidity. B. The symptoms in Criterion A have persisted for a minimum duration of approximately six months. C. The symptoms in Criterion A cause clinically significant distress in the individual. D. The sexual dysfunction is not better explained by a nonsexual mental disorder or as a consequence of severe relationship distress or other significant stressors and is not attributable to the effects of a substance/medication or another medical condition.	• The subject is unable to participate in a sexual relationship as he would wish. • The dysfunction occurs frequently, but may be absent on some occasions. • The dysfunction has been present for at least six months. • The dysfunction is not entirely attributable to any of the other mental and behavioural disorders in ICD-10, physical disorders (such as endocrine disorder) or drug treatment. • Erection sufficient for intercourse fails to occur when intercourse is attempted. The dysfunction appears as one of the following: ▸ Full erection occurs during the early stages of lovemaking but disappears or declines when intercourse is attempted (before ejaculation, if it occurs). ▸ Erection does occur but only at times when intercourse is not being considered. ▸ Partial erection, insufficient for intercourse, occurs, but not full erection. ▸ No penile tumescence occurs at all.

Source: Reprinted with permission from the Diagnostic and Statistical Manual of Mental Disorders (DSM), Fifth Edition, American Psychiatric Association (APA), 2013 and ICD-10 Classification of Mental and Behavioural Disorders: Diagnostic Criteria for Research, World Health Organisation (WHO), Geneva, 2007.

Male Erectile Disorder is associated with difficulty becoming physically aroused, although desire may be strong. Arousal disorders may be lifelong or acquired and may be generalised across sexual activities or situational depending upon the partner, and/or circumstances. Arousal disorders may be considered a greater impairment by men than by women. The prevalence of Male Erectile Disorder is high. Definitive worldwide prevalence data is lacking, but it is believed that percentages range from 7% to 58% of men (Brotto & Klein, 2007).

Male Hypoactive Sexual Desire Disorder

Diagnosis of this disorder must be based on two critical aspects, i.e. a low / absent desire for sex as well as the absence of sexual thoughts or fantasies (See Table 9.8).(APA, 2013). This disorder may often be associated, or caused by, other sexual or non-sexual disorders (e.g. Erectile Disorder, Major Depression, etc.) Men with this disorder of ten report that they do not initiate, or that they are unresponsive to partner's attempts to initiate sexual activity (APA, 2013).

Table 9.7: Diagnostic criteria for Male Hypoactive Sexual Desire Disorder as adapted from the DSM-5

DSM-5 Male Hypoactive Sexual Desire Disorder
A. Persistently or recurrecntly deficient (or absent) sexual/erotic thoughts or fantasies and desire for sexual activity. The judgement of deficiency is made by the clinician, taking into account factors that affect sexual functioning, such as age and general and sociocultural contexts of the individual's life. B. The symptoms in Criterion A have persisted for a minimum duration of approximately six months. C. The symptoms in Criterion A cause clinically significant distress in the individual. D. The sexual dysfunction is not better explained by a nonsexual mental disorder or as a consequence of severe relationship distress or other significant stressors and is not attributable to the effects of a substance/medication or another medical condition.

Source: Reprinted with permission from the Diagnostic and Statistical Manual of Mental Disorders (DSM), Fifth Edition, American Psychiatric Association (APA), 2013.

Orgasmic disorders

Research increasingly suggests that women's sexual excitement varies greatly. In the DSM-5, an attempt is made to reduce the normative stance in relation to how orgasms are perceived and what may constitute a 'normal excitement phase', especially in women. Also, it is increasingly recognised that orgasm is not an 'all or nothing' phenomenon. Severity and duration criteria are also being proposed to avoid pathologising normal variations and short-term changes in sexual functioning.

In the current DSM-5, however, the diagnosis of orgasmic disorders in both women and in men refers to the recurrent absence of orgasm or the unacceptable delay in orgasm following sexual excitement. This condition is also called 'anorgasmia' and refers to inhibited orgasm or the inability to achieve orgasm despite desire and arousal. In women this is called Female Orgasmic Disorder, and it is a common complaint in women seeking sexual therapy (Brotto & Klein, 2007). In the case of men there are two disorders that can be considered orgasmic disorders, Delayed Ejaculation or Premature Ejaculation. The partner variables and relationship functioning are furthermore emphasised in the DSM-5 (American Psychiatric Association, 2012).

Table 9.8: Diagnostic criteria for Female Orgasmic Disorder as adapted from the DSM-5 and the ICD-10

DSM-5	ICD-10 (Orgasmic Disorder)
A. Presence of either of the following symptoms and experienced in almost all or all (approximately 75 – 100%) occasions of sexual activity (in identified situational contexts or, if generalized, in all contexts): (1) Marked delay in, marked infrequency of, or absence of orgasm. (2) Marked reduced intensity of orgasmic sensations. B. The symptoms in Criterion A have persisted for a minimum duration of approximately six months. C. The symptoms in Criterion A cause clinically significant distress in the individual. D. The sexual dysfunction is not better explained by a nonsexual mental disorder or as a consequence of severe relationship distress (e.g. partner violence) or other significant stressors and is not attributable to the effects of a substance/ medication or another medical condition.	• The subject is unable to participate in a sexual relationship as he or she would wish. • The dysfunction occurs frequently, but may be absent on some occasions. • The dysfunction has been present for at least six months. • The dysfunction is not entirely attributable to any of the other mental and behavioural disorders in ICD-10, physical disorders (such as endocrine disorder) or drug treatment. • Orgasmic dysfunction (either absence or marked delay) appearing as one of the following: ▸ Orgasm has never been experienced in any situation. ▸ Orgasmic dysfunction has developed after a period of relatively normal response. • General: Orgasmic dysfunction occurs in all situations and with any partner. • Situational: ▸ For women: Orgasm does occur in certain situations (e.g. when masturbating or with certain partners). ▸ For men, one of the following can apply: Only during sleep, never during the waking state.Never in the presence of a partner. In the presence of a partner but not while inserted.

Source: Reprinted with permission from the Diagnostic and Statistical Manual of Mental Disorders (DSM), Fifth Edition, American Psychiatric Association (APA), 2013 and ICD-10 Classification of Mental and Behavioural Disorders: Diagnostic Criteria for Research, World Health Organisation (WHO), Geneva, 2007.

Premature (Early) Ejaculation

The most common male sexual disorder is Premature Ejaculation (PE). As indicated earlier, this is also one of the two sex-specific disorders, in that it only occurs in males. Premature Ejaculation is a dysfunction of the orgasm phase, as based on the classical theories of Masters and Johnson. The DSM-5 diagnostic criteria for Premature Ejaculation are those most often used, and are as follows: persistent or recurrent onset of orgasm and ejaculation with minimal sexual stimulation before, upon, or shortly after penetration and before the person wishes it. The disorder is also marked by emotional distress or interpersonal (romantic relationship) difficulty. The disorder should not be exclusively due to the direct effects of a substance, such as opiate withdrawal.

The DSM-5 cautions that mediating factors such as age, novelty of the situation or partner, and frequency of sexual activity need to be considered before making this diagnosis. Several features helpful in determining the severity of the problem are incorporated in the DSM-5 diagnostic parameters. These include the onset or duration (lifelong or acquired/episodic), the context as generalised (global or all situations) or situational (some circumstances), and the aetiology as psychological or combined (psychological and medical or substance use) (American Psyciatric Association, 2013).

Table 9.9: Diagnostic criteria for Premature (Early) Ejaculation as adapted from the DSM-5 and ICD-10

DSM-5	ICD-10
A. A persistent or recurrent pattern of ejaculation occurring during partnered sexual activity within approximately 1 minute following vaginal penetration and before the individual wishes it. **Note:** Although the diagnosis of premature (early) ejaculation may be applied to individuals engaged in nonvaginal sexual activities, specific duration criteria must not have been established for these activities. B. The symptom in Criterion A must have been present for at least six months and must be experienced in almost all or all (approximately 75 – 100%) occasions of sexual activity (in identified situational contexts or, if generalized, in all contexts). C. The symptoms in Criterion A cause clinically significant distress in the individual. D. The sexual dysfunction is not better explained by a nonsexual mental disorder or as a consequence of severe relationship distress or other significant stressors and is not attributable to the effects of a substance/medication or another medical condition.	• The subject is unable to participate in a sexual relationship as he would wish. • The dysfunction occurs frequently, but may be absent on some occasions. • The dysfunction has been present for at least six months. • The dysfunction is not entirely attributable to any of the other mental and behavioural disorders in ICD-10, physical disorders (such as endocrine disorder) or drug treatment. • Inability to delay ejaculation sufficiently to enjoy the sexual interaction manifests as either: ‣ Occurrence of ejaculation before or very soon after entry (before or within 15 seconds of entry) or ‣ Ejaculation in absence of sufficient erection to make entry possible. **Note:** Not due to prolonged abstinence of sexual activity.

Source: Reprinted with permission from the Diagnostic and Statistical Manual of Mental Disorders (DSM), Fifth Edition, American Psychiatric Association (APA), 2013 and ICD-10 Classification of Mental and Behavioural Disorders: Diagnostic Criteria for Research, World Health Organisation (WHO), Geneva, 2007.

Delayed Ejaculation

Men with this disorder are either unable to reach ejaculation or in cases where they do, this often delayed (APA, 2013). There is a problem with the concept of delayed ejaculation as there is no real norm for what a normal time period before reaching ejaculation is or should be (APA, 2013), Rather than defining this disorder in terms of time, the essential feature is rather to describe it in terms of a man's report that he has the inability to ejaculate despite adequate stimulation and the desire to ejaculate (APA, 2013).

Table 9.10: Diagnostic criteria for Delayed Ejaculation as adapted from the DSM-5

DSM-5 (Delayed Ejaculation)
A. Either of the following symptoms must be experienced in almost all or all (approximately 75 – 100%) occasions of partnered sexual activity (in identified situational contexts or, if generalized, in all contexts), and without the individual desiring delay: (1) Marked delay in ejaculation. (2) Marked infrequency or absence of ejaculation. B. The symptom in Criterion A must have persisted for a minimum duration of approximately six months. C. The symptoms in Criterion A cause clinically significant distress in the individual. D. The sexual dysfunction is not better explained by a nonsexual mental disorder or as a consequence of severe relationship distress or other significant stressors and is not attributable to the effects of a substance/medication or another medical condition.

Source: Reprinted with permission from the Diagnostic and Statistical Manual of Mental Disorders (DSM), Fifth Edition, American Psychiatric Association (APA), 2013.

Sexual pain disorders

In previous editions of the DSM-5, there were two disorders that could be considered to be sexual pain disorders, i.e. Dyspareunia and Vaginismus. Dyspareunia was disorder that could be made in either men or women, with Vaginismus was gender specific. The DSM-5 does not distinguish between these disorders, and they are now considered to be one disorder, i.e. Genito-Pelvic Pain/Penetration Disorder, and this disorder is limited to women only (APA, 2013). The ICD-10, however, does distinguish between these disorders.

Genito-Pelvic Pain/Penetration Disorder

This disorder is characterised by genital pain during sexual intercourse. The essential feature of this is the persistent or recurrent experience of genital pain before, during, or after engaging in sex (American Psychiatric Association, 2013). In women, this is experienced as vaginal pain that is either shallow or deep. People with this disorder do experience sexual desire and arousal, but the severe pain that is associated with this will in all likelihood disrupt their sexual behaviour.

Table 9.11: Diagnostic criteria for Genito-Pelvic Pain/Penetration Disorder as adapted from the DSM-5 and the ICD-10

DSM-5	ICD-10 (Dyspareunia)
A. Persistent or recurrent difficulties with one (or more) of the following: (1) Vaginal penetration during intercourse. (2) Marked vulvovaginal or pelvic pain during vaginal intercourse or penetration attempts. (3) Marked fear or anxiety about vulvovaginal or pelvic pain in anticipation of, during, or as a result of vaginal penetration. (4) Marked tensing or tightening of the pelvic floor muscles during attempted vaginal penetration. B. The symptom in Criterion A have persisted for a minimum duration of approximately six months. C. The symptoms in Criterion A cause clinically significant distress in the individual. D. The sexual dysfunction is not better explained by a nonsexual mental disorder or as a consequence of severe relationship distress (e.g. partner violence) or other significant stressors and is not attributable to the effects of a substance/medication or another medical condition.	• The subject is unable to participate in a sexual relationship as they would wish. • The dysfunction occurs frequently, but may be absent on some occasions. • The dysfunction has been present for at least six months. • The dysfunction is not entirely attributable to any of the other mental and behavioural disorders in ICD-10, physical disorders (such as endocrine disorder) or drug treatment. • In addition, for women: ‣ Pain during sexual intercourse, experienced at the entry of the vagina, throughout or only when deep thrusting of the penis occurs. ‣ Not attributable to vaginismus or failure of lubrication; dyspareunia due to organic pathology should be classified according to the underlying disorder. • In addition, for men: ‣ Pain or discomfort during sexual response. Careful recording should be established of the timing of the pain and the exact localisation. • Absence of local physical factors. If found, the dysfunction should be classified elsewhere.

Source: Reprinted with permission from the Diagnostic and Statistical Manual of Mental Disorders (DSM), Fifth Edition, American Psychiatric Association (APA), 2013 and ICD-10 Classification of Mental and Behavioural Disorders: Diagnostic Criteria for Research, World Health Organisation (WHO), Geneva, 2007.

Another feature of the disorder is the persistent or recurrent involuntary contraction of the muscles surrounding the opening of the vagina, thus preventing intercourse. This action is a spasm of muscles that closes the vagina and can occur as a result of attempted penetration with a penis, finger, tampon, or even a speculum (as in a medical examination). In the normal human sexual response cycle, a woman typically experiences a relaxing of the vaginal muscles with sexual arousal. A woman with this disorder, however, would experience a closing of these muscles that is involuntary, or not under her control. It can be diagnosed with reports of involuntary muscle spasms in the outer third of the vagina when intercourse or other types of vaginal penetration are attempted (McConaghy, 2005). The problem affects 1% to 6% of women (Hersen, Turner, & Beidel, 2007).

Table 9.12: Diagnostic criteria for Vaginismus as adapted from the ICD-10

ICD-10
• The subject is unable to participate in a sexual relationship as she would wish. • The dysfunction occurs frequently, but may be absent on some occasions. • The dysfunction has been present for at least six months. • The dysfunction is not entirely attributable to any of the other mental and behavioural disorders in ICD-10, physical disorders (such as endocrine disorder) or drug treatment. • Spasm of the perivaginal muscles is sufficient to prevent penile entry or make it uncomfortable. • The dysfunction appears as one of the following: ‣ Normal response has never been experienced. ‣ Vaginismus has developed after a period of relatively normal response.

Source: Reprinted with permission from the ICD-10 Classification of Mental and Behavioural Disorders: Diagnostic Criteria for Research, World Health Organisation (WHO), Geneva, 2007.

SECTION 2: GENDER DYSPHORIA

Previous editions of the DSM referred to this disorder as Gender Identity Disorder (GID), but DSM-5 refers to it as Gender Dysphoria (GD). The essential feature of the disorder is a psychological dissatisfaction with one's biological sex. GD is diagnosed when people believe that they are fundamentally people of the opposite sex. They may report the belief that they were born with the 'wrong' sex's genitals and experience so much distress from this misassignment that psychological problems result. People with Gender Dysphoria may dress in the clothes of the opposite sex simply in order to wear the clothes of the sex to which they feel they truly belong. This differs from the cross-dressing of transvestites. A transvestite man will wear women's clothing because this advances his sexual arousal and satisfactions, but a gender identity disordered man would dress as a woman, with no sexual arousal aims but because he feels that he is (or should be) 'a she', a woman.

Figure 9.1: Transgender rally

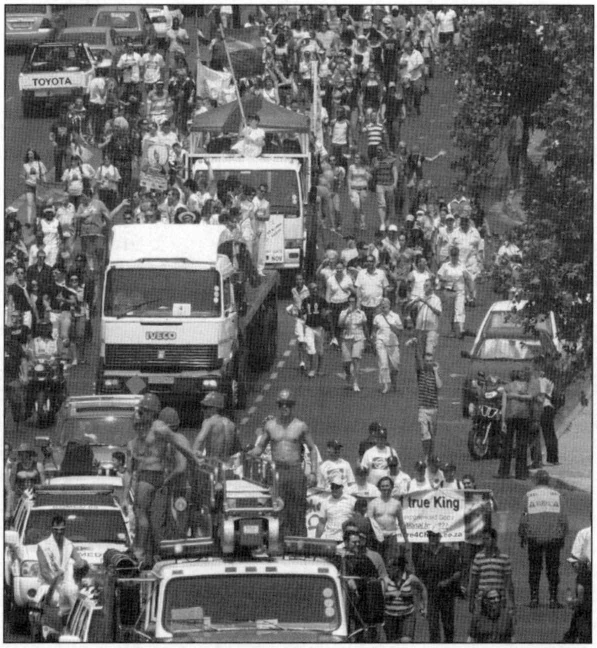

A fundamental component of most people's self-concept is their gender identity, or their sense of themselves as either male or female. This differs from their gender role, which instead refers to how they believe they should behave in society as either a male or female. Gender identity should also, importantly, be clearly distinguished from a person's sexual orientation, which is the emotional, romantic, and/or sexual attraction for either a male or female sexual partner. Also, a male with GD differs from the same-sex sexual arousal patterns of a male with so-called 'effeminate' behaviour. People with GD also differ from intersex individuals (or hermaphrodites). In some cultures, individuals with GD are held in esteem (Barlow & Durand, 2011).

Depending on the biological sex of the individual in question, GD results in an attraction to partners of either the same or opposite sex. For example, it is possible for a biological male to experience GD and feel convincingly that 'he' is in the 'wrong body' as 'his' sense of gender identity is strongly female, while still conforming to the historical masculine gender roles of pursuing a competitive career and playing aggressive sports, and having a man as 'his' romantic and sexual partner.

The DSM-5 acknowledge the developmental stages of a person with GD, and how this manifests differently in children and adolescents/adults, by describing different criteria for these age groups (see Table 9.13).

Table 9.13: Diagnostic criteria for Gender Dysphoria (DSM-5) and Gender Identity Disorder (ICD-10)

DSM-5 (Gender Dysphoria in children)	DSM-5 (Gender Dysphoria in adolescents	ICD-10
A. A marked incongruence between one's experienced/ expressed gender and assigned gender, of at least six months' duration, as manifested by at least six of the following (one of which must be Criterion A): (1) A strong desire to be of the other gender or an insistence that one is the other gender (or some alternative gender different to one's assigned gender).	A. A marked incongruence between one's experienced/expressed gender and assigned gender, of at least six months' duration, as manifested by at least two of the following: (1) A marked incongruence between one's experience/ expressed gender and primary and/ or secondary sex characteristics (or in young adolescents, the anticipated secondary sex characteristics).	• Desire to live and be accepted as a member of the opposite sex, mostly accompanied by the wish to transform one's body to closely as possible resemble that of the preferred sex through surgery and hormonal treatment. • Presence of the transsexual identity for a minimum of two years persistently.

DSM-5 (Gender Dysphoria in children)	DSM-5 (Gender Dysphoria in adolescents	ICD-10
(2) In boys (assigned gender), a strong preference for cross-dressing or simulating female attire; or in girls (assigned gender), a strong preference for wearing only typical masculine clothing and a strong resistance to the wearing of typical feminine clothing. (3) A strong preference for cross-gender roles in make-believe play or fantasy play. (4) A strong preference for the toys, games, or activities stereotypically used or engaged in by the other gender. (5) A strong preference for playmates of the other gender. (6) In boys (assigned gender), a strong rejection of typically masculine toys, games, and activities and a strong avoidance of rough-and-tumble play; or in girls (assigned gender), a strong rejection of typically feminine toys, games and activities. (7) A strong dislike of one's sexual anatomy. (8) A strong desire for the primary and/or secondary sex characteristics that match one's experienced gender. B. The condition is associated with clinically significant distress or impairment in social, school, or other important areas of functioning.	(2) A strong desire to be rid of one's primary and/or secondary sex characteristics because of marked incongruence with one's experienced/ expressed gender (or in young adolescents, a desire to prevent the development of the anticipated secondary sex characteristics). (3) A strong desire for the primary and/ or secondary sex characteristics of the other gender. (4) A strong desire to be of the other gender (or some alternative gender different to one's assigned gender). (5) A strong desire to be treated as the other gender (or some alternative gender different to one's assigned gender). (6) A strong conviction that one has the typical feelings and reaction of the other gender (or some alternative gender different to one's assigned gender). B. The condition is associated with clinically significant distress or impairment in social, occupational, or other important areas of functioning.	• Not a symptom of another mental disorder, such as Schizophrenia, or associated with chromosome abnormality.

Source: Reprinted with permission from the Diagnostic and Statistical Manual of Mental Disorders (DSM), Fifthe Edition, American Psychiatric Association (APA), 2013 and ICD-10 Classification of Mental and Behavioural Disorders: Diagnostic Criteria for Research, World Health Organisation (WHO), Geneva, 2007.

Issues with gender identity

The evolution of the social and legal position on same-sex orientation from that of 'sick' to just another aspect of human diversity is important to emphasise here, as it seems that an analogous process is occurring with gender identity disorders. However, Gender Identity Disorder, also known as 'gender dysphoria' and previously referred to as 'transsexuality', is still firmly considered psychopathology and included as a diagnostic category in the DSM-5 (American Psychiatric Association, 2013). Similarly, the ICD-10 lists 'transsexualism' and gender identity disorders as sexual deviations and disorders of adult personality and behaviour (MACGLH, 2002). However, many progressive psychotherapists who affirm lesbian, gay, bisexual, transgender, and intersexual (LGBTI) individuals do not consider transsexuality to be a mental illness (see the discussion of the abbreviation LGBTI in the section on cross-cultural and African perspectives). Recent criticisms against labelling gender dysphoria as mental illness have proposed that gender identity perception is a right. Critics argue that psychology and other health fields, for that matter, do not help people by pathologising what may be viewed as a normal variant of human sexuality and gender roles.

Most people (including transsexual people) feel that having a recognised gender identity accords with their sense of self. However, Dreger (2006) challenges the notion that everyone has a true, core, single, unchanging gender identity. Dreger suggests that, just as physical, sexual anatomies do not come in only two types that never change, neither do gender identities. A libertarian view of legal gender or sex identity advocates that, instead of the state adjudicating who is who in terms of sex and gender, people ought to have their own say about their genders, regardless of their anatomies (Dreger, 2006). LGBTI-affirmative therapists believe that transsexuality is not a mental illness and that there is no need for psychotherapeutic treatment for transsexuality per se (Nel, 2007).

Transitioning from one gender to another is often a complex and phased process. This involves adopting the appearance of the desired sex (that is, in clothing and grooming, treatment with cross-sex hormones, and surgical alteration of secondary sex characteristics). Many GID individuals, who have health insurance that would fund it or who can afford it themselves, may seek sex-reassignment surgery (SRS). This involves the so-called sex-change operations and treatments that aim to alter the genitals surgically (a GD woman may request that the uterus and ovaries be removed) and other sex-typing physical characteristics (breasts and facial hair) changed with the therapeutic use of medicines and hormones. Note, the overall goal of treatment, whether psychotherapeutic, endocrine, or surgical therapy, for people with gender dysphoria is lasting personal comfort with the gendered self in order to maximise overall psychological well-being and self-fulfilment (World Professional Association for Transgender Health [WPATH], 2001).

Transsexuals have, more often than not, been misunderstood and mis-diagnosed by their caregivers, who have frequently allowed personal prejudice to adversely affect their judgements (WPATH, 2001). In recognition of the scarcity of so-called 'qualified gender specialists', standards of care for GD were established as early as 1979, by WPATH (formerly known as HBIGDA, the Harry Benjamin International Gender Dysphoria Association) with the assistance of professionals in both the medical and psychological sciences. The standards of care (SOC), which are currently in their seventh version (WPATH, 2011), specify the minimum requirements for proper care and protection of both the person with GD and the professionals who provide treatment. The SOC articulate WPATH's professional consensus regarding the psychiatric, psychological, medical, and surgical management of GD. Included are requirements for determining a patient's suitability for hormone therapy and sex-reassignment surgery. The SOC specify the treatment goal of psychotherapy, and of endocrine and surgical therapies for people with GD, as lasting personal comfort with their gendered self in order to enhance their overall psychological well-being and self-fulfilment (WPATH, 2001).

Figure 9.2: Intersex people are indistinguishable from any other people.

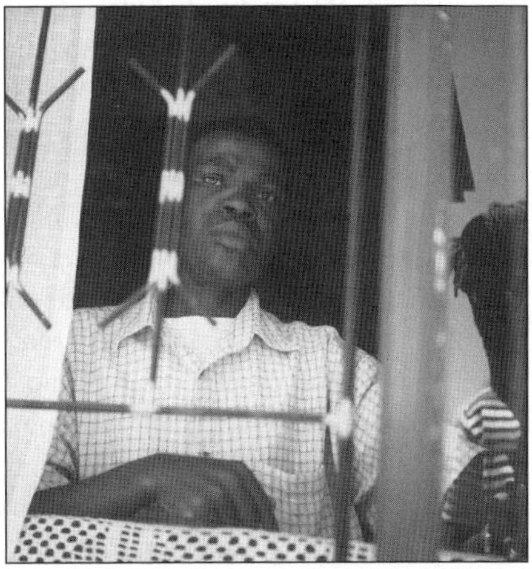

Importantly, in the 7th version of the SOC, gender dysphoria is the preferred term for GD and it is considered gender non-conformity, which is not pathological. The idea of mental health care is minimised and reparative therapies are considered unethical. The SOC promote a client-centred, and health-focussed (rather than clinician-centred) approach. Access to health care for medical treatment ought not to be reliant on a diagnosis, unless SRS is required (WPATH, 2011).

Lastly, intersex people (or hermaphrodites) are marginalised in the extreme and may become almost totally invisible in society, being regarded mostly as abnormal (Samelius & Wägberg, 2005). The standard protocol on the treatment of intersex children has been SRS and altering the genitals of the person in order to assign them to one of the two recognised biological sexes: male and female. Internationally, a small but growing intersex movement is lobbying against this practice, which it considers to be discriminatory, disrespectful, and at risk of causing both physical and psychological harm (Samelius & Wägberg, 2005). Increasingly, advocacy and lobbying efforts aim to ensure such choices are left to intersex individuals themselves to be made at a time when they can do so in an informed manner.

Informed by many of the aforementioned arguments, the DSM-5 includes a range of significant changes to this classification category. Among others, in response to the criticisms that the term was stigmatising, the initial proposal was to replace Gender Identity Disorder with 'Gender Incongruence'. Although removal of the 'disorder' label from the name of the diagnosis was welcomed, submitters of comments to the initial proposal, including members of WPATH, suggested the alternative term gender dysphoria as semantically more appropriate because it expresses an aversive emotional component.

Debates furthermore focused on the merit of placing this condition in a special category apart from (formerly Axis 1) psychiatric diagnoses to reflect its unusual status as a mental condition treated with cross-sex hormones, sex-reassignment surgery, and social and legal transition to the desired gender (particularly with regard to adolescents and adults). The Subworkgroup wished to avoid jeopardising either insurance coverage or treatment access. Finding a special placement for a condition in the developing organisational structure of the DSM-5 thus proved a challenge. It appears that gender diagnoses will in the final instance be separated from the sexual dysfunctions and paraphilias (American Psychiatric Association, 2012).

SECTION 3: PARAPHILIC DISORDERS

'Paraphilia' is the term used to describe the sexual disorders in which sexual arousal, behaviours, and satisfaction occur in the context of unusual or inappropriate objects including either non-human objects (or body parts, activities, or situations), and/or non-consenting adults or children (Love, 1995) (see Table 9.14 for an overview of the paraphilias). Paraphilias may include suffering or humiliation of self, partner, or children.

Figure 9.3: Fetish gear

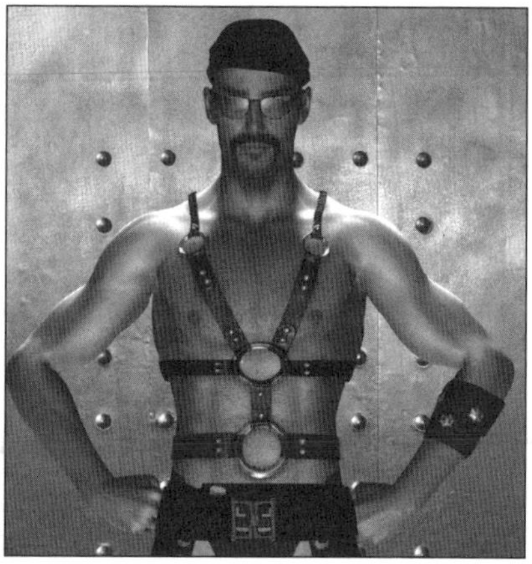

The paraphilias can be divided into those that involve consenting others (such as sadomasochism) or non-consenting others (such as in exhibitionism). They can also be divided into those that involve contact with others (such as frotteurism) or no contact with others (such as in some fetishes).

The associated recurrent, intense sexual urges, fantasies, or behaviours must bring about clinically significant distress or impairment in personal, social, academic, or occupational functioning, or in other important domains of an individual's life. To qualify for such a diagnosis, a person would also need to have acted on the urges and/or fantasies or to have experienced marked distress or interpersonal difficulties as a result of them (American Psychiatric Association, 2000).

The meaning of paraphilia, coined by Stekel in 1923, is 'love' for, or an attraction to, something beyond the usual (*para*: besides, going beside or beyond, amiss; *philia*: love or attachment to). Paraphilias are also, amongst other common terms, referred to as 'deviances', 'perversions', or 'sexual aberrations' (Love, 1995). It ought to be noted that the ICD-10 refers to Disorders of Sexual Preference, instead of referring to a Paraphilia (World Health Organisation, 2007).

Table 9.14: Summary of paraphilias

TYPE	DESCRIPTION
Fetishism	The use of inanimate objects as the preferred or exclusive source of sexual arousal. Fetishism may also refer to being sexually attracted to inanimate objects (or just a single body part) or a source of specific tactile stimulation (Love, 1995). People with a fetish most often focus their sexual activities on non-human objects and thus do not impose their desires on other people and may go unnoticed. Fetish objects include clothing (in particular, underwear), footwear, certain materials or fabrics (including leather, plastics, diapers, and gloves). Fetish behaviours commonly include fondling, smelling, and licking the object(s), but where the individual needs to acquire the object secretly from someone else (such as women's worn panties), they may also include having to steal the object(s).

TYPE	DESCRIPTION
Transvestic fetishism	In transvestic fetishism, sexual arousal in heterosexual men is associated with the act of cross-dressing in women's clothes (APA, 2000). This cross-dressing, from only one item of women's clothing to completely dressing as a woman with make-up and a wig, can go on to become the man's primary means of becoming sexually aroused. This condition also indicates a sexual attraction to the clothing of the opposite sex, but once orgasm occurs, sexual arousal typically declines and the man is strongly motivated to remove the items of women's clothing.
Sexual sadism	Sexual sadism involves the recurrent urge or behaviour to inflict (real, not simulated) pain or humiliation on a sexual partner for sexual arousal (APA, 2000). The person typically achieves their sexual satisfaction from inflicting pain and/or humiliation on a sexual partner. Sexual sadism often includes certain rituals (such as binding and handcuffing the partner) and clearly recognisable props (such as leather zip masks and whips) to be used in such encounters. More males than females engage in sadist and masochist sex and females not engaged in commercial sex work may become involved only in response to a male's wishes or as non-consenting victims.
Sexual masochism	Sexual masochism involves the recurrent urge or behaviour of wanting to be made to suffer (real, not simulated) pain or humiliation for sexual arousal (APA, 2000). It can be considered, to a great extent, to be the reverse of sexual sadism. In sexual masochism, an individual will also gain sexual gratification by having a sexual partner cause them to suffer pain and or humiliation.
Voyeurism	Voyeurism refers to the act of watching an unsuspecting individual undressing, naked, engaging in sex, or bathing, in order to become sexually aroused. The watching is done in secret, most often by a man, who may masturbate while watching the scene or shortly thereafter. The person being watched, most often a woman, must be unaware of the peeping and would be very distressed were she to find out; in other words, the woman is not a cooperative sexual partner, nor is the act consensual. While many people may engage in such behaviours at some point or another in their lives, they become a problem for individuals when the voyeurism develops into their primary sexual outlet or when these individuals clash with law-enforcement agencies as a result thereof (Love, 1995).

TYPE	DESCRIPTION
Exhibitionism	The recurrent urge or behaviour to gain sexual arousal from shocking others (most often unsuspecting strangers) by exposing one's genitals (APA, 2000). It can be considered, to a great extent, to be the reverse of voyeurism. There are many different degrees or levels of exhibitionism as well as reasons or benefits believed to be obtained from exposing. The observers are typically strangers who are quite involuntarily made witness to the exhibitionist's display. In almost all cases, a man will exhibit himself to a surprised woman. The exhibitionist's sexual arousal typically comes from observing the victim's response in terms of surprise, fear, or disgust or even from the fantasised notion that the woman was aroused by his actions. The viewer's reactions must provide sufficient perceived ego boost, novelty, embarrassment, defilement, or other discomfort to produce the high level of stimulus required for the exhibitionist's orgasm (Love, 1995).
Frotteurism	Frotteurism is the recurrent urge to or behaviour of touching or rubbing against a non-consenting person (APA, 2000). This leads to sexual arousal and will also result in sexual gratification through the pressing up against a stranger or even fondling parts of his or her body. The frotteur's behaviours are often opportunistic in nature, with the setting playing an important role. When many people are packed together in a crowded place, such as an underground subway, a train, elevator, or a queue, the frotteur's bumping or rubbing against another person may not be identified as sexual. Quite often the target or victim will not realise that the contact has anything to do with sexual behaviours (Love, 1995).
Paedophilia	Paedophilia, often erroneously understood to be synonymous with child molestation, involves sexual attraction to prepubescent or peri-pubescent children, most often girls (Love, 1995). People with paedophilia (who are typically adults, but are required to be at least 16 years of age in order to make the diagnosis) are sexually attracted to children (required to be less than 13 years of age, and at least 5 years younger than the perpetrator). Most troubling about this disorder is that it is the most common of the paraphilias and the non-consenting others are young people. The sexual acts that paedophiles most often engage in with children are those of exposing or touching the child's genitals, or oral and even penetrative sex.
Paraphilias Not Otherwise Specified	Other paraphilias not otherwise specified include disorders like: • telephone scatalogia (obscene phone calls) • necrophilia (sexual attraction to corpses) • partialism (exclusive focus on one part of the body) • zoophilia (sex with animals) • coprophilia (sexual attraction to faeces) • urophilia (sexual attraction to urine).

Source: American Psychiatric Association, 2000; Love, 1995.

Some people find numerous creative ways of enhancing their sexual satisfaction or fulfilling their sexual needs and desires. Most of the time, this can be done within the social limitations on sexual behaviour. Judgments about what sexual behaviours are acceptable have differed across historical periods and cultures and continue to be subjective and socioculturally constructed. Socially unacceptable sexual behaviours are those that are prohibited by modern cultural norms, and sometimes even by laws, in which case they become criminal. The DSM-5 uses the term 'paraphilias' to designate those atypical sexual behaviours that are considered to be disorders. When people with a paraphilia also violate laws, they would additionally be considered sex offenders or criminals. People with paraphilias rarely present voluntarily (American Psychiatric Association, 2000), until their actions attract the attention of law-enforcement agencies.

Although the paraphilias are often associated with sexual offending by the general public, this is not always the case. Those convicted of sexual offences represent the more severe end of the spectrum of the atypical sexual behaviours. Fetishism and transvestic fetishism are mostly considered benign, whereas sadism and masochism (S&M), although often practised between consenting adults, are less benign as they may result in injury. Frotteurism, voyeurism, and exhibitionism are not considered benign as they involve non-consenting others who may feel that they became 'victims'. Lastly, paedophilia is considered the most severe of the paraphilias and is clearly a punishable offence.

Several of the more recently written psychopathology text books are, however, beginning to acknowledge that the inclusion of atypical sexual behaviour in the DSM-5 is a contentious issue. As argued earlier in this chapter, the distinction between 'normal' and 'abnormal' sexual behaviour is a difficult one. Norms regarding sexual practices change considerably over time, because of the influence of changing cultural and religious beliefs and values (see the example of same-sex sexuality above). Norms regarding sexual practices also vary across and within cultures. For example, in Western cultures, women's breasts are eroticised, and revealing them is considered sexually arousing, while in many other cultures, breasts are viewed purely as a means to feed babies. Amongst many other norms, societal expectations for sexuality have changed with regard to masturbation and the virtuousness of suppressing sexual arousal. For example, in stark contrast to earlier times and their mores and values, the absence of sexual desire is today considered a clinical disorder. Also, we know the extent to which premarital heterosexual sexual behaviour has in recent years become culturally acceptable in many parts of the world.

In response to the abovementioned criticisms, the DSM-5 made two broad changes that affect several of the paraphilia diagnoses, in addition to various amendments to specific diagnoses. The first broad change follows from consensus that paraphilias are not per se psychiatric disorders. The DSM-5 makes a distinction between 'paraphilias' and 'paraphilic disorders', and notes that there are a number of paraphilias that are not listed under paraphilic disorders (APA, 2013). The implication is that a paraphilia, in and of itself, would not automatically justify or require psychiatric intervention. A paraphilic disorder, on the other hand, is a paraphilia that causes distress or impairment to the individual or harm to others.

A paraphilia is recognisable according to the nature of the associated urges, fantasies, or behaviours, but a paraphilic disorder is diagnosed on the basis of distress and impairment. In this conception, having a paraphilia would be a necessary but not sufficient condition for having a paraphilic disorder (American Psychiatric Association, 2012). According to the Paraphilias Subworkgroup, the abovementioned approach leaves intact the distinction between normative and non-normative sexual behaviour, which could be important for researchers, but resists automatically labelling non-normative sexual behaviour as psychopathological (American Psychiatric Association, 2012).

The second broad change applies to paraphilias that involve non-consenting persons, such as Voyeuristic Disorder, Exhibitionistic Disorder, and Sexual Sadism Disorder. In these instances, especially for uncooperative patients, it is suggested there be a minimum number of separate victims for diagnosing the paraphilia. Research indicates that a substantial proportion – perhaps a majority – of patients referred for assessment of paraphilias are referred after committing a criminal sexual offence. Such patients are typically neither truthful nor forthcoming about their sexual urges and fantasies. The criteria have therefore been modified to lessen the dependence of diagnosis on patients' self-reports regarding urges and fantasies (American Psychiatric Association, 2012).

In an attempt to obtain similar rates of false positive and false negative diagnoses for all the paraphilias, the suggested minimum number of separate victims varies for diagnosis of the different paraphilias in the DSM-5. For example, three different victims are required for a diagnosis of Voyeuristic Disorder, but only two different victims for a Sexual Sadism Disorder diagnosis. This is informed by the rationale that paraphilias differ in the extent to which they resemble behaviours in the typical adult's sexual repertoire (American Psychiatric Association, 2012).

CROSS-CULTURAL AND AFRICAN PERSPECTIVES

In this section, an overview of the needs and rights of South African sexual minorities, and in particular, LGBTI people and communities, provides a lens through which to comment on this specific context and on the sexuality and gender 'landscape'.

Sexuality and gender touch upon some of the most intimate and personal aspects of human existence. Sexuality is a core value and central to self, identity, culture, and nation (Pigg & Adams, 2005). Issues of sexuality and gender, moreover, carry much cultural weight and are, therefore, vulnerable to exploitation for political means (Human Rights Watch [HRW], 2003). Rape as an act of war is but one example of such exploitation. Most societies attempt to control the sexual behaviour of their members in some way or other (Goodwach, 2005). Sexuality is thus recognised as a powerful domain, in terms of both general social prejudice and stigmatisation, and more specifically, the pathologising of minority groups or 'deviant' categories of people (Hook, 2002).

The values, beliefs, and stereotypes of a psychotherapist (or researcher on sexual and gender functioning) are central in working with sexuality and sexual minorities. These values will directly influence the way in which problems are defined, formulated, and evaluated and the types of intervention that may be offered. While some experts understand sexuality as universal, there are others who view sexuality as context-specific in terms of meaning, practice, and outcome (Pigg & Adams, 2005).

However, sex and sexuality are often universalised in the name of health and well-being. Patriarchal Westernised ways of defining sexual 'norms', sexual orientation, and gender identity make the assumption that biological sex (which is essentially fixed) forms the basis for people's identities and determines their sexual expression (Pigg & Adams, 2005). The medical model is interested in objective knowledge that is unaffected by the health care recipient's values and meanings. Similarly, the contextual aspects of sex, race, and culture also do not feature significantly in the medical model. Thus, within the medical model, the assumption is that an expert can 'diagnose' objectively and apply a clearly linked solution (Hook, 2002).

Yet human sexuality is powerfully influenced by the specific sociocultural and temporal context within which it is found. Apartheid South Africa, for instance, was notorious for having been a particularly repressive society (Nel, 2005b; Seedat, Duncan, & Lazarus, 2001). Until the early 1990s, strong emphasis was placed on the legal restriction of sexuality, with several laws regulating sexual behaviour. For instance, sex 'across the colour line' was prohibited, sex between men was criminalised until as recently as 1996, and there were laws against all forms of pornography (Nel, 2005b; Potgieter, 1997). Sex work is still illegal in South Africa, but recently there were proposals to make prostitution legal during the 2010 Soccer World Cup, in order to serve the international sex trade market that was expected.

The freedom of political association, of speech, and of sexual expression that now exists in South Africa is new. Sexuality-related issues often elicit strong (negative) emotional responses, including feelings of guilt and shame, and are considered 'private' and 'personal', and 'not to be discussed'. The sexual behaviours of others still tend to be viewed in strict and rigid terms of 'rightness' or 'wrongness', and those behaviours departing from the norm are severely criticised. For these reasons, sexuality has more often than not been veiled in secrecy. However, following decades of Calvinist rule, the multibillion-rand South African sex industry (including upmarket entertainment venues, strip clubs, several chains of sex shops, house parties, and sex work) that has emerged post-1994 suggests that a sexual revolution has occurred (Geldenhuys, 2006).

Nonetheless, hetero-normative assumptions remain a core characteristic of contemporary South African culture. These assumptions and attitudes are pervasive in the media, religious teachings and practices, legal discourses, education, and health care. Neglect or deliberate exclusion of LGBTI people in gender analyses and policy discussions reflect the pervasiveness of hetero-normative assumptions (Samelius & Wägberg, 2005). The silencing of same-sex assumptions that occurs in this manner implies a taboo and undesirability, and perpetuates prejudice (Eliason, 1996).

The South African LGBTI community also has to contend with homoprejudice and transphobia (Du Plessis, 1999; Hattingh, 1994). Being lesbian or gay in South Africa has often been considered a 'sickness', a 'sin', 'criminal', or un-African. Today, there are restrictions against the public expression of these opinions. However, religious condemnation, harassment in the workplace and other places, public statements of homoprejudice, and violence towards LGBTI people are still rife. Moreover, internalised homoprejudice is prevalent within many LGBTI people (Isaacs & McKendrick, 1992; Nel, 2005a).

LGBTI identities in South Africa differ significantly along the designated 'racial' categories of black, 'coloured', Asian, and white. Given South Africa's history of apartheid and patriarchy, the most visible and vocal subsection of the LGBTI community was, until recently, white and predominantly male, many of whom are well positioned in the workplace and are affluent in comparison to other sectors of society. This group has been the most researched and is often considered the least vulnerable. However, this group is not a true reflection of the community as a whole. The vast majority of LGBTI individuals in South Africa are black, unemployed, and poor, and have low literacy levels (Reid & Dirsuweit, 2002).

Owing to the multiplicity of contributions to their minority status in terms of gender, sexual orientation, socio-economic status, and race, under-resourced black lesbians are assumed to be the most vulnerable subsection of the community (Reid & Dirsuweit, 2002). For a variety of reasons, this subsection of the community is also severely under-researched. However, recent research indicates disproportionately high levels of risk of victimisation, including 'corrective rape' (Polders, 2006; Reid & Dirsuweit, 2002; Rich, 2006; Wells, 2006).

As in Europe and America, and for very much the same reasons, use of the abbreviation LGBTI in reference to sexual minorities is common practice in South African activist circles. Use of this abbreviation is, however, not a true reflection of representation or inclusion in decision-making. In fact, participation of bisexual, transsexual, and intersexual people in the so-called 'LGBTI' sector or movement is very limited, partly because numbers are relatively small. As a consequence, knowledge of issues related to bisexual, transgender, and especially intersex people is also very limited.

The paucity of referenced accounts of bisexual life (specifically) in South Africa, and the under-representation of bisexual concerns in lesbian and gay organisations in general, is striking. Bisexual people's greater invisibility, as well as the preconceived ideas that bisexual people are fence-sitters and fearful of disclosing their sexual orientation, has been suggested as a possible reason (Nicholas, Daniels, & Hurwitz, 2001, in Francoeur, 2001).

Internationally, activism within the LGBTI community attaches a very high premium to the notions of inclusion and representation. Use of the abbreviation LGBTI in reference to sexual minorities, not only on the basis of alternative sexual orientation but also gender non-conformity and biological variance, is an indication of this inclusive stance. This position is a corrective measure in response to lifelong experiences of marginalisation, exclusion, and disqualification; it is also politically informed by the need for solidarity among minorities in the face of discrimination at the hands of a vast majority. However, in terms of academic research, the abbreviation LGBTI minimises theoretical distinctions drawn between biological variance, gender, and sexual orientation. This may not be helpful in either research endeavours or psychosocial intervention programmes. As the transgender community in South Africa becomes more organised, they are also resisting being clustered together with the LGB community (GenderdynamiX, n.d.).

The formal training of psychologists and psychology professionals is currently not sufficiently inclusive of the issues and needs of the sexually diverse. It is inexcusable for professionals not to consciously counteract notions of same-sex sexuality as psychopathology or criminal behaviour. Representatives at a 2007 South African conference on teaching psychology at universities, held at the University of the Free State, acknowledged that content related to sexual orientation and gender identity is often restricted to subfields such as social and abnormal psychology (Nel, 2007).

The 2007 conference referred to above, considered the considerable challenges in addressing these issues. These challenges include an inherent conservatism and patriarchy in South Africa, as well as resistance to addressing themes of sexuality and gender within the profession of psychology. In addition, related terminology, such as sexual orientation, gender identification, LGBTI, MSM (men who have sex with men), WSW (women who have sex with women), and homosexuality versus same-sex sexuality, is often confusing, poorly understood, and controversial. Conventional labelling and stereotypes require careful 'unpacking' in terms of meaning, as well as problemetisation that acknowledges fluidity instead of linear descriptions (Nel, 2007).

Large parts of Africa have been devastated by the effects of sexual ill-health and suffering brought about by, amongst other things, a lack of sexual rights and education, a culture of sexual coercion, and limited access to professional sexual health care. South Africa is no exception in this regard. Whilst South Africa has one of the most progressive constitutions in the world, which includes freedom of sexual orientation in its Bill of Rights, unfortunately, the incidence of rape in South Africa is one of the highest in the world and South Africa is 'second only to India with regard to the endemic prevalence of HIV/AIDS' (Nel, 2007, p. 133).

In South Africa, the field of sexology is poorly developed, and specialised health care, including sex therapy, is available only to a select few, almost exclusively at private health care facilities in urban centres. Until recently in South Africa, very limited funds and support were made available for research and education on sexuality issues. Only a limited number of medical professionals, psychologists, and other therapists can consider themselves to be well-versed sexologists, and most have no recognised formal qualification in this speciality (Nel, 2007; SASHA, n.d.).

The arrival of oral treatments for erectile dysfunction changed the lack of funding for sexuality research in South Africa. Pharmaceutical companies that produce related treatments, such as Viagra, Cialis, and Levitra have prioritised the provision of credible information and education on sexual health issues from a multidisciplinary perspective. This information is made available to the general public, the media, and health care professionals.

The endemic prevalence of HIV/AIDS, as well as of rape and of women and child abuse (De la Rey & Eagle, 1997), may be partly related to the lack of sexuality education and inadequate understandings of gender issues. Until the mid-1990s, very little emphasis was placed on sexual rights, and it is only recently that public campaigns and debates on sexuality issues, and the responsibilities that go with freedom, have been introduced. Despite strong recommendations in this regard, sex education and gender awareness are yet to be comprehensively introduced in schools (OUT, 2006).

South Africa, as a signatory of the International Agreement reached at the Fourth World Conference on Women held in Beijing in 1995, subscribes to the rights contained in the Sexual Health Charter and is therefore obliged to ensure that the sexual rights of all people are respected, protected, and fulfilled. Furthermore, several sexual and reproductive rights are included as human rights in the South African Constitution. These include the right to expression of sexual orientation without interference from others, equality and equity for all, the right to make choices free from gender-based discrimination, freedom from sexual violence or coercion, and the right to privacy (The Gender Manual Consortium, 1999).

However, South Africa is far from translating these 'paper rights' into practice. The relentless HIV pandemic and also the very high levels of rape, domestic violence, incest, and teenage pregnancy suggest that many people are not able to claim their sexual and reproductive rights (The Gender Manual Consortium, 1999).

BOX 9.1: WHAT ARE SEXUAL RIGHTS?

Sexual rights derive from human rights (see Chapter 14) that are recognised in national, regional, and international human-rights laws. Sexual rights include the right of all persons, free of coercion, discrimination, and violence, to:

- The highest attainable standard of sexual health, including access to sexual and reproductive health-care services.
- Seek, receive, and impart information related to sexuality.
- Sexuality education.
- Respect for bodily integrity.
- Choice of one's partner or partners.
- Decide whether to be sexually active or not.
- Consensual sexual relations.
- Consensual marriage.
- Decide whether or not, and when, to have children.
- Pursue a satisfying, safe, and pleasurable sexual life.

Source: PAHO & WHO, 2000. Promotion of Sexual Health: Recommendations for Action. Proceedings of a regional consultation convened by Pan-American Health Organisation (PAHO) and World Health Organisation (WHO), in collaboration with the World Association for Sexology (WAS), Antigua, Guatemala, May 19-22, 2000, pp. 37-38. Available online: http://www.paho.org/english/hcp/hca/promotionsexualhealth.pdf

HIV and AIDS have contributed significantly to the current state of the public health care system in South Africa being overstretched, with state hospitals bearing the brunt as they attempt to accommodate people suffering from HIV/AIDS-related illnesses (Boyle, 2006). However, LGBTI issues are virtually non-existent in the Department of Health (DoH), and also in HIV prevention and care. Similarly, reports on HIV transmission mostly do not adequately differentiate between male-to-male and male-to-female modes of transmission (Samelius & Wägberg, 2005). As indicated, HIV prevention and treatment programmes initiated by the government insufficiently recognise the diversity of sexual expressions, behaviours, and needs of LGBTI groups and generally target only the mainstream. It is only with the 2005-2011 South African National Strategic Plan (NSP) for HIV/AIDS and STIs that the vulnerabilities of LGBTI people and men who have sex with men (MSM) have been recognised.

While the LGBTI sector in South Africa (including organisations such as OUT LGBT Well-Being, Triangle Project, and Men4Health) renders (sexual) health and psychosocial services, recognition is seldom given to LGBTI clients in government and civil society initiatives. No specific health-care service for LGBTI clients is provided by government. Increasingly, clients demand the services of LGBTI-affirming health care workers, and although the number of these providers has significantly increased in recent years, not many qualify as LGBTI affirmative when the American Psychiatric Association guidelines (2000) are used as yardstick.

BOX 9.2: TRANSGENDER RIGHTS

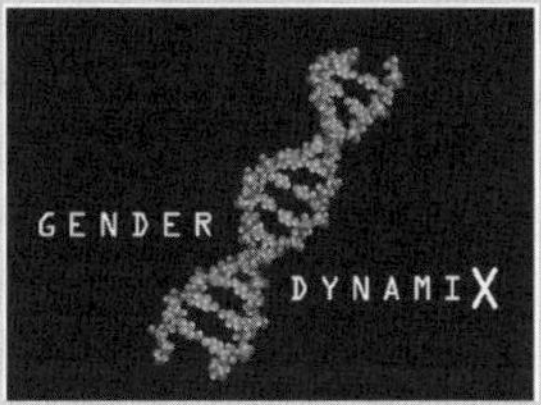

The first specifically transgender organisation on the continent, Gender DynamiX, located in Cape Town, South Africa, was launched only in 2005. While transgender rights are now protected, and it is possible legally to change gender on birth certificates and in identity documents (Samelius & Wägberg, 2005), bureaucratic procedures and state official ignorance and prejudice render many of these rights useless.

Current practice in mainstream health care in South Africa is, more often than not, to render services with an assumption of sameness, rather than with respect for difference or diversity (Nel, 2007). It goes without saying that everyone has the right to be treated as equal and to health care services that adhere to the minimum standards. However, because of the diverse people who inhabit South Africa, it is erroneous and inappropriate to believe that 'one size fits all'. On the rare occasion that sexuality issues are addressed in professional contexts or in public forums in South Africa, it is often from a hetero-normative (Potgieter, 1997), and until recently also a patriarchal, perspective (De la Rey & Eagle, 1997).

This is set to change somewhat in the foreseeable future: The Psychological Society of South Africa (PsySSA), with the guidance of the International Network on Lesbian, Gay and Bisexual Concerns and Transgender Issues in Psychology (INET), of which PsySSA has been a member since 2007, aims to:

- Develop a PsySSA/University of South Africa post-graduate psychology course in African perspectives on sexuality and gender to be presented as a pilot in 2013. The focus of the envisioned course will be on sexuality, not limited to sexual minorities, and specifically on the various roles of psychology within the field of sexology.
- Develop detailed programming and planning meetings to bring together psychology professionals and psychological associations, in particular from Africa, at the International Congress of Psychology (ICP) Sexuality Stream to be held during July, 2012.
- Establish a Sexuality and Gender Division within PsySSA.
- Develop (South) African psychological guidelines for LGBTI-affirmative practice.
- Produce position statements to ensure the rights of LGBTI persons in Africa are observed (PsySSA, 2011).

AETIOLOGY

Scientific enquiry to establish causality is an enduring feature of conventional psychology. This also applies with regard to the sexual disorders and gender dysphoria. Ongoing debates highlight 'nature' on the one hand and 'nurture' on the other, or suggest a combination of both. Inherent qualities, such as biochemistry and the prenatal influences of hormones and nutrition feature in the biological theories of causality or predisposition that support nature as cause. The psychological theories suggest that intrapsychic factors, such as early childhood experiences or belief systems, can cause disorders. The social and interpersonal theories of causality would then look to interpersonal relationships and the impact of the social environment on a person.

Sexual and gender identity problems are usually associated with other presenting symptoms as well. Thus, most sexual dysfunctions include a combination of both physical and psychological causes. An individual's specific biological predispositions may interact with psychological factors to produce a dysfunction in what we call the diathesis-stress model (see Chapter 2). This model proposes that it takes both a predisposition (or vulnerability) to a disorder and a life stressor (or trigger) to create the disorder. Vulnerabilities may be found in various biological factors (genes or brain anomalies), psychological factors (maladaptive beliefs, poor skills, or unconscious conflicts), and social factors (maladaptive upbringing, poor relationships, or chronic stress). Stressors may include biological triggers (onset of a disease or exposure to toxins), psychological triggers (violation of trust or perceived loss of control), and social triggers (major loss or traumatic event).

Clinical assessment of sexual behaviour consists of interviewing, medical evaluation, psychological assessment, and physiological assessment. Clinicians must be sensitive to patients' discomfort with discussing sexual issues and a possible lack of understanding of clinical terminology. Physiological assessment may include techniques such as use of a penile plethysmograph (penile strain gauge) for men or a vaginal photoplephysmograph for women. Measurements of arousal may be taken concurrent with exposure to erotic stimuli. Measurement of nocturnal penile tumescence may also be useful in showing whether erection can occur.

Biological factors

A number of biological factors may play a role in either predisposing an individual to sexual disorders and gender dysphoria or triggering such a disorder. These include organic factors (such as diabetes; neurological, vascular, thyroid, pituitary, renal or liver disease; depression; and fatigue), medications (such as antihypertensive and psychotropic drugs), and the use or abuse of other substances (such as alcohol and drugs).

In terms of organic factors, neurological diseases and chronic illness may interfere with sexual functioning. Vascular disease, such as arterial insufficiency and venous leakage, has been associated with erectile problems in males (McConaghy, 2005). The use of certain drugs, recent surgery, and other medical conditions may all affect sexual functioning. Drug and alcohol abuse also suppresses sexual arousal. In addition, a major physical cause of sexual dysfunction is the use of antihypertensive or antidepressant medications (SSRIs) and tranquillisers.

Biological mechanisms of sexual arousal and orgasm in women are poorly understood at present (Brotto & Klein, 2007). For example, the neurophysiology of the female sexual response has not been adequately studied. This includes the role of neurotransmitters and local vaso-active substances in determining vascular smooth muscle tone, vasodilatation, and vaginal lubrication. Likewise, the role of steroid hormones in the modulation of sexual desire and arousal in women is not well understood. The effects of aging and menopause on female sexual functioning are important areas for further research.

Another good example of the many organic causal factors behind a sexual dysfunction is that of premature ejaculation. Among the numerous organic conditions that may lead to abnormalities of emission and ejaculation are acute or chronic polyneuropathy, endocrine disorders, serological disorders, and the side effects of other drug therapies (McConaghy, 2005). In the aetiology of gender dysphoria, exposure to certain hormones at critical periods *in utero* has been suggested as an important contribution to the development of this disorder (McConaghy, 2005).

If we refer back to the distinctions in Orgasmic Disorder as being either primary (having never experienced an orgasm) or secondary (had previous orgasms), we see that secondary Orgasmic Disorder is more frequently due to underlying organic disease or medication (and, at times, underlying relationship difficulties) (Sarason & Sarason, 1993).

More attention should be also be focused on aetiology of sexuality issues in the aging. Risk factors such as the normal aging process, chronic illness, a history of surgery or physical trauma, drugs, and other modifiable factors may be important in sexual dysfunction in the elderly. Other risk factors include chronic illness, and systemic diseases such as atherosclerosis, diabetes, cardiovascular disease, and renal and liver failure. Neurogenic conditions such as Alzheimer's disease, multiple sclerosis, tumours, and brain trauma may also play a role in sexual dysfunctions. Psychiatric disorders such as depression and anxiety, as well as endocrine disorders such as hyper- and hypothyroidism, hypogonadism, and hyperprolactinaemia, have also been implicated.

As biological factors are strongly implicated in some sexual dysfunctions, effective medical treatments have been developed for some of them, for example erectile dysfunction. Vaso-active therapy involves injection of papaverine into the penis immediately before intercourse, which facilitates erection. This method may cause discomfort or pain, and studies have reported high attrition rates. Penile implants and vascular procedures are surgical alternatives. Also, vacuum device therapy creates a vacuum that draws blood into the penis, which is then trapped by placing a ring around the base of the penis.

Psychological factors

Psychological factors can play a major role in causation, with anger, stress, and anxiety frequently implicated in the sexual dysfunctions. Current theory suggests that cognitive processes are heavily involved in sexual problems (Sarason & Sarason, 1993). Learning theory implicates early learning or 'erotophobia' in sexual disorders. Within the individual, dysfunctional attitudes (such as sexual guilt), past experience, and traumatic experiences (such as rape or incest) may become problematic for sexual functioning.

The aetiology of Vaginismus provides us with examples of fear and trauma factors that can play a role in sexual dysfunction. Sexual traumas such as rape, incest, molestation, and painful, coercive, or unsatisfactory first sexual intercourse experience can lead to this. More general fears of pregnancy or infertility, sexually transmitted infections (including HIV), intimacy, penetration, or loss of control, and other factors such as misinformed beliefs that a woman is 'too small', or that sex results in pain, may be problematic. Poor body image or poor self-esteem and performance anxiety may also lead to difficulties in sexual functioning. An individual who experiences sexual orientation-related distress may also be more at risk of sexual dysfunction.

Ignorance of sexual functioning and even basic ignorance of anatomy may lead to sexual problems. For example, a very young or uninformed individual may believe that he may 'get lost' in his sexual partner, and that this may result in losing his penis. Much in the way of societal faulty beliefs regarding sex and sexual functioning may be carried over to the individual in myths and misinformation from any number of sources. This can result in unrealistic expectations that serve only to impede the individual's sexual functioning and satisfaction. On the other hand, the fear of losing control of feelings and behaviour, in someone who is sexually responsive, is often at the core of the problem. The resulting defensive behaviour of 'holding back' and over-control may prevent some women letting go to orgasm. Fear of losing control over bladder function, or fear of losing consciousness if becoming too highly aroused, may further inhibit and prevent orgasm.

Freud contributed an important example in the way of myth or unrealistic expectations with his views on vaginal versus clitoral orgasm, with the former being considered the preferable, and only 'mature', form of sexual pleasure for women. Today it is accepted that there is no superior form of orgasm. The epidemiological data varies, but it is accepted that more than 50% of women need direct clitoral stimulation to orgasm (Brotto & Klein, 2007). Unfortunately, this medical knowledge is not always carried over to the beliefs held in society. Many media sources, such as popular men's and women's magazines, still back the idea that some forms of sexual expression are 'must-do' and are readily achievable by anyone, if they just try hard enough.

A further myth is that of the simultaneous orgasm. In modern sexology, this is seen as a sign of male dominance or control instead of a sign of couple closeness. Such expectations create performance pressure in the female partner that would definitely further inhibit sexual enjoyment and freedom to orgasm. Many popular sexual myths (some of which are more strongly held in some population groups) include the following: men know everything about sex; the woman should not initiate sex; men are always in the mood; a person who does not enjoy sex does not love their partner; women should not ask for what they want; the man will know best how to please the woman, etc.

Body-image problems might be a reason for primary anorgasmia, but could also be present in the woman who is orgasmic with solo masturbation but not in the presence of a partner. As suggested above, a related factor is that of performance anxiety. In women who have normal sexual arousal but fail to orgasm, performance pressures and anxieties are very often to blame. Regardless of whether these pressures are self-imposed or due to scrutiny from the male partner, the result is often a pattern of 'spectatoring' (that is, detailed self-monitoring during sexual activity). This leads to a loss of spontaneity and inhibits the woman's responsiveness. This inhibition leads to further sexual 'failure', thereby reinforcing expectation in a self-perpetuating cycle. Men may also have difficulties with spectatoring.

Masters and Johnson (1970) revolutionised sex therapy with a brief, direct, therapeutic programme that first excluded physical or organic causes of dysfunction (which would be treated medically if indicated) and offered the psychological and interpersonal treatment strategies for which they are still well known today. The therapy includes basic education about sexuality and emphasises improving communication and reducing performance anxiety. The methods of 'sensate focus' and non-demand pleasuring are also used. The success of the programme is widely documented (Sarason & Sarason, 1993), and sex therapies have evolved and expanded upon these pioneering methods.

Social and interpersonal factors

Interpersonally, we need to look to social issues such as sexual myths and misinformation, covered extensively in the previous section, and interpersonal factors such as relationship failure and poor communication as causal factors in sexual dysfunctions. Current theory suggests that numerous social and interpersonal factors are likely to interact in contributing to sexual function problems (Sarason & Sarason, 1993). The distinction between primary and secondary Orgasmic Disorder can be a useful example in understanding this, and we see that primary Orgasmic Disorder is often the result of sexual guilt due to a strictly conservative sexual upbringing, for instance.

In the aetiology of Vaginismus, social and interpersonal factors may cause problems for an individual. These include socially learned sexual inhibitions or sexual aversion due to conflict or trauma, as well as guilt, which may be due to religious orthodoxy or negative parental attitudes to nudity, masturbation, or sex in general (Sarason & Sarason, 1993).

Script theory postulates that behaviours are demonstrated in accordance with scripts that reflect social and cultural expectations (McConaghy, 2005). Sexual guilt can play havoc with otherwise healthy people and their otherwise healthy sexual functioning. The origins of sexual guilt are numerous and often complex. Very often, such guilt is the result of religious or cultural upbringing which portrays sex in a negative light. Many anorgasmic women were brought up to feel that sex is inherently sinful and bad, that their genitals are dirty, and that masturbation is evil or perverted (McConaghy, 2005). A further, closely linked contributor is that women with negative attitudes towards sex typically feel that sexual fantasies are improper, and they actively fight off such fantasies when they occur. This creates an impediment to natural sexual arousal and release.

Deterioration in personal relationships and poor social skills may also play a role. Although tensions in relationships are quite normal and do not necessarily result in sexual dysfunction, it is striking that anorgasmia can be a sign of underlying relationship problems. Common problems are power struggles, poor communication and conflict resolution, dysfunction, it is striking that anorgasmia can be a sign of underlying relationship problems. Common problems are power struggles, poor communication and conflict resolution, gender-role conflicts, jealousies, or retribution for real or perceived injustices between partners. It is not difficult to see why physical or emotional abuse may prevent a person from relaxing sexually in order to orgasm. Even minor issues in a relationship, however, can create resentment or frustration that interferes with sexual enjoyment.

The aetiology of the paraphilias often includes learning and experience with others in an interpersonal setting. The development of unusual or inappropriate sexual arousal patterns may occur in the context of other sexual and social difficulties, although not all adults with sexual and social difficulties develop unusual or 'deviant' sexual patterns (McConaghy, 2005). Early experience and the nature of an individual's sexual fantasies appear to play a role. According to an operant conditioning paradigm, a learning process may occur (often in early childhood psychosexual development) in which a deviant sexual behaviour is reinforced through association with pleasure. An alternative theory is suggested by those who believe that 'unusual' sexual attraction patterns are acquired, often in later life, and are indicative of sexual sophistication, and not pathology (Baldwin, 1993; Moser, 1999).

There is no convincing evidence for any particular explanation for gender dysphoria (McConaghy, 2005). Researchers with a biological orientation provide explanations pointing to genes or sex hormone fluctuations in intrauterine development. Researchers with other orientations implicate social and interpersonal learning experiences. In developmental terms, the period between approximately 18 months and three years of age may be critical for gender identity development, and 'learning' of gender roles may furthermore be influenced by family experiences (McConaghy, 2005).

CONCLUSION

This chapter makes it apparent that there is a large degree of variability in the diagnostic features and presumed aetiologies of the sexual dysfunctions in men and women. As complaints tend to be highly co-morbid within an individual, and between partners in a couple, a comprehensive biopsychosocial assessment of both partners may be required for accurate diagnoses with the aim of effective treatment.

It is also important to bear in mind some of the challenges and concerns regarding the sexual disorders and gender dysphoria as raised by activists, academics, and researchers who in their work prioritise the needs and rights of females, sexual minorities, and the sexually diverse. The responsiveness of the compilers of the DSM (and seemingly also the ICD) to these issues, as is evident from current revisions that are underway, is to be welcomed.

MULTIPLE-CHOICE QUESTIONS

1. Gender Dysphoria is diagnosed when:
   a) a person's physical gender is inconsistent with the person's gender identity
   b) a person's physical gender is consistent with the person's gender identity
   c) an individual is born with ambiguous genitalia
   d) All of these are correct.

2. Paraphilia is defined as:
   a) a dysfunction
   b) an attraction to inappropriate individuals or objects
   c) an attraction to machines
   d) a desire that dominates the personality

3. The main feature of sexual arousal disorders is:
   a) lack of desire for sex despite normal physical sexual response
   b) sexual arousal to inappropriate stimuli
   c) the experience of pain during sex
   d) lack of physical sexual response despite desire for sex

PARAGRAPH AND ESSAY QUESTIONS

1. Describe the impact of culture on the definition of a sexual disorder. What cross-cultural evidence suggests that 'normal' sexual behaviour is culturally defined?

2. Describe the symptoms of three different forms of paraphilia. What do all paraphilias have in common?

3. Name three gender differences that exist in sexual attitudes and sexual behaviours.

10 SUBSTANCE-RELATED AND ADDICTIVE DISORDERS

Gale Ure

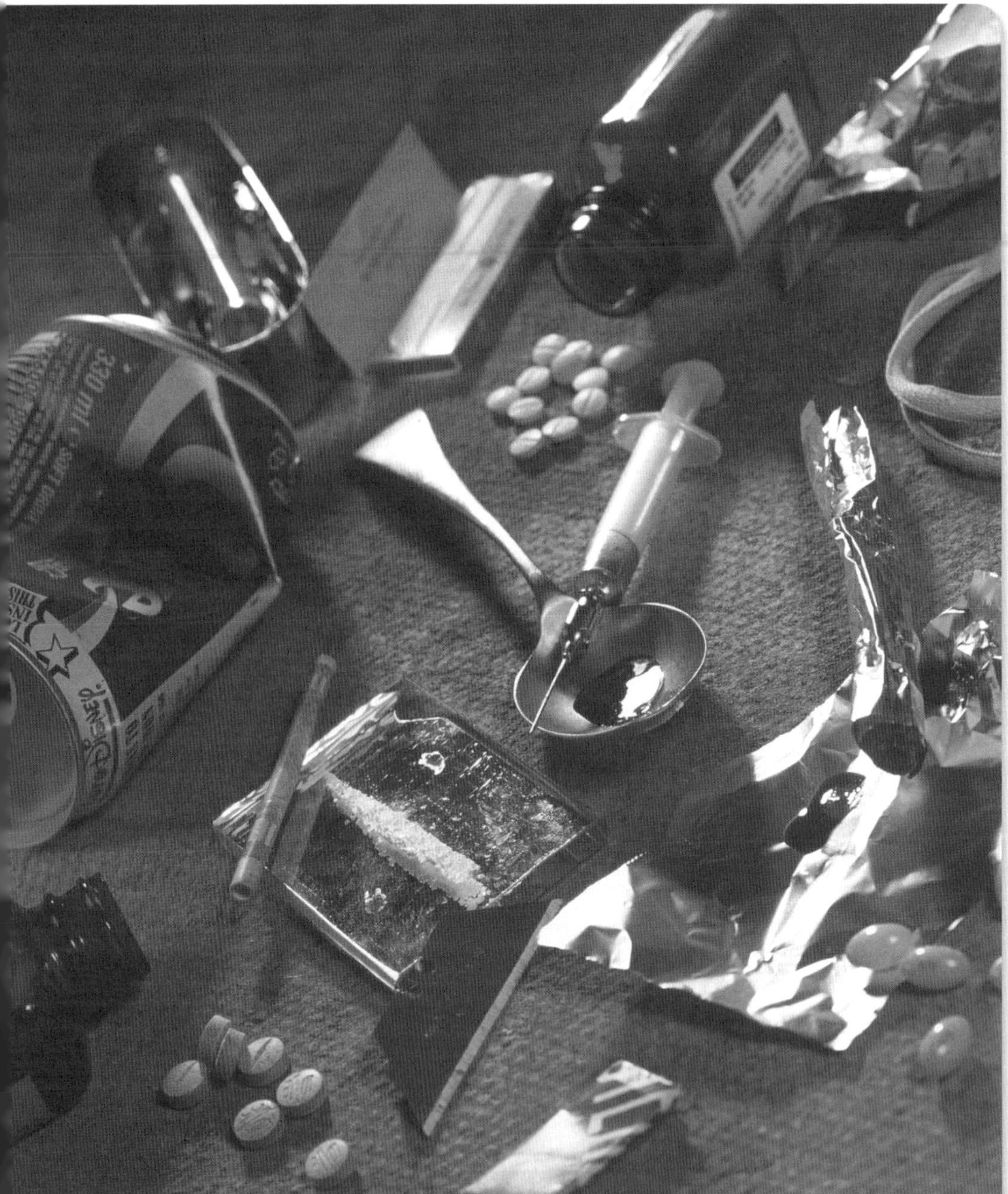

10 CHAPTER OUTLINE

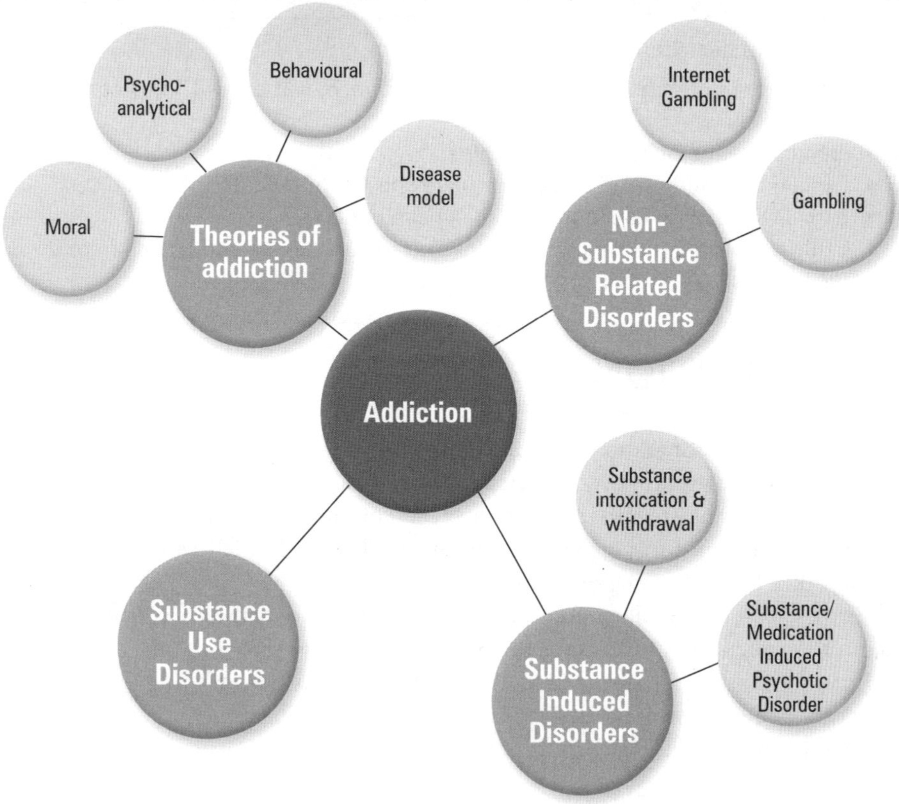

LEARNING OUTCOMES

At the end of this chapter you should be able to:

- Identify the difference between use, dependence, withdrawal, intoxication, and addiction.
- Identify groups of substances by type.
- Explain the aetiology of substance buse and the potential for addiction.
- Explain substance use in the South African context.
- Explain the similarities between addiction to substances and addiction to behaviours.

INTRODUCTION

When you think about addiction, what comes into your mind first – a picture of a drunk person weaving down the street or watching Tiger Woods baring his soul on Oprah about his 'disease', about his 'treatment' programme, and his hope for a 'full recovery' (Martinez, 2010)? This difference in perception of what an addict is has led us to a crossroads in the path that understanding addiction has taken through the ages. Public declarations of what used to be a hidden disorder take place with increasing frequency, and as a result, acceptance of previously unacceptable behaviour has become common. The public war against drugs shows us pictures of people who are unwitting drug smugglers being executed in some countries, while celebrity users of the same illegal substances are forgiven in public media.

Figure 10.1: The two faces of addiction

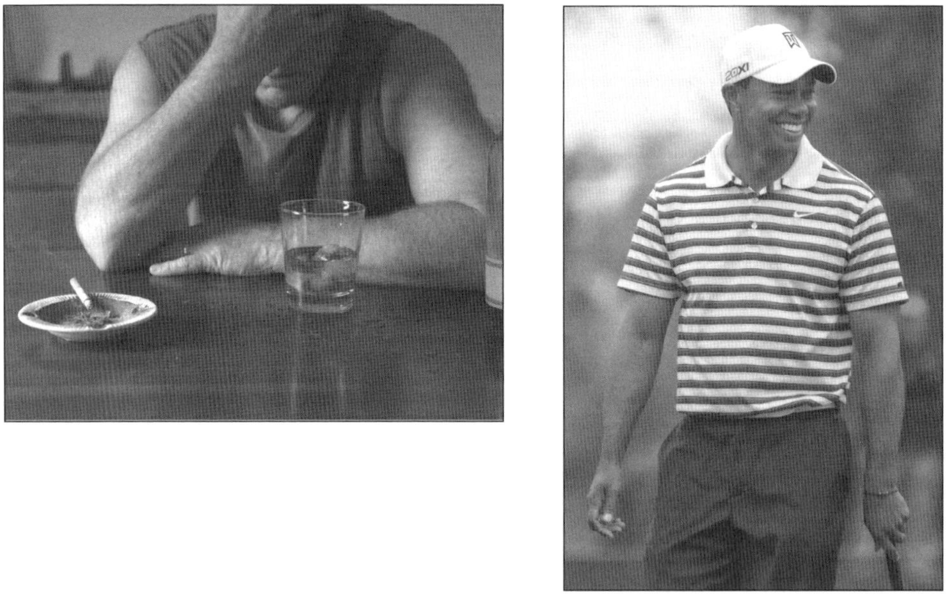

Substance use is often listed as a symptom under other disorders, for example, Antisocial Personality Disorder and Conduct Disorder. Other addictions which are of sufficient clinical concern presently fall under the DSM-5 and IDC-10 categories of impulse-control disorders, although, in light of the present thinking around addiction, this may change in the near future. These addictions include those involving food, the Internet, pathological gambling, and sex. Disorders categorised in the DSM-5 under Disruptive, Impulse-Control, and Conduct Disorders sometimes have components of addictive behaviour listed in the ICD-10 as, for example, kleptomania and pyromania (fire-starting), as well as some of the Eating Disorders (American Psychiatric Association, 2000; World Health Organisation, 2007).

Disorders of this nature have as their specific identifier the compulsive failure to control, or extreme difficulty in controlling, impulses, in spite of the negative consequences which may be attached to acting on these impulses. This can include the failure to stop gambling even if one realises that not doing so will result in a significant negative consequence, for example, that one's wife could leave. This failure to control impulses can also refer to the impulse to engage in violent or destructive behaviours (e.g. road rage, sexual behaviour, pyromania, stealing, and self-abusive behaviours) (Lemonick, 2007; World Health Organisation, 2007).

The most significant recent development in medical thinking around addiction is a press release adopted by the Board of the ASAM (American Society of Addiction Medicine, 2011) which formalises the following definition of addiction:

> *Addiction is a primary, chronic disease of brain reward, motivation, memory, and related circuitry. Dysfunction in these circuits leads to characteristic biological, psychological, social, and spiritual manifestations. This is reflected in an individual pathologically pursuing reward and/or relief by substance use and other behaviours.*
>
> *Addiction is characterised by inability to consistently abstain, impairment in behavioural control, craving, diminished recognition of significant problems with one's behaviours and interpersonal relationships, and a dysfunctional emotional response. Like other chronic diseases, addiction often involves cycles of relapse and remission. Without treatment or engagement in recovery activities, addiction is progressive and can result in disability or premature death.*

This definition does not necessarily provide a revolutionary definition of addiction but it does cement medicine's acceptance of addiction as a disease. It does this by noting the role of the brain in the aetiology and prognosis of the disease. It also attempts to consolidate previous psychological, behavioural, moral, and biological models under one umbrella interpretation. This formalisation of the definition appears to be in response to the difficulties which have surfaced in the development of the DSM-5, and which were the cause of a number of obstacles in interpretation of addiction (Robinson & Wilson, 2011). It is hoped that incorporation of all of the elements in a formal definition will provide a holistic picture of how to provide appropriate care and resources.

HISTORICAL PERSPECTIVE

Prior to 1914 and the implementation of the Harrison Act in the USA (Clausen, 1957; Reid & Sheeby, 1990), there was no formalised concept of addiction. Following this Act, the addiction concept was adopted in various guises across the Western world. Descriptions of addiction were linked to the social notion that behavioural excesses were related to morbid appetites, vices, or habits. With the introduction of various categories of diagnostic labelling, there were challenges around how to align the disease concept of addiction with psychological theories, cultural relevance, and social practices. A substantial amount of the literature from the late 1960s until well into the 1980s rejected outright the medical model of mental illness and the usefulness of hospitalisation and medication for addiction. Use of clinical diagnostic criteria was seen as medicalisation of violations of social norms rather than clinical symptoms (Levine & Troiden, 1988). Despite this, the medical/disease model has retained its popularity. A number of other conceptions which have gained in popularity over the years include the moral model, behavioural theories, psychological theories, and combinations of these.

As far as substances are concerned, historical references to substances of use and dependence have been made as far back as 3000 BCE. There is evidence of the first wine industry along the banks of the Nile. There are over 400 biblical references to wine, and also warnings against the excessive use of alcohol. In 1492, Christopher Columbus arrived in America to find Native Americans smoking tobacco. In the 1600s, marijuana was cultivated by the Jamestown Settlers who utilised the fibres to make ropes and clothing (Lemonick, 2007). Many of the sailors treated for mental illness in the Cape Colony in the early 1900s demonstrated symptoms of alcohol and substance use psychosis (Minde, 1974).

The acceptability of substance use, as well as the types of substances which have been declared substances of use, has changed over time. The use of alcohol was prohibited in the United States in the 1920s, for example, and both possession and use was punishable with a jail sentence (Dreyer, 2006). Also in the United States, LSD (lysergic acid diethylamide) was legally used in the 1960s as a mind-expanding substance in psychedelic psychotherapy. LSD was discovered accidentally in 1943 by Dr Albert Hofmann, a researcher at Sandoz Laboratories in Switzerland. During its heyday as a wonder drug, it was used for, amongst others, treating alcoholics (Hofmann, 1980). A community of 'hippies' lived in a Los Angeles suburb called Haight-Ashbury, many using LSD openly in what was effectively a social experiment in peaceful, stoned co-existence. It turned out to be an unsuccessful existence (Smith, 1969). Timothy Leary, a psychology professor at Harvard University in the 1960s, reported that the drug could not only alter behaviour, prevent criminal behaviours, and act as an aphrodisiac, but could also provide profoundly mystical experiences. He is famously quoted as saying: 'Turn on, tune in, and drop out'.

Tobacco use was acceptable and even fashionable until the health risks over time became obvious and costly. Governments in many countries have taken action to reduce tobacco use in their citizens. In the United States, many states have banned smoking in public places. For example, tobacco use in public was prohibited in Arizona as far back as 1973. Smoking has been banned in public places in South Africa for a number of years (Tobacco Products Control Act 1993; Tobacco Products Control Amendment Bill 2007). Both France and the United Kingdom implemented their legislation to ban smoking in all public places in January 2008.

CASE STUDY

TRADITIONAL BEER IN AN UNTRADITIONAL WORLD

In the apartheid years (from around the end of the 1940s to 1994), many black families lived below the poverty line. In order to supplement or provide the household income, many black women took to working in the informal sector, becoming prostitutes, laundry women, or beer brewers (SA History Online, 2009).

A traditional South African institution, the shebeen, also came into being to during the apartheid years. The lack of formal entertainment and amenities in South Africa townships gave birth to a colourful public drinking culture which remains today. The operation of shebeens was originally illegal, but is now legal. Shebeen queens manufactured and sold alcohol to patrons from their houses in the townships, along with cigarettes and stew. Musicians provided music to ensure relaxation at the end of the week. The shebeens catered to different classes and levels of clientele, with the better shebeens providing armchairs for a more relaxed social environment. Violence was not uncommon, with brawls, stabbings, and injuries occurring regularly. This shebeen culture was in reaction to prohibitions, firstly, on the drinking of alcohol by Africans, and secondly, on the prohibition of black people from possessing or selling liquor (Van Onselen, 1982).

Traditional beer (*utshwala* or *mqombothi*) was brewed in the rural districts. It was usually made from sprouted corn, maize meal, and water, which are all readily available and grown in the area for food. This beer's effect was mild as it had a low alcohol content. It was predominantly brewed for special occasions as it took a long time to brew. It formed the foundation of traditional community celebrations, for example, weddings and coming-of-age celebrations.

The towns had a different beer production profile. The beer was required as a social drink for use after the working week. This beer was made more quickly from ingredients which were purpose bought. The speed of brewing meant that there was less chance of beer being discovered in police raids during the apartheid era, and it also meant that if the beer was discovered and confiscated or destroyed, more could be brewed in time to meet customer demand. These 'concoctions' often had additions like methylated spirits – which is poisonous – to increase the intoxication potential. This beer formed the foundation of the suburban beer hall culture. This beer's effect was more intoxicating than that of rural beer. Its effects could sometimes be lethal (SA History Online, 2008).

Some other examples of home-brewed alcoholic drinks are (SA History Online, 2008):

- *Isiqataviki (isikilimiqiki)* was made from porridge, bread, sugar, and syrup. It got its name from its strength and its ability to intoxicate.
- *Isishimiyana (shimeya)* was made from yeast, sugar, syrup, and

potatoes. It was named after the gait which people exhibit when drunk.

- *Babaton* (buckshot or *Mbamba*) was made from malt, yeast, stale bread, and sugar. It got its name from the workers who worked on the Barberton gold mines in the late 1800s.
- *Gavine (tototo)* was a very strong drink, often containing additional dangerous ingredients such as car-battery acid.

The working of modern shebeen remains similar. These facilities are seldom regulated, and shebeen beer often contains additives which are added to increase the intoxication value. These additional substances, while certainly intoxicating, are usually poisonous and may cause blindness and death (SA History Online, 2008).

THEORIES OF ADDICTION

Moral theory

This model has its foundations in the social thinking that certain people either have deficits in their ability to take personal responsibility for their lives and/or they lack spiritual strength to deal with events in their lives. While this thinking may seem old-fashioned and quite blaming, many present-day spiritually based programmes rely on this maxim, including those of Alcoholics Anonymous and Narcotics Anonymous (Alcoholics Anonymous World Services, Inc, 2012; Narcotics Anonymous, Inc., 2012). A spiritual guide or religious teacher is required to assist the person back to the right moral path.

The judicial system takes a similar position. Substance use is not a justifiable defence for a crime and individuals are held accountable for their actions. This means that using substances – or not attempting to get help in controlling an addiction – is regarded as 'wilful misconduct' and requires law enforcement to punish offenders. Driving under the influence of alcohol is a crime, regardless of whether the person is diagnosed as an alcoholic or not, for example (Maatz, 2005; Reid & Sheeby, 1990). Correctional services intervention may be required to ensure that the person remains accountable and to impose punitive consequences, if considered necessary.

Psychoanalytic theories

Models of addiction based on individual character trait differences came into being after World War II and were grounded in psychoanalytic understandings of people. Psychoanalysis postulated that addiction was the result of a person's developmental stasis at a significant stage of their personality development. In the case of addiction, this has been regarded as being at the oral phase. This has been linked over time to sex-role conflicts, latent homosexuality, and low self-esteem (Meyer, Moore, & Viljoen, 1993; Reid & Sheeby, 1990), amongst others. Contemporary psychoanalytic theory views addiction as a result of an individual's attempts to reduce anxiety (Thombs, 2006). Use of substances and/or the continuous use of pornography, for example, are ways for the person to protect him- or herself against debilitating and painful emotions such as loneliness and depression. In this situation, intervention by a trained professional is required (Gumbiner, 2010).

Behavioural theories

In the past, the term addiction referred exclusively to the use of substances. Today, it has come to include any and all behaviours which are habitual. Addiction can also be described as compulsive participation in pleasurable behaviours which becomes pathological, for example, pathological gambling. Thus, addictions can be seen as persistent and repetitive behaviours in the face of negative consequences (National Institute on Drug Abuse, 2007). An addiction could be considered to be a persistent behaviour pattern characterised by:

- A powerful desire to continue the activity, which places it out of voluntary control.
- A tendency to increase the frequency, duration, or amount of the activity over time.
- A psychological or physical dependence on the gratification which is derived from participating in the activity.
- A potentially detrimental effect on both the individual and society. For example, if a person steals money from his or her family to sell and/or purchase drugs, the family may become economically deprived by the loss of funds, a sense of trust may be lost, etc.

The disease model

The American disease model has been in existence since 1935 (Reid & Sheeby, 1990) and has not changed substantially since then (see the Board of the American Society of Addiction Medicine definition in the Introduction to this chapter). The central assumption was that addiction is an irreversible, progressive condition typified by loss of control over substance use. It is not considered to be curable and can only be controlled with complete abstinence. Denial of substance addiction is a symptom of the disease often carried out in spite of observable collapse of the person's social and interpersonal structures. The liquor industry has been supportive of this model as it suggests that only *some* people will become alcoholics and the rest of the population is able to drink without long-term consequence. This model has resulted in more benevolent treatment of substance users, diversion from prison into rehabilitation facilities, and less rejection by the community.

TYPES OF ADDICTION

Typically, in the past, addiction to substances was thought of as being the only form of addiction. to The DSM-5 views addiction as extending beyond substances alone to include a wide array of other behaviours, both in the current classification (i.e. Gambling Disorder) as well as in the section that includes condition that require further study (i.e. Internet Gaming Disorder). The ICD-10, however, does not list or describe non-substance related addictions. The comparison between DSM-5 and ICD-10 disorders is represented in Table 10.1

Table 10.1: Summary of substance- and non-substance related disorders in DSM-5 and ICD-10

DSM-5		ICD-10
Category	Disorders	
Substance-Related Disorders	Alcohol	Mental and behavioural disorders due to use of alcohol

	Caffeine	*Note: ICD-10 lists this as a stimulant*
	Cannabis	Mental and behavioural disorders due to use of cannabinoids
	Hallucinogen	Mental and behavioural disorders due to use of hallucinogens
	Inhalant	Mental and behavioural disorders due to use of volatile solvents
	Opioid	Mental and behavioural disorders due to use of opioids
	Sedative, Hypnotic or Anxiolytic	Mental and behavioural disorders due to use of sedative hypnotics
	Stimulant	Mental and behavioural disorders due to use of other stimulants, *including caffeine* Mental and behavioural disorders due to use of cocaine
	Tobacco	Mental and behavioural disorders due to use of tobacco
	Other / Unknown	Mental and behavioural disorders due to multiple drug use and use of other psychoactive substances
Non-Substance Related	Gambling	No provision for behavioural addictions as an independent spectrum of mental disorders.
Conditions for Further Study	Caffeine use Disorder	
	Internet Gaming	

CLINICAL PICTURE

The description of this category of disorders has become complicated since the introduction of the DSM-5. This is due, in large, to the ongoing debates regarding the constructs that underlie these disorders, such dependence, addiction, use, abuse, etc. In the past only substance-related disorders were included in this category, whereas the DSM-5 also makes provision for non-substance related addictions. Furthermore, in the past the DSM made a distinction between *abuse* and *dependence,* whereas the DSM-5 does not make this distinction. Furthermore, the DSM-5 now describes the substance-related disorders in terms of use, intoxication and withdrawal, and the ICD-10 describes them in terms of acute intoxication, harmful use, dependence and withdrawal. The "addictive" component of substance-related disorders is subsumed in the diagnostic criteria where reference is made to "craving" or "a strong desire or urge to use a substance" (APA, 2013). A further way in which this is addressed is by means of severity specifiers (e.g. mild, moderate or severe).

This group of disorders can be divided into three categories, i.e. substance induced disorders, substance use disorders, and non-substance related disorders.

SECTION 1: SUBSTANCE-INDUCED DISORDERS

This section includes intoxication, withdrawal and other substance/medication induced disorders (e.g. psychotic, bipolar, depressive, anxiety, obsessive compulsive, sleep, and neurocognitive disorders as well as sexual dysfunctions and delirium) (APA, 2013).

Substance intoxication and withdrawal

In previous editions of the DSM, general criteria for intoxication and withdrawal were provided; however, due to the differences between these states for different substances, the DSM-5 has opted to include them within the substance specific sections. The ICD-10, however, still provides general criteria for these states. Due to practical constraints, only the general criteria for substance intoxication and withdrawal will be discussed.

Acute intoxication is the state which follows administration, ingestion, or exposure to a psychoactive substance. The administration results in changes and disturbances in consciousness, cognition, perception, mood, or behaviour. These cause maladaptive changes in behaviour or psychological states and responses which are of clinical significance. These can be, for example, belligerence, mood disturbance, cognitive impairment, impaired judgment, and impaired social or occupational functioning. These changes can be directly attributed to the immediate pharmacological effects of the substance and will resolve over time. These symptoms are reversible and differ between substances. There is usually a complete recovery, except in cases of long-term use, where there is residual damage, for example, to brain structure or where complications may have been caused. Consequences of Substance Intoxication may include delirium, coma, trauma, convulsions, and vomiting (American Psychiatric Association, 2000; World Health Organisation, 2007).

Table 10.4: Diagnostic criteria for Substance Intoxication as adapted from the ICD-10

ICD-10
• A transient condition following the administration of alcohol or other psychoactive substance, resulting in disturbances in level of consciousness, cognition, perception, affect, or behaviour, or other psychophysiological functions and responses. • This should be a main diagnosis only in cases where intoxication occurs without more persistent alcohol- or drug-related problems being concomitantly present. Where there are such problems, precedence should be given to diagnoses of harmful use, dependence syndrome, or psychotic disorder.

Source: Reprinted with permission from the ICD-10 Classification of Mental and Behavioural Disorders: Diagnostic Criteria for Research, World Health Organisation (WHO), Geneva, 2007.

After prolonged and persistent use of a substance, there might be an attendant group of symptoms which develop when the person either terminates the use of the substance completely, or when the drug is reduced. These symptoms may vary in intensity and severity. These symptoms are time limited, that is, they last for a specific period of time which is related to the type of substance and dosage being utilised immediately before the reduction or termination of use. These symptoms cause clinically significant distress or impairment in functioning. Convulsions and delirium are relatively common during cessation of use of a substance (American Psychiatric Association, 2000; World Health Organisation, 2007).

Table 10.5: Diagnostic criteria for Substance Withdrawal as adapted from the ICD-10

ICD-10
• A group of symptoms of variable clustering and severity occurring on absolute or relative withdrawal of a substance after repeated, and usually prolonged, and/or high-dose use of that substance. Onset and course of the withdrawal state are time limited and are related to the type of substance and the dose being used immediately before abstinence. The withdrawal state may be complicated by convulsions. • Withdrawal state is one of the indicators of dependence syndrome and this latter diagnosis should also be considered. • Withdrawal state should be coded as the main diagnosis if it is the reason for referral and sufficiently severe to require medical attention in its own right. • Physical symptoms vary according to the substance being used. Psychological disturbances (e.g. anxiety, depression, and sleep disorders) are also common features of withdrawal. Typically, the patient is likely to report that withdrawal symptoms are relieved by further substance use.

Source: Reprinted with permission from the ICD-10 Classification of Mental and Behavioural Disorders: Diagnostic Criteria for Research, World Health Organisation (WHO), Geneva, 2007.

Substance/Medication-induced Psychotic Disorder

Psychosis caused by substance use may also mimic some of the psychiatric disorders; for example, substance abuse psychosis can be confused with Schizophrenia. Substance use psychosis includes a group of symptoms which may occur following psychoactive substance use and which are not merely symptoms of intoxication produced by that substance. These symptoms also do not form part of a withdrawal state. Hallucinations are typically present and these, while most often auditory, can also be found in more than one sensory modality. There may be delusions (which are often paranoid), perceptual disturbances, psychomotor disturbances, and abnormal mood (World Health Organisation, 2007).

Table 10.6: Diagnostic criteria for Substance/Medication-Induced Mental Disorders (DSM-5) and Substance-Induced Psychotic Disorder (ICD-10)

DSM-5	ICD-10
A. The disorder represents a clinically significant symptomatic presentation of a relevant mental disorder. B. There is evidence from the history, physical examination, or laboratory findings of both of the following: (1) The disorder developed during of within one month of a substance intoxication or withdrawal or taking a medication; and (2) The involved substance/medication is capable of producing the mental disorder. C. The disorder is not better explained by an independent mental disorder (i.e. one that is not substance- or medication-induced). Such evidence of an independent mental disorder could include the following: (1) The disorder preceded the onset of severe intoxication or withdrawal or exposure to the medication, or (2) The full mental disorder persisted for a substantial period of time (e.g. at least one month) after the cessation of acute withdrawal or severe intoxication or taking the medication. This criterion does not apply to substance-induced neurocognitive disorders or hallucinogen persisting perception disorder, which persist beyond the cessation of acute intoxication or withdrawal. D. The disorder does not occur exclusively during the course of a delirium. E. The disorder causes clinically significant distress or impairment in social, occupational, or other important areas of functioning.	• A cluster of psychotic phenomena that occur during or immediately after psychoactive substance use and are characterised by vivid hallucinations (typically auditory, but often in more than one sensory modality), misidentifications, delusions and/or ideas of reference (often of a paranoid or persecutory nature), psychomotor disturbances (excitement or stupor), and an abnormal affect, which may range from intense fear to ecstasy. The sensorium is usually clear but some degree of clouding of consciousness, though not severe confusion, may be present. The disorder typically resolves at least partially within one month and fully within six months. • Psychoactive substance-induced psychotic disorders may present with varying patterns of symptoms. These variations will be influenced by the type of substance involved and the personality of the user. For stimulant drugs such as cocaine and amphetamines, drug-induced psychotic disorders are generally closely related to high dose levels and/or prolonged use of the substance. • A diagnosis of psychotic disorder should not be made merely on the basis of perceptual distortions or hallucinatory experiences when substances having primary hallucinogenic effects (e.g. lysergic acid diethylamide (LSD), mescaline, cannabis at high doses) have been taken. In such cases, and also for confusional states, a possible diagnosis of acute intoxication should be considered.

DSM-5	ICD-10
	• Particular care should also be taken to avoid mistakenly diagnosing a more serious condition (e.g. Schizophrenia) when a diagnosis of psychoactive substance-induced psychosis is appropriate. Many psychoactive substance-induced psychotic states are of short duration provided that no further amounts of the drug are taken (as in the case of amphetamine and cocaine psychoses). False diagnosis in such cases may have distressing and costly implications for the patient and for the health services.

Source: Reprinted with permission from the Diagnostic and Statistical Manual of Mental Disorders (DSM), Fifth Edition, American Psychiatric Association (APA), 2013 and ICD-10 Classification of Mental and Behavioural Disorders: Diagnostic Criteria for Research, World Health Organisation (WHO), Geneva, 2007.

SECTION 2: SUBSTANCE USE DISORDERS

The pattern of substance use in this disorder is maladaptive, leading to clinical impairment or distress as described below. These maladaptive patterns continue for a period of twelve months or more, and are demonstrated by one or more of the following:

- Ongoing use which results in a failure to meet important role obligations as required by home, work, or school. This can include being repeatedly absent from work or school, poor work performance, suspensions, expulsions from school, neglect of children or household, all of which are directly attributable to the substance use.
- Recurrent use of substances in places where this could be hazardous. This would include driving a car while under the influence or operating heavy machinery, for example.
- Legal problems that may arise because of substance use. These can include being arrested for disorderly conduct or for criminal behaviours, for example, petty theft due to substance use.
- Continued use of the substance, despite experiencing problems in interpersonal or vocational situations which are either caused, or made worse, by the use of substances. These problems may include arguments and physical fights with a spouse about consequences of intoxication (American Psychiatric Association, 2000).

Furthermore, substance use encompasses a group of behavioural, cognitive, and physiological phenomena which occur after a period of repetitive and prolonged substance use. It involves a difficulty in controlling the use of a substance and an associated desire to continue its use. There are a number of symptoms which would indicate dependence:

- 'Tolerance' describes the need for ever-increasing amounts of a substance to produce intoxication or the desired effect. Use of increased amounts of the substance can sometimes cause tolerance to levels that would be lethal to a non-user.
- 'Withdrawal' is the development of a substance-specific syndrome due to the termination of, or reduction in, substance use which has been heavy and prolonged. It is a maladaptive behavioural change which occurs in the blood and cells when use of a substance of dependence is terminated. These changes can be either physical or cognitive, or both, and are acute and unpleasant. Depending on the substance being removed, they can include convulsions, shaking, difficulty sleeping, and perceptual difficulties. Delirium, confusion, and hallucinations may also occur. In alcohol withdrawal, delirium tremens may occur. There is a time limit to the period of withdrawal, and this is related to the type and the amount of substance being used at the time of removal. The person is likely to resume using the substance to relieve or reduce the symptoms.
- 'Compulsive use' describes the pattern of taking the substance in larger amounts or over a longer period than was originally intended, for example, if a person decides to have one or two drinks when socialising but instead ends up drinking until they are intoxicated.
- There are often numerous and unsuccessful attempts to decrease or discontinue use. The person continues to express a desire to stop or cut down on the use of the substance.
- There is a time component, where the person's life is taken over by substance-related activities. There would be, for example, excessive time spent on:
  - Acquiring the substance
  - Using the substance
  - Recovering from its effects.
- A person may, for example, take leave from work on days when he or she has a hangover from excessive alcohol consumption the night before.
- The person's life begins to revolve around the use of the substance. There is a corresponding reduction in other activities of daily life, for example vocational activities, sport, and socialising.
- Psychological and physiological symptoms which can be directly attributed to use of the substance, for example depression, do not contribute to a desire or attempts to stop. This occurs even if the cause of the problem is directly related to substance use, for example, damage to organs due to alcohol use (American Psychiatric Association, 2000; World Health Organisation, 2007).

Table 10.5: Summary of general symptoms of substance use (DSM-5) and Substance Dependence (ICD-10

<table>
<tr><th colspan="2">DSM-5 (adapted from text)</th><th>ICD-10</th></tr>
<tr><th>Grouping</th><th>Criterion</th><th></th></tr>
<tr><td rowspan="2">Impaired control</td><td>Gradual increase of dosage over time than was initially intended</td><td>• A definite diagnosis of dependence should usually be made only if three or more of the following have been present together at some time during the previous year:
‣ A strong desire or sense of compulsion to take the substance.
‣ Difficulties in controlling substance-taking behaviour in terms of its onset, termination, or levels of use.
‣ A physiological withdrawal state when substance use has ceased or been reduced, as evidenced by: the characteristic withdrawal syndrome for the substance or use of the same (or a closely related) substance with the intention of relieving or avoiding withdrawal symptoms.
‣ Evidence of tolerance, such that increased doses of the psychoactive substances are required in order to achieve effects originally produced by lower doses (clear examples of this are found in alcohol- and opiate-dependent individuals who may take daily doses sufficient to incapacitate or kill intolerant users).
‣ Progressive neglect of alternative pleasures or interests because of psychoactive substance use; increased amount of time necessary to obtain or take the substance or to recover from its effects.
Persisting with substance use despite clear evidence of overtly harmful consequences, such as harm to the liver through excessive drinking, depressive mood states consequent to periods of heavy substance use, or drug-related impairment of cognitive functioning. Efforts should be made to determine that the user was actually, or could be expected to be, aware of the nature and extent of the harm.</td></tr>
<tr><td>Despite intention, the individual is unable to cut down or regulate use</td><td></td></tr>
</table>

Impaired control	Spends a a great deal of time obtaining the substance and recovering from the effects of use	
	In more serious cases all daily activities revolve around the substance	
	Craving, which is characterised by strong urges for the drug	
Social impairment	Use results in inability in fulfilling obligations at school, work or home	
	Continues use despite it causing interpersonal problems, or interpersonal problems are worsened by use	
	Reduced, or withdrawal from, social, occupational or recreational activities	
Risky use	Recurrent use in situations which are physically hazardous	
	Use despite of knowledge of recurrent physical or psychological problems caused or worsened by the substance	
Pharma-cological	Tolerance: Increased dosage to achieve effects that were previously achieved by lower dosages	
	Withdrawal: Adverse symptoms when substance is not consumed, and which only disappear when substance is taken	

Source: Reprinted with permission from the Diagnostic and Statistical Manual of Mental Disorders (DSM), Fifth Edition, American Psychiatric Association (APA), 2013 and ICD-10 Classification of Mental and Behavioural Disorders: Diagnostic Criteria for Research, World Health Organisation (WHO), Geneva, 2007.

SECTION 3: NON-SUBSTANCE-RELATED DISORDERS

In addition to the substance-related disorders, the DSM-5 also considers other forms of addiction, such as Gambling Disorder (APA, 2013). During the development of the DSM-5 excessive behavioural patterns, such as Internet Gaming Disorder, sex, exercise and shopping addiction were also considered for inclusion; however, due to a lack of scientific evidence, these disorders were not included. Internet Gaming Disorder was however included in the section for disorders that need further investigation. The reason for considering the behavioural addictions is due to evidence that suggests that certain repetitive behaviours activate the reward systems similar to those activated by drugs, and that the resulting behaviours are comparable to those produced by substance use disorders (APA, 2013).

Gambling Disorder

For most people, gambling is a form of recreation, but for some, gambling becomes an addiction with far-reaching personal and social consequences. Compulsive gambling affects people from all cultures, ethnicities, ages, genders, and socio-economic groups. A definition of compulsive gambling would be:

> *A progressive condition characterised by increasing preoccupation with gambling, a need to bet increasing amounts of money with increasing frequency. Restlessness and mood changes when the person attempts to stop gambling. 'Chasing' losses – or trying to make up for money lost by gambling more in an attempt to win to cover these. The person experiences a general inability to stop gambling even when the person is confronted by serious negative consequences. (Compulsive Gambling, 2012)*

South Africa has a well-developed research entity run by the Casino Association of South Africa, which monitors the gambling behaviours in the national context. Findings of this group demonstrate that only 12% of the gambling population use regulated gambling institutions, while 19% gamble in informal venues. The gambling population is also analysed according to socio-economic status: more people in low to middle socio-economic groups choose to gamble in informal venues. Informal gambling is linked to problem gambling on a larger scale than formal gambling (Casino Association of South Africa, 2011).

Table 10.6: DSM-5 criteria for Gambling Disorder

DSM-5 Gambling Disorder
A. Persistent and recurrent problematic gambling behaviour leading to clinically significant impairment or distress, as indicated by the individual exhibiting four (or more) of the following in a 12-month period: (1) Needs to gamble with increasing amounts of money in order to achieve the desired excitement. (2) Is restless or irritable when attempting to cut down or stop gambling. (3) Has made repeated unsuccessful efforts to control, cut back, or stop gambling.

(4) Is often preoccupied with gambling (e.g. having persistent thoughts of reliving past gambling experiences, handicapping or planning the next venture, thinking of ways to get money with which to gamble).
(5) Often gambles when feeling distressed (e.g. helpless, guilty, anxious, depressed).
(6) After losign money gambling, often returns another day to get even ('chasing' one's losses).
(7) Lies to conceal the extent of involvement with gambling.
(8) Has jeopardised or lost a significant relationship, job, or educational or career opportunity because of gambling.
(9) Relies on other to provide money to relieve desperate financial situations caused by gambling.

B. The gambling behaviour is not better explained by a manic episode.

Source: Reprinted with permission from the Diagnostic and Statistical Manual of Mental Disorders (DSM), Fifth Edition, American Psychiatric Association (APA), 2013

The symptoms, as described in Table 10.6 usually has an onset during adolescence or early adulthood, but may have a first onset during later adulthood (APA, 2013). Typically the disorder has a slow onset that gradually increases over time (interestingly more rapidly in women than men) and the gambling patterns may either be regular or episodic (APA, 2013). An interesting phenomena is that most individuals with this disorder report one or two types of gambling, however, some individuals participate in a wide range of gambling activities. There is some evidence of a genetic component in this disorder as supported by the fact that it is more frequent in monozygotic than dizygotic twins and first degree relatives. It also has a high comorbidity with antisocial personality disorder, depressive and bipolar disorders, and other substance use disorders (APA, 2013).

Internet Gaming Disorder

Internet addicts display similar brain changes to those seen in substance users and other impulse-control disorders. This is one of the findings of a series of MRI scans done by a group of Chinese researchers on 35 participants (Briggs, 2012). The scans indicated that there was a disruption to white matter connections in the orbital frontal cortex, the same areas as those involved in substance se (Fowler, Volkow, Kassed, & Chang, 2007). These white matter connections are the bridge between regions of the brain involved in generating emotion, executive functioning (e.g. sustaining attention), cognition, self-control, and decision-making. Comparable similarities have been found in video game addicts.

CROSS-CULTURAL AND SOUTH AFRICAN PERSPECTIVES

The Alcohol and Drug Abuse Research Unit of the Medical Research Council in Cape Town maintains ongoing research into trends of substance use in South Africa. The SACENDU (South African Community Epidemiology Network on Drug Use) project monitors the use, changes in consumption patterns, and general developments in alcohol and other drug usage. The system operates in the centres of Cape Town, Durban, Port Elizabeth, East London, Mpumalanga, and

Gauteng, which includes Johannesburg and Pretoria. The project has been operational since 1996 and provides updated information every six months. The information is acquired from numerous sources, including mortuaries, hospitals, specialist substance treatment facilities, and police forensic services. The data is then analysed and distributed to interested parties and organisations. Community studies are included when available (SACENDU, 2006).

Alcohol

South Africa's relationship with alcohol is complex, and is linked to both the political and socio-economic history of the country. It has a specific historical significance in South Africa which pre-dates the implementation of formal apartheid. From the late 1800s, alcohol imported from Mozambique and bottled in Pretoria was one of the most important sources of income for the burgeoning population of the Transvaal. This population provided hospitality services for the influx of miners drawn to the province by the promise of gold and instant wealth (Van Onselen, 1982).

In the Cape wine regions, the workers on the wine-producing farms were provided with alcohol instead of wages. This is still called the 'dop system'. As recently as 1998, some farms in the area still provided their workers with alcohol as part of their conditions of service (Te Water Naude, 1998). This practice is illegal, as it promotes the excessive and ongoing use of alcohol as a functional norm. Extremely high numbers of children and adults with Foetal Alcohol Syndrome (FAS) are found in many of the small communities in the Cape as a long-term result of this practice.

Alcohol use has a number of significant consequences:

- Alcohol continues to be a significant cause of death in South Africa. Figures from 2003 show that in Cape Town, Durban, Gauteng, and Port Elizabeth, 45% of all people who died unnatural deaths had blood alcohol concentrations greater than or equal to 0.05g/100ml (the legal limit for driving). Levels of alcohol were particularly high for transport-related deaths and homicides, with 63% of transport-related deaths and 69% of homicides in Port Elizabeth, for example, having levels above 0.05g/100ml (Medical Research Council, 2006).
- Trauma unit statistics from the Medical Research Council in 2001 show that in Cape Town, Durban, and Port Elizabeth, 39% of trauma patients had breath alcohol concentrations greater than or equal to 0.05g/100ml. Levels of alcohol were particularly high for transport- and violence-related injuries with, for example, 73% of patients with violence-related injuries in Port Elizabeth and 46% of patients with transport-related injuries in Cape Town having levels above the legal limit for driving (Medical Research Council, 2006).
- FAS is of increasing concern in South Africa. In research conducted in the Western Cape, the prevalence of FAS among Grade 1 learners was found to be 4.6% in 1997 and 7.5% in 1999. Comparable research carried out in Gauteng and De Aar in 2001, and Upington in 2003, found FAS frequency rates of 1.9%, 10.3%, and 7.5% (estimate) respectively (Medical Research Council, 2006).
- Alcohol use is linked to high-risk behaviours, which often involve impaired judgment and can lead to exposure to life-threatening situations. Risky sex, for example, may lead to exposure to HIV and unwanted pregnancy. In 2003, the Medical Research Council research conducted in Atteridgeville among people aged 25–44 years found a significant positive association between various measures of alcohol use (past month use, frequency, and problem use) and having multiple sexual partners or sexual relations in the past three

months that are regretted (Medical Research Council, 2006).

- There are correlations between alcohol use and family violence, according to Medical Research Council findings in 2000. Between one-third and a half of arrestees in Cape Town, Durban, and Johannesburg charged with offences categorised as 'family violence' reported being under the influence of alcohol at the time of the alleged offence.
- Academic failure and absenteeism: Among Grade 8 and Grade 11 learners in Cape Town, a significant association was found between past month use of alcohol, the number of days absent from school, and repeating a grade. For example, the odds of repeating a grade at school were found to be 60% higher for learners who consumed alcohol (Medical Research Council, 2006).

Tik (methamphetamine)

Described by many as the world's most dangerous drug, methamphetamine ('meth') was developed by the Japanese over a hundred years ago. At the time, it did not have a clear use. However, with the advent of the Second World War, troops on both sides used the drug to overcome the effects of reduced sleep and limited food so that they could keep fighting. Kamikaze pilots are reputed to have used the substance to maintain their courage and motivation to perform their famous suicide missions. Sixty years later, Asia still has more than 60% of the world's meth users (Castro, 2006).

Meth is illegal, but in economies which put a high premium on the amount of work done, the drug is not utilised for recreational purposes. Instead, it is used by working people to give an energy boost which increases the amount of work that can be done and the speed at which it can be done, so that they can get ahead in an increasingly competitive environment. Workers can earn more money if they can work more shifts. It is such a feature of Thai work culture that employers often hand out meth to their employees to increase and maintain production. However, after a number of public and violent meth-fuelled hostage dramas in which ordinary people were negatively affected after ongoing cycles of too much meth and too little sleep, the government of Thailand took extreme action to stamp out meth use. Government operatives were involved in killing 2000 dealers and users in just three months. However, they were not successful in cutting the use to any noticeable degree (Castro, 2006).

Meth is an 'upper', which means that initially, users feel euphoric, confident, and energetic when they use the drug. As described above, meth was designed to deceive the brain into keeping awake, stop eating, and promote feelings of bravery. These feelings of well-being are produced by dopamine, a neurotransmitter produced in the brain. Initial use of the drug produces up to two-thirds more dopamine than the body produces naturally. However, with sustained use, tolerance is built up. This tolerance forces the body to seek more and more of the drug to achieve the feelings of well-being which were experienced at the first use of the drug. Eventually, the body stops producing dopamine altogether, which plunges the user into depression. The body's ability to restore its dopamine production systems may be impaired or permanently damaged by ongoing use of meth.

Methamphetamine is an inexpensive drug, and is three-and-a-half times more powerful than cocaine. The duration of the high is from six to twelve hours, compared to the half-an-hour to three hours of some other substances like cocaine. It can be made in a normal domestic kitchen. It is used by people of all ages in all communities. It is also more common in rural environments which are not commonly associated with substance use, although use is spreading rapidly to major centres around the world. It was estimated that in 2006, 26 million people globally were using the drug. In American jails, one in four inmates tests positive for meth on arrest (Castro, 2006).

'Meth mouth' is an identifying feature of long-time meth users. The users suffer from tooth loss due to decay. The decay is caused by meth's capacity to impede the flow of saliva in the mouth. Meth addicts commonly do not keep themselves adequately hydrated, and this causes natural acids and bacteria to build up around the base of the teeth, eating away at the gums and the enamel of the teeth. Poor hygiene, and a corresponding lack of oral care, exacerbates the problem. The money which could be spent on attending to dental problems is spent on acquiring the drug. Users also report a 'crawling' sensation on their skin, which they often pick at until they cause lesions, producing a distinctive bleeding and scarred facial picture of the addiction (Castro, 2006).

Table 10.7: Primary substances of use by race January to June 2010

Centre	Alcohol	Cannabis	Cannabis/ mandrax	Crack/ cocaine	Ecstasy	Heroin	Metham-phetamine
WESTERN CAPE							
Black	24%	17%	14%	7%	0%	3%	5%
Coloured	48%	73%	83%	28%	40%	82%	87%
Asian/Indian	<1%	<1%	0%	2%	0%	1%	<1%
White	27%	10%	3%	64%	60%	15%	8%
GAUTENG							
Black	41%	71%	67%	24%	29%	54%	31%
Coloured	8%	15%	17%	16%	43%	3%	31%
Asian/Indian	3%	2%	3%	7%	0%	3%	3%
White	49%	12%	14%	53%	29%	39%	34%
EASTERN CAPE							
Black	31%	38%	31%	7%	0%	4%	4%
Coloured	31%	47%	65%	30%	50%	7%	68%
Asian/Indian	2%	1%	2%	7%	0%	7%	2%
White	36%	14%	3%	55%	50%	82%	27%
KWAZULU-NATAL							
Black	56%	66%	95%	11%	50%	50%	67%
Coloured	9%	10%	5%	19%	50%	11%	33%
Asian/Indian	16%	15%	0%	36%	0%	30%	0%
White	18%	9%	0%	33%	0%	8%	0%
NORTHERN REGION							
Black	54%	81%	50%	12%	0%	66%	-
Coloured	19%	4%	0%	27%	0%	3%	-
Asian/Indian	0%	<1%	0%	4%	0%	2%	-
White	32%	16%	50%	58%	0%	30%	-
CENTRAL REGION							
Black	50%	63%	25%	14%	-	22%	-
Coloured	19%	18%	42%	14%	-	0%	50%
Asian/Indian	0%	0%	33%	0%	-	0%	-
White	32%	19%	0%	73%	-	78%	50%

Source: South African Community Epidemiology Network on Drug (SACENDU), 2010.

As suggested above, there are racial and provincial differences in the substances chosen by users in South Africa at present. These are often along the lines of historically black, white, and coloured area divisions which go back to the apartheid years. These traditional areas maintain social structures which either promote substance use, or reject it on community and cultural grounds. Different racial groups show a propensity for different drugs, often depending on the economic and social circumstances of the geographic area. It will be of interest for researchers to compare these usage trends in the next 10 to 20 years to discover if the blurring of historical social, geographic, and economic lines correlates with a similar blurring in substance use trends.

AETIOLOGY

Despite wide coverage in the media and many psychoeducational programmes, substance use and addiction continue to be psychosocial problems. Internationally, governments have tried to curb smoking in public, and in many countries cigarette advertising has been banned. The use and distribution of many substances have been outlawed in many countries. Furthermore, many people are aware of the negative effects of short- and long-term use of substances; however, none of this seems to prevent people from starting or continuing the use of substances. In order to understand this, we have to take a closer look at the causes of substance use, as this may offer some explanation as to why preventive strategies have been largely unsuccessful.

Substance use is problematic because it poses many health problems and it is seen as a challenge across many areas of social and community life. This means that treatment needs to include many varied aspects, some not necessarily directly to related to health care, but which might be required to assist the person recover. An example would be vocational training, amongst others.

As suggested earlier, there has been much discussion around what could cause substance use and addiction, and whether the causes indicate or affect what treatment should be used. In the past, there have been two prominent theories: the first is that substance use is an illness and needs to be medically treated, and the second is that it is a habit and needs willpower to be cured.

Biological factors

Genetic predisposition

There is a growing body of evidence that genetic factors play a significant role in both substance dependence and substance use. Scientists believe that these may influence as much as 40% to 60% of a person's predisposition to addiction (American Society of Addiction Medicine, 2011). While there is no obvious Mendelian gene transmission, it would not be unreasonable to assume that addictions may be polygenic (determined or influenced by many genes), which would certainly increase the possibility of addiction heritability (Goldman, Orozi, & Ducci, 2006).

According to gene studies, addictions are moderately to highly hereditable. A person's risk is mediated by the degree of relationship to an addicted relative (Bevilacqua & Goldman, 2009). This means that if an immediate family member has an addiction to a substance, the children will be significantly more prone to addictive behaviour.

People with a predisposition to a mental disorder also appear to run a significantly higher risk of substance use and addiction than the broader populace. This is possibly because of the attendant lack of insight which is symptomatic of a number of psychiatric disorders like Schizophrenia, for example (National Institute on Drug Abuse, 2007).

The influence of environmental and social factors which interact with this biological inheritance will affect how much these genetic factors will be expressed in a person's life. Nurture factors, for example, parenting and life experiences, will affect the person's resilience, and will have a direct influence on whether or how these indications of addiction will appear. Resilience (Akst, 2011; Wallace, 1999) and cultural factors will also play a role in how addiction manifests in people with a genetic susceptibility (Rodgers, 2011) (see Chapters 2 and 3). Environmental and genetic variables combine to trigger, firstly, the initial use of an addictive agent, and secondly, to press the transition from use to addiction.

Brain structures

The structures of the brain affected by addiction are those generally associated with reward. These structures, which include the nucleus accumbens, anterior cingulate cortex, basal forebrain, and amygdala, are all part of the motivational hierarchy and which are modified by the addiction. Overarousal of these areas, which reward our normal behaviours, produces the euphoric results which are constantly being sought by people who use substances. This cycle teaches them to repeat the behaviour. Other biological variances may have an effect on addictions. Stress has been shown to increase the desire for drugs. Hormones also play a role in addictions. Research has shown, for example, that some women crave nicotine more during certain phases of their menstrual cycle (National Institute on Drug Abuse [NIDA], 2007).

Brain imaging studies have been valuable in identifying neurobiological effects of substance addiction. They have also been useful in providing explanations for vulnerability and have been able to provide insight into users' struggles with recovery and their subjective experiences.

Figure 10.2: Major brain regions with roles in addiction

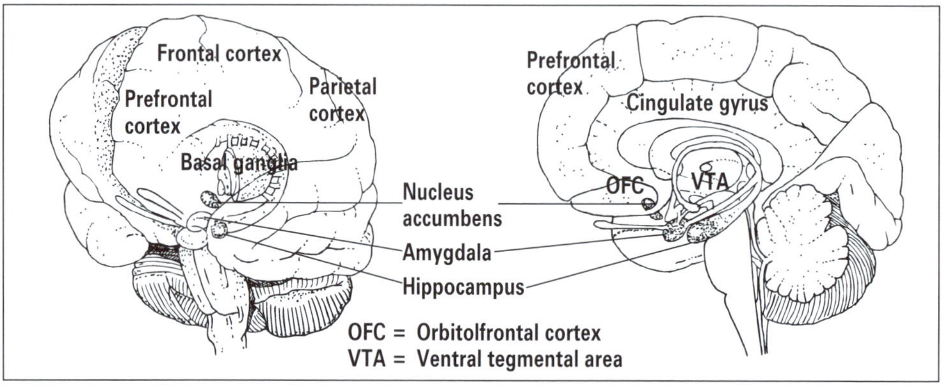

The prefrontal cortex is the focal area for cognition and planning. The ventral tegmental area (VTA) and nucleus accumbens (NAc) are key components of the brain's reward system. The VTA, NAc, amygdala, and hippocampus are major components of the limbic system, which coordinates and drives, emotions, and memories.

Source: Fowler et al., 2007.

Neurotransmission and interconnection between the hippocampal and cortical systems, which are brain reward structures, are also affected by addiction. When there has been a previous experience of reward, be it food, sex, alcohol, or other substances, these structures will trigger cravings for the substance, and the subsequent participation in addictive behaviours (Fowler, Volkow, Kassed, & Chang, 2007).

Long-term use of substances may disturb the way important brain structures cooperate to influence behaviour particularly that which is linked to the substance use. In particular, ongoing use may lead to tolerance of a substance. Tolerance to a drug means that the user will need to take more and more of the substance to recreate the original dopamine high (National Institute on Drug Abuse, 2007). Thus, increased dosages are required to produce the same intoxication effect. In turn, brain changes might lead to addiction – or the need to seek out substances and to take them compulsively. Addiction removes a person's ability to maintain control over their own behaviour. It also reduces their ability to make appropriate decisions, while at the same time it produces intense pressure to take the substance.

The neurobiological component of addiction goes far beyond being simply the neurochemistry of reward (see next section). Altered impulse control, impaired judgement, and the pathological quest for rewards are all the result of dysfunction of memory, motivation, and reward functions of the white matter connections between the frontal cortex and reward circuits. The ability to delay gratification and control impulsivity is housed in the frontal lobes. Early-life exposure of the frontal lobe, connective tissue, and functioning to substance use while these structures are maturing plays a significant role in the development of addiction.

Neurotransmitters

The rewards produced by substances are often more pleasurable than those produced naturally. When some substances are used, this can lead to the release of two to ten times the quantity of dopamine than a natural reward. If the substance is inhaled during smoking, or injected straight into a vein, the resulting high is also virtually immediate and the effects can be sustained for extended periods, unlike those of many natural rewards which produce pleasure like eating and sex. The brain remembers this pleasure, as the extreme nature of the high leaves an enduring memory of the experience. This memory drives the person to seek the same pleasure over and over, and this compulsion is effectively addiction (National Institute on Drug Abuse, 2007).

The brain operates using chemicals, and, as substances are chemicals, they work along with the brain's neurotransmitters to disrupt normal functioning. The chemical make-up of some substances, for example marijuana and heroin, closely resembles that of neurotransmitters naturally found in the brain. This allows these substances to initiate neurotransmitter activity. However, these triggers are not the same as normal activation, and the neurons then convey aberrant information to various brain centres (National Institute on Drug Abuse, 2007).

This close resemblance in structure tricks the receptors and permits the substance to attach to and activate the nerve cells 'under false pretences'. Deviant messages are then sent via the neural network. Methamphetamine and cocaine are two substances which trigger the neurons to release excessive quantities of naturally produced neurotransmitters, or which alter the usual re-uptake process which manages these chemicals. This interference can lead to vastly amplified neural messages. These messages then disturb the usual communication pathways. The magnitude of the altered effect is comparable to the difference between having someone sit in the dark with candlelight and someone sitting in a room with a halogen searchlight (National Institute on Drug Abuse, 2007).

Dopamine

All substances which are used either directly or indirectly home in on the brain's reward system by flooding the circuit with dopamine. Dopamine is a neurotransmitter found in the areas of the brain which control movement, emotion, cognition, motivation, and feelings of pleasure.

The brain responds to these floods of dopamine by adjusting its natural production of the chemical, either by producing less or by shutting down the number of receptors which are involved in the reception or transmission of this information. The production of natural dopamine is reduced and the supply becomes depleted, thus reducing the person's own ability to feel pleasure without the drug. Users often become anhedonic or emotionally 'flat' and unable to enjoy what they would have found pleasant before. Use of the substance is therefore maintained simply to elevate their dopamine levels to normal.

There are a number of physical effects which can be experienced when substances are used continuously and, usually, in the long term. The same processes which are involved in producing tolerance to a substance can cause structural changes which in turn alter brain function. These changes may lead to irreversible damage and deterioration in the long term. Glutamate, a neurotransmitter also found in the brain, aids in the process of learning and is also affected by changes to the reward system. When the amount of glutamate in the brain is changed by the use of substances, attempts by the brain to counterbalance the changes can lead to impairment of cognitive processes (National Institute on Drug Abuse, 2007).

Ongoing use can also lead to changes in habits or subconscious memory systems, for example conditioning. This type of learning, during which contextual triggers are associated with the pleasurable substance experience, can lead to cravings. These cravings are then activated when the person is exposed to the triggers, even if the substance is not always associated directly with them. This learned response is long lived, and can re-surface after long periods of abstinence (National Institute on Drug Abuse, 2007).

Psychological and social factors

A basic human desire is to feel good. Substances of use produce overwhelming feelings of pleasure and well-being. Once this euphoria has died away, however, it is usually followed by other, often negative, effects. These may vary from substance to substance. Cocaine, a stimulant, is one such example. The initial 'high' is accompanied by feelings of power, increased self-confidence, and improved energy levels. In a different drug cluster, the results may be radically different. The exhilaration caused by an opiate, for example heroin, is usually followed by the sensation of calm. Clearly, it would not make sense to become addicted to a substance which initially produces unpleasant effects (National Institute on Drug Abuse, 2007).

Secondly, people may want to make themselves feel less anxious or more capable in circumstances they believe are difficult. People who are shy and nervous in social situations may use substances to give them courage and to reduce their social anxiety. In addition, stress has been identified as a key factor in initiating substance use, maintaining substance use, and causing relapse in people attempting to rehabilitate from addiction. Those who suffer from stress and related disorders, and those who suffer from depressive illness, may begin abusing substances to reduce their general feelings of being unable to cope (National Institute on Drug Abuse, 2007).

Thirdly, people may want to improve their performance in work, social, sexual, or sporting spheres. The increasing demands that are put on individuals to achieve in all spheres of human life may create a need in some people to utilise substances just to keep up with the rest of the human race. In addition, they may use these to augment or increase their sporting or mental performance beyond their natural talent. This pressure to perform above one's capacity can play a role both in initiating experimentation with substances and in maintaining substance use behaviour (National Institute on Drug Abuse, 2007).

Curiosity and peer pressure add a fourth, social, dimension. Adolescents and young people are particularly susceptible to the significant effects of peer pressure and media exposure. This exposure tells people that they should not be anything other than thin (hence the use of chemical appetite suppressants), 'cool' (add the use of alcohol and/or drugs when socialising), and fashionable (smoking was seen as being very sophisticated right up to the 1980s). These behaviours are driven by the person's own need to fit in with others of the same age and social groups. These people are more prone to participate in dangerous and risk-taking behaviours when they are with others, for example, speeding while driving a vehicle, or having unprotected sex with strangers while intoxicated (National Institute on Drug Abuse, 2007).

Many people experiment to see what effect substances will have on them, and they do this with little coercion. When substance use becomes the sole focus of a person's life, however, it reduces a person's capacity for containing their desires and exercising self-control. Because there are physical changes to the brain in individuals addicted to substances (see previous section), their ability to make appropriate judgments and decisions may be impaired. Studies also show that this damage results in the reduction in the ability to learn and remember, and in the ability to control and moderate behaviour. These changes are believed to modify the way the brain functions in the long term and may go a long way towards explaining the apparently irrational, obsessive, and detrimental patterns of behaviour which are seen in addiction (National Institute on Drug Abuse, 2007).

However, not all substance use, or even ongoing use, can be diagnosed as pathological or clinically significant. This means that not all people using a substance will require professional assistance to reduce usage or terminate usage of the substance. These people may show little or no visible interference or alteration in their level of functioning. Thus, even if the person uses the substance regularly, it does not reduce their ability to work, to bring up a family, or to behave appropriately in social interactions. For example, many people drink heavily on weekends, or utilise sleeping pills to sleep, sometimes for their whole lives, or smoke dagga (marijuana) every day but they appear to experience no marked side effects. Other useful examples are smoking and drinking coffee, both of which are considered substances of use (National Institute on Drug Abuse, 2007), but neither of which is considered to impact on normal daily functioning. Long-term health disruption and the harm done, if any, may become clinically significant only once physical consequences like emphysema or cancer occur.

Social and environmental factors can have a compounding effect on the likelihood of substance use. A lack of parental supervision which provides appropriate discipline and structure, and contact with friends or social situations where drugs are freely available and in open use may desensitise one to the potential harm of substance use. Early aggressive behaviours and poor social skills may also predispose a person to future substance problems. Conversely, people who exhibit personal self-control, who have positive relationships with their families, and who are academically competent are less likely to turn to substances. Attending schools with firm anti-substance policies and monitoring processes may also prevent early exposure to substance use.

Substance use is a significant community problem because it has an observable impact on the social environment. A substantial amount of research in the United States has linked substance use to crime (National Institute on Drug Abuse, 2007), loss of ability to work, harm to self and others while under the influence of alcohol, and loss of inhibitions, which might lead to indiscriminate sexual practices (Strong, Bancroft, Carnes, Davis, & Kennedy, 2005), or to self-harm behaviours (Roy, 2001). Communities with high levels of poverty and which may be marginalised from participating in community structures pose more risk to their members than those with strong neighbourhood connections and inclusion.

CONCLUSION

Countries, societies, and cultures differ in their attitude to substance use. Some view it as a personal choice to be tolerated and regulated (e.g. in Holland, where marijuana can be acquired and smoked in some licensed and controlled establishments), whereas others view it as a potentially harmful habit which not only threatens the mental and physical health of the individual, but also the broader social system.

Use of 'gateway' drugs like marijuana is believed to lead to hard drug use and addiction, and yet court cases take place where people fight for their rights to use marijuana in religious ceremonies or as an individual freedom – something which the Constitution of South Africa upholds. Use of alcohol is not illegal, and yet the news media highlight how many accidents and deaths are caused by people who were under the influence of alcohol.

Criminal behaviour is associated with the use of substances, either directly or indirectly, and this has a significant economic impact. Based on this, many countries try to eradicate the production and sale of substances in order to reduce their use and thus reduce accidents, crime, health care costs, and loss of productivity. The costs of these attempts are vast. Suppliers and dealers spend as much (if not more) on providing these substances as governments spend on trying to stop them (DeGrandpre, 2006). Poverty is often perceived to be a catalyst both for substance use and for the accompanying supply and distribution of substances in areas where poverty is rife (DeGrandpre, 2006; London, 1999; Rogerson, 1986; Van Onselen, 1982).

Substance use is implicated in around 50% of diagnoses of mental disorders. The general population of the United States demonstrated the following in terms of substance use: 15% of the population will qualify for a diagnosis of alcohol dependence in their lifetimes, 80% to 85% of adults consume at least 200mg of caffeine every day, and 42% of all college students had used cannabis at some time during their attendance at college (American Psychiatric Association, 2000).

The social questions which arise around substance use are usually those around the individual's personal responsibility for their behaviour and the state's regulation of what is available to the individual by way of recreational drugs. The laws in place making it illegal to use these substances do not allow South Africans freedom to choose, which is a foundational principle of the South African constitution (see Chapter 14). If we have the right to autonomy, and the right to security in and control over our bodies, what we put into them should be our personal choice. If our choice to use substances has repercussions which impact on our families and the broader social sphere, is that not also our responsibility? If the long-term use may cause harm, should we be permitted to use the substance simply because we choose to? Who takes responsibility for when we suffer the harm and perhaps need long-term care? Do we perhaps have a responsibility to choose *not* to take substances because of the impact on our communities and families?

There are many discussions which can arise out of the social context of substance use and these will continue for as long as there are a bigger high and an easier thrill to be had. What we should bear in mind at the end of this chapter is that there is a very human story behind each incidence of substance use or addiction.

MULTIPLE-CHOICE QUESTIONS

1. In terms of substance-related disorders, the word *addiction* is most closely associated with:
   a) substance use
   b) intoxication
   c) substance dependence
   d) polysubstance abuse

2. Consequences of long-term excessive drinking include:
   a) liver disease and/or pancreatitis
   b) cardiovascular disorders
   c) brain damage
   d) all of these

3. Foetal Alcohol Syndrome (FAS) is a combination of problems that can occur in a child whose mother drank alcohol while pregnant. Symptoms of FAS include all of the following EXCEPT:
   a) cognitive deficits and behaviour problems
   b) distorted facial features
   c) learning difficulties
   d) excessive foetal growth

PARAGRAPH AND ESSAY QUESTIONS

1. What four reasons are given to explain why people use substances?

2. Describe the general effects of each of the following:
   a) Cannabinoids
   b) Opiates
   c) Benzodiazepines
   d) Stimulants
   e) Hallucinogens

3. Name six negative results of alcohol use in South Africa today.

4. List three harmful effects which substance abuse can have on others

5. Name and describe three forms of therapy used to treat addiction.

6. Describe the three phases of rehabilitation which would benefit from the addition of medication to the treatment protocol.

7. Name and describe the five areas of functioning which need to be addressed in a comprehensive treatment programme.

8. Name the brain structures which are involved in the process of addiction.

9. List four behaviours which are commonly associated with addiction.

10. Describe how MRI, MRS, PET, and SPECT scans contribute to our knowledge of the brain's function in relation to addiction.

11 EATING AND FEEDING DISORDERS

Elsabe Jordaan

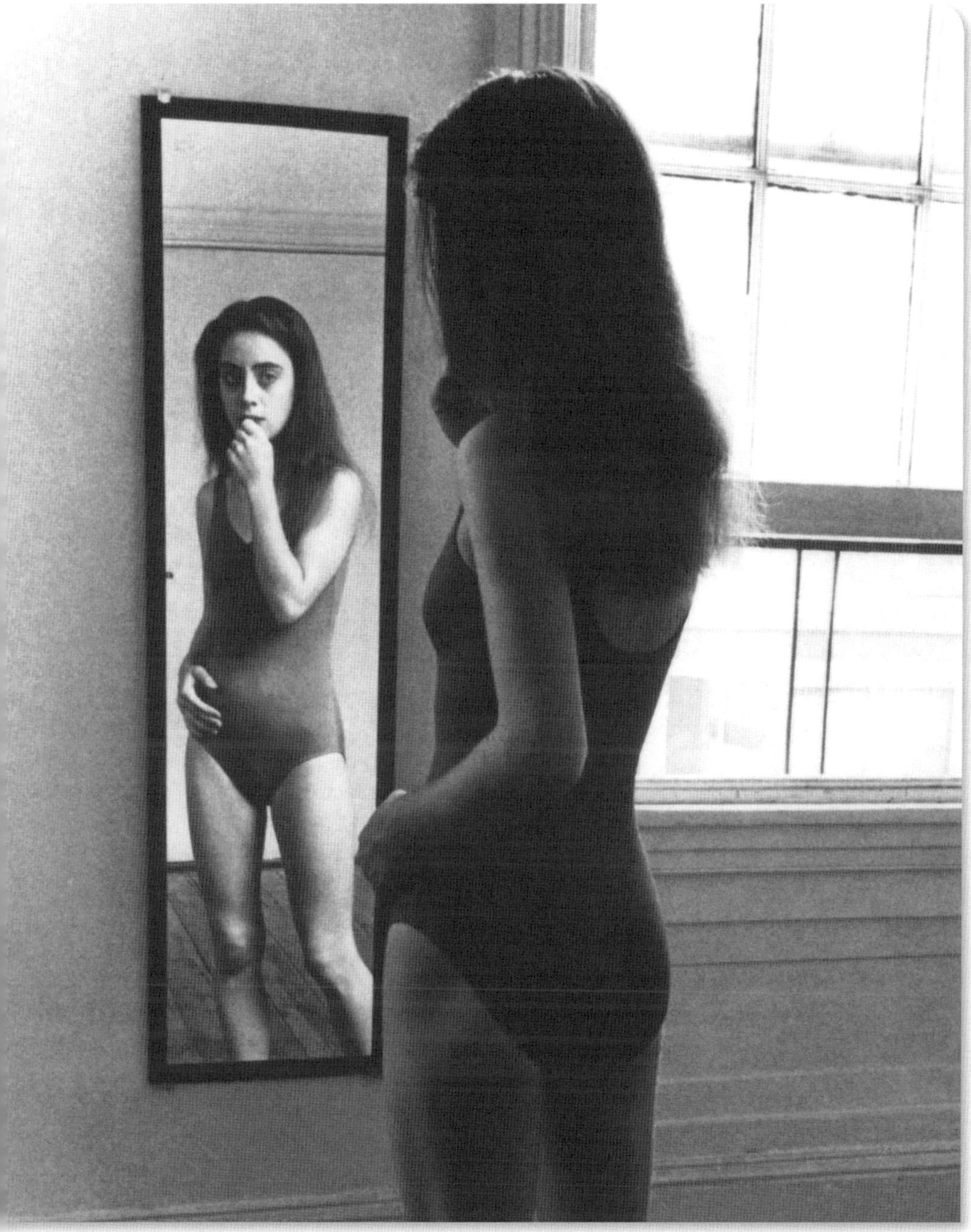

11 CHAPTER OUTLINE

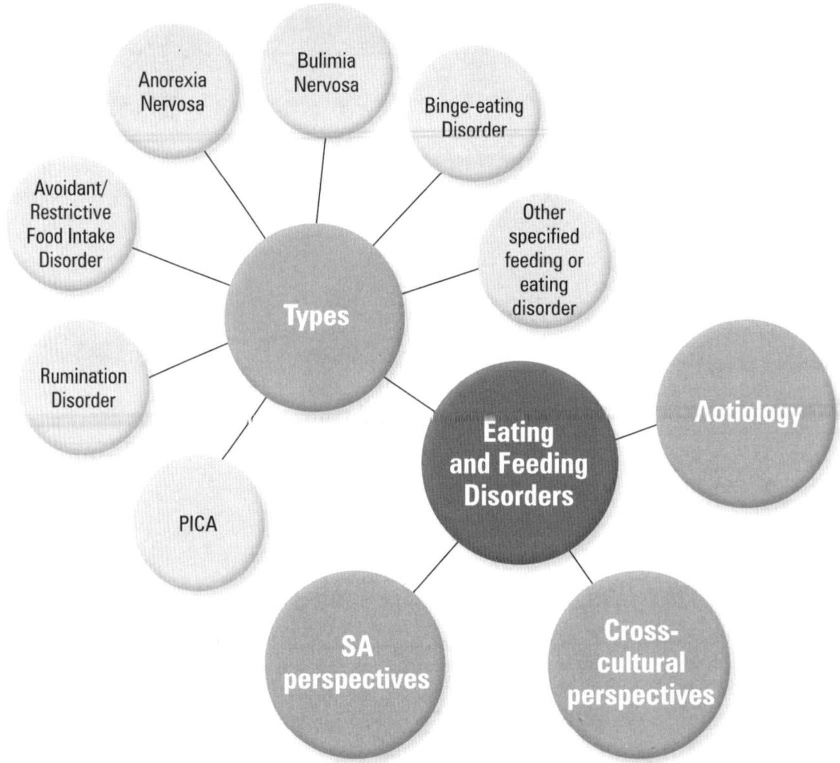

Introduction

History of eating disorders

Types of Feeding and Eating disorders

PICA

Rumination Disorder

Avoidant/Restrictive food intake disorder

Anorexia Nervosa

Prevalence and course

Specific cultural, gender, and age features

Clinical picture

Anorexia Nervosa subtypes

Bulimia Nervosa

Prevalence and course

Specific cultural, gender, and age features

Clinical picture

Binge-eating disorder

Other specified feeding or eating Disorder

Aetiology

Biological factors

Genetic factors

Neurobiological factors

Psychological factors

Developmental factors

Psychological theories

Personality factors

Role of the family context

Child abuse

Sociocultural factors

Sociocultural ideals for physical beauty

Gender and the eating disorders

Cross-cultural perspectives

South African perspective

Conclusion

LEARNING OUTCOMES

After studying this chapter you should be able to:

- Show a general understanding of Feeding and Eating Disorders and distinguish them from each other.
- Distinguish between Anorexia Nervosa subtypes.
- Describe the intrapersonal aspects of the aetiology of the eating disorders.
- Describe the role of cultural and gender features in the aetiology of the eating disorders.
- Identify cross-cultural, more specifically South African, aspects that are relevant to the prevalence of eating disorders.

INTRODUCTION

The discussion in this chapter will focus on one of the aspects of human physiology that is a basic requirement for our survival (and well-being), namely, eating. This is something that most of us take for granted, but for some, eating can become disordered.

Extreme disruptions in eating behaviour characterise the eating disorders. The DSM-5 has expanded on this section from previous editions by including Pica, Rumination Disorder and Avoidance/Restrictive Food Intake Disorder in addition to the more traditional eating disorders, i.e. Anorexia Nervosa and Bulimia Nervosa (American Psychiatric Association, 2013). Anorexia Nervosa can be described as 'a refusal to maintain a minimally normal body weight' (American Psychiatric Association, 2000, p. 583). Bulimia Nervosa comprises recurrent episodes of binge-eating, together with compensatory behaviours that can be regarded as inappropriate. Examples of compensatory behaviours are the use of laxatives to purge and excessive exercise. In both Anorexia and Bulimia, the person's experience and perception of their own body weight and shape appear to be disturbed. Both these disorders are associated with an extreme drive to be thin.

The changes of the eating disorders diagnostic category in the DSM-5, from the DSM-IV-TR, include changing the name of this category to 'Feeding and Eating Disorders'. This change reflects the inclusion of the Feeding Disorders (Disorders Usually First Diagnosed in Infancy, Childhood, or Adolescence, in DSM-IV-TR terms).

Obesity, after much contemplation and debate, was not included in the DSM-5, since it has not been linked to a consistent psychological or behavioural syndrome. Simple obesity is included as a general medical condition in the *International Classification of Diseases* (ICD-10) (American Psychiatric Association, 2000).

Binge-Eating Disorder was not formally included in the DSM-IV-TR, but is now included in the DSM-5. This disorder is characterised by excessive eating in a hort period of time, and people with this disorder report a sense of lack of control during an episode (APA, 2013).

Although Anorexia Nervosa has been described in Western culture since the eleventh century, it appears that both Anorexia Nervosa and Bulimia Nervosa have shown dramatic increases in Western countries in the past 60 years (Hay & Hall, 1991; Lacey, 1992). Similarly, in the South African context, an increase in the prevalence of eating disorders has been noted, particularly among sections of the population that espouse Western values (Szabo, 1998).

Another defining aspect of Anorexia and Bulimia Nervosa is that these disorders are mostly highly population specific. Initially, these disorders appeared to be almost exclusive to young females and almost exclusive to Western groups (or groups that have assimilated Western values). People from a higher socio-economic class were also thought to be more at risk; however, recent prevalence data suggests that these trends may be changing (Kaplan, Saddock, & Grebb, 1994). Data that includes the entire age span puts the gender ratio at between 1:29 and 1:10 of male to female, but small-scale studies of clinical populations of children suggest that as many as 19%–30% are boys (Wenar & Kerig, 2006).

Figure 11.1: Eating disorder types and subtypes

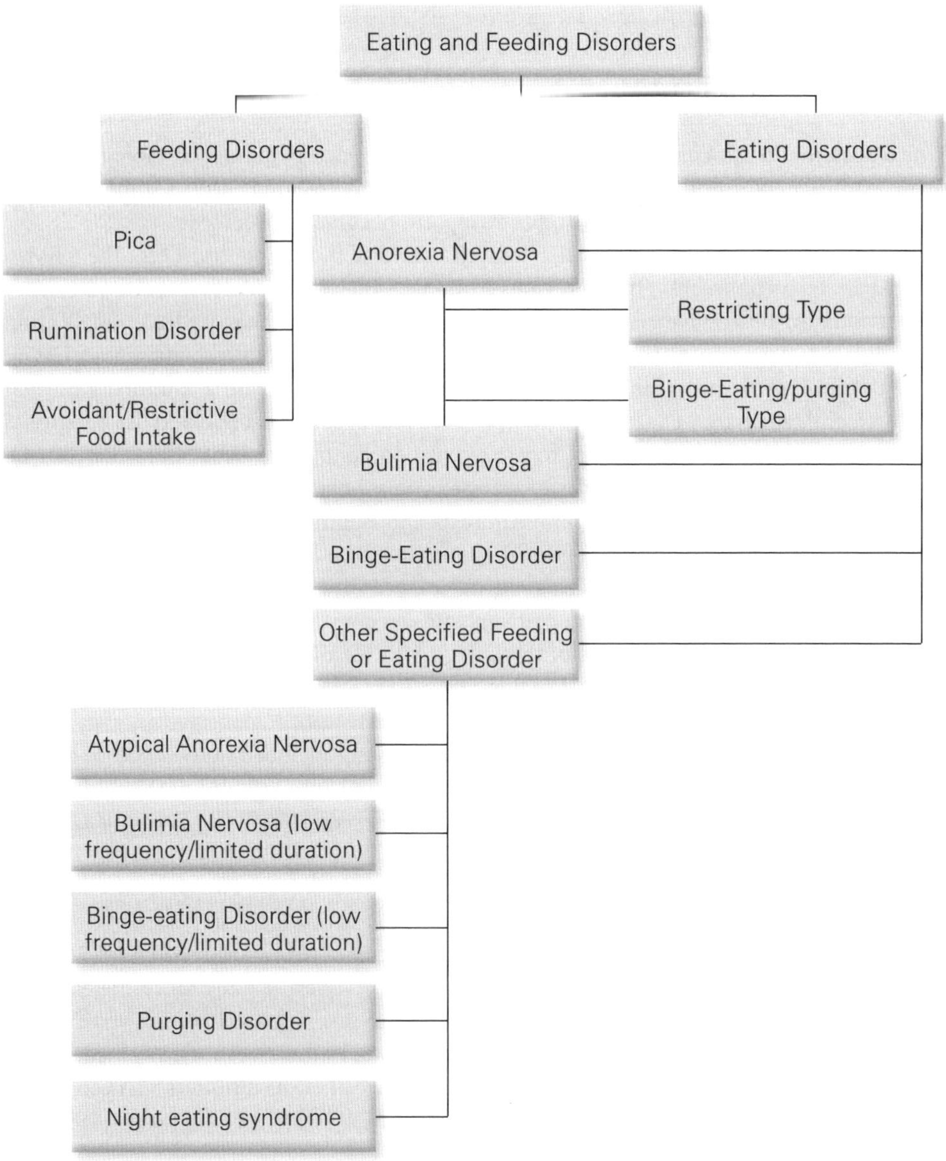

The assumption that the eating disorders are exclusive to Western groups is also not supported by recent data (Lake, Staiger, & Glowinski, 2000). Some studies have also failed to support the association between social class and the eating disorders (Wenar & Kerig, 2006). Nevertheless, these disorders seem to have a very strong sociocultural aetiological component. It appears then that disorders of eating are increasing in both Western society and in South Africa.

The eating disorders and obesity have significant impact on human life and well-being. The mortality rate for Anorexia Nervosa is the highest of all the psychological disorders. A woman with Anorexia Nervosa is twelve times more likely to die than a woman of the same age in the general population without Anorexia Nervosa (Miller & Golden, 2010). The mortality rates for Anorexia Nervosa are between 5% and 18%, while obesity is associated with increased morbidity and mortality (Kaplan et al., 1994; Schwartz & Brownell, 2007).

HISTORY OF EATING DISORDERS

In the Middle Ages (as early as 1242), the actions of fasting female saints were well documented. These could well be the earliest known examples of Anorexia Nervosa. Examples include Princess Margaret of Hungary, who is described as outstanding in all her studies, in her duties in the convent, and as always being industrious. She died at the age of 28 years, her body being described as 'wasted'. Catherine of Sienna is described as using a reed to induce vomiting, also for religious reasons. These two examples may represent Anorexia Nervosa, Restricting Type and Anorexia Nervosa, Purging Type, respectively (Halmi, 2000). The restricted eating of the female saints was for religious reasons, and not for the sake of appearance, as is the case of current eating disorders. However, an argument can be made that the girls and women diagnosed with eating disorders in our time are dieting for the sake of the 'religion of appearance', which is prevalent in current Western society (Halmi, 2000).

The first case descriptions of self-starvation are documented in the second half of the seventeenth century. An 18-year-old English girl by the name of Martha Taylor was described by John Reynolds. She refused all solid food, had stopped menstruating, and became emaciated. Reynolds wrote at that time that most young women who fell into this state were between 14 and 20 years of age, implying that the condition was known even then. At about the same time, Richard Morton described two cases with symptoms typical of Anorexia, and distinguished them from consumptive disease (tuberculosis) (Halmi, 2000).

In France, in the nineteenth century, Dr Louis-Victor Marce described cases of 'young girls' who carried their refusal to eat to 'the utmost limits' (Halmi, 2000). In 1873, two papers were published virtually simultaneously by Sir William Gull and Ernest Charles Laseque, discussing the description and treatment of 'hysterical anorexia'. Although this period saw little publication of cases describing 'fasting women' in the United States, two neurologists did describe cases of extreme self-starvation. Common usage of the term 'Anorexia Nervosa' arose after the publication of Gull's work (Halmi, 2000).

In the early twentieth century, pituitary insufficiency and Anorexia Nervosa were confused with one another. The pituitary gland and the hypothalamus are brain areas involved in the control of eating behaviour. Destruction of these areas results in emaciation and starvation (Kaplan et al., 1994). However, endocrine studies, together with the clinical histories and psychological descriptions of Anorexia Nervosa, showed pituitary insufficiency and Anorexia Nervosa to be different disorders (Halmi, 2000).

By the 1950s, Bruch described the central psychological aspect of Anorexia Nervosa as a sense of inadequacy that pervades the person's behaviour and cognition. She also described methods for intervening in the cognitive processes of these patients, creating a foundation for cognitive therapy with this disorder (Halmi, 2000).

Bulimia Nervosa was first described as a distinct syndrome in 1979 by Gerald Russell (Halmi, 2000). Bulimia Nervosa was first recognised as a disorder in the DSM-III in 1980 (American Psychiatric Association, 1980). Historical accounts exist of self-induced vomiting in ancient Egypt, Greece, Rome, and Arabia. In Ancient Egypt, purging was a medical practice. Roman and other practices were driven by hedonism. Thus, wealthy Romans would overeat at banquets, and then practice self-induced vomiting. These practices were clearly not driven by a fear of gaining weight, thus distinguishing them from Bulimia Nervosa (Miller & Pumariega, 2001).

TYPES OF FEEDING AND EATING DISORDERS

In this section we will be exploring all the disorders that are characterised by a persistent disturbance of eating, or eating-related behaviours, that impacts physical health and/or psychosocial functioning.

PICA

This disorder typically has a childhood onset, but may occur during childhood, adolescence or adulthood. The essential feature of the disorder is the eating of one or more non-nutritional or non-food substances (e.g. soil, paper, chalk, etc.). Typically there is no aversion to normal or healthy food and the non-nutritional substances that are eaten must be developmentally and culturally inappropriate (APA, 2013). One would not diagnose this disorder before the age of 2 years, as children before this age often eat non-food substances as part of their exploration of their world. This disorder is often associated with other mental disorders such as intellectual disabilities, autism spectrum disorders or schizophrenia (APA, 2013).

Rumination Disorder

This disorder may occur at any stage of human development, but the onset is usually between the ages of 3 and 12 months. It is characterised by the repeated regurgitation of food after feeding or eating which is characterised by previously digested or swallowed food being brought up into the mouth. This occurs in the absence of nausea, retching or disgust, and is not due to any identifiable medical reason. Although the disorder frequently remits spontaneously it may, in severe cases result in medical emergencies and may even be fatal, especially during infancy (APA, 2013).

Avoidant/Restrictive food intake Disorder

This disorder usually develops in infancy or early childhood and may, or may not, persist into adulthood. The main diagnostic feature is the avoidance, or restriction, of food intake to such an extent that healthy nutritional requirements are not met (APA, 2013). The key features of this disorder include (APA, 2013, p. 334):

- Significant weight loss
- Significant nutritional deficiency
- Dependence on enteral feeding or nutritional supplements
- Marked interference with psychosocial functioning

The symptoms of this disorder occur in the absence of any clear medical reasons, cultural practices or excessive concern about body weight. It seems as if in many cases the restriction may be based on the characteristics of food such as appearance, colour, smell, texture or taste. Given the fact that the restriction may be due to the sensory characteristics of food, it should not come as a surprise that it is often associated with disorders where heightened sensory sensitivities, such as in the case of autism, is a characteristic (APA, 2013). The DSM-5 (APA, 2013, p.335) suggests that the food restriction may be due to different reasons during different developmental stages, i.e.:

- Young infants: Too sleepy, agitated or distressed
- Infancy and young childhood: May not engage with caregiver or be distracted by other activities
- Older children and adolescents: General emotional problems.

Anorexia Nervosa

Prevalence and course

The DSM-5 describes the prevalence of Anorexia Nervosa as about 0.4% among females, while the prevalence among males appears to be in the vicinity of one-tenth of that in females (American Psychiatric Association, 2013).

A variety of sources indicate that the incidence of Anorexia Nervosa has increased in recent times (Critser, 2003). Studies from different Western countries reiterate this trend, including Switzerland, where a four-fold increase over a period of 30 years was found. In Scotland, a six-fold increase over 30 years was noted. Various studies were done in the United States with similar findings of increased incidence (Halmi, 2000; Jones, Fox, Babigan, & Hutton, 1980; Lucas, Beard, O'Fallon, & Kurlan, 1991; Willi & Grossman, 1983). In addition, it also appears that partial eating disorders (individuals who do not meet the full criteria for Anorexia Nervosa) occur in even greater frequency (between 5% and 10% of the young female population) (American Psychiatric Association, 2000; Halmi, 2000).

The onset of Anorexia Nervosa is usually between 14 and 18 years of age. Onset may be associated with a life stressor. A poor prognosis and greater disturbance appears to be associated with onset earlier than adolescence (American Psychiatric Association, 2000). Onset after 40 years of age appears to be rare. In terms of course and outcome, a high degree of variability appears to characterise Anorexia Nervosa. Some individuals make a full recovery subsequent to one episode; others exhibit a pattern of weight gain and relapse, while the course appears to be chronic and deteriorating over many years for a third group.

The eating disorders are notable for the great deal of diagnostic overlap that occurs between categories of disorder. One group of people initially diagnosed with the Restricting Type of Anorexia, will probably shift to a Binge-Eating/Purging subtype presentation within five years of diagnosis, and may eventually have a diagnosis of Bulimia Nervosa (American Psychiatric Association, 2000). Miller & Golden (2010) estimate that 30% of patients with a diagnosis of Anorexia Nervosa on intake will cross over to Bulimia Nervosa, but are also likely to relapse into Anorexia Nervosa. A smaller group (about 14%) is likely to cross over from an intake diagnosis of Bulimia Nervosa to Anorexia Nervosa. While the DSM-5 rates long-term mortality associated with Anorexia Nervosa as about 5%, due to starvation, electrolyte imbalance, or suicide, some studies indicate that this figure may be as high as 20% (American Psychiatric Association, 2013; Eisler, Szmuhter, & Russell, 1991). Suicide accounts for up to half of these mortalities (Agras, 1987).

Specific cultural, gender, and age features

The eating disorders are arguably the group of disorders where age, culture, and gender features come together in the most obviously significant way. The occurrence of Anorexia Nervosa is almost exclusively in females (approximately 90%). It is most prevalent in countries that are industrialised and where thinness is associated with attractiveness. In addition, the disorder increases in prevalence in immigrant groups where ideals of thinness are adopted from their new context (American Psychiatric Association, 2000). It appears that recent immigrants are at a greater risk for developing an eating disorder (Van Den Broucke & Vandereycken, 1986).

Clinical picture

The term 'Anorexia Nervosa' means 'nervous loss of appetite'. It is distinguished by three core criteria, namely: (1) behaviour aimed at achieving significant weight loss; (2) a great fear of becoming fat; and (3) disturbance in perception of body shape or size. An additional feature is evidence of cessation of menstruation in females past puberty (American Psychiatric Association, 2000; Halmi, 2000).

Table 11.1: Diagnostic criteria for Anorexia Nervosa as adapted from the DSM-5 and ICD-10

DSM-5	ICD-10
A. Restriction of energy intake relative to requirements, leading to a significantly low body weight in context of age, sex, developmental trajectory, and physical health. Significantly low weight is defined as weight that is less than minimally normal or, for children and adolescents, less than that minimally expected.	• For a definite diagnosis, all the following are required: ▸ Body weight is maintained at least 15% below that expected (either lost or never achieved), or Quetelet's body-mass index is 17.5 or less. Prepubertal patients may show failure to make the expected weight gain during the period of growth. ▸ The weight loss is self-induced by avoidance of 'fattening foods' and one or more of the following: self-induced vomiting; self-induced purging; excessive exercise; use of appetite suppressants and/or diuretics.

DSM-5	ICD-10
B. Intense fear of gaining weight or of becoming fat, or persistent behaviour that interferes with weight gain, even though at a significantly low weight. C. Disturbance in the way in which one's body weight or shape is experienced, undue influence of body weight or shape on self-evaluation, or persistent lack of recognition of the seriousness of the current low body weight.	▸ There is body-image distortion in the form of a specific psychopathology whereby a dread of fatness persists as an intrusive, over-valued idea and the patient imposes a low weight threshold on himself or herself. ▸ A widespread endocrine disorder involving the hypothalamic-pituitary-gonadal axis is manifest in women as amenorrhoea and in men as a loss of sexual interest and potency. (An apparent exception is the persistence of vaginal bleeds in anorexic women who are receiving replacement hormonal therapy, most commonly taken as a contraceptive pill.) There may also be elevated levels of growth hormone, raised levels of cortisol, changes in the peripheral metabolism of the thyroid hormone, and abnormalities of insulin secretion. ▸ If onset is prepubertal, the sequence of pubertal events is delayed or even arrested (growth ceases; in girls the breasts do not develop and there is a primary amenorrhoea; in boys the genitals remain juvenile). With recovery, puberty is often completed normally, but the menarche is late.

Source: Reprinted with permission from the Diagnostic and Statistical Manual of Mental Disorders (DSM), Fifth Edition, American Psychiatric Association (APA), 2013 and ICD-10 Classification of Mental and Behavioural Disorders: Diagnostic Criteria for Research, World Health Organisation (WHO), Geneva, 2007.

CASE STUDY

Mary is a fifteen-year-old girl who is currently an inpatient in a private hospital that has a special unit for the treatment of eating disorders. Mary was admitted to the unit urgently because her body weight had dropped to dangerously low levels. At the time of her admission, Mary was an award-winning gymnast, who was planning to make this sport her career.

It transpired that Mary was severely restricting her intake of food. She was allowing herself half a can of creamed corn every second day. Mary was proud of her ability to control her appetite. Although an attractive girl, Mary's problems with eating and weight were affecting her appearance. Her hair was dull and thinning. She wore several layers of shapeless clothing, and she always seemed to be cold. Mary's skin was also dull and breaking out in a rash. Mary was painfully thin. She admitted that she might be a little underweight, but the staff at the unit had the feeling that she was just saying this to pacify them. While being in the unit, Mary got into trouble several times for breaking the unit rules. Once, she was found in the bathroom drinking a lot of water before she was due to be weighed, and on another occasion, she was discovered quietly doing push-ups in her room in the middle of the night.

Mary's treatment was complicated by the fact that the staff on the unit were at their wits' end about how to deal with Mary's mother. Mary's mother was extremely demanding of all the staff members on the unit. She repeatedly told the treating team that she loved her daughter and had her best interests at heart. According to Mary's mother, she knew exactly what was best for Mary. Her mother felt that Mary had to get back to gymnastics as soon as possible, because she was such a gifted athlete. This meant that she had to gain some weight so that she could be discharged and attend gymnastics practice with a top coach. Mary's mother once showed the team a picture of the cabinet that she had specially ordered for all her daughter's trophies. Mary's mother regularly telephoned Mary's psychotherapist after sessions to tell the therapist what Mary had thought of the session, and to inform the therapist whether it had been a useful session or not. Her mother also insisted on attending all Mary's consultations with the dietician. The treatment team never met Mary's father, who frequently worked away from home. He had a high-paying job which supported the family's very comfortable lifestyle. The treatment team got the impression that the relationship between Mary's parents was strained, but this was never openly acknowledged. Mary's mother described their family as loving, caring, and 'very close'.

Mary had a sister who was three years younger. Both girls were being home-schooled by their mother at the time of Mary's admission. All of the family members claimed that an extremely positive and close relationship existed between Mary and her sister. Mary's sister accompanied her mother on most visits to the unit. On two occasions, they were dressed in very similar outfits.

During a session with her therapist, Mary said that Victoria Beckham was her idol. She also stated that her problem with eating started during a gymnastics practice session three years ago when her male coach told her that she was three kilograms overweight, and that she had to lose the weight before the next practice session in four days time, if she wanted to be any good at the sport at all.

The weight loss which characterises Anorexia Nervosa is primarily achieved by means of restricting food intake. This may take the form of initially excluding foods that the individual perceives to be 'fattening' and gradually lead to a diet that includes a very limited number of foods. Attempts to aid weight loss can take the form of purging (self-induced vomiting or use of laxatives or diuretics) or excessive exercise (American Psychiatric Association, 2000).

The intense fear of weight gain or 'becoming fat' experienced by these individuals usually continues despite successful attempts at weight loss. In addition, the self-esteem of the individuals diagnosed with Anorexia Nervosa appears to depend greatly upon their weight and body shape. Their experience of their own body shape is typically unrealistic, in that they invariably see themselves as 'fat', even when they appear very thin to an objective observer. They also tend to have unrealistic views about the significance of weight fluctuations. Weight loss is regarded as a great achievement, while weight gain is seen as unacceptable and a loss of self-control (American Psychiatric Association, 2000).

Denial and lack of insight are often associated with a diagnosis of Anorexia Nervosa. People with this diagnosis may verbalise an acknowledgement of being too thin, but do not believe this within themselves. They often deny the medical consequences of their state of starvation. Indeed, people with a diagnosis of Anorexia Nervosa seldom seek help or medical attention of their own accord, and seldom complain of weight loss. It is more likely that pressure from family will bring the person to seek medical help. The person with Anorexia Nervosa may be unreliable when it comes to the history of the problem, and it is advisable for practitioners to obtain collateral information (Agras, 1987; American Psychiatric Association, 2000). The 'lack of insight' associated with Anorexia Nervosa can also be seen in the phenomenon of 'ProAna' websites, discussed later in this chapter.

In the case of Mary described above, Mary restricted her food intake to just half a can of creamed corn per day. She also used purging behaviours in that she exercised in the middle of the night. In the case study, Mary appears to lack insight into her condition, since she violates rules designed to help her gain weight and she attempts to deceive unit staff into thinking that she has gained weight, which was not the case.

Features associated with Anorexia Nervosa include obsessive-compulsive behaviours related to food, such as hoarding food, collecting recipes, and thinking constantly of food and cooking. These features appear to be related to the undernutrition in the person diagnosed with Anorexia Nervosa.

Other aspects associated with Anorexia Nervosa include a strong need for control and perfectionism, issues relating to eating in public, a rigid thinking style, as well as limited social and emotional behaviour (American Psychiatric Association, 2000). Some of these personality aspects are illustrated in the case study of Eva.

CASE STUDY

Eva is an attractive woman in her early forties. She takes care of her appearance, even though she looks too thin. When Eva was in her mid-teens, she was diagnosed with Anorexia Nervosa. Eva denies that she is currently anorexic; however, she continues to exhibit some of the behaviours associated with this condition. Eva works seven days a week, even though her job as an estate agent is not that demanding. She insists on doing everything perfectly and spends long hours in the office to achieve this. Eva's hobby is cake-baking and decorating. She even gets special requests for functions and parties. Eva has many acquaintances, but few friends. Eva has never been married and is not in a relationship currently. She ascribes this to the fact that she is only attracted to tall, blue-eyed men between the ages of 20 and 30 years.

Depressive symptoms and Obsessive-Compulsive Disorder (also with content unrelated to food), personality disorders, and problems relating to impulse control (particularly in the Binge-Eating/Purging subtype) frequently occur co-morbidly with Anorexia Nervosa. The associated presence of depressive symptoms in Anorexia Nervosa is thought to be the consequence of starvation (Agras, 1987; American Psychiatric Association, 2000).

The cessation of menstruation in post-pubertal females is a sign of physiological (endocrine) dysfunction due to weight loss in the individual diagnosed with Anorexia Nervosa. Other medical consequences are dry skin and brittle hair and nails, cold sensitivity, and the growth of downy body hair called lanugo on the face and body (American Psychiatric Association, 2000).

Anorexia Nervosa subtypes

The DSM-5 describes two subtypes of Anorexia Nervosa: Restricting Type and Binge-Eating/Purging Type. These subtypes are identified according to the presence or absence of binge-eating and purging behaviour during an episode of Anorexia Nervosa (American Psychiatric Association, 2013).

Restricting Type

Weight loss in this subtype is typically achieved by means of restricting food intake or engaging in excessive exercise. Binge-eating or purging behaviour is not regularly present during the episode in question (American Psychiatric Association, 2013).

Binge-Eating/Purging Type

This subtype is characterised by the use of purging techniques such as self-induced vomiting, the use of laxatives (medication that relieves constipation), diuretics (medication that increases the frequency of urination so that the body loses fluids), or enemas, subsequent to ingesting any amount of food. These occur on a frequent basis, possibly at least weekly (American Psychiatric Association, 2013).

Bulimia Nervosa

CASE STUDY

Sindi is a 19-year-old student who has presented at the student counselling centre of the large university where she is a first-year student in the Commerce Faculty. She is a pretty girl of slightly above average weight. The problems that she describes to her counsellor are a low mood, feelings of self-disgust, and being out of control. Sindi describes herself as 'fat, worthless, and pathetic'.

Sindi confides in her counsellor that she has problems in maintaining her weight. She has picked up a lot of weight since the beginning of her first year at university. Sindi tells her counsellor that she sometimes resorts to self-induced vomiting in order to control her weight.

Sindi describes her introduction to university life as a shock. She initially experienced being away from home as very difficult. Sindi describes the situation at home as problematic. She says that she often feels guilty because she has left her two younger siblings to cope on their own. Sindi's mother suffers from a bipolar disorder, and her mood sometimes affects her ability to cope with the two younger children. Sindi's father tries his best, but he just can't stand up to her mother when she gets 'into one of her states'.

Sindi describes her pattern of eating and vomiting as occurring more and more often. Sometimes food is all she can think about. She spends large amounts of money on junk food such as ice cream, cakes, and burgers. She usually can't wait to get to her room so that she can eat all the food at once. She then induces vomiting to get rid of the large amount of food that she has consumed. After this she weighs herself to make sure that she hasn't gained any weight from her session of overeating.

Prevalence and course

Bulimia Nervosa appears to exhibit a prevalence of approximately 1%–1.5% of females in industrialised countries, while the prevalence among males appears to be one-tenth of that in females (American Psychiatric Association, 2013; Halmi, 2000).

A review of 50 prevalence studies of Bulimia Nervosa indicates consistency of this prevalence rate at about 1% of young adult and adolescent females over a period of nine years (1981–1989) in Europe and the United States (Halmi, 2000). As with Anorexia Nervosa, the male-to-female ratio in clinical populations remains steady at between 1:10 and 1:20 (Halmi, 2000).

The course of Bulimia Nervosa typically has its onset in late adolescence or early adulthood, often during or after a period of dieting. The pattern of disturbed eating appears to be maintained for several years. The course could be chronic or be marked by remissions and relapses into binge-eating behaviour. Over the longer term, the symptoms appear to dissolve to an extent. Remissions of a year or longer appear indicative of a better long-term prognosis (American Psychiatric Association, 2013).

Specific cultural, gender, and age features

The incidence of Bulimia Nervosa appears to be similar for most industrialised countries. As with Anorexia Nervosa, at least 90% of cases are female. In addition, as with Anorexia Nervosa, the race group in which this disorder occurs appears to be mainly white, although cases from other groups have been reported. In males, a higher rate of premorbid obesity appears to have been present than in females (American Psychiatric Association, 2000).

In terms of specific culture, gender, and age features, it appears that younger, better-educated females who may be from a variety of cultural and racial backgrounds, but who identify with white, middle-class values, are at a greater risk of developing both Anorexia Nervosa and Bulimia Nervosa (Halmi, 2000).

Clinical picture

The literal translation of 'Bulimia' is 'ox-hunger', which means any great, ravenous hunger and it refers to the binging behaviour associated with this disorder. The three pivotal aspects of the diagnosis of Bulimia Nervosa can be described as: (1) an overwhelming urge to overeat, which culminates in episodes of overeating; (2) evading weight gain by means of self-induced vomiting and/or purgative use; and (3) an extreme fear of becoming fat (Halmi, 2000). The use of purgatives could include abusing laxatives or diuretics.

The central characteristics of Bulimia Nervosa are binge-eating episodes, together with compensatory behaviours aimed at preventing weight gain. The person's evaluation of themselves is typically focused, to an inappropriate degree, on body shape and weight (American Psychiatric Association, 2013).

A binge can be defined as eating an amount of food that is certainly more than most people would eat in a similar situation, in a restricted period of time (typically less than two hours) (American Psychiatric Association, 2000; Vitousek & Gray, 2005). In addition, the eating behaviour is out of control during a binging episode. In the early stages of this disorder, the lack of control may manifest as ravenous eating. As the disorder progresses, a lack of control of behaviour, such as irresistible impulses to binge or inability to stop the course of the binge, appear to become evident. Some individuals report dissociative experiences as part of the binge-eating episode, as well as during the post-binge period (American Psychiatric Association, 2013).

Binge-eating and compensatory behaviour must take place at least twice a week for a period of three months in order to warrant a diagnosis of Bulimia Nervosa. A diagnosis of Bulimia Nervosa cannot be made where the binge-eating and purging occur exclusively during episodes of Anorexia Nervosa (Halmi, 2000).

The inappropriate compensatory behaviours to avoid gaining weight involve purging, for instance self-induced vomiting (in about 80%–90% of cases), laxative use (one-third of cases), or extremely restrictive dieting. Alternative behaviour in this disorder involves binge-eating behaviour without purging. Some individuals utilise more than one purging technique. Apart from laxative use, purging techniques include use of diuretics (33% use these occasionally), enemas (7%), and excessive exercise.

It appears that about two-thirds of people diagnosed with Bulimia Nervosa use purging techniques (American Psychiatric Association, 2000; McCann, Rossiter, King, & Agras, 1991; Pyle, Neuman, Halvorson, & Mitchell, 1991). The vomiting behaviour typically has the effect of immediately relieving the physical discomfort and fear of weight gain, and this relief becomes a goal in itself in some cases. In some individuals, vomiting occurs even after a small amount of food has been consumed (American Psychiatric Association, 2013).

Table 11.2: Diagnostic criteria for Bulimia Nervosa as adapted from the DSM-5 and ICD-10

DSM-5	ICD-10
A. Recurrent episodes of binge eating. AN episode of binge eating is characterised by both of the following: (1) Eating, in a discrete period of time (e.g. within any two-hour period), an amount of food that is definitely larger than what most individuals would eat in a similar period of time under similar circumstances. (2(A sense of lack of control over eating during the episode (e.g. a feeling that one cannot stop eating or control what or how much one is eating). B. Recurrent inappropriate compensatory behaviours in order to prevent weight gain, such as self-induced vomiting; misuse of laxatives, diuretics, or other medications; fasting; or excessive exercise. C. The binge eating and inappropriate compensatory behaviours both occur, on average, at least once a week for three months. D. Self-evaluation is unduly influenced by body shape and weight. E. The disturbance does not occur exclusively during episodes of anorexia nervosa.	• For a definite diagnosis, all of the following are required: ▸ There is a persistent preoccupation with eating, and an irresistible craving for food; the patient succumbs to episodes of overeating in which large amounts of food are consumed in short periods of time. ▸ The patient attempts to counteract the 'fattening' effects of food by one or more of the following: self-induced vomiting; purgative abuse, alternating periods of starvation; use of drugs such as appetite suppressants, thyroid preparations or diuretics. When bulimia occurs in diabetic patients they may choose to neglect their insulin treatment. ▸ The psychopathology consists of a morbid dread of fatness and the patient sets herself or himself a sharply defined weight threshold, well below the premorbid weight that constitutes the optimum or healthy weight in the opinion of the physician. There is often, but not always, a history of an earlier episode of Anorexia Nervosa, the interval between the two disorders ranging from a few months to several years. This earlier episode may have been fully expressed, or may have assumed a minor cryptic form with a moderate loss of weight and/or a transient phase of amenorrhoea.

Source: Reprinted with permission from the Diagnostic and Statistical Manual of Mental Disorders (DSM), Fifth Edition, American Psychiatric Association (APA), 2013 and ICD-10 Classification of Mental and Behavioural Disorders: Diagnostic Criteria for Research, World Health Organisation (WHO), Geneva, 2007.

In terms of impact on body weight, people diagnosed with Bulimia Nervosa who do not purge appear to exhibit a tendency towards obesity. Purging is also not an effective way in which to restrict the intake of calories, since vomiting results in a reduction of only about 50% of calories consumed, while laxative use has very little impact on weight (Kaye, Weltzin, Hsu, McConaha, & Bolton 1993). It appears that people with a diagnosis of Bulimia Nervosa are usually within the range of normal weight, although some may be under- or overweight to a slight degree. People diagnosed with Bulimia Nervosa appear to tend to restrict their food intake ('diet') between binges and thus avoid food that they regard as 'fattening' or that is likely to trigger a binging episode (American Psychiatric Association, 2013).

In the case of Sindi, she is described as being slightly overweight and she overemphasises the aspects of weight and appearance when describing herself to her counsellor. Binging behaviour is present in her buying large amounts of junk food and consuming it in a short period of time. Sindi vomits to purge herself of the food, and her fear of gaining weight is illustrated by her weighing herself after every binging and purging session.

Features associated with Bulimia Nervosa are medical consequences such as enlarged salivary glands in chronic Bulimia Nervosa (which, ironically, result in a 'chubby' facial appearance) and electrolyte imbalances. With vomiting, the dental enamel of the teeth may be eroded and calluses on the fingers or backs of the hands may develop as a result of stimulating the gag reflex. Frequent laxative abuse can lead to intestinal problems such as permanent colon damage or severe constipation.

Co-morbid features include increased mood and anxiety symptoms, with the Purging Type exhibiting more depressive symptoms. An increased likelihood of substance abuse or dependence involving alcohol or stimulants (used to suppress appetite) appears to be present. A significant number of people (between 28% and 77%) diagnosed with Bulimia Nervosa meet the criteria for one of the personality disorders, most frequently Borderline Personality Disorder (American Psychiatric Association, 2013; Halmi, 2000).

Table 11.3: Comparison of eating disorders

ANOREXIA NERVOSA	BULIMIA NERVOSA
Age of onset: 14	Age of onset: 18
Excessive thinness	Average or overweight
Intense fear of weight gain	Fear of losing control of eating
Disturbance of body image	Self-evaluation unduly impacted weight
Amenorrhea	Normal menstruation
Voluntary food restriction, binging and purging in Binge-Eating/Purging Type	Binging and purging
Family enmeshed, rigid, overprotective, poor conflict resolution	Family history of psychological problems, substance abuse, family discord, overt hostility
Socially isolated and insecure	Low self-esteem, sensitive to rejection
Not interested in sex	Sexually active with little enjoyment
Over-controlled	Emotionally labile
Co-morbid with depression and anxiety disorders (including Social Phobia and OCD)	Co-morbid with depression, anxiety, substance abuse, and personality disorders
Maternal history of anorexia	Family history of obesity
Ego-syntonic	Ego-dystonic

Source: Wenar & Kerig, 2006, p. 378.

Binge-eating disorder

Binge-Eating Disorder is characterised by episodes of binge-eating which cause significant distress for the individual, but the person does not engage in compensatory behaviours. This disorder has been included in the DSM-5 as a new disorder.

CASE STUDY

Gertrude is a 42-year-old woman who presented for treatment at a specialised ward for eating disorders. She is visibly overweight, but very well groomed and well dressed. Gertrude has a career as a successful attorney and she also takes excellent care of her husband and her two primary-school children from her previous marriage. Her husband has been unemployed for a few years due to his disabling Major Depressive Disorder. His symptoms are so severe that he can do little more than spend his days on the couch. Gertrude describes spending large amounts of money on food or snacks which she consumes in her car after work. She says this usually happens on her way home from a busy day at work when she feels guilty because she knows that her children need her at home to help them with their homework and to prepare the evening meal. She then stops off at an expensive shop to buy the food or snacks (roast chicken is her favourite). Gertrude then usually drives to the parking lot of another shopping centre and eats all the food or snacks in her car. She does this very fast and is terrified that someone might notice or recognise her. She then drives home feeling devastated by guilt and remorse. What makes it worse is that her husband keeps on telling her that she is not physically attractive to him anymore because she has gained so much weight. Gertrude feels that he may leave her because of this. She is desperate not have another failed marriage and presented for treatment for this reason. Her episodes of binge-eating became much worse after her husband was diagnosed with depression and withdrew from her.

In the case study of Gertrude, the pattern of rapid eating is clearly present, as is the aspect of eating alone because of embarrassment, as well as the feelings of guilt present after an episode of binging. Comparisons between Binge-Eating Disorder and Anorexia and Bulimia Nervosa have found a number of similarities. For example, for all three disorders, there is typically distress on the part of the 'sufferer', as well as a decrease in quality of life and a similar pattern of co-morbidity. However, Binge-Eating Disorder seems to be associated with an older age of onset, as well as with a greater prevalence in males than the other eating disorders. The course of Binge-Eating Disorder is also distinctive. While Anorexia and Bulimia Nervosa are characterised by frequent crossover between the two disorders during the course of the disturbance, Binge-Eating Disorder appears less likely to shift in symptomology (Wonderlich, Gordon, Mitchell, Crosby, & Engel, 2009).

People with Binge-Eating Disorder experience greater discomfort about body shape and weight and lower quality of life than those with obesity. Co-morbidity with the personality disorders and the mood and anxiety disorders is more likely in Binge-Eating Disorder than in obesity. Binge-Eating Disorder appears to respond to antidepressant treatment and to specialised treatment programmes rather than to weight loss programmes, which also distinguished the condition from obesity (Wonderlich et al., 2009). Finally, Binge-Eating Disorder probably runs in families, indicating that it is not just a variation of obesity (American Psychiatric Association, 2010). Despite Binge-Eating Disorder often occurring with obesity, it appears to be associated with different aetiological factors compared to obesity without Binge-Eating Disorder (Hudson et al., 2006).

Figure 11.2: Summary of outcomes for Anorexia Nervosa and Bulimia Nervosa after a six-year follow-up

Summary of outcomes for Anorexia Nervosa over a six-year period

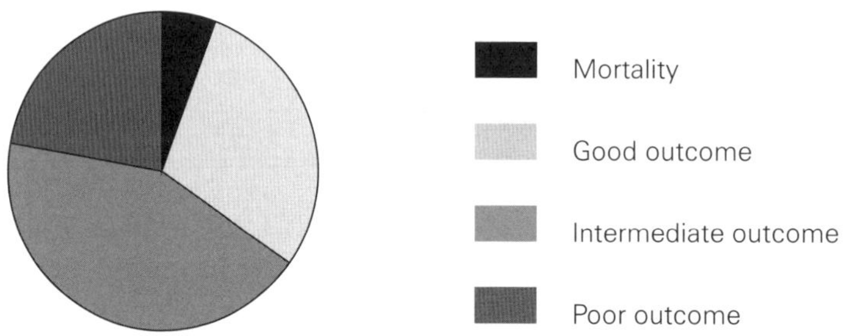

Summary of outcomes for Bulimia Nervosa over a six-year period

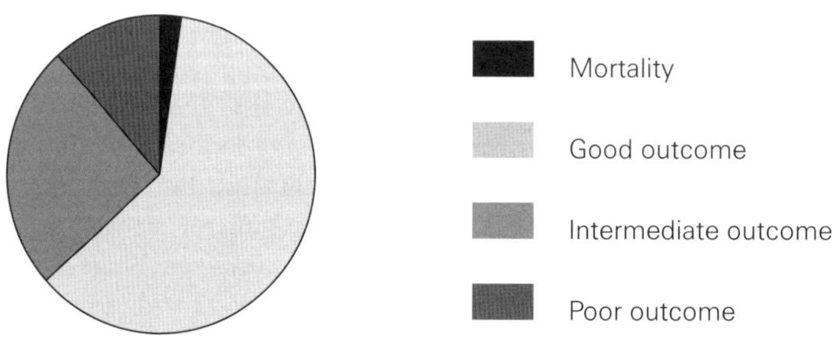

Source: Fichter & Quadflieg, 1997; 1999).

Other Specified Feeding or Eating Disorder

The DSM-5 provides the category of Other Specified Feeding or Eating Disorder for disordered eating that does not meet the full criteria of Anorexia or Bulimia Nervosa or other patterns of disordered eating, such as Purging Disorder and Night Eating Syndrome. Cases where all the criteria for Anorexia Nervosa are met, with the exception where the person's weight remains in the normal range despite significant weight loss, are diagnosised in this category as Atypical Anorexia Nervosa. This diagnosis is also made when all the criteria for Bulimia Nervosa are met, except the frequency or duration criteria (American Psychiatric Association, 2013).

Another disorder in this category is that of Purging Disorder where a person displays recurrent purging behaviour, in the absence of binge eating, in order to influence body weight or shape (APA, 2013). The last disorder in this category is referred to Night Eating Syndrome, where a person either eats after awakening from sleep, or where the person continues to eat excessively after an evening meal (APA, 2013).

These disorders account for 60% of patients seeking treatment for an eating disorder in clinical settings, yet it is the diagnostic category that has been the least researched (Miller & Golden, 2010). A study conducted by Fairburn et al. (2007) found that most cases that meet the criteria for these disorders are of a 'mixed' nature and are not merely subclinical forms of Anorexia Nervosa or Bulimia Nervosa. In this study, the conditions that received a diagnosis of one of these disorders were typically as severe as Bulimia Nervosa in terms of the nature, duration, and severity of pathology, and could not be regarded as representing less severe forms of Anorexia Nervosa and/or Bulimia Nervosa. These authors concluded that atypical eating disorders are common, severe, and persistent.

South African research on subclinical eating disorders (defined as the presence of some eating disorder symptoms, but not enough to meet DSM-5 diagnostic criteria) echo the conclusions of international research described above. Subclinical eating disorders were found to be associated with themes of personal brokenness and shame, experiences of personal inadequacy and body image difficulties, as well as perceptions of social pressure and isolation (Kirsten & Du Plessis, 2008). These researchers conclude that the impact of subclinical eating disorder symptoms is underestimated and that the presence of these symptoms represents a significant risk factor for developing a full-blown eating disorder.

Table 11.4: Diagnostic criteria for Other Specified Feeding or Eating Disorder as adapted from the DSM-5

DSM-5
This category applies to presentations in which symptoms characteristic of a feeding and eating disorder that cause clinically significant distress or impairment in social, occupational, or other important areas of functioning predominate but do not meet the full criteria for any of the disorders in the feeding and eating disorders diagnostic class. The other specified feeding or eating disorder category is used in situations in which the clinician chooses to communicate the specific reason that the presentation does not meet the criteria for any specific feeding and eating disorder. This is done by recording 'other specified feeding and eating disorder' followed by the specific reason (e.g. 'bulimia nervosa of low frequency'). Examples of presentations that can be specified using the 'other specified' designation include the following: 1. **Atypical anorexia nervosa:** All of the criteria for anorexia nervosa are met, except that despite significant weight loss, the individual's weight is within or above the normal range. 2. **Bulimia nervosa (of low frequency and/or limited duration):** All of the criteria for bulimia nervosa are met, except that the binge eating and inappropriate compensatory behaviours occur, on average, less than once a week and/or for less than three months. 3. **Binge-eating disorder (of low frequency and/or limited duration):** All of the criteria for binge-eating disorder are met, except that the binge eating occurs, on average, less than once a week and/or for less than three months. 4. **Purging disorder:** Recurrent purging behaviour to influence weight or shape (e.g. self-induced vomiting; misuse of laxatives, diuretics, or other medications) in the absence of binge eating. 5. **Night eating syndrome:** Recurrent episodes of night eating, as manifested by eating after awakening from sleep or by excessive food consumption after the evening meal. There is awareness and recall of the eating. The night eating is not better explained by external influences such as changes in the individual's sleep-wake cycle or by local social norms. The night eating causes significant distress and/or impairment in functioning. The disordered eating pattern is not better explained by binge-eating disorder or another mental disorder, including substance use, and is not attributable to another medical disorder or to an effect of medication.

Source: Reprinted with permission from the Diagnostic and Statistical Manual of Mental Disorders (DSM), Fifth Edition, American Psychiatric Association (APA), 2013

AETIOLOGY

The circumscribed population that eating disorders have high prevalence rates in young, white, middle-class females from industrialised societies is suggestive of the aspects that must be considered in the aetiology of these disorders. As in the case of other psycho-pathologies, it appears unlikely that a single causal factor can give rise to these disorders. Issues that will be considered in this discussion of the aetiology of the eating disorders include intrapersonal aspects such as genetics, biological and psychological functioning, as well as interpersonal considerations, such as cultural expectations, the changing role of women in Western society, the role of the media, and the impact of family dynamics.

Biological factors

When considering the biological or medical dimensions in the aetiology of the eating disorders, two aspects are typically in the forefront. These are genetics and neurophysiological considerations.

Genetic factors

Both Anorexia Nervosa and Bulimia Nervosa appear to run in families. First-degree female relatives of women with eating disorders are more likely to be diagnosed with an eating disorder (Kasset, Gwirtsman, Kaye, Brandt, & Jimerson, 1987; Strober, Lampert, Morrell, Burroughs, & Jacobs, 1990). Relatives of people with a diagnosis of an eating disorder are also more likely to exhibit eating disorder symptoms that do not meet the full criteria for diagnosis (Lilienfeld, Kaye, Greenco, Merikangas, & Plotniciv, 1998). In addition, twin studies have found significantly higher concordance rates for monozygotic than for dizygotic twins in both Anorexia Nervosa and Bulimia Nervosa (Fichter & Naegel, 1990; Holland, Hall, Murray, Russell, & Crisp, 1988; Kendler, MacLean, Neale, & Kessler, 1991).

There has been speculation about the nature of the heritable genetic predisposition to eating disorders. Researchers such as Hsu (1990) suggest that more general aspects of personality, such as poor impulse control and emotional instability, may constitute the heritable aspects involved in the causality of eating disorders. The implication is that an inherited disposition to react to any source of stress in a particular way represents the genetic vulnerability associated with the eating disorders. These reactions include a more emotional response and engaging in impulsive eating behaviour as a way of alleviating the experience of stress and anxiety.

A general vulnerability to psychological difficulties associated with eating disorders is suggested by several studies. Rutherford, McGuffin, Katz, and Murray (1993) found genetic influences on eating attitudes in a normal female twin population. A greater frequency of mood disorders and anxiety disorders, specifically Obsessive-Compulsive Disorder, was found in first-degree relatives of people diagnosed with eating disorders, when compared to first-degree relatives of the control participants (Halmi, 2000).

Overall, the available research suggests a general genetic predisposition. This, of course, still needs to be clarified by more, and more sophisticated, research.

Neurobiological factors

The hypothalamus is the part of the brain associated with the regulation of hunger and eating. It appears obvious therefore to look to this area when considering biological possibilities in the causation of eating disorders. Hypothalamic lesions in animals are associated with weight loss in these animals, but they do not parallel what we know of the clinical picture of Anorexia Nervosa. The animals in question become indifferent to food, whereas Anorexia Nervosa is characterised by both hunger and an interest in food (Hoebel & Teitelbaum, 1966). The levels of some hormones (e.g. cortisol and norepinephrine) regulated by the hypothalamus are found to be abnormal in people diagnosed with Anorexia Nervosa, but these abnormalities appear to be the result, rather than the cause, of self-starvation (Doer, Fichter, Pirke, & Lund, 1980; Liebowitz, 1983). In addition, it appears that a raised level of dopamine in the hypothalamus leads to decreased eating; however, there is as yet no evidence that links dopamine levels and the eating disorders (Fava, Copeland, Schweiger, & Hertzog 1989; Hsu, 1990).

Another set of evidence suggests links between levels of serotonin and eating disorders. Serotonin is involved in the modulation of appetite in that increased serotonin causes feelings of satiety while starvation decreases serotonin activity. In addition, increased serotonin levels are associated with anxiety. The hypothesis is therefore that individuals with innately high levels of serotonin experience high levels of anxiety and employ excessive dieting as a strategy to reduce anxiety (Kaye et al., 2003). These researchers experimentally reduced serotonin levels in groups of anorexics and non-anorexic controls and were able to confirm this hypothesis.

Bulimia Nervosa is, in turn, associated with insufficient serotonin levels. Smith, Fairburn, and Cowen (1999) utilised the same procedure as Kaye et al. (2003) to deplete serotonin levels in a group of recovered bulimics and a normal control group. They found that lowered serotonin levels in the group of recovered bulimics caused depressive symptoms, difficulties with body-image, and fear of losing control of eating behaviour.

Some research has found low levels of serotonin metabolites in people diagnosed with Bulimia Nervosa, as well as decreased responses to serotonin agonists, again implicating an underactive serotonin system (Jimerson, Wolfe, Metzger, Finkelstein, & Cooper, 1997). Finally, antidepressant medications that boost serotonin levels have met with some success in the treatment of Bulimia Nervosa. From the available information, serotonin appears to be implicated in Bulimia Nervosa, at least to a certain extent.

Endogenous opioid peptides (EOPs) are also hypothesised to be involved in a vicious cycle related to the starvation–binge behaviour of people with an eating disorder diagnosis (Marrazzi & Luby, 1986). More specifically, the EOPs occur naturally within our bodies and are produced by the body as a response to starvation. The opiate system is involved in decreasing the body's experience of pain, and the EOPs are involved with the experience of pleasure in eating. The theory put forward by some researchers is that people diagnosed with eating disorders become 'addicted' to the body's opiates during a period of self-starvation, and that patterns of starvation–binging stimulate EOP production in the body. In addition, opioids are increased by the pattern of excessive exercise present in some people with a diagnosis of an eating disorder (Davis, 1996). However, evidence for an addiction model for the eating disorders still has to be established (Marrazzi & Luby, 1986; Wilson, 1991).

In summary, in terms of neurobiological factors and the eating disorders, it appears that the issue of cause and effect constitutes the greatest current challenge to researchers in this area. Biochemical factors do not account for some aspects of the eating disorders such as a fear of gaining weight and the specific population involved. In order to gain some understanding of aspects that could influence these factors, we will look to the psychological and interpersonal aspects discussed in the following section.

Figure 11.3: The possible role of serotonin in Anorexia and Bulimia Nervosa

Innate excessive serotonin → Anxiety Dieting → Lowered serotonin → Temporary decreased anxiety
Dieting → Lowered serotonin → Depressed mood and urge to binge → Binge and purge

Source: Adapted from Kerig & Wenar, 2006.

Psychological factors

The discussion in this section will focus on individual factors. These individual factors are described in the context of the developmental demands associated with adolescence. The section on factors involving the family is also contextualised by the adjustments that families have to make when children enter adolescence. The broader social aspects that impact individuals will be discussed in the following section.

Developmental factors

Adolescence can be regarded as a time of great transition. The shift from childhood to adulthood brings with it changes in every sphere of a person's life (Ebata, Peterson, & Conger, 1990). The arena for this transition is the body itself. The physical changes that happen during adolescence include the development of mature size and body shape, hormonal changes, and the start of adult sexuality (Wenar & Kerig, 2006). Because of the physical changes that occur during adolescence, the adolescent's body image (psychological representation of the body) becomes much more central than during childhood (Wenar & Kerig, 2006).

Adolescence also marks a time during which a person experiences further cognitive development. Society increases its demands during this time, and a person is expected to take responsibility for decisions about their future (most importantly regarding romantic relationships and career choice). Relationships with peers also take on increased importance during this developmental phase (Wenar & Kerig, 2006).

The main developmental task of adolescence can be seen as finding the answer to the question 'Who am I?' In terms of Erik Erikson's theory of human development, this stage represents the struggle between 'identity' and 'role confusion' and it occurs from the age of eleven years through to the end of adolescence. Erikson viewed this stage as a time during which a person struggles to develop ego identity (a sense of inner sameness or continuity). Difficulties during this stage result in role confusion (not having a sense of self or one's place in the world). The ability to separate from the parent and leave home represents important challenges during this stage. Many of the disorders of adolescence can be linked to identity confusion, for example, Conduct Disorder and the psychotic disorders (Kaplan et al., 1996).

The family system also becomes an arena where change plays out, because parents are required to adapt their expectations and their parenting styles to accommodate the increased needs for independence and autonomy that adolescence brings with it (Wenar & Kerig, 2006).

The eating disorders typically emerge during adolescence. However, there are few studies that have produced data that view the eating disorders from a developmental perspective (Steiner & Lock 1998). Some theorists regard the eating disorders as normative developmental processes 'gone awry' (Wenar & Kerig, 2006, p. 360). A few of the psychological theories and social factors discussed in the following sections describe how normative developmental processes 'go awry' in the areas of body-image and emerging sexuality (Bruch's psycho-analytical theories), cognitive styles (cognitive-behavioural theories), the personality, and the family (the family systems approach). The consequences of these skewed developmental processes play out in the bodies of people diagnosed with an eating disorder.

Psychological theories

The various psychological theories regarding the aetiology of Anorexia Nervosa and Bulimia Nervosa centre on psychodynamic formulations, cognitive and learning approaches, views of the family dynamics, and descriptions of personality functioning. Aspects regarding family dynamics will be discussed in the section on interpersonal causal factors.

Early psychodynamic views on the causality of Anorexia Nervosa focused on phobic mechanisms. According to this view, the physical changes associated with puberty cause sexual and social tension. Anorexia Nervosa is described as a phobic avoidance of food as a consequence of these tensions. In this view, the tensions described are usually characterised by feelings of aggression and ambivalence towards the mother (as the primary supplier of food), while the relationship with the father is seductive and dependent. The fathers are themselves warm, but passive. All of these dynamics result in the Anorexia sufferer experiencing guilt (Halmi, 2000). These dynamics are evident in the case study of Mary, described earlier in this chapter, where her mother appears to be over-involved in her daughter's life, while her father is often away from home.

Other psychodynamic views describe eating disorder symptoms as a need fulfilment; for example, the experience of success in dieting bolsters the individual's experience of personal efficacy. Avoiding sexual maturation and its consequences by maintaining a child-like body shape through dieting is also a psychodynamic view (Goodsitt, 1997).

Hilde Bruch (1904–1984) was considered a world authority on the eating disorders. She theorised that Anorexia and Bulimia Nervosa were psychologically similar phenomena. Her view of the aetiology of the eating disorders was that the person with this diagnosis has an underdeveloped sense of personal effectiveness and personal power, which they attempt to rectify through their symptoms by being 'different' and 'independent'. In her view, a sense of personal helplessness and powerlessness is fostered by an approach to parenting in which the wishes and views of the parent are imposed on the child.

In this approach, the parents fail adequately to take into account the child's actual needs. For instance, the parents decide when the child is hungry or tired. Individuals brought up in this manner fail to learn to recognise their own internal states and do not develop independence from others. The developmental demands of adolescence, including developing a sense of identity and achieving independence (as discussed above), push the person towards the societal values of being thin. The individual uses dieting as a means to experience a sense of personal control, power, and independence.

Psychodynamic views of Bulimia Nervosa describe food as symbolic of a chaotic mother–daughter relationship. In this view, the daughter does not develop an adequate sense of self and thus expresses ambivalence towards her mother in binging (bringing her closer) and purging (rejecting her) (Goodsitt, 1997).

Attachment theory emphasises the importance of early relationships for later psychological functioning. The nature of the attachment formed by an infant is determined by the interactions between the caregiver and the infant. The infant learns to regulate emotional experiences on the basis of the caregiver's sensitivity and responsiveness to the infant's communication behaviours (e.g. clinging and crying). Attachment theory postulates a connection between disrupted attachment and the development of an eating disorder (O'Shaughnessy & Dallos, 2009). Women with eating disorders often report disrupted attachments. Extreme separation anxiety and unresolved loss and trauma have been identified as issues of concern in the treatment of eating disorders from the perspective of attachment theory. However, conflicting data complicates attempts to find associations between subgroups of eating disorder and attachment style.

Cognitive-behavioural views of the aetiology of the eating disorders regard weight loss and the experience of successful dieting as strong reinforcing factors. These, in turn, are motivated by fear of weight gain and faulty perceptions of body image. Dieting and successful weight reduction are positively reinforced since they become associated with feelings of control, while dieting behaviours are negatively reinforced because they are associated with decreased anxiety about gaining weight (Fairburn, Shafran, & Cooper, 1999). Faulty perceptions of body image, and an extreme desire to be thin, also appear to be linked to experiences of negative comments about weight by parents or peers (Paxton, Schutz, Wertheim, & Muir, 1999; Thompson, Coovert, Richards, Johnson, & Cattarin 1995).

The cognitive-behavioural view of the aetiology of Bulimia Nervosa involves a vicious cycle that starts with the individual experiencing low self-esteem and high levels of negative affect. In an attempt to influence one of the few aspects of self that are within a person's control, they diet in an attempt to feel better. In the course of this attempt, intake of food is restricted unrealistically, which leads to an inevitable breaking of the diet. This break grows into a binge. Binging behaviour in turn creates a fear of gaining weight, which is alleviated by compensatory behaviours (purging). These actions relieve some of the anxiety associated with the binging behaviour, but also negatively impact the person's self-esteem, which initiates the vicious cycle again (Fairburn, 1997). Various studies support the link between purging behaviour and anxiety reduction, also explaining the apparent tendency of people diagnosed with Bulimia Nervosa to binge and purge particularly during times of stress and emotional difficulties (Jarrel, Johnson, & Williamson, 1986; Stice, 1998).

Personality factors

The earlier section on genetics has suggested that more general, inherited aspects of personality may be involved in the aetiology of the eating disorders. This section will focus on the more specific personality traits associated with the eating disorders.

Assessment of the personality traits associated with the eating disorders is a difficult undertaking for a number of reasons. For example, the physical semi-starvation associated with an eating disorder can, in itself, impact on personality functioning. This was shown in studies of male conscientious objectors done in the 1940s, which aimed to replicate concentration camp conditions (Keys, Brozek, Hsu, McConoha, & Bolton, 1950). On the other hand, retrospective reports of a person's personality functioning prior to diagnosis are usually collected from the diagnosed person and family members and could be influenced by pre-existing biases.

The personality aspects that appear to be central to the functioning of individuals with a diagnosis of eating disorders are low self-esteem (Garner, Vitousek, & Pike, 1983), lack of confidence in their personal abilities, and a decreased experience of control over their environment (Bruch, 1985; Dyken & Gerrard, 1986). In addition, particularly negative and distorted views of personal body image characterise these disorders (Klemchuck, Hutchinson, & Frank, 1990). Perfectionism also appears to play a role in these disorders (Pliner & Haddock, 1996) and may be related to the poor body image of people diagnosed with eating disorders (Davis, 1997).

In terms of relating to others, people diagnosed with eating disorders are usually described as agreeable or compliant, and shy, prior to diagnosis (Vitousek & Manke, 1994). A combination of increased social anxiety and a heightened proccupation with how others perceive the self appear to be at play in causality of the eating disorders (Striegel-Moore, Silberstein, & Rodin, 1993).

Some research has attempted to describe the current personality functioning of people diagnosed with eating disorders utilising personality questionnaires such as the MMPI (Minnesota Multiphasic Personality Inventory) (Vitousek & Manke, 1994). This study reports that people with these diagnoses measure high on neuroticism and anxiety, with low scores on self-esteem. High scores on traditionalism (ascribes strongly to family and social standards) have been reported. Differences between people diagnosed with Anorexia Nervosa and those diagnosed with Bulimia Nervosa include high scores for depression, anxiety, and social isolation associated with Anorexia Nervosa, while a diagnosis of Bulimia Nervosa was associated with a greater variety of serious psychopathology on MMPI scores (Vitousek & Manke, 1994).

In terms of risk factors for developing an eating disorder identified by prospective studies, low scores on measures of interoceptive awareness (ability to identify own physical state) appeared to be predictors of risk for eating disorders (Leon, Fulkerson, Perry, & Early-Zald, 1995).

Aspects of personality functioning that appear to be associated with Bulimia Nervosa specifically, are qualities such as histrionic traits, affective instability, and extraversion (Vitousek & Manke, 1994). People with a diagnosis of Bulimia Nervosa can be described as angrier, more impulsive, and more outgoing than those who are anorexic. Dependence on alcohol and other substances, shoplifting, and self-destructive sexual relationships are also associated with the difficulties in impulse control associated with Bulimia Nervosa (Kaplan et al., 1994).

People with a diagnosis of Bulimia Nervosa also appear to experience increased anxiety associated with eating, and an experience of intense relief associated with purging. This experience of relief may create a vicious cycle, because it reinforces the binging and purging cycle (Rosen & Leitenberg, 1985). Other studies place less emphasis on the reinforcing effect of anxiety relief as they emphasise the tendency to restrict food intake and associated negative attitudes towards body image in structuring treatment for Bulimia Nervosa (Fairburn, Agras, & Wilson, 1992).

The way in which personality manifests is also influenced by the co-morbid disorders often found with the eating disorders, discussed in an earlier section. Mood disorders and anxiety disorders (specifically Obsessive-Compulsive Disorder), and the personality disorders which are frequently co-morbid with the eating disorders, influence the expression of personality in people with this diagnosis (American Psychiatric Association, 2000; Halmi, 2000). Indeed, some researchers suggest that the eating disorders are an expression of the mood disorders, while others maintain that depression is a consequence of the eating disorder (Rutter, Bolton, Harrington, & Couteur, 1990; Vanderlinden, Norre, & Vandereycken 1992).

Finally, assessments of people diagnosed with an eating disorder in recovering phases of the disorders continue to show rigid and obsessional thinking patterns, shyness, feelings of insecurity, minimisation of feelings, compliance with convention, and rigid behaviour patterns (Halmi, 2000).

Role of the family context

The family provides the context for the developmental tasks that face family members. Aetiological aspects that address the role of the family context include family characteristics and the Family Systems approach. The so-called 'typical' anorexic family and their associated patterns of interaction have been the focus of numerous studies from both the psychodynamic and Family Systems perspectives.

The following characteristics are associated with a family context where eating disorders may develop: The mothers of the families have the role of being 'society's messengers'. They tend to transmit messages about the desirability of thinness to their daughters and are likely to be dieters themselves (see section on sociocultural factors). The mothers appear to be more 'perfectionistic' and the family as a whole is ambitious and places great emphasis on appearances (Bruch, 1985; Hsu, 1990; Minuchin, Rosman, & Baker, 1978; Pike & Rodin, 1991).

The psychodynamic view on aetiology was discussed in the previous section. The psychodynamic view of the family's involvement is that people with eating disorders often experience their bodies as being under the control of their parents. They regard their mothers as intrusive and unempathic, but are unable to separate from their mothers psychologically. The self-starvation of the anorexic patient is regarded as an attempt to attain a sense of autonomy and selfhood (Kaplan et al., 1994).

It appears likely that differences exist in the enmeshment patterns of families of anorexics and families of bulimics (Evans & Street, 1995). The families of bulimics appear more likely to exhibit high levels of conflict and to be less close than those of anorexics. Bulimia Nervosa patients often describe their parents as neglectful and rejecting (Kaplan et al., 1994).

A Family Systems Theory view of the eating disorders was formulated by Salvador Minuchin and his co-workers (1975). This view proposes that the symptoms of eating disorders are inseparable from the family context in which they arise. Minuchin is regarded as the father of Structural Family Therapy. In this view, the symptoms of the eating disorders are understood to be related to the dysfunctional structure of the family in which they occur. The symptoms are regarded as serving a function in the family.

In the case of eating disorders, one possible function of the symptom is to assist the family in escaping other conflicts and to distract attention from other problems within the family. From this perspective, the families of people diagnosed with an eating disorder are characterised by the following:

- ***Enmeshment:*** A dynamic characterised by diffuse boundaries within the family, resulting in family members being overly involved with, and responsive to, one another. An example is parents who speak for their children since they believe that they know how their children feel.
- ***Overprotectiveness:*** Members of the family exhibit excessive concern for one another's well-being. In an overprotective family, criticism is softened by pacifying behaviour. The effect is that children of such a family do not move towards autonomy, and in turn, feel responsible for protecting the family from distress.
- ***Rigidity:*** Members attempt to maintain balance and try to escape change. During times of normal growth and transition (such as adolescence), they increase their attempts to hold on to their usual patterns.
- ***Lack of conflict resolution:*** Conflict is avoided, denied, or is engaged in constantly but in an ineffective way. An example is a father who leaves the house every time conflict threatens.

Minuchin and his colleagues describe the family of the future anorexic as being very concerned with diet, appearance, and control. The family is intrusive to the point of scrutinising the adolescent's bodily and psychological functions, with the effect that their autonomy is blocked. Because adolescence is a developmental phase that requires separation, it is a particularly stressful time for the enmeshed family. The identified patient, in response to the stress, responds with self-starvation. This allows the anorexic to remain overtly dependent on the parents, while enabling them to engage in covert rebellion (Minuchin et al., 1978).

Once a family member has been diagnosed with an eating disorder, this is also likely to impact negatively on family relationships. Parents may experience high levels of frustration and guilt as a result of their child's symptoms. Levels of conflict can escalate to the point of physical violence when parents have to deal with the struggle to persuade their daughter or son to eat.

Child abuse

There are indications that higher incidences of reported childhood physical and sexual abuse are found among people diagnosed with eating disorders (Everill & Waller, 1995). In particular, childhood sexual abuse among this population has been the focus of research, with some studies indicating higher rates of reported sexual abuse in this population (Deep, Lilenfeld, Plotnicov, Pollice, & Kaye 1999; Welch & Fairburn, 1994). Schmidt, Evans, Tiller, and Treasure (1995) reported that 22%–31% of eating disorder patients included in their study had been sexually abused as children.

Other research has not confirmed this suggested causal connection (Connors & Morse, 1993; Pope & Hudson, 1992). It should be noted that childhood sexual abuse is associated with a number of diagnostic categories, and that the experience of abuse is a general variable, making it difficult to establish a definite causal link between physical or sexual abuse and the eating disorders.

Sociocultural factors

As mentioned earlier in this chapter, the eating disorders are unique in that they are found most often among one of the most specific population groups, i.e. middle- and upper-class young females from industrialised settings. The specific nature of the population diagnosed with these disorders is thought to have aetiological implications. Aspects of these aetiological implications will be discussed in the following section.

Sociocultural ideals for physical beauty

The increased incidence of the eating disorders in industrialised settings has been associated with other sociocultural developments in these contexts. Among other aspects, the role of women in society has been changing at the same time as the incidence of the eating disorders has increased. This will be discussed further in the following section.

In industrialised settings, a preoccupation with thinness has emerged and the ideal for beauty has become increasingly thin over time. There has been an emergence of an entire industry associated with dieting and weight loss (and health and fitness), and all of these aspects have been developing against the background of a population that has been becoming increasingly heavy (Brownell & Fairburn, 1995). Fortunately, however, there are indications that women's striving towards an unrealistically thin body ideal has begun to abate in recent years (Cash, Morrow, Hrabosky, & Perry, 2004).

Ideals for beauty do not apply only to females. An increasing drive for muscularity in men has been identified as impacting on adolescent boys. Exposure to sports, health, and fitness magazines in adolescent boys, together with critical body-image processing and social comparisons, have been identified as predictors for body-image disturbances and eating disturbances in adolescent males (Botta, 2003)

The tension between the cultural ideal and the actual body shape and size of the population has steadily increased as the ideal has become thinner and the population bigger. The human species has been becoming bigger in terms of weight and height over a number of centuries. Coupled with better nutrition and availability of food, and a less active life style, the average American female (aged 17–24 years) became 3 kg heavier between 1960 and the early 1980s (Bureau of Census, 1983). The prevalence of obesity in American society has doubled since 1900, with 20%–30% of the population being overweight in the mid-1980s (Killen et al., 1986). By 2004, this rate had reached 32.2% (Ogden et al., 2006).

Research focusing on the media found that comparisons between ideals for feminine beauty have shown a steady decrease in size since the 1950s. Compare the iconic Marilyn Monroe with current film stars, for instance (Brownell, 1991). Various studies have investigated the feminine ideal by comparing shifts in the size of the women featured in *Playboy* centrefolds (Wiseman, Gray, Mosimann, & Arhens, 1992) and beauty pageant contestants (Moser, 1989). This trend towards thinness continued into the 2000s (Seifert, 2005).

Other studies have recorded the number of weight-loss and diet-related articles in women's magazines and have found steady increases in the number of these articles while the cultural ideal has been becoming thinner. Some studies indicate that this tendency may have levelled off, but body-image dissatisfaction appears to continue to increase (Garner, 1997; Paquette, & Raine, 2004). However, it is clear that the media plays a role in the transmission of the cultural standards of ideal beauty and in the promotion of thinness (Bessenhof, 2006; Botta, 2003, 2006; Vaughan & Fouts, 2003).

As suggested above, one of the effects of the tension between the cultural ideal and the actual increase in body size has been women's dissatisfaction with their own bodies. Killen et al. (1986) found that one-third of normal tenth-grade girls saw themselves as fat (even when they were not). By 1999, 44% of American women were on a diet (Serdula et al., 1999). Research by Fallon and Rozin (1985) indicates that women tend to assume that the body shape most attractive to the opposite sex is much thinner than the weight which males actually considered to be most attractive. In addition, they tended to view their own current size as much heavier than the most attractive or the ideal. Other studies mirrored the tendency in women to overestimate their own body size (Thompson, 1986). By 1988, a survey of 2000 women found that they wished to weigh about 4.5 kg less than their actual body weight (Drewnowski, Yee, & Krahn, 1988).

Emerging research demonstrates that children as young as five years old experience anxiety about their bodies and want to be thinner (Andrist, 2003). Bessenhof (2006) found that exposure to thin-ideal advertisements was associated with increased body dissatisfaction, negative moods, and depression, as well as lower self-esteem in female undergraduates, confirming the link between the cultural ideal, the media, and body-image dissatisfaction. Similarly, a study investigating the relationships between mass media, self-esteem, body-image, and tendencies to disordered eating found that greater exposure to fashion and beauty magazines was related to overall dissatisfaction with appearance and greater eating disorder tendencies in females (Kim & Lennon, 2007).

A type of media exposure that is enjoying increasing attention from researchers is the rise of Internet websites that promote Anorexia (so-called 'pro-Ana' sites). Sites that promote Bulimia (pro-Mia sites) are not as numerous, but can also be found in cyberspace. These types of Internet sites provide social support for beliefs and behaviours that generally would be considered unacceptable. Examples of similar 'extreme communities' also include pro-suicide and pro-amputation groups (Bell, 2007).

BOX 11.1 'THE THIN COMMANDMENTS'

1. If you aren't thin, than you aren't attractive.
2. Being thin is more important than being healthy.
3. You must buy clothes, cut your hair, take laxatives, starve yourself, and do anything to make yourself look thinner.
4. Thou shall not eat without feeling guilty.
5. Thou shall not eat fattening food without punishing thyself afterwards.
6. Thou shall count calories and restrict intake accordingly.
7. What the scale says is the most important thing.
8. Losing weight is good; gaining weight is bad.
9. You can never be too thin.
10. Being thin and not eating are signs of true willpower and success.

Discussion: The 'Thin Commandments' are published on many of the pro-Ana websites and are well known in the extreme communities that regard Anorexia Nervosa and Bulimia Nervosa as lifestyle choices rather psychological disorders. Discuss.

Pro-Ana websites typically share 'tips and tricks' for weight loss, 'thinspiration' (quotes and photos that are motivation for weight loss), as well as lifestyle descriptions and advice on concealing symptoms (Harshbarger, Ahlers-Schmidt, Mayans, Mayans, & Hawkins, 2009; Norris, Boydell, Pinhas, & Katzman, 2006). Some of the common themes of the pro-Ana websites are concerned with control, success, and perfection (Harshbarger et al., 2009). The Internet has significant global reach and young people are most likely to be Internet users. Considering the typical age of onset of Anorexia Nervosa, the phenomenon of pro-Ana (and pro-Mia) websites begs further investigation. Some researchers suggest that clinicians use pro-Ana sites to develop a greater empathy for and understanding of clients and patients with a diagnosis of Anorexia Nervosa (Overbeke, 2008).

BOX 11.2 EXAMPLES OF 'HINTS AND TIPS' FROM PRO-ANA WEBSITES

- Brush your teeth constantly so you won't be tempted to eat.
- Put a rubber band around your wrist. Snap it when you feel like eating 'bad' food.
- Clean something gross (toilet, litter box, boyfriend's closet) when you want to eat. You will not want to eat after cleaning a litter box.
- Keep your hair in good condition so no one will suspect anything.
- Get a job so you'll have to work through mealtimes.
- You don't want food! Food is disgusting, and if you eat it now, you WILL regret it later. You're not even hungry! Don't give in. All it will do is make you bigger and further away from your goal weight. You want to be skinny and beautiful, don't you?

Source: Pro ana tips & tricks, n.d.

In terms of commerce, the diet industry (selling medication, books, and special foods) has blossomed in relation to the changes in cultural ideals. Similarly, the related health-and-fitness industry has expanded exponentially. The diet industry alone was estimated in the early 1990s to be have been worth about $30 billion per year (about the same amount as the US government budget for education, training, social services, and employment at that time) (Brownell & Rodin, 1994).

One of the factors associated with the sociocultural value placed on thinness is the meaning attributed to being 'fat' in industrialised societies. 'Fat' is associated with being 'lazy', being 'unsuccessful', and having little self-control. In a study by Silverstein and Perdue (1988), women tended to equate thinness not only with attractiveness, but also with intelligence and professional success. This aspect comes into play when the changing role of women in society is considered.

Gender and the eating disorders

Women appear to internalise the societal ideal of thinness to a greater extent than do men. Evidence exists that physical attractiveness is at the centre of the female sex-role stereotype. This is not the case for the masculine sex-role stereotype. This may be one aspect that explains the fact that fewer males are diagnosed with an eating disorder (Meyer, Blisset, & Oldfield, 2001). Also, males who endorse feminine sex-role characteristics are at greater risk for developing an eating disorder. This is also true for the gay community, where greater emphasis is placed on physical attractiveness (Meyer et al., 2001). In addition, Western cultural norms (that have a greater impact on females) associate more positive attributes (unrelated to body size) with a slim figure. These norms dictate that 'fat' is 'ugly' and 'bad', while 'thin' is 'beautiful', and beautiful is 'good' (Wenar & Kerig, 2006).

On the other hand, the ideal body-image portrayed in the media for males emphasises an increasingly muscular appearance. Men may typically strive for more body mass, whereas women attempt to attain thinness (Harvey & Robinson, 2003). While males who experience body dissatisfaction may attempt to exercise weight control, they are also likely to utilise muscle development behaviours such as exercise and the use of anabolic steroids and untested dietary supplements as body change strategies (Labre, 2002). The interplay between body-image, disturbance in body-image, and body change strategies is probably different in males. Increased research and clinical attention directed to disordered body change strategies in males may well result in additional eating disorder diagnoses in future DSM editions.

Some authors suggest that the increased incidence of eating disorders in the latter half of the twentieth century is associated with the changing role of women in Western society (Bemporad, 1997). Traditionally, women were expected to be compliant, unassertive, and respectful (Miller & Pumariega, 2001). Changes in society have resulted in greater opportunities for women, but also in greater demands. These demands are often in conflict with traditional role demands. Women now have to juggle pressures to conform with pressures to compete (Miller & Pumariega, 2001). Examples of these pressures are expectations from professional roles, nurturing demands, and social expectations (Halmi, 2000). Dieting and the eating disorders may represent one way in which women respond to the conflicting demands of success and attractiveness (Miller & Pumariega, 2001). Feminist views on the eating disorders can be summarised in the following four hypotheses:

- Thinness may be a way to attempt to balance demands between traditional femininity and achievement, as discussed above.
- Western patriarchal society may oppress women through a culture of thinness (Miller & Pumariega, 2001). More militant feminist authors have criticised the diet industry as a male strategy to ensure the continued oppression of women (Wolf, 1990). As long as women are starving themselves and are expending their energies on their appearance, they represent no real threat to male power.
- Weight may represent power and control for women. It may constitute the one aspect of their lives that is within their control (Miller & Pumariega, 2001).
- Weight and eating disorders may represent a way for women to establish their own identities and self-definition by using their bodies. The roles of woman as wife and mother are devalued by Western society. This may create a situation where women use dieting and weight loss as a means to define an identity (Miller & Pumariega, 2001).

The feminist theories summarised above can be integrated with transcultural theories. In this view, the changing roles of women in Western society represent an example of 'straddling two worlds'. Other examples of this are groups in which acculturation takes place, such as immigrant groups. Research findings of increased incidence of the eating disorders in such groups lend some support to the idea that a situation of cultural change or conflict creates a breeding ground for the eating disorders (Miller & Pumariega, 2001).

A significant aspect of the relationship between gender and the eating disorders is the developmental view. The developmental demands of adolescence (the resolution of issues pertaining to identity, sexuality, achievement, and independence) were discussed in a previous section. These developmental demands intersect with gender in the case of young girls. An increase in body fat due to puberty occurs at a time when attractiveness, popularity, and success become more important to them. If self-worth becomes equated with physical appearance, a preoccupation with weight and dieting may develop (Strober, 1995).

It appears that a preoccupation with thinness emerges in early adolescence in young girls, with some research indicating that many girls between the ages of 10 and 15 years wished for a thinner body shape, but did not report significant body dissatisfaction, and did not regard themselves as fat (Cohn et al., 1987). By their early twenties, women's standards of thinness were much higher than those of young girls, suggesting that the desire to be thin becomes firmly established in women as they move from adolescence to adulthood (Walsh & Devlin, 1998).

CROSS-CULTURAL PERSPECTIVES

Cultural beliefs and attitudes are significant contributing factors in the development of eating disorders, as is social class. Prevalence rates of eating disorders vary among racial or ethnic groups and nationalities. These rates also shift as cultures undergo changes. Eating disorders appear to be prevalent across a greater variety of cultural groups than was believed in the past (Miller & Pumarierga, 2001).

As discussed in the previous section, cultural change itself may be associated with increased risk for developing eating disorders, particularly when values related to physical attractiveness are affected. This change may occur over time within a specific society or may take place within an individual when an immigrant moves to a new culture (Miller & Pumarierga, 2001).

Race and social class previously appeared to be very strongly associated with the incidence of eating disorders. In the United States, eating disorders have traditionally been less prevalent among African Americans, as well as among ethnic minority groups (Miller & Pumarierga, 2001). Thus, the incidence in white American girls is eight times that in their counterparts of other races (Dolan, 1991). Recent research, however, suggests a trend among African Americans towards an increased risk for eating disorders, as well as among young females in other ethnic minority groups.

One hypothesis to explain this trend is that thinness is gaining more value within African-American culture (Hsu, 1987). It also appears that the cultural beliefs that may have served as protective factors lose their potency as teenagers experience pressure to move towards mainstream American culture (Miller & Pumarierga, 2001). Research done in the United States suggests that recent immigrants may be at particular risk for eating disorders. It has been hypothesised that the stress of experiencing a culture clash may trigger the development of an eating disorder (Kope & Sack, 1989).

Outside the United States, some studies suggest that the prevalence of eating disorders is not significant in cultures where the ideal for attractiveness places less emphasis on being thin (Furnham & Baguma, 1994). In many non-Western societies, plumpness is associated with prosperity, success, and fertility, and is regarded as attractive. In these cultures, eating disorders are less prevalent than in Western-oriented countries, which appear to have prevalence rates comparable to those of the United States (Miller & Pumarierga, 2001).

This picture appears to be changing, however. During the 1990s, reports of the increasing presence of eating disorders in the developing world emerged (Rittenbaugh, Shisslak, & Prince, 1992). Outside the United States, research also suggests that women who move from a culture where thinness is not valued to a culture where it is are at greater risk of developing an eating disorder (Yates, 1989).

In addition to the impact of culture and cultural transition, class differences in the incidence of eating disorders appear to be diminishing (Root, 1990). Some recent studies have not supported the link between social class and the eating disorders (Wenar & Kerig, 2006). Indeed, epidemiological surveys do not show a greater distribution of the eating disorders among the upper classes, as was initially thought (Kaplan et al., 1994)

The eating disorders clearly have important variations in their incidence and patterns. Our knowledge of the role of culture remains unclear and is not supported by adequate empirical evidence. The study of the cultural variations, however, may hold one of the keys to understanding the aetiology of these disorders (King, 1993). The South African context, which can be regarded as a microcosm involving all the variables above, will be considered in the following section.

South African perspective

As suggested in the introductory section, international research indicates an increase in the prevalence of eating disorders, with between 1% (Anorexia Nervosa) and 1%–4% (Bulimia Nervosa) of young women being affected. In the South African context, it is to be expected that similar rates will occur amongst young women of settler descent. However, as suggested in the previous section, research has been emerging both locally and internationally that implies that ethnic groups, age groups, and social classes, other than the white, middle-class, young females traditionally associated with the eating disorders, are also at risk (Dirks, 2001).

Eating disorders have been described in South Africa since the 1970s (Norris, 1979); however, early descriptions related only to white females. In 1995, the first descriptions emerged of eating disorders in black females in South Africa (Szabo, 1999; Szabo, Berk, Tlou, & Allwood, 1995). Subsequent cross-cultural community-based studies of eating attitudes, and behaviours associated with eating disorders, were conducted in mainly urban settings. Eating disorder pathology was found in South African women from a range of ethnic backgrounds (Wassenaar, Le Grange, Winship, & Lachenicht, 2000). In a student population, black students scored significantly higher than other ethnic groups on measures of the presence and severity of eating disorder pathology (Le Grange, Telch, & Tibbs, 1998).

In 2001, eating attitudes were surveyed in a sample of South African schoolgirls from different ethnic backgrounds, who were drawn from five schools in the greater Cape Town area. Findings suggested equal prevalence of disordered attitudes towards eating in schoolgirls from different ethnic backgrounds, although white girls reported greater concerns about body image (Caradas, Lambert, & Charlton, 2001). In summary, these findings implied that prevalence of eating disorders among the black community was on the increase and that eating disorders in other communities would emerge to the same extent as in the white ('settler') community (Szabo & Allwood, 2004).

Indeed, it appears that increasing numbers of black women have presented for treatment of eating disorders, although these numbers have not reached equivalence with those presenting for treatment from the white community (Szabo & Allwood, 2004). Other surveys have indicated that disordered eating is equally common among black female students and white female students (Le Grange, Louw, Breen, & Katzman, 2004).

Body-image dissatisfaction is closely linked to the eating disorders. A South African investigation of body-image satisfaction among black female students found that the majority of participants were satisfied with their body-image. However, a minority of participants were dissatisfied with their body-image and reported engaging in pathological eating behaviours (Mwaba & Roman, 2009).

A recent study was conducted by Mould, Grobler, Odendaal, and Jager (2011) of the ethnic differences in age of onset and prevalence of disordered eating attitudes and behaviours among girls in a South African school. This research found no differences between white and black schoolgirls on measures of disordered eating attitudes and behaviours between Grades four and six. In Grades seven to nine, no differences were found, with the notable exception that black students reporting more Bulimia-associated behaviours than white students. Ethnic differences in Bulimia-associated behaviours disappeared in Grades ten to twelve, with white students emerging with significantly higher drives for thinness, body-image dissatisfaction, and poorer eating attitudes than black students. The Bulimia scale was the only scale that did not indicate a significant difference between the two groups in Grades ten to twelve. The findings of this study have implications for the development of prevention and early intervention programs in the South African context (Mould et al., 2011).

Goedeke et al. (2006) describe South Africa as a country in the process of epidemiological transition, comparable to Mexico and some South American countries. These authors acknowledge that public health issues such as HIV/AIDS prevention and treatment and the health problems associated with undernutrition and poverty are pressing difficulties facing South Africa. However, obesity and its associated consequences for health negatively affect the lives of many South Africans and add to health care expenses, both in the private and public sectors. These authors reviewed the available South African research on obesity and concluded that obesity is increasing in prevalence in all population sectors in South Africa, but especially among children and urbanised black women. These authors recommend the development and implementation of culturally specific prevention programmes aimed at changing the dietary and behavioural aspects associated with obesity in South African women and children.

Interestingly, the rural-urban distinction emerges as a significant factor mediating risk for the eating disorders and for obesity. In the South African context, urban females have an increased risk for developing both obesity and an eating disorder. Furthermore, in terms of the distinction between urban and rural populations in the South African setting, lower prevalence of abnormal eating attitudes was found in rural settings, implying a lower risk for eating disorders. It must be pointed out that risk was nonetheless found in rural settings (Szabo & Allwood, 2004).

Further cross-cultural research into the body-figure preference in South African female adolescents confirmed the distinction between rural and urban populations, with both white and black respondents in urban areas expressing the desire to be smaller, while significantly fewer rural respondents desired to be smaller (Szabo & Allwood, 2004). It also seems that the meaning of 'self-starvation' and its related symptoms may differ for young black females in impoverished circumstances. This emphasises the need for care when conducting cross-cultural research, since a variety of culturally related aspects may change the meaning of standard measures (Le Grange et al., 2004).

Intriguing research done in the United States on the cultural differences in Expressed Emotion (EE) between white and ethnic minority families has found no significant differences, implying that white families and families from other cultural backgrounds may share a number of similarities when it comes to the eating disorders (Hoste & le Grange, 2008). A South African study similarly found no significant differences in clinical presentation or reported symptoms between white and black participants in a hospital setting. These findings are representative of an increasing body of research suggesting that there are more similarities than differences between patients from different ethnic groups when it comes to the eating disorders (Delport & Szabo, 2008).

As suggested at the beginning of this section, it does appear that in the South African context, as in the rest of the world, indications are emerging that challenge the notion of eating disorders as a mainly Western, white phenomenon. Thus, the risk of eating disorders in developing societies like South Africa appears to be increasing. The South African context provides a backdrop of rapid and dramatic political and social change for the emergence of eating disorders in black, urban females (Szabo & Allwood, 2004).

CONCLUSION

The eating disorders present us with a puzzling and intriguing aspect of human behaviour. This chapter discussed the variety of disorders that can impact on an aspect of our lives that is essential to our survival, namely eating. The eating disorders represent a divergent range of aetiological factors. The aetiological factors associated with the eating disorders are impacted by human genetics and human development, as well as by human culture and society. These factors play out in the arena of the human body and are further complicated by the constant flux of society and culture.

The eating disorders and obesity represent great costs to individuals and families in terms of distress and suffering, and great costs to society in terms of lost potential. Indeed, the eating disorder mortality rate (especially Anorexia Nervosa), is the highest for any psychological disorder (Keel et al., 2003). Obesity (which is not currently a psychological disorder) is associated with high rates of morbidity and lower quality of life (Neumark-Stainer & Haines, 2004). The potential threat to human life associated with the eating disorders and obesity implies that these disorders and conditions warrant continued attention and awareness.

MULTIPLE-CHOICE QUESTIONS

1. What does 'Bulimia Nervosa' mean?
   a) ox hunger
   b) nervous loss of appetite
   c) nervousness or fear of fat
   d) split mind

2. Which of the following is the central feature of the eating disorders?
   a) fear of becoming fat
   b) significant and steady weight loss
   c) unrealistically negative body-image
   d) severe restriction of kilojoule intake

3. Which Family Systems theorist made a significant contribution to our understanding of Anorexia Nervosa?
   a) Satir
   b) Bruch
   c) Szabo
   d) Minuchin

4. Which South African researcher first described Anorexia Nervosa among black South African women?
   a) Satir
   b) Bruch
   c) Szabo
   d) Minuchin

5 The main symptom of Anorexia Nervosa is:
   a) refusal to maintain body weight
   b) food restriction
   c) binging and purging
   d) binging and compensating

6. The 'typical' anorexic family is:
   a) successful and hard driving
   b) chaotic
   c) warm and caring
   d) unconcerned about appearances

7. The age, culture, and gender features of the eating disorders are significant because:
   a) they are so variable and diverse
   b) in the eating disorders, these factors are not suggestive of aetiology
   c) they come together in an obviously significant way
   d) the age, culture, and gender features are non-specific

8. Mothers of daughters diagnosed with Anorexia Nervosa are more likely to be:
   a) obese
   b) focussed on their own careers
   c) emotionally distant and uninvolved
   d) on diet themselves

PARAGRAPH AND ESSAY QUESTIONS

1. Describe the age, culture, and gender features of the eating disorders. Comment on the significance of these features.

2. The courses of Anorexia Nervosa and Bulimia Nervosa are characterised by high 'crossover' between the disorders. Discuss this statement.

3. Discuss some of the causative factors of the eating disorders including genetic influences, neurotransmitter imbalances, and psychological stressors.

4. ProAna and ProMia websites promote Anorexia Nervosa and Bulimia Nervosa as lifestyle choices. Discuss the arguments for and against this point of view.

12 PERSONALITY DISORDERS

Beate von Krosigk

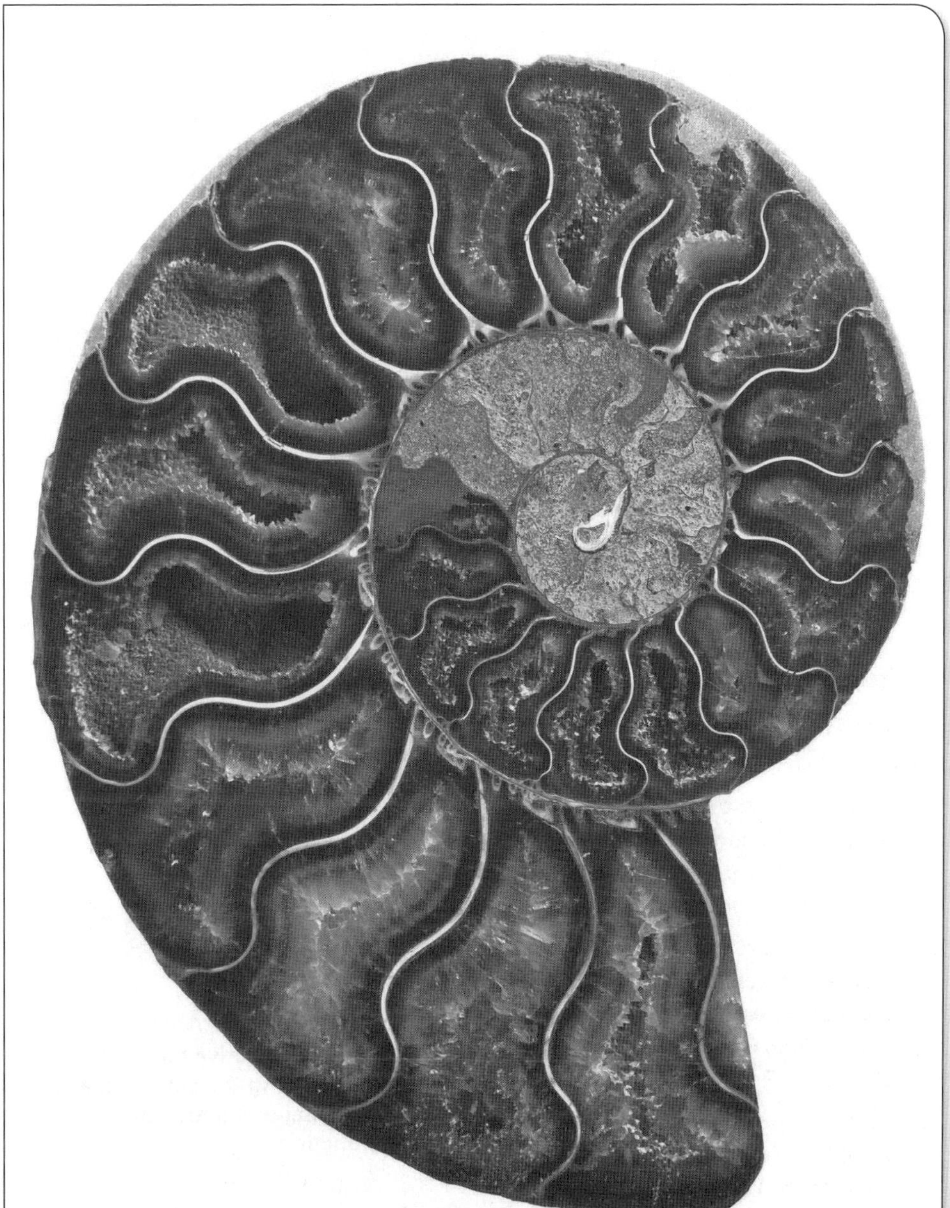

12 CHAPTER OUTLINE

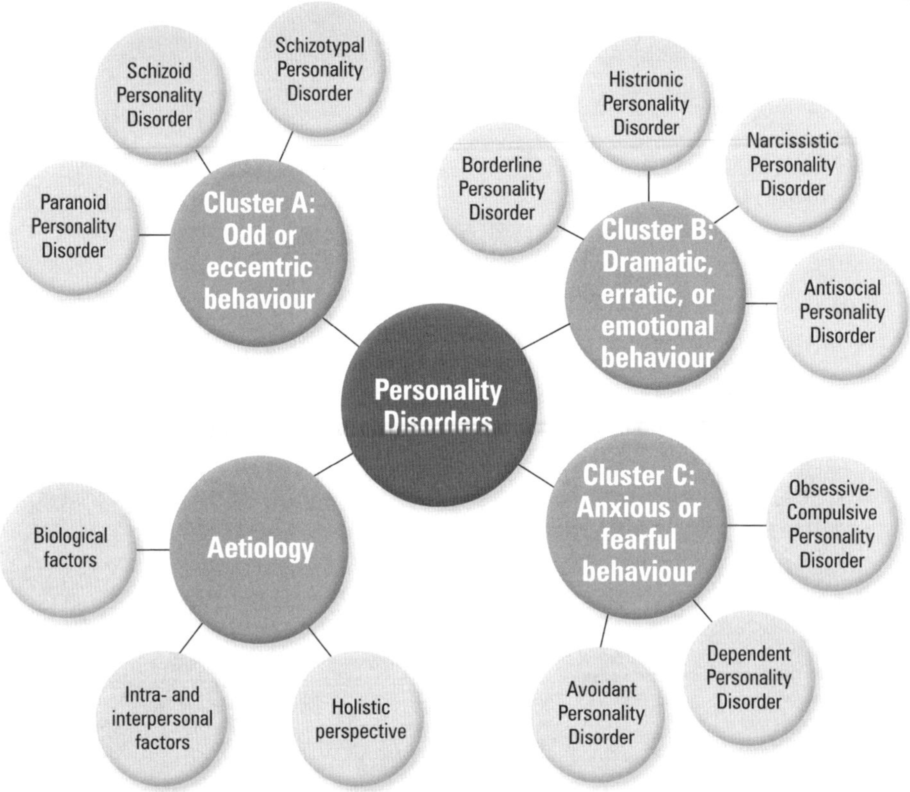

LEARNING OUTCOMES

After studying this chapter, you should be able to:

- Describe the personality disorders according to the *Diagnostic and Statistical Manual of Mental Disorders* (DSM-5) and the *International Classification of Diseases* (ICD-10).
- Demonstrate an understanding of the problems with regard to diagnosing personality disorders.
- Demonstrate an understanding for the high degree of overlap between the personality disorders.
- Describe the clinical pictures of the different personality disorders.
- Identify the main aetiological factors for the different personality disorders.

INTRODUCTION

It is thought that each of us has a unique personality made up of traits that come from both our genetic make-up and our life experiences; our personality is a vital part of what makes us who we are and how we interact with others. A person is known through their personality. Personality traits are the characteristics that distinguish someone from others. These characteristics include how a person thinks, feels, behaves, and relates to their environment. When someone's traits are rigid, not adaptive to new situations, and cause significant difficulty in their work and social life, then that individual may have a personality disorder.

Someone may be diagnosed as having a personality disorder if their pattern of behaviour, mood, social interaction, or impulsiveness causes distress to them, or to other people in their lives. Many of these behaviours can cause severe disturbance in the individual's personal and work life. In general, individuals with personality disorders may have difficulty sustaining close or intimate relationships. They may experience chronic interpersonal problems, or have difficulties in establishing a coherent sense of self or identity. Others may perceive them to be impulsive, irritable, fearful, demanding, hostile, manipulative, or even violent. Problem alcohol or substance use, mood disorders, certain anxiety or eating disorders, self-harm, suicidal thoughts or attempts, and sexual problems often accompany personality disorders.

In order to understand personality disorders, we have to start with a definition of personality. This, in itself, is problematic as it is extremely difficult to define something as complex as personality. For the purposes of this chapter, we will adopt the definition of personality as formulated by Larsen and Buss (2002, p. 4), who state that personality 'is the set of psychological traits and mechanisms within the individual that are organised and relatively enduring and that influence his or her interactions with, and adaptation to, the environment (including the intrapsychic, physical, and social environment)'. The elements of this definition can be described briefly as follows (Larsen & Buss, 2002):

- ***Psychological traits:*** These are the characteristics that describe the way in which people are different from each other and which include aspects such as values, attitudes, motives, styles, sentiments, beliefs, and goals.

- ***Psychological mechanisms:*** The processes of personality include three essential aspects: inputs, decisions, and outputs. Inputs refer to perception and perceptual biases, that is, people differ in terms of the information that they are sensitive to (input). This information influences the cognitive interpretation of the environment (decisions), which in turn influences the person's behaviour (output).
- ***Within the individual:*** According to Larsen and Buss (2002), personality is 'something' that people typically carry with themselves over time from one situation to the next; thus personality refers to the stability and consistency of a person.
- ***Organisation:*** The psychological traits and mechanisms are not a random collection of elements; rather, they form a coherent whole because the traits and mechanisms are interlinked in an organised way. The personality is organised in the sense that it contains decision rules which determine which traits are activated in given circumstances.
- ***Influence:*** Personality traits and mechanisms influence people's behaviour, self-image, moods, interpersonal relationships, and goals, as well as their selection of, and adaptation to, their environments.
- ***Person–environment interaction:*** Interactions with the environment include perception (how a person interprets the environment), selection (the manner in which a person chooses situations, e.g. friends, hobbies, careers, etc.), evocations (the reactions a person elicits from, or produces in, others), and manipulations (the way in which people attempt to influence others).
- ***Adaptation:*** Adaptive functioning refers to the way in which people accomplish their goals, as well as the way in which they adjust to, and deal with, life challenges.
- ***Environment:*** This refers to a person's physical, social, and intrapsychic environments. All these environments, individually and collectively, pose challenges to people on a continuous basis.

Because of how fundamental personality is to people's functioning in the world, one can assume that if a person's personality is deemed to be 'disordered', it would imply a relatively pervasive disorder. The DSM-5 (American Psychiatric Association, 2013, p. 645) defines personality disorders 'as enduring patterns of perceiving, relating to, and thinking about the environment and oneself that are exhibited in a wide range of social and personal contexts and are inflexible and maladaptive, and cause significant functional impairment or subjective distress'.

We can expect that a person who is considered to have a personality disorder to experience difficulties in the following areas:

- Self-image
- Relationships with others
- Understanding themselves, others, and the environment
- Impulse control.

Many people may display certain symptoms of a personality disorder; however, it is only individuals who demonstrate enduring personality traits and difficulties as described above who can be diagnosed with a personality disorder. According to the DSM-5 (American Psychiatric Association, 2013) and ICD-10 (World Health Organisation, 1992), people can be diagnosed with a personality disorder only if they fulfill certain general criteria (see Table 12.1).

When deciding whether or not a person has a personality disorder, it is imperative to keep two aspects in mind: firstly, one has to compare the person's behaviour to cultural norms and, secondly, one has to decide whether the behaviour is extreme enough to warrant such a diagnosis. In terms of extreme behaviour, the judgement is not always clear as many personality disorders are an extreme form of a personality style (see Table 12.4.). It is only once a personality style becomes pervasive and extreme that one can consider a diagnosis of a personality disorder.

Table 12.1: General symptoms of personality disorders as adapted from the DSM-5 and ICD-10

DSM-5	ICD-10
A. An enduring pattern of inner experience and behaviour that deviates markedly from the expectations of the individual's culture. The pattern is manifested in two (or more) of the following areas: (1) Cognition (i.e. ways of perceiving and interpreting self, other people, and events). (2) Affectivity (i.e. the range, intensity, lability, and appropriateness of emotional response). (3) Interpersonal functioning. (4) Impulse control. B. The enduring pattern is inflexible and pervasive across a broad range of personal and social situations. C. The enduring pattern leads to clinically significant distress or impairment in social, occupational, or other important areas of functioning.	• A personality disorder is a severe disturbance in the characterological constitution and behavioural tendencies of the individual, usually involving several areas of the personality, and nearly always associated with considerable personal and social disruption. A personality disorder tends to appear in late childhood or adolescence and continues to be manifest into adulthood. It is therefore unlikely that the diagnosis of a personality disorder will be appropriate before the age of 16 or 17 years. General diagnostic guidelines applying to all personality disorders are that the condition is not directly attributable to gross brain damage or disease, or to another psychiatric disorder, meeting the following criteria: ▸ Markedly disharmonious attitudes and behaviour, usually involving several areas of functioning, e.g. affectivity, arousal, impulse control, ways of perceiving and thinking, and style of relating to others. ▸ The abnormal behaviour pattern is enduring, of long standing, and not limited to episodes of mental illness. ▸ The abnormal behaviour pattern is pervasive and clearly maladaptive to a broad range of personal and social situations. ▸ The above manifestations always appear during childhood or adolescence and continue into adulthood. ▸ The disorder leads to considerable personal distress but this may only become apparent late in its course. The disorder is usually, but not invariably, associated with significant problems in occupational and social performance.

DSM-5	ICD-10
	• For different cultures it may be necessary to develop specific sets of criteria with regard to social norms, rules, and obligations. For diagnosing most of the subtypes, clear evidence is usually required of the presence of at least three of the traits or behaviours given in the clinical description.

Source: Reprinted with permission from the Diagnostic and Statistical Manual of Mental Disorders (DSM), Fifth Edition, American Psychiatric Association (APA), 2013 and ICD-10 Classification of Mental and Behavioural Disorders: Diagnostic Criteria for Research, World Health Organisation (WHO), Geneva, 2007.

The prevalence of personality disorders may vary according to the specific type of disorder. It is estimated that 9.1% of the general population would meet the criteria for a personality disorder. The prevalence rates of the different clusters of personality disorders differ, e.g. 5.7% for disorders in Cluster A, 1.5% for disorders in Cluster B and 6% for disorders in Cluster C (American Psychiatric Association, 2013). It is, however, difficult to establish the exact prevalence of personality disorders in the general population as these disorders rarely present to psychiatric and psychological services in isolation. In addition, they are frequently associated with alterations of eating behaviour, and alcohol and substance abuse, as well as other mental disorders, antisocial behaviour, and sexual promiscuity.

BOX 12.1: MYTHS ABOUT PERSONALITY DISORDERS

It is commonly believed that people with personality disorders are dangerous. This is probably due to the fact that the term psychopath is often wrongly ascribed to criminals. Board and Fritzon (2005) found in their study of senior business managers that so-called 'psychopaths' can and do function quite effectively in mainstream society. After subjecting the managers to a variety of psychometric tests (e.g. the MMPI), she found evidence of three personality disorder profiles:

- Histrionic Personality Disorder: including superficial charm, insincerity, egocentricity, and manipulation.
- Narcissistic Personality Disorder: including grandiosity, self-focused lack of empathy for others, exploitativeness, and independence.
- Obsessive-Compulsive Personality Disorder: including perfectionism, excessive devotion to work, rigidity, stubbornness, and dictatorial tendencies.

When comparing these profiles to incarcerated criminals, she found that the above-mentioned profiles were more common in the managers than in the criminals, thereby dispelling the myth that all psychopaths are necessarily criminals.

HISTORY OF PERSONALITY DISORDERS

The category of personality disorders is one category in the DSM classification system which has undergone significant changes over the years. The changes can be summarised as follows (see Table 12.2):

- ***Changes in the names of the disorders:***
  - In DSM-I, there is reference to an Emotionally Unstable Personality Trait disturbance, which changed to a Hysterical Personality Disorder in DSM-II, which finally changed to a Histrionic Personality Disorder in DSM-III and DSM-IV and DSM-5.
  - The Obsessive-Compulsive Personality Disorder in DSM-5 was initially called a Compulsive Personality Disorder in DSM-I.
  - Antisocial and Dyssocial Personality Disorders in DSM-I have been called different disorders over the years, but are now known as Antisocial Personality Disorder in DSM-IV and DSM-5.

Table 12.2: History of DSM classification of personality disorders

DSM-I (1952)	DSM-II (1968)	DSM-III (1980)	DSM-IV (1994)
Personality Pattern Disturbance Inadequate Paranoid Cyclothymic Schizoid	Inadequate Paranoid Cyclothymic Schizoid	**Cluster A** Paranoid Schizoid Schizotypal	**Cluster A** Paranoid Schizoid Schizotypal
Personality Trait Disturbance Emotionally Unstable Passive-Aggressive: • Dependent type • Aggressive type Compulsive	Hysterical Passive-Aggressive Obsessive-Compulsive	**Cluster B** Histrionic Antisocial Borderline Narcissistic	**Cluster B** Histrionic Antisocial Borderline Narcissistic
Sociopathic Personality Disturbance Antisocial Dyssocial	Asthenic Antisocial Explosive	**Cluster C** Compulsive Avoidant Dependent Passive-Aggressive	**Cluster C** Obsessive-Compulsive Avoidant Dependent

- ***Termination of disorders:***
  - Inadequate Personality Disorder, first described in the DSM-I, was last used in the DSM-II.
  - Passive-Aggressive Personality Disorder was first described in the DSM-I, and appeared in the DSM-II, as well as in the DSM-III. Although it does not appear in the main text in DSM-IV, it was described in the appendix as a disorder that needed further investigation. This personality disorder has disappeared from the DSM altogether and is not mentioned or described in the DSM-5.
- ***Inclusion of new disorders:***
  - Schizotypal, Borderline, and Narcissistic Personality Disorders first appeared in the DSM-III.
  - In all likelihood, Depressive Personality Disorder will appear for the first time in DSM-5.
- ***Change from Axis II to Axis I:***
  - The Cyclothymic Personality Disorder that appeared in DSM-I and DSM-II was moved to Affective/Mood Disorders in DSM-III and still appears as such in the DSM-IV and DSM-IV-TR. This disorder is now described in the Bipolar and Related Disorders section of the DSM-5.
  - The Explosive Personality Disorder, as was described in DSM-II, was a variant of the Antisocial Personality Disorder as described in DSM-I, has subsequently been moved to the Impulse Control Disorders, and is currently referred to as the Intermittent Explosive Disorder.

Castillo (1998) argues that although there are many aetiological factors that are shared between personality disorders and other mental disorders, this notion is not reflected in the organisational system of the DSM. According to Castillo (1998), the DSM-IV made some strides towards a more postmodern way of classifying personality disorders, but this move was neither new, nor was it sufficient. This statement is based on the fact that, in both DSM-I and DSM-II, the distinction between different disorders was much more fluid. This is because the DSM-I and DSM-II were based on a psychodynamic paradigm which holds the view that mental illnesses exist on a continuum. The transition from DSM-II to DSM-III marked a change in the underlying paradigm in the DSM from a psychodynamic to a biopsychosocial paradigm, which was carried through to both the DSM-IV and the DSM-IV-TR. This shift had the following implications (Castillo, 1998):

- The spectrum, continuum, or dimensional approach to mental illnesses was mostly abandoned.
- Mental disorders were split into narrow disease entities, each with their own biological causes and narrowly defined symptoms.
- Disorders that were thought to be of a specific kind of pathology with no connection to personality development were placed on Axis I.
- Those disorders that were assumed to be the result of abnormal personality development were placed on Axis II.

It is important to note that although the spectrum, continuum, or dimensional approach fell out of use, the disorders that were assumed to be the result of abnormal personality development were provided a place on Axis II. These disorders can be seen as occurring along a continuum from normal to maladaptive variants of personality traits. The problem that arose was a practical diagnostic problem. Despite the fact that abnormal personality development is acknowledged as a dimensional process of change, it was diagnosed as a categorical disorder, similar to the way Axis I disorders were conceptualised and diagnosed, while the positive and negative changes of development during the course of childhood, adolescence, and early adulthood were ignored. Instead, personality functioning was classified as if it were a discrete category of a fixed abnormal personality style, rather than fluid, dimensional, continually evolving ways of being and becoming.

The fact that the diagnostic process was based on the paradigm of the biopsychosocial approach made this shift away from a dimensional approach even more bewildering, since biological evidence is often intermingled with psychoanalytic/dynamic interpretations within a single explanation of the behavioural aspects of a personality disorder. Since evidence and interpretations are qualitatively different from each other, and since the psychoanalytic/dynamic approach lacks empirical verification, interpretation of a character trait from the psychoanalytic/dynamic perspective should not be a part of an evidence-based diagnostic syndrome required for diagnosing a specific personality disorder. The process of identifying a cluster of specific symptoms (syndrome) together with a certain way of personality functioning that can be recognised as a personality disorder according to the DSM-IV-TR classification system on Axis II was therefore much more difficult than was initially assumed.

The DSM-5 introduced a number of paradigmatic and structural changes which impacted on the classification and description of personality disorders in a number of ways. In previous editions of the DSM, a multi-axial diagnostic system was used where a distinction was made between "Clinical Disorders" (Axis I) and "Personality Disorder" (Axis II). In the DSM-5 there is no longer a distinction between Axis I and Axis II disorders, with the result that Personality Disorders are coded as any other disorder. DSM-5 recognises the complexity of these disorders by adopting three different approaches (See Figure 12.1) to classifying and describing these disorders, i.e.:

- Noting some of the Personality Disorders in the categories where they fit best etiologically. Schizotypal Personality Disorder is noted in the category of Schizophrenia Spectrum Disorders, and Antisocial Personality Disorder in the Disruptive, Impulse-Control, and Conduct Disorder category.
- The "traditional" categorical description in the Personality Disorder section where the personality disorders are grouped together in three clusters and described in terms of their clinical pictures.
- A trait approach where personality disorders are described in terms of personality functioning and pathological personality traits (APA, 2013).

Figure 12.1: Summary of different approaches and types of Personality disorders according to the DSM-5

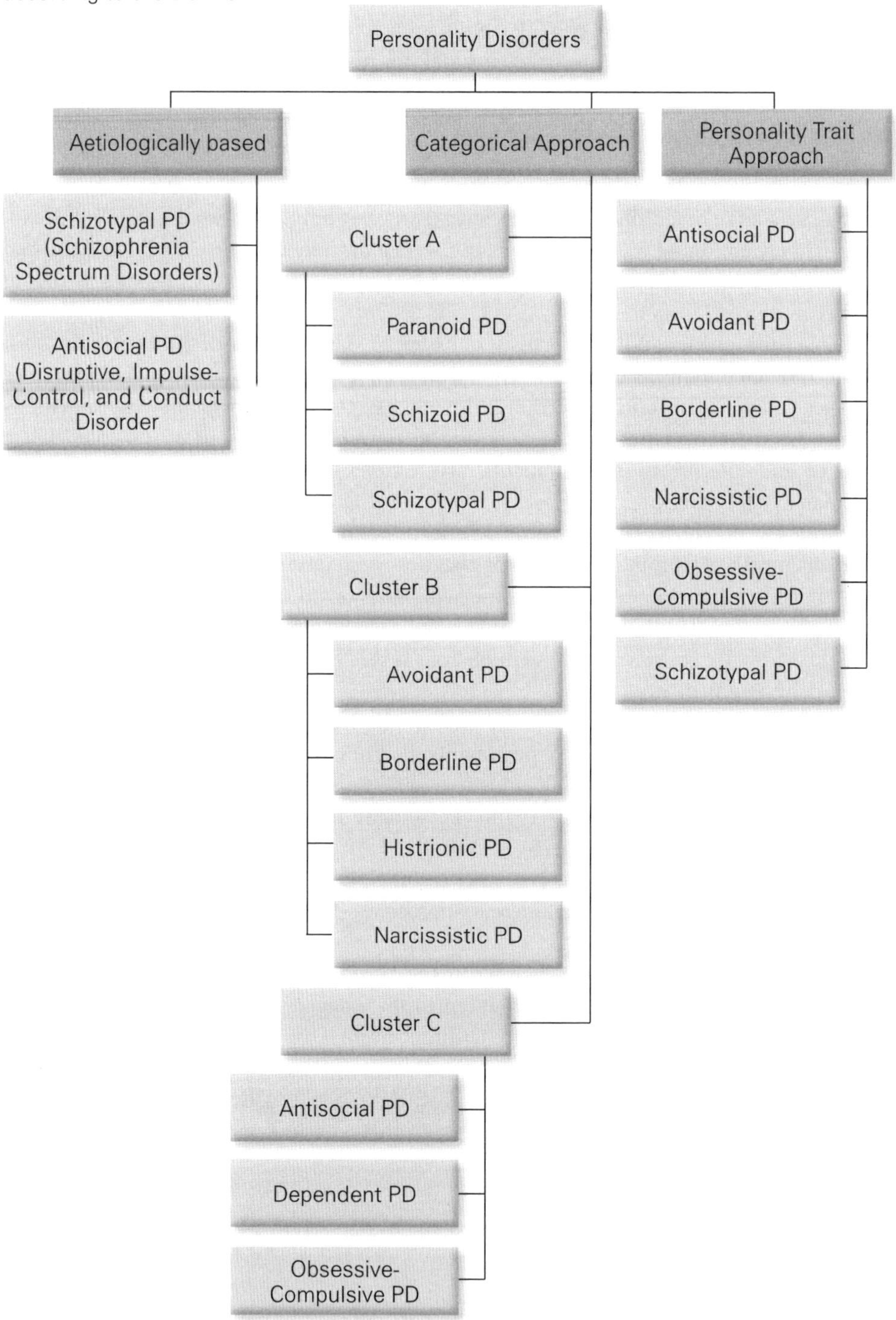

Source: Diagnostic and Statistical Manual of Mental Disorders (DSM), Fifth Edition, American Psychiatric Association (APA), 2013.

CLINICAL PICTURE

In general, patients with personality disorders have wide-ranging problems in social relationships and mood regulation. These problems have usually been present throughout their adolescent and adult lives (see Table 12.1). These patients' patterns of perception, thought, and behavioural responses are fixed and inflexible, although their behaviour is often unpredictable. These patterns deviate markedly from their specific culture's expectations. To meet the DSM-5 threshold for making a clinical diagnosis, the pattern of symptoms (syndrome) must result in clinically significant distress or impairment in social, occupational, or other important areas of functioning. Note that the disorder should occur in all settings (e.g. social as well as occupational) and is not limited to one sphere of activity.

The abovementioned general criteria for identifying personality functioning as a possible personality disorder need to be supplemented by another set of diagnostic criteria for each specific personality disorder in order to make a valid clinical diagnosis for a specific personality disorder. Both sets, general and specific, of DSM-5 diagnostic criteria need to be taken into account when the individual's syndrome is compared to the number of required criteria to reach the threshold for making a diagnosis. However, that process is also fraught with difficulties. According to Meyerson et al. (2009, in Phend, 2009), making a diagnosis requires the presence of general criteria of personality disorders as well as from two to five (out of eight or nine) specific criteria for the different personality disorders. By applying the abovementioned freedom of various diagnostic options, 200 to 250 different ways of labeling personality functioning and behaviours are possible, which can all have the possible outcome of diagnosing one individual with more than one personality disorder (Meyerson et al., 2009, in Phend, 2009).

This diversity of symptom manifestation for individuals diagnosed with personality disorders may in some cases result in two entirely different syndromes although both individuals are diagnosed with the same disorder. For example, two individuals can each manifest five out of nine different symptoms with one symptom common to both, but will be diagnosed according to the DSM-5 criteria as having the same personality disorder. Theoretically they have the same personality disorder because they manifest five out of nine possible symptoms, despite the fact that their behavioural profiles look like two different disorders. Under such circumstances, it is extremely difficult to identify individuals with personality disorders by observing their symptomatic behaviour.

Another factor that contributes to the difficulty in diagnosing an individual with a personality disorder is the high rate of symptom overlap amongst all the personality disorders, in conjunction with a high rate of co-morbidity with other disorders. This is demonstrated by the fact that personality disorders are often misdiagnosed (Gunderson, 2009; Meyerson et al., 2009, in Phend, 2009). Since misdiagnosing leads to administering the wrong kind of medications, which are thus ineffective in assisting the individual to get better, stigmatisation may follow (Oldham, 2009). For example, if an individual is misdiagnosed several times and treated ineffectively with multiple medications for every incorrect diagnosis, they might be reluctant to try further medications upon being given yet another diagnosis (Oldham, 2009). Such an individual might refuse further treatment, and on account of refusing to comply with the clinician's instructions may be labelled as difficult, uncooperative, or resistant. Indeed, both the patient and the clinician might thus become stigmatised, the individual for being difficult, uncooperative, and resistant, and the clinician for failing to treat his or her clients successfully.

The abovementioned difficulties involved in diagnosing personality disorders and their high rate of misdiagnosis makes patients and caregivers of almost adult children shy away from taking the arduous road through multiple diagnoses and ineffective treatments. Clinicians, on the other hand, dislike working with clients who are classified with a personality disorder due to the high failure rate in treating these disorders. In addition, these difficulties may lead to a refusal by medical insurance companies to pay for ineffective treatments over long periods of time, sometimes up to five years, according to Kernberg and Michels (2009).

It has been mentioned previously that DSM-5 approaches personality disorders in three different ways, however, for the purposes of this book, we will only focus on the main category, and not on the aetiologically based category, nor the trait approach of personality disorders. As is the case with other disorders, the personality disorder category is also divided into subcategories. Figure 12.1 illustrates the different clusters and diagnostic categories of personality disorders, according to DSM-5 classification system.

In comparing the ICD-10 and DSM-5 classifications of personality disorders, quite a few differences are apparent. The DSM-5 distinguishes between ten different personality disorders arranged in three clusters (see Figure 12.1) and one category for personality disorders not otherwise specified. In contrast, the ICD-10 lists eight different personality disorders and one category for personality disorders not otherwise specified (see Table 12.3).

As illustrated in Figure 12.1, the DSM-5 groups the personality disorders into three clusters, based on their 'descriptive similarities' (American Psychiatric Association, 2013). The main reason for doing this is the enormous overlap in the diagnostic criteria for the various personality disorders in the DSM-5. Most people who are diagnosed with one disorder also tend to meet the diagnostic criteria for at least one other disorder as we discussed above (Nolen-Hoeksema, 2008; Oldham, 2009; Kernberg & Michels, 2009). However, the DSM-5 acknowledges that, although the clustering system is useful in some research and educational contexts, it has serious limitations and has not been consistently validated. It also acknowledges that it is possible, in some instances, for individuals to present with symptoms from two different clusters of personality disorders (American Psychiatric Association, 2000; Oldham, 2009; Kernberg & Michels, 2009).

Despite the difficulties with the DSM-5 classification system mentioned above, the DSM-IV-TR cluster system will be used for systematically describing the typical syndromes (clusters of necessary symptoms) for making a diagnosis for each personality disorder in the three clusters.

Table 12.3: Comparison between ICD-10 and DSM-5 categories of Personality Disorders

DESCRIPTION	ICD-10	DSM-5
Suspicious; believes that other people will treat them wrongly; insists on own rights.	Paranoid PD	Paranoid PD
Shows great social detachment and is restricted in emotional expressions; is indifferent to emotional expressions of others and not interested in social relationships.	Schizoid PD	Schizoid PD
Social and interpersonal deficits marked by acute discomfort with, and reduced capacity for, close relationships.		Schizotypal PD
History of non-compliance with social norms and victimising others.	Dissocial PD	Antisocial PD
Characterised by instability, impulsivity, recklessness, and explosiveness.	Emotionally Unstable PD • Explosive type • Borderline type • Aggressive type	Borderline PD
People who show exaggerated emotional expressions and have an extremely strong longing for attention.	Histrionic PD	Histrionic PD
Difficulty in performing work because of an obsession about making everything perfectly right. (Not the same as Obsessive-Compulsive Disorder).	Anankastic PD	Obsessive-Compulsive PD

DESCRIPTION	ICD-10	DSM-5
People with a basic fear of being judged; shyness and constant social discomfort (embarrassed; avoid social situations); unwilling to commit themselves to a relationship.	Anxious (avoidant) PD	Avoidant PD
Not able to make day-to-day decisions; afraid of being rejected or abandoned; put aside own wishes and needs, while doing what others want.	Dependent PD	Dependent PD
Strong sense of self-importance; exaggerate own capabilities and achievements.	Other specific PDs • Eccentric • 'Unstable' type • Narcissistic • Passive-Aggressive • Psychoneurotic • Immature	Narcissistic PD

Source: http://www.web4health.info, n.d.

CLUSTER A PERSONALITY DISORDERS

This cluster of personality disorders share a common theme of withdrawal from others due to fear and anxiety of people, and an indifference to people which is based on perceptions of the social environment that differ from cultural or social expectations. Furthermore, these disorders share symptoms with Schizophrenia, but without psychotic symptoms, and are often considered to reflect the personality processes that underlie, or predispose people to, Schizophrenia. This cluster includes Paranoid, Schizoid, and Schizotypal Personality Disorders.

Paranoid Personality Disorder

The typical symptom that characterises this disorder is a perception that other people, and the world at large, are hostile (American Psychiatric Association, 2013); this leads to extreme distrust and hypervigilance. According to Castillo (1998), typical symptoms include beliefs that:

- Other people want to exploit or deceive them and that even friends and significant others are untrustworthy.
- All personal information shared with others may be used maliciously.
- There is hidden meaning in remarks or events which others perceive as benign.
- The spouse or partner is unfaithful.

Table 12.4: The relationship between personality style and personality disorders

PERSONALITY STYLE	PERSONALITY DISORDER
Conscientious, diligent	Obsessive-Compulsive (**Note:** Obsessive-Compulsive PD is not the same as OCD.)
Ambitious, self-confident	Narcissistic
Expressive, emotional	Histrionic
Alert, suspicious	Paranoid
Erratic, spontaneous	Borderline
Affectionate, loyal	Dependent
Independent, secretive, chary, lonely	Schizoid
Self-critical, careful	Anxious; Avoidant
Full of foreboding, sensitive	Schizotypal
Adventuresome, likely to take risks	Antisocial (diagnosis)

Source: http://www.web4health.info, n.d.

Because of these perceptions, one can generally expect that people with this disorder will be cold and distant in their interpersonal relationships. They tend to react with suspicion to changes in situations and to find hostile and malevolent motives behind other people's trivial, innocent, or even positive acts (Barlow & Durand, 2005). Bernstein, Useda, and Siever (1993) provide an interesting description of the everyday behaviour of people with a paranoid disorder. According to them, these people tend to be either overtly or passively hostile towards others. They tend to be very argumentative, they complain, are very sensitive to criticism, and they have an excessive need for autonomy. The implications are that this type of behaviour will elicit rejection from others, which then reinforces their distrust of others; in this way, their interpersonal style (see Table 12.4), and the disorder, are reinforced.

Castillo (1998) warns that although paranoid tendencies may develop among people who feel particularly alienated because of physical defects (e.g. deafness) or social factors (e.g. being an immigrant), one should be cautious not to diagnose the disorder too quickly and, as is the case with most other disorders, be mindful of the social context of the person.

There is close congruence between the DSM-5 and ICD-10 criteria for this disorder (see Table 12.5).

Table 12.5: Diagnostic criteria for Paranoid Personality Disorder as adapted from the DSM-5 and ICD-10

<table>
<tr><th>DSM-5</th><th>ICD-10</th></tr>
<tr><td>
A. A pervasive distrust and suspiciousness of others such that their motives are interpreted as malevolent, beginning by early adulthood and present in a variety of contexts, as indicated by four (or more) of the following:
(1) suspects, without sufficient basis, that others are exploiting, harming, or deceiving him or her
(2) is preoccupied with unjustified doubts about the loyalty or trustworthiness of friends or associates
(3) is reluctant to confide in others because of unwarranted fear that the information will be used maliciously against him or her
(4) reads hidden demeaning or threatening meanings into benign remarks or events
(5) persistently bears grudges, i.e. is unforgiving of insults, injuries, or slights
(6) perceives attacks on his or her character or reputation that are not apparent to others and is quick to react angrily or to counterattack
(7) has recurrent suspicions, without justification, regarding fidelity of spouse or sexual partner
B. Does not occur exclusively during the course of Schizophrenia, a Mood Disorder With Psychotic Features, or another psychotic disorder and is not due to the direct physiological effects of a general medical condition.
Note: If criteria are met prior to the onset of Schizophrenia, add 'Premorbid', e.g. 'Paranoid Personality Disorder (Premorbid)'.
</td><td>
• Personality disorder characterised by at least three of the following:
‣ Excessive sensitiveness to setbacks and rebuffs.
‣ Tendency to bear grudges persistently, i.e. refusal to forgive insults and injuries or slights.
‣ Suspiciousness and a pervasive tendency to distort experience by misconstruing the neutral or friendly actions of others as hostile or contemptuous.
‣ A combative and tenacious sense of personal rights out of keeping with the actual situation.
‣ Recurrent suspicions, without justification, regarding sexual fidelity of spouse or sexual partner.
‣ Tendency to experience excessive self-importance, manifest in a persistent self-referential attitude.
‣ Preoccupation with unsubstantiated 'conspiratorial' explanations of events both immediate to the patient and in the world at large.
• Includes: expansive paranoid, fanatic, querulant, and sensitive paranoid personality (disorder)
• Excludes: Delusional Disorder, Schizophrenia
</td></tr>
</table>

Source: Reprinted with permission from the Diagnostic and Statistical Manual of Mental Disorders (DSM), Fifth Edition, American Psychiatric Association (APA), 2013 and ICD-10 Classification of Mental and Behavioural Disorders: Diagnostic Criteria for Research, World Health Organisation (WHO), Geneva, 2007.

Schizoid Personality Disorder

One way of describing people with this disorder would be to say that they are extreme introverts; however, this would not be accurate as it is more extreme than 'mere' introversion. According to the American Psychiatric Association (2013), the key features of this disorder include both a pervasive detachment from social relationships, as well as a restricted range of emotions. Castillo (1998) describes these people as extremely self-absorbed, with little or no contact with their social or physical environment. They tend to show very little emotional response to events and they tend to have a lack of emotional motivation for engaging in activities that others seem to enjoy (e.g. intimate relationships, relationships with family and colleagues). According to Barlow and Durand (2005), other people tend to experience them as being 'cold', 'indifferent', or 'aloof'. Due to their lack of emotional responsiveness, they seem to be untouched by social feedback such as praise or criticism. As is the case with Paranoid Personality Disorder, the DSM and ICD criteria for this disorder are similar (see Table 12.6).

Table 12.6: Diagnostic criteria for Schizoid Personality Disorder as adapted from the DSM-5 and ICD-10

DSM-5	ICD-10
A. A pervasive pattern of detachment from social relationships and a restricted range of expression of emotions in interpersonal settings, beginning by early adulthood and present in a variety of contexts, as indicated by four (or more) of the following: (1) neither desires nor enjoys close relationships, including being part of a family (2) almost always chooses solitary activities (3) has little, if any, interest in having sexual experiences with another person (4) takes pleasure in few, if any, activities (5) lacks close friends or confidants other than first-degree relatives (6) appears indifferent to the praise or criticism of others (7) shows emotional coldness, detachment, or flattened affectivity	• Personality disorder characterised by at least three of the following: ‣ Few, if any, activities, provide pleasure. ‣ Emotional coldness, detachment or flattened affectivity. ‣ Limited capacity to express either warm, tender feelings or anger towards others. ‣ Apparent indifference to either praise or criticism. ‣ Little interest in having sexual experiences with another person (taking age into account). ‣ Almost invariable preference for solitary activities. ‣ Excessive preoccupation with fantasy and introspection. ‣ Lack of close friends or confiding relationships (or having only one) and of desire for such relationships. ‣ Marked insensitivity to prevailing social norms and conventions. • *Excludes:* ‣ Asperger's Syndrome ‣ Delusional Disorder ‣ Schizoid Disorder of Childhood ‣ Schizophrenia ‣ Schizotypal Disorder

DSM-5	ICD-10
B. Does not occur exclusively during the course of Schizophrenia, a Mood Disorder With Psychotic Features, another psychotic disorder, or a Pervasive Developmental Disorder and is not due to the direct physiological effects of a general medical condition. **Note:** If criteria are met prior to the onset of Schizophrenia, add 'Pre-morbid', e.g. 'Schizoid Personality Disorder (Pre-morbid)'.	

Source: Reprinted with permission from the Diagnostic and Statistical Manual of Mental Disorders (DSM), Fifth Edition, American Psychiatric Association (APA), 2013 and ICD-10 Classification of Mental and Behavioural Disorders: Diagnostic Criteria for Research, World Health Organisation (WHO), Geneva, 2007.

Schizotypal Personality Disorder

This disorder shares some of the characteristics of Schizoid Personality Disorder, such as emotional detachment and social isolation. However, it differs from Schizoid Personality Disorder in that in addition to anxiety in social relationships, people with this disorder also display eccentricities such as superstitiousness, preoccupation with paranormal phenomena, magical thinking, and rituals (Castillo, 1998). The symptoms of this disorder can be summarised as follows:

- Ideas of reference, that is, the belief that random events have some special meaning for them (Nolen-Hoeksema, 2004).
- Paranoia or extreme suspiciousness, that is, as is the case with Paranoid Personality Disorder, the tendency to view other people as hostile and deceitful (Nolen-Hoeksema, 2004).
- Odd beliefs or magical thinking, for example, believing that they are clairvoyant or telepathic (Barlow & Durand, 2005).
- Illusions, which can be described as the misperception or misinterpretation of real external sensory stimuli (Kaplan, Sadock, & Grebb 1994). An example of this would be feeling the presence of another person when they are alone (Barlow & Durand, 2005).
- Vague, circumstantial, or stereotyped speech (Nolen-Hoeksema, 2004).

Table 12.7: Diagnostic criteria for Schizotypal Personality Disorder as adapted from the DSM-5

DSM-5
A. A pervasive pattern of social and interpersonal deficits marked by acute discomfort with, and reduced capacity for, close relationships as well as by cognitive or perceptual distortions and eccentricities of behaviour, beginning by early adulthood and present in a variety of contexts, as indicated by five (or more) of the following: (1) ideas of reference (excluding delusions of reference) (2) odd beliefs or magical thinking that influences behaviour and is inconsistent with subcultural norms (e.g. superstitiousness, belief in clairvoyance, telepathy, or 'sixth sense'; in children and adolescents, bizarre fantasies or preoccupations) (3) unusual perceptual experiences, including bodily illusions (4) odd thinking and speech (e.g. vague, circumstantial, metaphorical, over-elaborate, or stereotyped) (5) suspiciousness or paranoid ideation (6) inappropriate or constricted affect (7) behaviour or appearance that is odd, eccentric, or peculiar (8) lack of close friends or confidants other than first-degree relatives (9) excessive social anxiety that does not diminish with familiarity and tends to be associated with paranoid fears rather than negative judgments about self
B. Does not occur exclusively during the course of Schizophrenia, a Mood Disorder With Psychotic Features, another psychotic disorder, or a Pervasive Developmental Disorder.
Note: If criteria are met prior to the onset of Schizophrenia, add 'Pre-morbid', e.g. 'Schizotypal Personality Disorder (Pre-morbid)'.

Source: Reprinted with permission from the Diagnostic and Statistical Manual of Mental Disorders (DSM), Fifth Edition, American Psychiatric Association (APA), 2013

Some of these symptoms are very similar to those of Schizophrenia, but are not severe enough to warrant a diagnosis of Schizophrenia. It is for this reason that DSM-5 also notes this disorder in the Schizophrenia Spectrum Disorders. The similarities are such, however, that there is clearly a strong link between this disorder and Schizophrenia. The main difference between DSM-5 and ICD-10 is that the ICD-10 does not make provision for a Schizotypal Personality Disorder, and sees this as a variant of Schizoid Personality Disorder.

CLUSTER B PERSONALITY DISORDERS

The core feature of people with personality disorders in this cluster is that they tend to engage in dramatic, impulsive behaviour with little regard for their own safety or the safety of others. They may also act in a hostile and, in some cases, violent way and show very little empathy for others (Nolen-Hoeksema, 2005). This cluster includes Borderline, Histrionic, Narcissistic, and Antisocial Personality Disorders.

Borderline Personality Disorder

According to Castillo (1998), the core feature of this disorder is a persistent instability in social relationships, self-image, and emotions. It seems as if fear of rejection and abandonment, as well as intense unmet needs for affection and closeness, are central to this instability. It is clear that there is some tension between these two core features: on the one hand, people with this disorder have an intense need for affection; however, on the other hand, they have an intense fear of being rejected or abandoned.

The key clinical features of this disorder include:

- Unstable mood, which is characterised by severe depression, anxiety, and anger, with no obvious environmental triggers (Nolen-Hoeksema, 2005).
- Unstable self-concept, which can range from episodes of extreme self-doubt to episodes of grandiose self-importance (Nolen-Hoeksema, 2005).
- Feelings of emptiness which are often described as chronic boredom (Barlow & Durand, 2005); however, this may be due to difficulties with their own identities, in other words, a global lack of knowing who or what they are (Nolen-Hoeksema, 2005).
- Impulsive, self-mutilating, and suicidal behaviour (Barlow & Durand, 2005).
- Unstable interpersonal relationships, which are characterised by switching from idealising a person to despising them for no apparent reason (Nolen-Hoeksema, 2005).

This disorder produces significant impairment in social, academic, and occupational functioning. Borderline Personality Disorder's high co-morbidity with other disorders, such as major depression, Bipolar Disorder, eating and substance disorders (Barlow & Durand, 2005), and with other personality disorders, makes Borderline PD rather difficult to identify and deal with.

Table 12.8: Diagnostic criteria for Borderline Personality Disorder as adapted from the DSM-5 and for Emotionally Unstable (Borderline) Personality Disorder as adapted from ICD-10

DSM-5	ICD-10
A pervasive pattern of instability of interpersonal relationships, self-image, and affects, and marked impulsivity beginning by early adulthood and present in a variety of contexts, as indicated by five (or more) of the following: (1) frantic efforts to avoid real or imagined abandonment. **Note:** Do not include suicidal or self-mutilating behaviour covered in Criterion 5. (2) a pattern of unstable and intense interpersonal relationships characterised by alternating between extremes of idealisation and devaluation (3) identity disturbance: markedly and persistently unstable self-image or sense of self	• A personality disorder in which there is a marked tendency to act impulsively without consideration of the consequences, together with affective instability. The ability to plan ahead may be minimal, and outbursts of intense anger may often lead to violence or 'behavioural explosions'; these are easily precipitated when impulsive acts are criticised or thwarted by others. Two variants of this personality disorder are specified, and both share this general theme of impulsiveness and lack of self-control. • **Impulsive type:** The predominant characteristics are emotional instability and lack of impulse control. Outbursts of violence or threatening behaviour are common, particularly in response to criticism by others.

DSM-5	ICD-10
(4) impulsivity in at least two areas that are potentially self-damaging (e.g. spending, sex, substance abuse, reckless driving, binge-eating). **Note:** Do not include suicidal or self-mutilating behaviour covered in Criterion 5. (5) recurrent suicidal behaviour, gestures, or threats, or self-mutilating behaviour (6) affective instability due to a marked reactivity of mood (e.g. intense episodic dysphoria, irritability, or anxiety usually lasting a few hours and only rarely more than a few days) (7) chronic feelings of emptiness (8) inappropriate, intense anger or difficulty controlling anger (e.g. frequent displays of temper, constant anger, recurrent physical fights) (9) transient, stress-related paranoid ideation or severe dissociative symptoms	• *Includes:* explosive and aggressive personality (disorder) • *Excludes:* Dissocial Personality Disorder • **Borderline type:** Several of the characteristics of emotional instability are present; in addition, the patient's own self-image, aims, and internal preferences (including sexual) are often unclear or disturbed. There are usually chronic feelings of emptiness. A liability to become involved in intense and unstable relationships may cause repeated emotional crises and may be associated with excessive efforts to avoid abandonment and a series of suicidal threats or acts of self-harm (although these may occur without obvious precipitants). • *Includes:* borderline personality (disorder)

Source: Reprinted with permission from the Diagnostic and Statistical Manual of Mental Disorders (DSM), Fifth Edition, American Psychiatric Association (APA), 2013 and ICD-10 Classification of Mental and Behavioural Disorders: Diagnostic Criteria for Research, World Health Organisation (WHO), Geneva, 2007.

Histrionic Personality Disorder

The main characteristics of this disorder include 'excessive' emotionality and attention-seeking (American Psychiatric Association, 2013). Although this seems relatively clear, Castillo (1998) points out that it may be difficult to define 'excessive' as this definition may vary from one culture to another. One may add that this definition may also be influenced by gender.

Castillo (1998), Nolen-Hoeksema (2005), and Barlow and Durand (2005) describe the core features of this disorder as follows:

- People with this disorder are overly dramatic, enthusiastic, and flirtatious. Although they may dress and appear to be overly sexual in social situations, this apparent seductiveness is often not to be taken seriously as it is often only used to attract attention.
- They show active and purposeful seeking of attention. They constantly want approval and reassurance from others, and if they do not get this, they may get upset or angry.
- They are typically very concerned about their physical appearance.
- They tend to exaggerate medical problems, make more frequent doctor's appointments, and have more suicidal gestures than the average person.
- Other people may experience them as being shallow, self-centred, demanding, and dependent.

Table 12.9: Diagnostic criteria for Histrionic Personality Disorder as adapted from the DSM-5 and ICD-10

DSM-5	ICD-10
A pervasive pattern of excessive emotionality and attention-seeking, beginning by early adulthood and present in a variety of contexts, as indicated by five (or more) of the following: (1) is uncomfortable in situations in which he or she is not the centre of attention (2) interaction with others is often characterised by inappropriate, sexually seductive, or provocative behaviour (3) displays rapidly shifting and shallow expression of emotions (4) consistently uses physical appearance to draw attention to self (5) has a style of speech that is excessively impressionistic and lacking in detail (6) shows self-dramatisation, theatricality, and exaggerated expression of emotion (7) is suggestible, i.e. easily influenced by others or circumstances (8) considers relationships to be more intimate than they actually are	• Personality disorder characterised by at least three of the following: ‣ Self-dramatisation, theatricality, exaggerated expression of emotions; ‣ Suggestibility, easily influenced by others or by circumstances; ‣ Shallow and labile affectivity; ‣ Continual seeking for excitement, appreciation by others, and activities in which the patient is the centre of attention; ‣ Inappropriate seductiveness in appearance or behaviour; ‣ Over-concern with physical attractiveness. • Associated features may include egocentricity, self-indulgence, continuous longing for appreciation, feelings that are easily hurt, and persistent manipulative behaviour to achieve own needs. • *Includes:* ‣ hysterical and psychoinfantile personality (disorder)

Source: Reprinted with permission from the Diagnostic and Statistical Manual of Mental Disorders (DSM), Fifth Edition, American Psychiatric Association (APA), 2013 and ICD-10 Classification of Mental and Behavioural Disorders: Diagnostic Criteria for Research, World Health Organisation (WHO), Geneva, 2007.

Narcissistic Personality Disorder

Whereas people with a Histrionic Personality Disorder actively seek attention, people with a Narcissistic Personality Disorder do so in a more passive way. Their whole demeanour tends to portray a quiet sense of knowing that they are more important than others. Nolen-Hoeksema (2005) and Barlow and Durand (2005) describe these people as follows:

- They are preoccupied with thoughts of their self-importance and fantasies of power and success.
- They make unreasonable demands of others.
- They have little empathy, and ignore the needs and wants of others.
- They exploit others to gain power.
- They can be arrogant and demean others.
- They require (and expect) a great deal of special attention.
- When in the presence of truly successful people, they tend to become envious and arrogant.
- They can be very boastful and exaggerate their own talents and accomplishments and, at the same time, downplay, or blame others, for their failures.

Table 12.10: Diagnostic criteria for Narcissistic Personality Disorder as adapted from the DSM-5 and ICD-10

DSM-5	ICD-10
A pervasive pattern of grandiosity (in fantasy or behaviour), need for admiration, and lack of empathy, beginning by early adulthood and present in a variety of contexts, as indicated by five (or more) of the following: (1) has a grandiose sense of self-importance (e.g. exaggerates achievements and talents, expects to be recognised as superior without commensurate achievements) (2) is preoccupied with fantasies of unlimited success, power, brilliance, beauty, or ideal love (3) believes that he or she is 'special' and unique and can only be understood by, or should associate with, other special or high-status people (or institutions) (4) requires excessive admiration (5) has a sense of entitlement, i.e. unreasonable expectations of especially favourable treatment or automatic compliance with his or her expectations (6) is interpersonally exploitative, i.e. takes advantage of others to achieve his or her own ends (7) lacks empathy: is unwilling to recognise or identify with the feelings and needs of others (8) is often envious of others or believes that others are envious of him or her (9) shows arrogant, haughty behaviours or attitudes	• While the ICD-10 does not specifically define the characteristics of this personality disorder, it is classified in the category other specific personality disorders. • ICD-10 states that Narcissistic Personality Disorder is a personality disorder that fits none of the specific criteria of the other personality disorders.

Source: Reprinted with permission from the Diagnostic and Statistical Manual of Mental Disorders (DSM), Fifth Edition, American Psychiatric Association (APA), 2013 and ICD-10 Classification of Mental and Behavioural Disorders: Diagnostic Criteria for Research, World Health Organisation (WHO), Geneva, 2007.

Antisocial Personality Disorder

The essential diagnostic feature of Antisocial Personality Disorder is a pervasive pattern of violation of, and disregard for, the rights of others without showing remorse or guilt for one's behaviour. This pattern of disrespect begins in childhood or early adolescence and continues into adulthood. Antisocial Personality Disorder is also referred to as 'psychopathy', 'sociopathy', or 'Dissocial Personality Disorder' (ICD-10) and it can only be diagnosed when an individual has reached the age of 18. Because deceit and manipulation are central features of this disorder, it is best to assess the individual systematically by collecting information from collateral sources.

In terms of their personal history, the individual must have had some symptoms of Conduct Disorder before the age of 15. Conduct Disorder involves four groups of persistent and repetitive patterns of behaviour that violate the norms, rules, or basic rights of others, such as aggression towards people and animals, destruction of property, deceit, or theft (see Chapter 13). The pattern of Conduct Disorder continues into adulthood as Antisocial

Personality Disorder through an intensification of repetitively performed acts that become grounds for arrest, such as destruction of property, harassing others, stealing, lying, and pursuing illegal occupations.

Table 12.11: Diagnostic criteria for Antisocial Personality Disorder as adapted from the DSM-5 and ICD-10

DSM-5	ICD-10
A. There is a pervasive pattern of disregard for and violation of the rights of others occurring since the age of 15, as indicated by three (or more) of the following: (1) failure to conform to social norms with respect to lawful behaviours as indicated by repeatedly performing acts that are grounds for arrest (2) deceitfulness, as indicated by repeated lying, use of aliases, or conning others for personal profit or pleasure (3) impulsivity or failure to plan ahead (4) irritability and aggressiveness, as indicated by repeated physical fights or assaults (5) reckless disregard for safety of self or others (6) consistent irresponsibility, as indicated by repeated failure to sustain consistent work behaviour or honour financial obligations (7) lack of remorse, as indicated by being indifferent to or rationalising having hurt, mistreated, or stolen from another B. The individual is at least 18 years old. C. There is evidence of Conduct Disorder with onset before the age of 15. D. The occurrence of antisocial behaviour is not exclusively during the course of Schizophrenia or a Manic Episode.	• Personality disorder, usually coming to attention because of a gross disparity between behaviour and the prevailing social norms, and characterised by at least three of the following: ‣ Callous unconcern for the feelings of others. ‣ Gross and persistent attitude of irresponsibility and disregard for social norms, rules, and obligations. ‣ Incapacity to maintain enduring relationships, though having no difficulty in establishing them. ‣ Very low tolerance for frustration and a low threshold for discharge of aggression, including violence. ‣ Incapacity to experience guilt and to profit from experience, particularly punishment. ‣ Marked proneness to blame others, or to offer plausible rationalisations, for the behaviour that has brought the patient into conflict with society. • There may also be persistent irritability as an associated feature. Conduct Disorder during childhood and adolescence, though not invariably present, may further support the diagnosis. • *Includes:* amoral, antisocial, asocial, psychopathic, and sociopathic personality (disorder) • *Excludes:* conduct disorders, emotionally unstable personality disorder

Source: Reprinted with permission from the Diagnostic and Statistical Manual of Mental Disorders (DSM), Fifth Edition, American Psychiatric Association (APA), 2013 and ICD-10 Classification of Mental and Behavioural Disorders: Diagnostic Criteria for Research, World Health Organisation (WHO), Geneva, 2007.

The typical clinical picture of people with an Antisocial Personality Disorder includes features such as the following:

- There is a pattern of impulsive behaviour that indicates their lack of planning ahead; their decision-making is often executed on the spur of the moment without forethought and consideration for the consequences to others and themselves. This impulsivity often leads to sudden changes of job, location, and relationship, and may manifest as irritability and aggressiveness, accompanied by fights and physical assaults on their spouse and/or children.
- There is a total disregard for their own safety and the safety of others, as displayed by driving recklessly, speeding excessively while intoxicated, and engaging in sexual behaviour or substance use with a high risk of harmful consequences.
- In order to gain personal profit or pleasure in the form of sex, money, or power, such individuals use manipulative and deceitful means to obtain their desires, often with much charm and by repeatedly lying to and deceiving others.
- Financial and occupational irresponsibility are indicated by truancy from work without explanation or future planning for the payment of debts, and failure to support their dependants.
- People with this disorder rarely compensate or make amends for their deliberately harmful behaviour, frequently lacking empathy, and they can be excessively callous, cynical, and contemptuous with regard to the feelings of others.
- An inflated and unrealistic self-appraisal.

CLUSTER C PERSONALITY DISORDERS

This cluster includes the Avoidant, Dependent, and Obsessive-Compulsive Personality Disorders. This cluster of personality disorders differs quite significantly from the other personality disorders in that anxiety and fearfulness are quite evident in these disorders. This feature makes it difficult to distinguish these disorders from other disorders and they also have, for this reason, a high co-morbidity with anxiety-related disorders.

Avoidant Personality Disorder

The key features of this disorder are social anxiety, low self-esteem, and hypersensitivity to criticism (Castillo, 1998). People with this disorder are so fearful of social interactions that they actively avoid any social contact that may result in rejection, humiliation, or criticism. Kaplan et al. (1994) highlight the following features shown by people with this disorder:

- They have a need for interpersonal contact. However, their fear of rejection prevents them from establishing interpersonal relationships. They are generally unwilling to enter into relationships unless there is a guarantee of uncritical acceptance.
- In conversations with others, they may express uncertainty and a lack of self-confidence.
- They have a fear of speaking in public or making requests from others.
- They have a tendency to interpret others' comments as derogatory or ridiculing.

This disorder, on face value, is similar to Schizoid Personality Disorder, as people with the latter diagnosis also display patterns of social inhibition, feelings of inadequacy, and hypersensitivity to rejection. However, unlike people with a Schizoid Personality Disorder, people with Avoidant Personality Disorder actually desire relationships with others but are paralysed by their fear and sensitivity into social isolation.

Table 12.12: Diagnostic criteria for Avoidant Personality Disorder as adapted from the DSM-5 and ICD-10

DSM-5	ICD-10
A pervasive pattern of social inhibition, feelings of inadequacy, and hypersensitivity to negative evaluation, beginning by early adulthood and present in a variety of contexts, as indicated by four (or more) of the following: (1) avoids occupational activities that involve significant interpersonal contact, because of fears of criticism, disapproval, or rejection (2) is unwilling to get involved with people unless certain of being liked (3) shows restraint within intimate relationships because of the fear of being shamed or ridiculed (4) is preoccupied with being criticised or rejected in social situations (5) is inhibited in new interpersonal situations because of feelings of inadequacy (6) views self as socially inept, personally unappealing, or inferior to others (7) is unusually reluctant to take personal risks or to engage in any new activities because they may prove embarrassing	• Personality disorder characterised by at least three of the following: ‣ Persistent and pervasive feelings of tension and apprehension. ‣ Belief that one is socially inept, personally unappealing, or inferior to others. ‣ Excessive preoccupation with being criticised or rejected in social situations. ‣ Unwillingness to become involved with people unless certain of being liked. ‣ Restrictions in lifestyle because of need to have physical security. ‣ Avoidance of social or occupational activities that involve significant interpersonal contact because of fear of criticism, disapproval, or rejection. • Associated features may include hypersensitivity to rejection and criticism.

Source: Reprinted with permission from the Diagnostic and Statistical Manual of Mental Disorders (DSM), Fifth Edition, American Psychiatric Association (APA), 2013 and ICD-10 Classification of Mental and Behavioural Disorders: Diagnostic Criteria for Research, World Health Organisation (WHO), Geneva, 2007.

Dependent Personality Disorder

While many people exhibit dependent behaviours and traits, those with Dependent Personality Disorder have an excessive need to be taken care of which results in submissive and clinging behaviour, regardless of consequences (American Psychiatric Association, 2013). The disorder may be characterised by the following:

- People with this disorder, because they feel inadequate to cope with the demands of life, may be very passive and indecisive concerning their own lives (Castillo, 1998).
- As a result, they may become overly dependent on others to make decisions for them and are generally unable to make decisions for themselves without advice and reassurance from others (Kaplan et al., 1994).

- Because of their dependency on others, they tend to deny their own thoughts, feelings, and needs that may upset others, and ultimately may lead to rejection (Nolen-Hoeksema, 2004).
- According to Kaplan et al. (1994), these people tend to avoid positions of responsibility and become anxious when asked to take a leadership role.
- Unlike people with Avoidant Personality Disorder, who cannot function in a relationship, people with Dependent Personality Disorder can *only* function in a relationship (Nolen-Hoeksema, 2004). Kaplan et al. (1994) state that they do not like to be alone and actively seek out others on whom they can depend.

Dependency may be a symptom of other personality disorders. The dependency in other personality disorders may, however, be less evident due to the other, more dramatic, symptoms of such disorders.

Table 12.13: Diagnostic criteria for Dependent Personality Disorder as adapted from the DSM-5 and ICD-10

DSM-5	ICD-10
A pervasive and excessive need to be taken care of that leads to submissive and clinging behaviour and fears of separation, beginning by early adulthood and present in a variety of contexts, as indicated by five (or more) of the following: (1) has difficulty making everyday decisions without an excessive amount of advice and reassurance from others (2) needs others to assume responsibility for most major areas of his or her life (3) has difficulty expressing disagreement with others because of fear of loss of support or approval **Note:** Do not include realistic fears of retribution (4) has difficulty initiating projects or doing things on his or her own (because of a lack of self-confidence in judgment or abilities rather than a lack of motivation or energy) (5) goes to excessive lengths to obtain nurturance and support from others, to the point of volunteering to do things that are unpleasant	• Personality disorder characterised by at least three of the following: ‣ Encouraging or allowing others to make most of one's important life decisions. ‣ Subordination of one's own needs to those of others on whom one is dependent, and undue compliance with their wishes. ‣ Unwillingness to make even reasonable demands on the people one depends on. ‣ Feeling uncomfortable or helpless when alone, because of exaggerated fears of inability to care for oneself. ‣ Preoccupation with fears of being abandoned by a person with whom one has a close relationship, and of being left to care for oneself. ‣ Limited capacity to make everyday decisions without an excessive amount of advice and reassurance from others. • Associated features may include perceiving oneself as helpless, incompetent, and lacking stamina.

DSM-5	ICD-10
(6) feels uncomfortable or helpless when alone because of exaggerated fears of being unable to care for himself or herself (7) urgently seeks another relationship as a source of care and support when a close relationship ends (8) is unrealistically preoccupied with fears of being left to take care of himself or herself	

Source: Reprinted with permission from the Diagnostic and Statistical Manual of Mental Disorders (DSM), Fifth Edition, American Psychiatric Association (APA), 2013 and ICD-10 Classification of Mental and Behavioural Disorders: Diagnostic Criteria for Research, World Health Organisation (WHO), Geneva, 2007.

Obsessive-Compulsive Personality Disorder

The name of this disorder is problematic in that it often leads to confusion between this disorder and the Obsessive-Compulsive Disorders. It must be noted that these two disorders have very little in common other than their names. In Obsessive-Compulsive Personality Disorder, there are neither obsessions nor compulsions (Nolen-Hoeksema, 2004). The key features of this disorder include a marked preoccupation with order, perfection, attention to detail, rules, and control (Castillo, 1998). People with this disorder tend to be inflexible and lack openness, which leads to poor interpersonal relationships (Nolen-Hoeksema, 2004). The characteristics of this disorder include:

- Their preoccupation with rules and procedures interferes with efficiency, according to Castillo (1998), and their dysfunctional belief that things can only be done according to their 'correct' way, makes them anxious and prone to develop a fear of making mistakes which prevents them from seeing the 'big picture'.
- They tend to be serious, control their emotions excessively, and lack spontaneity (Millon, Davis, Millon, Escovar, & Meagher, 2000).
- Others experience them as being stubborn, stingy, possessive, moralistic, and officious (Nolen-Hoeksema, 2004).
- They are workaholics and seemingly have very little need for leisure activities or friendships (Nolen-Hoeksema, 2004).
- They are bound by their self-created personal rules which reflect their own rigid standards of control; when they try to transfer these to others in an overly inflexible interpersonal style, this often leads to being ostracised by others.

Table 12.14: Diagnostic criteria for Obsessive-Compulsive Personality Disorder as adapted from the DSM-5 and for Anankastic Personality Disorder as adapted from ICD-10

<table>
<tr><th>DSM-5
Obsessive-Compulsive Personality Disorder</th><th>ICD-10
Anankastic Personality Disorder</th></tr>
<tr><td>A pervasive pattern of preoccupation with orderliness, perfectionism, and mental and interpersonal control, at the expense of flexibility, openness, and efficiency, beginning by early adulthood and present in a variety of contexts, as indicated by four (or more) of the following:
(1) is preoccupied with details, rules, lists, order, organisation, or schedules to the extent that the major point of the activity is lost
(2) shows perfectionism that interferes with task completion (e.g. is unable to complete a project because his or her own overly strict standards are not met)
(3) is excessively devoted to work and productivity to the exclusion of leisure activities and friendships (not accounted for by obvious economic necessity)
(4) is over-conscientious, scrupulous, and inflexible about matters of morality, ethics, or values (not accounted for by cultural or religious identification)
(5) is unable to discard worn-out or worthless objects even when they have no sentimental value
(6) is reluctant to delegate tasks or to work with others unless they submit to exactly his or her way of doing things
(7) adopts a miserly spending style toward both self and others; money is viewed as something to be hoarded for future catastrophes
(8) shows rigidity and stubbornness</td><td>• Personality disorder characterised by at least three of the following:
‣ Feelings of excessive doubt and caution.
‣ Preoccupation with details, rules, lists. order, organisation, or schedule.
‣ Perfectionism that interferes with task completion; excessive conscientiousness, scrupulousness, and undue preoccupation with productivity to the exclusion of pleasure and interpersonal relationships.
‣ Excessive pedantry and adherence to social conventions.
‣ Rigidity and stubbornness.
‣ Unreasonable insistence by the patient that others submit to exactly his or her way of doing things, or unreasonable reluctance to allow others to do things.
‣ Intrusion of insistent and unwelcome thoughts or impulses.
• Includes:
‣ compulsive and obsessional personality (disorder).
‣ Obsessive-Compulsive Personality Disorder.
• Excludes:
‣ Obsessive-Compulsive Disorder</td></tr>
</table>

Source: Reprinted with permission from the Diagnostic and Statistical Manual of Mental Disorders (DSM), Fifth Edition, American Psychiatric Association (APA), 2013 and ICD-10 Classification of Mental and Behavioural Disorders: Diagnostic Criteria for Research, World Health Organisation (WHO), Geneva, 2007.

CO-MORBIDITY

Co-morbidity is of interest from the viewpoint of a diathesis-stress approach to personality development. The diathesis-stress approach argues that development of a disorder depends on the interaction of an individual's vulnerability, due to an innate genetic predisposition and factors in the environment and stressful life experiences (Walker, Downey, & Bergman, 1989). When we apply the diathesis-stress model to the development of personality traits, personality functioning, personality dysfunction, and other disorders, we can see that continuous interactional processes between genetic vulnerabilities and environmental stressors are at work throughout life. These continuous interactional processes can emerge as a continuous developmental range of personality functioning that manifests as personality functioning/dysfunction or personality traits/disorders. According to this view, one should find some pre-existing personality disturbance in most clinical disorders, although the manifestations may not always be strong enough to meet the diagnostic criteria for personality disorders. It follows that the pattern of association between particular 'clinical' and personality disorders is not a random one, and clinical disorders are likely to be associated with particular personality disorders or classes of disorders (see Figure 12.2). In clinical practice, the 'clinical' disorders are often, initially, the most evident disorders; however, as these are treated and the symptoms are contained, the underlying personality disorder becomes more evident.

Figure 12.2: Relationship between 'Clinical' and Personality disorders

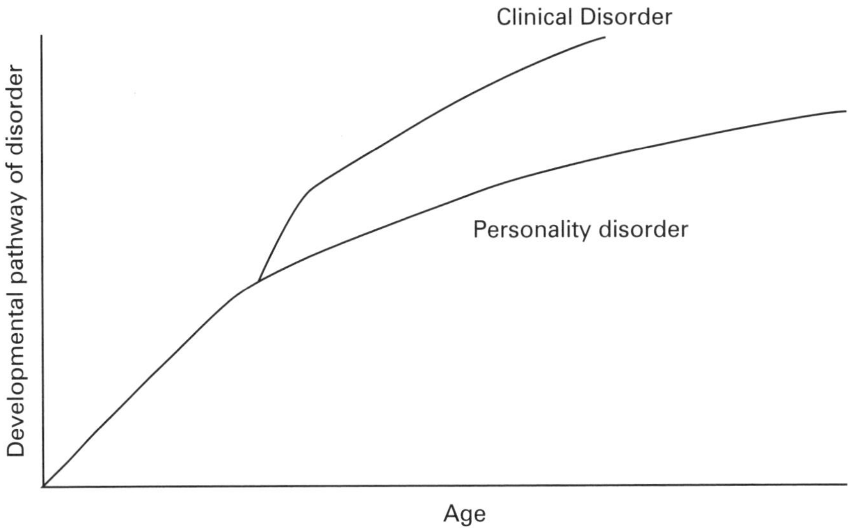

Source: © Burke, 2009.

AETIOLOGY

It is useful to return to the definition of personality disorders in order to distinguish them from other forms of psychopathology (specifically clinical syndromes). Unlike the clinical syndromes, personality disorders are always defined by enduring, inflexible, and maladaptive patterns of perceiving and responding to the environment and oneself. Individuals with personality disorders are seldom aware of their problematic cognitions and behaviours. The aetiology of personality disorders is unclear; however, a combination of personal history and biology appears to play a role in most personality disorders (see Figure 12.3).

Figure 12.3 illustrates the intricacies of the aetiology of personality disorders, and shows that the factors in the development of a personality disorder may vary from one type of disorder to another or from one individual to another. It is important to remember that one cannot view personality disorders from a purely medical model, as having a sudden onset with a specific trigger. Rather, they need to be viewed from a developmental perspective, as disorders that develop gradually from an early predisposition. The figure illustrates that there is most likely some genetic or biological vulnerability to a personality disorder, but this will develop into a disorder only if a person is exposed to adverse life events. The main aetiological factors in the personality disorders include biological, and intra- and interpersonal vulnerabilities. These will be discussed in the following sections.

Figure 12.3: Illustration of interaction of causal factors for personality disorders

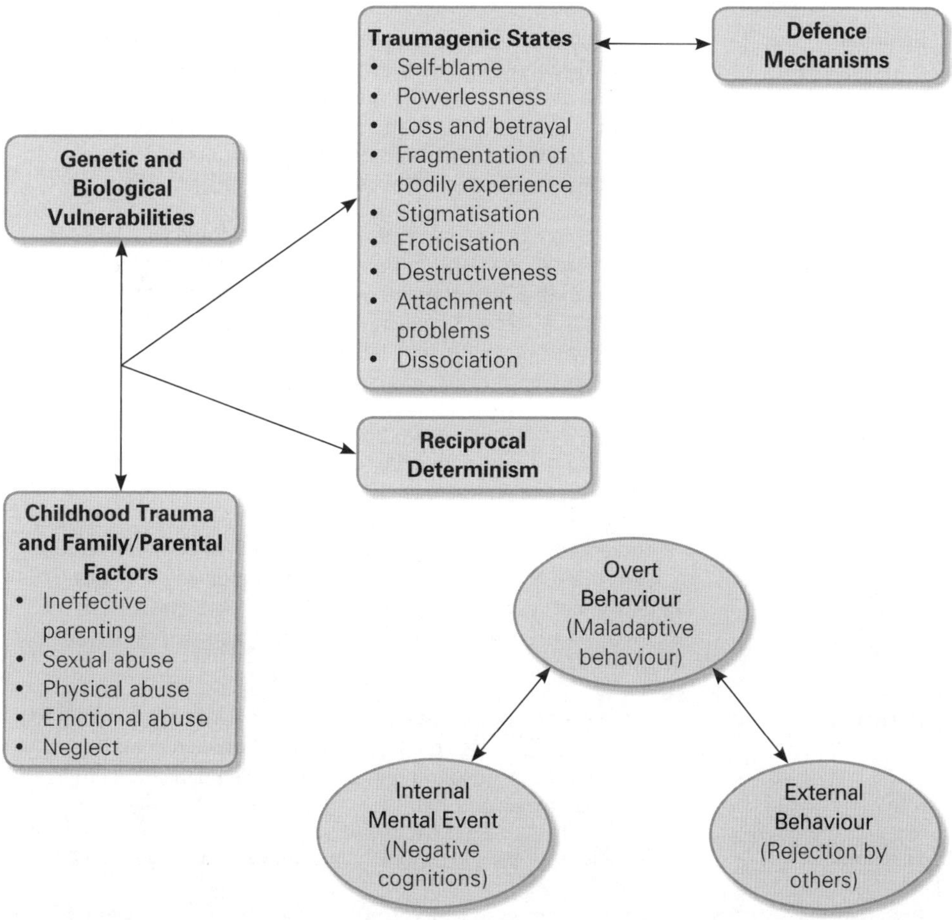

Biological factors

Genetic vulnerability

Kaplan et al. (1994) state that the concordance rate for personality disorders is significantly higher in monozygotic than in dizygotic twins, suggesting that genetics play a role in the development of a personality disorder. However, the role of genetic factors in the cause of various personality disorders varies depending on the specific disorder. The role of genetics for the different personality disorders is summarised in Table 12.15.

Table 12.15: Summary of the underlying genetic aetiological factors in personality disorders

Personality disorder	Genetic link
Schizotypal	According to Barlow and Durand (2005), this disorder could be viewed as the phenotype of a Schizophrenia genotype. Nolen-Hoeksema (2005) states that family history and adoption and twin studies indicate that this disorder may, to some degree, be transmitted genetically.
Schizoid	Although there is a suspected link between this disorder and Schizophrenia, the link is less clear than in the case of Schizotypal Personality Disorder (Kendler, Neale, Kessler, Heath, & Eaves, 1993). Twin studies of personality traits that are associated with this disorder indicate that traits such as low sociability and warmth may be partially inherited.
Paranoid	As in the previous disorders, there may be some link between this disorder and Schizophrenia, which suggests that it may be part of the Schizophrenia-spectrum disorders (Kendler et al., 1993). Genetic studies have not been able to separate the genetic and environmental influences on the development of this disorder.
Antisocial	There is substantial support for genetic influence on antisocial behaviours, particularly criminal behaviour. For example, Cloninger and Gottesman (1987) found in an adoption study that the criminal records of adopted sons are more similar to the records of the biological fathers than their adoptive fathers. Perry (1993) maintains that family history studies show that family members of people with Antisocial Personality Disorder have an increased predisposition for this disorder, alcoholism, and criminality.
Borderline	There are no conclusive findings that this disorder is transmitted genetically. There is an unexplained link between a family history of mood disorder and Borderline Personality Disorder (Nolen-Hoeksema, 2005).
Histrionic	No clear evidence for genetic cause (Barlow & Durand, 2005; Nolen-Hoeksema, 2005).

Personality disorder	Genetic link
Narcissistic	No clear evidence for genetic cause (Barlow & Durand, 2005; Nolen-Hoeksema, 2005).
Avoidant	Dahl (1993) states that this disorder is more common in first-degree relatives of people with the disorder than in the relatives of normal control groups. It is, however, not clear whether this is due to genetic or environmental factors.
Dependent	Dahl (1993) states that this disorder is more common in first-degree relatives of people with the disorder than in the relatives of normal control groups. It is, however, not clear whether this is due to genetic or environmental factors. However, children with histories of separation anxiety or chronic illnesses are more prone to develop this disorder (American Psychiatric Association, 2000).
Obsessive-Compulsive	According to Nolen-Hoeksema (2005), no family history, twin or adoption studies have been done for this disorder.

Neurobiological vulnerability

Children with Attention-Deficit/Hyperactivity Disorder and/or minimal brain damage have been found to be at risk for personality disorders, particularly for Antisocial Personality Disorder. Central nervous system dysfunction associated with soft neurological signs is particularly common in individuals with Antisocial Personality Disorder and Borderline Personality Disorder (Kaplan & Sadock, 1998). According to Gurvits, Koenigsberg, and Siever (2000), the frontal lobes, which control emotion and planning, show slight abnormalities in some cases of Borderline Personality Disorders. Low levels of behavioural inhibition may be mediated by serotonergic dysregulation in the septo-hippocampal system. There may also be developmental or acquired abnormalities in the prefrontal brain systems and reduced autonomic activity in Antisocial Personality Disorder. This may underlie the low arousal, poor fear-conditioning, and decision-making deficits described in Antisocial Personality Disorder.

Biological factors like neurobiological vulnerability may be intensified or perpetuated by familial interactional styles or broader environmental factors. For example, an unavailable or neglectful parent may not respond to either positive or negative behaviour that the child may display. Thus, there is neither consistent positive reinforcement for positive behaviour nor punishment for destructive behaviour. As a result, the child internalises the belief that any behaviour is acceptable as long as there are external personal gains. On the other hand, the parent who responds to the child's behaviour inconsistently gives the child mixed messages with regard to which behaviour is acceptable and which is unacceptable. Family factors will be discussed further in the next section. The role of neurobiological factors in the different personality disorders is summarised in Table 12.16.

Table 12.16: Summary of the underlying neurobiological factors in personality disorders

Personality disorder	Neurobiological factors
Schizotypal	According to Nolen-Hoeksema (2005), this disorder shares similar factors with Schizophrenia, such as: • Problems with sustained attention. • Low levels of monoamine oxidase which could lead to increased levels of dopamine. • Similar structural abnormalities of the brain as in Schizophrenia.
Schizoid	There seems to be a general lack of information on the causes of this disorder (Phillips, Yen, & Gunderson, 2003). It is postulated that it may share some of the neurobiological factors with autistic spectrum disorders such as a lower density of dopamine receptors (Wolff, 2000).
Paranoid	There is limited evidence of biological causes (Barlow & Durand, 2005).
Antisocial	According to Barlow and Durand (2005), there are two main theories: *Underarousal hypothesis:* According to this hypothesis, people with Antisocial Personality Disorder present with abnormally low levels of cortical arousal (lower skin conductance activity, lower heart rate during rest periods, slow frequency brain wave activity, etc). In order to boost arousal to more optimal levels, these individuals engage in stimulation-seeking behaviour. Furthermore, it has been found that people with Antisocial Personality Disorder frequently have excessive theta waves while awake, like those found in children. It has therefore been hypothesised that people with Antisocial Personality Disorder may have a cerebral cortex which is at an earlier stage of development than in other individuals, thus accounting for certain 'childlike' and impulsive behaviours. *Fearlessness hypothesis:* People with this disorder have a higher threshold for experiencing fear than most other people. Nolen-Hoeksema (2005) also lists the following possible neurobiological causes: • Elevated levels of testosterone; however, there is little evidence that ties this in with Antisocial Personality Disorder. • Low levels of serotonin, which may lead to impulsive and aggressive behaviour. • Deficits in executive functions of the brain, which may also contribute to poor impulse control.

Personality disorder	Neurobiological factors
Borderline	Weston and Siever (1993) maintain that impulsive behaviours associated with this disorder could be a result of low levels of serotonin. Further support for this lies in the fact that people with this disorder also show the same abnormalities as people with mood disorders.
Histrionic	Millon et al. (2000) maintain that people with this disorder were born with high levels of energy and a need for stimulation, which may lead to an intolerance for boredom.
Narcissistic	Halgin and Whitbourne (2003) maintain that this disorder does not have a neurobiological cause and seems to have mainly psychosocial causes.
Avoidant	There are high levels of physical arousal and hypersensitivity to the environment (Millon, et al. 2000).
Dependent	There is no evidence of neurobiological causes.
Obsessive-Compulsive	There is no evidence of neurobiological causes.

Intra- and interpersonal factors

According to Millon & Everly (1985, p. 18), 'early experiences are not only ingrained more pervasively and forcefully, but their effects tend to persist and are more difficult to modify than the effect of later experiences'. It has been hypothesised that early life experiences are intertwined with biological factors and that these experiences set the structure and tone for subsequent learning throughout the lifespan.

Ineffective parenting, sexual abuse, physical abuse, and emotional abuse and neglect have been extensively researched and found as significant factors with respect to the development of various personality disorders, as well as other forms of psychopathology (Millon et al., 2000). However, not all children who have endured any of the abovementioned traumas develop personality disorders or other forms of psychopathology. This reminds us that each child experiences, integrates, and copes with trauma uniquely and individually. The trauma cannot be viewed in isolation but should rather be viewed in dynamic interaction with various other factors, such as the biological and other factors already discussed.

Porter (1996) suggests an interesting link between trauma and personality disorders (see Figure 12.3), more specifically Antisocial Personality Disorder. According to him, there is sufficient clinical and empirical evidence supporting the hypothesis that negative childhood experiences can profoundly affect emotional functioning in adulthood. If a person is severely traumatised or disillusioned by significant others, such a person may ultimately learn to cope by 'turning off' their emotions. This could eventually lead to an 'underactive conscience', later emerging as an Antisocial Personality Disorder.

Psychoanalytic theory

In accordance with psychoanalytic theory, many clinicians view personality disorders through the lens of psychological defences. Historically, this is a vestige of the time when all individuals who were diagnosed with a personality disorder were treated from the psychoanalytic and/or psychodynamic approach (Gunderson, 2009). According to the psychoanalytic perspective, defences are the 'unconscious mental processes that the ego uses to resolve inner conflicts' (Kaplan & Sadock, 1998, p. 778).

We all use various defences and in most cases, we have a wide variety of these defence mechanisms at our disposal as ways of coping with our daily lives. Unconsciously, according to the psychoanalytic perspective, we select different defences in different situations, which enables us to adapt to our environments in a 'functional' way. However, individuals with personality disorders use particularly effective, but self-destructive, defence mechanisms in order to abolish anxiety and depression. If they were to abandon these defences, their conscious experience of anxiety and depression would increase, which is why these individuals are often reluctant to alter their behaviour. In addition, these defence mechanisms are considered to be immature and maladaptive by the dominant discourses in society, as the socially constructed myths that parents and/or caregivers have acquired and believe are used to uphold a particular social order (Walker, 2006).

In order to increase our understanding of personality traits with regard to the use of maladaptive defence mechanisms, it is imperative to consider and integrate theories with the latest brain research findings. Without such integration, there will always be individuals who continue to associate dominant defences with certain personality disorders (see Table 12.17).

Table 12.17: The relationship between coping styles/defence mechanisms and personality disorders

Common coping mechanisms			
Mechanism	**Definition**	**Result**	**Personality disorders involved**
Projection	Attributing one's own feelings or thoughts to others	Leads to prejudice, suspiciousness, and excessive worrying about external dangers	Typical of paranoid and schizotypal personalities Used by people with borderline, antisocial, or narcissistic personality when under acute stress
Splitting	Use of black-or-white, all-or-nothing thinking to divide people into groups of idealised all-good saviours and vilified all-bad evildoers	Allows a person to avoid the discomfort of having both loving and hateful feelings for the same person as well as feelings of uncertainty and helplessness	Typical of borderline personality

Common coping mechanisms			
Mechanism	**Definition**	**Result**	**Personality disorders involved**
Acting out	A direct behavioural expression of an unconscious wish or impulse that enables a person to avoid thinking about a painful situation or experiencing a painful emotion	Leads to acts that are often irresponsible, reckless, and foolish Includes many delinquent, promiscuous, and substance-abusing acts, which can become so habitual that the person remains unaware and dismissive of the feelings that initiated the acts	Very common in people with antisocial or borderline personality
Turning aggression against self	Expressing the angry feelings one has toward others by hurting oneself directly (e.g. through self-mutilation) or indirectly (e.g. in Body Dysmorphic Disorder) When indirect, it is called passive aggression	Includes failures and illnesses that affect others more than oneself and silly, provocative clowning	Dramatic in people with borderline personality
Fantasising	Use of imaginary relationships and private belief systems to resolve conflict and to escape from painful realities, such as loneliness	Is associated with eccentricity, avoidance of interpersonal intimacy, and avoidance of involvement with the outside world	Used by people with an avoidant or schizoid personality, who, in contrast to people with psychoses, do not believe (and thus do not act on) their fantasies
Hypochondriasis	Use of health complaints to gain attention	Provides a person with nurturing attention from others May be a passive expression of anger toward others	Used by people with dependent, histrionic, or borderline personality

Source: Gunderson, 2006. From The Merck Manual Home Health Handbook, edited by Robert Porter. Copyright (2009) by Merck Sharp & Dohme Corp., a subsidiary of Merck & Co., Inc., Whitehouse Station, NJ. Available online (accessed April 27, 2012): http://www.merckmanuals.com/home/mental_health_disorders/personality_disorders/personality_disorders.html

Language as a medium of communication

How do we understand each other? People most commonly use signs and symbols for thinking alone, for trying to understand each other and for reaching out to and communicating with each other. The signs we make with our body (body language) are as much a way of communicating our thoughts, feelings, motivations, and intentions as using the spoken or written word (language). However, it is not always easy to correctly interpret the body language or spoken words of others since we do not know for certain what they are thinking, feeling, and doing that motivates them to communicate with us in a certain way about a specific topic.

Indeed, the way we interpret the words or the behaviour of others is often far removed from the internal reality of these individuals. Therefore, there needs to be continual change and reinforcement within the process of communication and feedback in order to assist us to accurately assess the inner landscape of another individual (Tomm & Lannamann, 1988; Watzlawick, Beavin & Jackson, 1967). Ultimately, we can only assess the thoughts and feelings of others by questioning and verifying the intended meaning of their behavioural or verbal

Figure 12.4: Holistic representation of reciprocal interactions within and between an individual and others, the environment, physical world, structures, culture, and society.

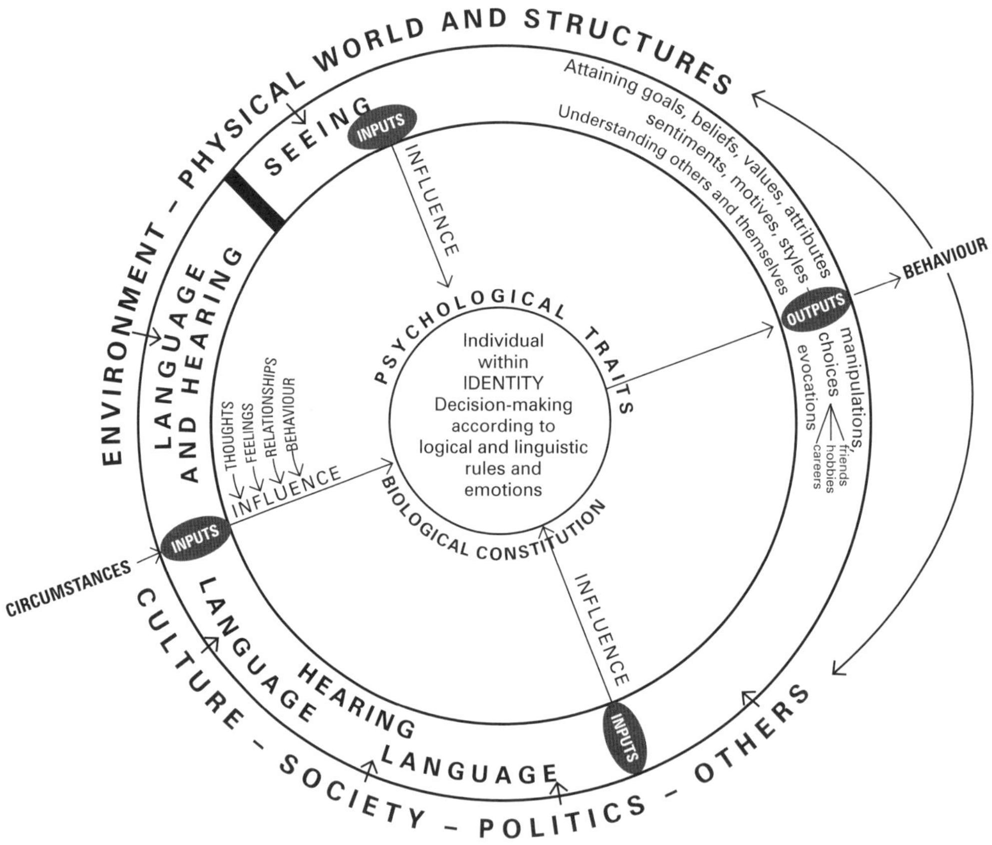

Source: © Von Krosigk, 2012.

symbols. This facilitates a better understanding of the internal aspects of both individuals and therefore a better understanding between them (Tomm & Lannamann, 1988).

In the previous section, we noted how individuals diagnosed with personality disorders tend to use immature and maladaptive defences. However, it does not necessarily follow that they use these kinds of defences when they are not under stress. In addition, their response to stressors might not be consistent and uniform, as the psychoanalytic paradigm suggests; rather, it may be the result of a complex interactional process between their biological heritage, their present physical health status, and their psychological development and health, all of which exist in the context of the presence (or absence) of a loving support system that practises effective and healthy patterns of communication (see Figure 12.4).
In the outer circle, Figure 12.4 illustrates how all input, output, and interactional processes have to pass through the medium of language; this happens through hearing and/or seeing others speak or by means of reading (seeing the written word in the physical world). Language therefore influences, creates, and shapes our thoughts, feelings, relationships, behaviours, as well as our identity.

But language and media are also situated within the context of time and culture which are also critical in the shaping of personality (see Figure 12.5A). Note how media, through

Figure 12.5: The use of language and media in the context of time and culture: Reciprocal processes between authority figure(s) (parents, teachers, adults) and others (peers, friends, enemies, e.g. bullies) and the growing child.

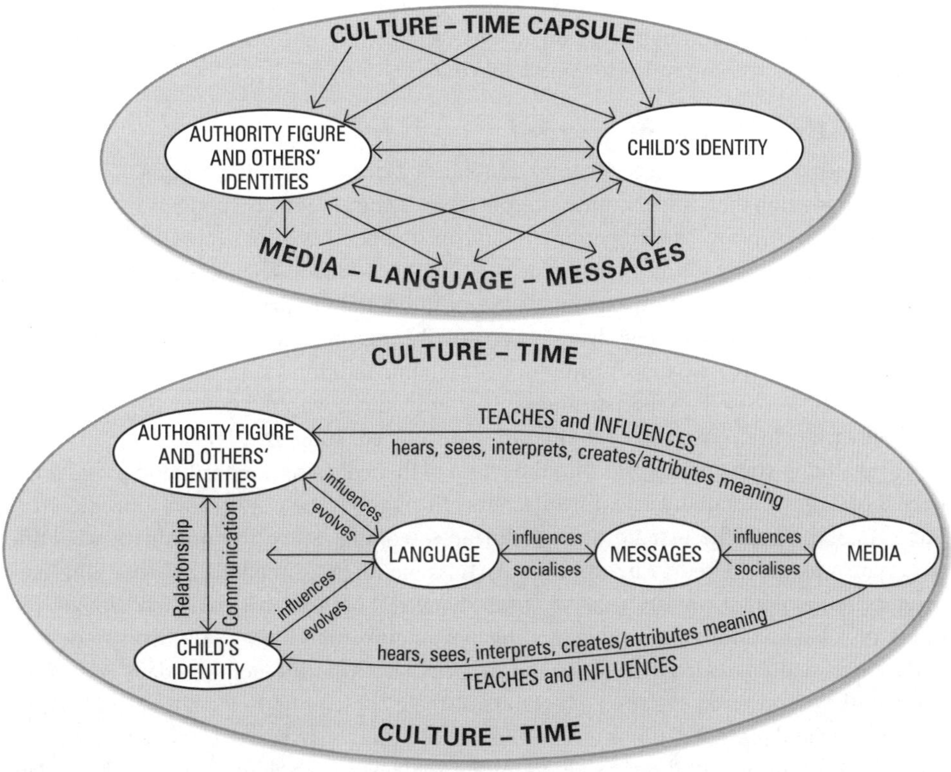

Source: © Von Krosigk, 2012.

messages expressed in the language of our culture and within our time, influences, creates, and shapes our and our authority figures' thoughts, feelings, and identity. Note also how the identities of authority figures and other identities such as peers, friends, and enemies and the growing child are reciprocally influenced through each others' messages and the messages of the media. These messages are expressed through the medium of the language of the culture, and/or the language of the dominant culture of the time.

Family systems theory

Another way of understanding personality disorders is through the lens of family systems theory, in which clinicians direct their focus on the quality of the multiple relationships within the context of nuclear and larger family systems. According to family theorists, the nature of symptoms and the type of behaviours that individuals exhibit under stressful circumstances can only be understood by observing the family members' reciprocal interactions within the context of their family system (Keeney, 1983; Watzlawick, Beavin, & Jackson, 1967; Weakland, Fish, Watzlawick, & Bodin, 1974).

From a family systems perspective, personality traits are internal aspects (that are only part of the whole person) which function in conjunction with the person's external components of functioning within a larger pattern of relationships of reciprocal communication with others. According to Keeney (1983), this can be considered a 'double description' of relationships in which internal personality attributes are conceptualised as the invisible half of a larger pattern of relationships and behaviours, which are seen as fulfilling a function within the interactional and communicational exchanges. The rules of this large interactional pattern of relationships are continually reinforced, changed, revised and adapted, according to the circular patterns of communication and behaviour.

The diathesis-stress model

The diathesis-stress model (see Chapter 2) follows a linear reasoning approach, based on the presupposition that, under conditions of stress, in the absence of support, a pre-existing vulnerability can move towards and/or result in a sudden breakdown of functioning by manifesting as clinical syndromes and/or personality disorders. The diathesis-stress model was developed as an attempt to explain why some individuals under the same environmental conditions develop a disorder while others do not. By presupposing an inherent vulnerability that would lead to a disease or disorder under certain conditions, such as cumulative stress, this model is also based on the assumption that individuals who did not develop a disorder were either free from such vulnerabilities or had sufficient support.

The diathesis-stress model falls into the realm of the biological/medical model, and it has been a part of the dominant scientific discourse throughout the last decades, thus directing our thinking along these same lines of linear reasoning. Since the dominant scientific paradigm was considered to be the only permissible research method for obtaining new insights, our attention was drawn away from theoretical options that could have uncovered other possible solutions for understanding personality functioning. Unfortunately, new researchers seldom referred back to the original scientific method for data collection. Instead, they built upon the research results of their contemporaries without questioning the premises and presuppositions upon which these results were based. Had they questioned their contemporaries' philosophical premises, the phenomenological approach to data collection may possibly have emerged as a deep, subjective method for uncovering the internal landscape of diverse ways of human thinking, feeling, behaving, and making decisions. Dialogical exchange with continual feedback could have uncovered the ways in which certain individuals came to be dysfunctional while others seemed to have developed character strengths and resilience (see Chapter 3).

Originally, phenomenology was considered to be the basis for all scientific research, for observing the object/subject of investigation in its natural surroundings, for collecting data (meticulously recording all observations), and particularly for investigating human consciousness (Husserl, 1989; published posthumously). Phenomenological philosophers like Husserl (1859-1938) based their thinking on the presupposition that we can only get to know other individuals by observing and recording what the observed individuals do, feel, and think without interpreting or judging their thoughts, feelings, and behaviour.

All scientific investigation was built on this process, together with hypothetical reasoning processes, the testing of hypotheses, and conclusions (Husserl, 1989). However, if the phenomenological method, with its detailed observations, its extensive sets of observational data, and longitudinal research studies had been employed for understanding the developmental trajectories from functional to dysfunctional behaviour over time, personality disorder research could have yielded rich data.

In addition, personality researchers should have placed the findings of these individual research studies into the context of environmental, social, cultural, and biological factors by means of a grounded research design. A grounded research design refrains from making assumptions with regard to the theoretical basis for the research. Instead, it bases the construction of a theory on the overt aspects of the collected data which forms the ground or basis from which the theory is constructed. Using this approach, this research might have uncovered categories of personality functioning that would have acknowledged all factors in interaction with each other on a dimensional continuum.

Sociocultural influences

As argued above, and as with various other forms of psychopathology, personality disorders are to some extent defined by the context within which they are found. Varying contexts exert differing expectations and pressures on the individual, thus triggering differing vulnerabilities and responses. In addition, there are other possible ways in which the broader context impacts upon the aetiology of personality disorders. Some examples of the role of contextual factors will be given in this section.

Individuals with Antisocial Personality Disorder were found to come from high-risk backgrounds, which may include poor, first-time, and single mothers (Freeman & Reinecke, 2007). Mothers from such backgrounds often have poor parenting skills and may experience poor nutrition themselves. The resulting inadequate pre- and post-natal care of their children in the context of ineffective parental care, discipline, and supervision can lead to delinquency and later Conduct Disorder and Antisocial Personality Disorder (Dishion & Patterson, 1997). From the perspective of sociocultural norms, Antisocial Personality Disorder can also be the negative outcome of an attempt by an individual to function in a personally meaningful way from within a dysfunctional family and larger sociocultural context.

Individuals with Borderline Personality Disorder tend to report an inordinate number of negative and traumatic events in childhood. These experiences range from abandonment, neglect, separation, rejection, and loss, to physical, emotional, and sexual abuse. Since Borderline Personality Disorder shows a high rate of co-morbidity with other disorders such as Posttraumatic Stress Disorder, Dissociative Disorder, eating disorders, and mood disorders, the possibility exists that socialisation and relational interactions between primary caregivers and these individuals may have been dysfunctional throughout childhood and adolescence, or during critical periods of development.

A holistic perspective for understanding the development of personality functioning/ dysfunction

HOLISM AND UBUNTU

Holism recognises that all life is connected, interdependent, and developing to fulfil its potential, and welcomes and celebrates diversity of culture and belief (as described in the Holistic Manifesto). Holism is also something which underpins our understanding of *ubuntu*. Holism and *ubuntu* go hand in hand.

Archbishop Emeritus Desmond Tutu has the following to say about *ubuntu*: 'A person with *ubuntu* is open and available to others, affirming of others, does not feel threatened that others are able and good, for he or she has a proper self-assurance that comes from knowing that he or she belongs in a greater whole and is diminished when others are humiliated or diminished, when others are tortured or oppressed.'

Tutu also said: 'One of the sayings in our country is *ubuntu* – the essence of being human. *Ubuntu* speaks particularly about the fact that you can't exist as a human being in isolation. It speaks about our interconnectedness. You can't be human all by yourself, and when you have this quality – *ubuntu* – you are known for your generosity. We think of ourselves far too frequently as just individuals, separated from one another, whereas you are connected and what you do affects the whole world. When you do well, it spreads out; it is for the whole of humanity.'

As the Zulu maxim states, '*Umuntu ngumuntu ngabantu*', a person is (only) a person through other persons. In the concept of *ubuntu* (as described by Tutu), a person with *ubuntu* is open and available to others and affirming of others.

Source: http://en.wikipedia.org/wiki/Ubuntu_(philosophy)

An inclusive, holistic approach to finding a way for understanding, identifying, diagnosing, treating, and dealing with the phenomenon known as personality disorders has become essential in the light of the high rate of misdiagnoses, co-morbid factors, overlapping symptoms amongst many personality disorders, as well as between clinical syndromes and personality disorders. The concept of holism was first introduced by Jan Smuts in his book *Holism and Evolution* (Smuts, 1926). Holism is built upon the premise of life's complexity and diversity. It presupposes that the parts of a whole cannot live or exist divorced from that whole. It also presupposes that parts of that whole cannot be understood separately (e.g. if they are divorced from the whole). Separate parts can only be understood by viewing them in relation to the whole, and in interaction with all other parts of the whole. Thus one needs to include their relationships and communicational patterns, in the light of their circular feedback and reciprocal response patterns (Becvar & Becvar, 2009). From this perspective, all aspects of the whole should be taken into account in the quest for understanding human functioning and dysfunction.

The five dimensions of human life include the biological, psychological, social, cultural, and environmental dimensions of life and functioning. Some of these dimensions have been involved in the long-standing nature versus nurture debate which has been ongoing since the inception of psychology and psychotherapy around 1900. Cause-effect reasoning processes within the context of dichotomous (either/or) thinking have proved to be of little value in finding a solution to the complex question of whether our naturally inherited biological nature/constitution, or the way we were nurtured/raised and what we learnt from our families and communities, determines our functioning or our dysfunction.

However, the linear reasoning inherent in this debate risks severely restricting our view with regard to finding explanations for our functional/dysfunctional development. By assuming that people can only be influenced by either the biological dimension or the psychosocial dimension, but never by both, we exclude other important and available aspects that could also have played a role in our development.

Viewing the same complex question from the holistic perspective yields a more comprehensive way of looking at the possibilities for developing functional and dysfunctional behaviour. Figure 12.6 is a diagrammatic representation of the five dimensions and their possible pathways of reciprocal influence with interactive feedback in a complex, living system. It is important to note that the system changes, adapts to those changes, and initiates new areas of development. It does this by responding over time to coaxing, admonishing, neglect, or receiving incongruent feedback during the developing years of childhood, adolescence, and early adulthood. This happens in interaction with the dimensions of the self or individual, the family, social community, cultural community, and the environmental aspects that recursively provide input, feedback, mishaps, and misfortunes for individuals, all in the context of their biological vulnerabilities.

We have already described some of the possible factors on the five dimensions that could negatively influence the development of a young person and which could, over time, emerge as one or more difficulties in functioning effectively. Once these difficulties become rigid patterns of behaviour by having been learnt and rehearsed, the use of inappropriate thinking and emotional strategies, personality dysfunction, and/or behavioural, cognitive, or emotional dysfunction can appear for a while. If these rigid patterns of behaviour are then changed by learning appropriate thinking and emotional strategies, the personality dysfunction or behavioural, cognitive, or emotional dysfunction may disappear again.

Figure 12.6: The five dimensions and their possible pathways of influence: A holistic process model for understanding the development of personality functioning and personality dysfunction

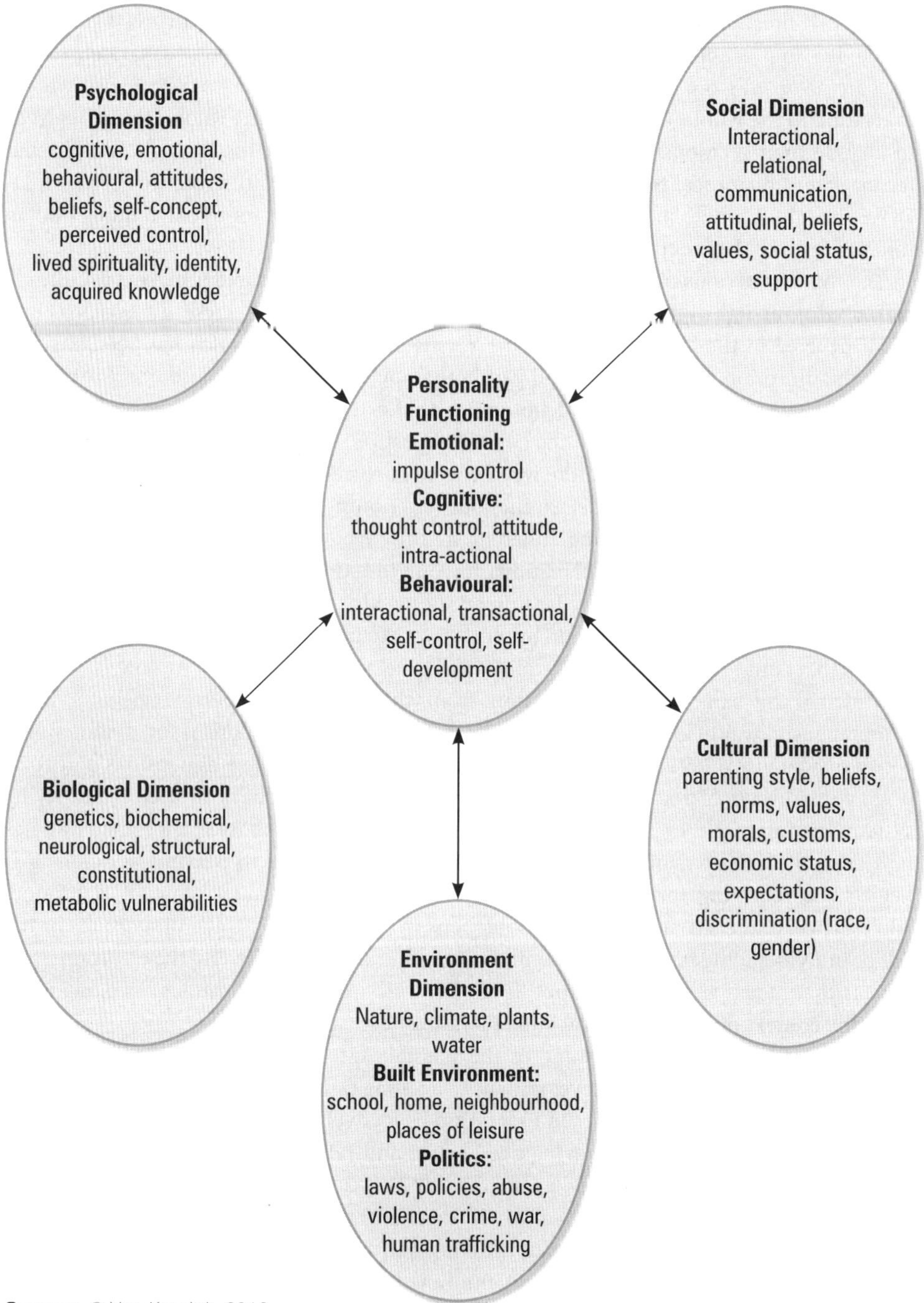

Source: © Von Krosigk, 2012.

PROBLEMS AND CONTROVERSIES

CASE STUDY

Dorothy, who was a child in the 1950s, was cared for by a subservient mother and disciplined by an authoritarian father. She was taught to respect and defer to her superiors (parents, teachers, other adults). Dorothy was allowed to speak only when she was directly addressed and was taught to model herself on her mother, who was openly considered to be irrational, emotional, and incapable of making decisions on the grounds that she lacked knowledge about the ways of the world.

As a young girl, Dorothy observed how her brothers were allowed to engage in further studies, while she was consigned to learning to look after the household by imitating her mother. She was told that every young girl needed to learn to be proficient in the home because it was necessary for becoming a good wife. Dorothy left school at the age of 16 and, when she was about 18, she married a socially acceptable man chosen by her father.

A few years later, Dorothy, who had been totally dependent on her parents, was becoming totally dependent on her husband. After giving birth to three children in quick succession, she lost her husband in a car accident. Without financial backing or education, and with three small children, she was left destitute. She had no life skills, or decision-making ability since her father, mother, and later her husband, failed to understand that even women needed to learn these life-enhancing skills.

Dorothy's grief following the death of her husband, coupled with a lack of life skills, made her deeply depressed and eventually drove her to move back to her father's house. Her father still considered her to be too inexperienced and too emotional (she was still grieving for her late husband) to manage her financial affairs. As Dorothy had previously allowed her husband to make all her decisions, she now allowed her father to make all the decisions again.

Many years after the death of her husband, Dorothy was even more dependent on her parents than before. She regularly asked her mother to help her make decisions with regard to her three children, her personal life, her personal appearance, and even her choice of friends.

The personality profile of the young woman in the case study above would closely resemble the diagnosis of Dependent Personality Disorder according to the DSM-5 criteria. However, as we can see from the case study, this woman was taught to be submissive, dutiful, subservient, and dependent. Between 1900 and 1960, these character traits were highly desirable for Western women in general, while today they are considered to be dysfunctional in many different contexts. Despite changes with regard to what is considered to be desirable and undesirable behaviour as time goes by, the criteria for Dependent Personality Disorder have remained the same for both men and women; however, they reflect a much higher statistical frequency for women than for men. Due to the different socialisation processes for boys and girls, this could have been expected. The statistical frequency for Antisocial Personality Disorder is, however, much higher for men than for women. Could that perhaps also have something to do with child-rearing practices? Or does it perhaps reflect a dysfunctional society?

Although the DSM-5 and ICD-10 distinguish between different personality disorders, and describe each of these in detail, these disorders are not without controversy. One of the main criticisms against the present classification systems regarding personality disorders is the organisation and categorisation of these disorders. Both the DSM and ICD classification systems make a distinction between personality disorders and other mental disorders. According to Castillo (1998), there are three main reasons for this:

- Personality disorders are viewed as being enduring patterns of subjective experience and behaviour.
- They are based on personality development rather than some specific disease entity.
- These disorders generally do not have significant periods of remission, improvement over time, or changes in the type or severity of symptoms.

There seem to be two major schools of thought on the approach to the classification of personality disorders. One is the categorical approach, as reflected in both the DSM and ICD classification system, while the other is a dimensional approach to classification.

The dimensional approach takes the view that personality disorders are maladaptive variants of personality traits that merge with adaptive variants of personality traits. This view sees personality traits as existing on a continuum which allows for a person to function anywhere within the full range from low to high functioning. The attempt to fit the dimensional approach of a personality trait continuum into the qualitatively distinct categories of clinical syndromes (the categorical approach) is like trying to fit every uniquely comprised individual person's personality traits into a single, predetermined, fixed, and acceptable formal category. This implies that there is a normative or acceptable, formal category of personality that requires everybody to think, feel, behave, and respond in the same way to specific situations, while ingenuity, creativity, intuitiveness, and new ways of coping are discounted.

According to the DSM-5, personality disorders are first diagnosed by applying a set of six general diagnostic criteria for identifying the possibility of the presence of a personality disorder (see Table 12.1), after which another specific set of diagnostic criteria is applied for diagnosing the particular personality disorder. When we examine the six general diagnostic criteria for a personality disorder, we find that Criterion A refers to a marked deviation from the expectations of a person's culture. Criterion A is manifested as a pattern of behaviour in the areas of cognition, affectivity or emotional response, interpersonal functioning, and impulse control.

On account of the general criteria for personality disorders, everyone who is compared to these theoretical, general diagnostic criteria will necessarily need to fit into the statistical norm of what is considered to be 'normal' (by the clinician) at the time of identifying and classifying the client's symptoms and syndrome. This means that the diagnostic criteria are not differentiated enough for specific disorders to emerge, which increases the possibility of overlapping diagnoses of a number of disorders. It is assumed that we can make a clear, categorical distinction between the presence and absence of a personality disorder, but this assumption is false, due to the poorly differentiated criteria and because of dynamic changes within individual behaviour, as well as changes in society, over time.

One of the major challenges that face the classification of personality disorders is the dynamic nature of personality and the factors that influence personality development. If personality is static, or reaches a point of homeostasis, as was initially thought, classification of 'normal' and 'abnormal' personality would be relatively simple. Human development is, however, multifaceted and complex, and occurs on a number of levels simultaneously without a predetermined path. Recently, genetic vulnerabilities and other biological factors have been found to play a role in the causes of personality disorders such as Schizotypal Personality Disorder. In addition, biological and psychosocial factors have been identified as possible causes for the development of high levels of impulsivity and affective instability, which may lead to a diagnosis of Borderline Personality Disorder in high-risk individuals (Gurvits et al., 2000). A linear cause-effect research strategy unfortunately fails to consider the complex and mutually interactive factors and communications in dysfunctional family systems for example.

Responses to stressors, including internal and external expectations and limited internal and external resources, often seem dysfunctional from the functional perspective of society, but they may be functional from the perspective of the dysfunctional environment in which the individual is embedded. When clinicians are evaluating individuals for possible personality disorder diagnoses, they often compare them to the 'ideal' characteristics of a statistically normal personality. However, in a constantly changing and culturally diverse society, these mutually exclusive categories for personality disorders are problematic for clinicians. Diagnosticians thus find themselves trying to fit their clients, who are dynamically evolving and who are in dynamic reciprocal interaction with their environments, into these static categories.

Misdiagnoses and overlapping symptoms of personality disorders are therefore partly the result of describing such wide variations of what may be idiosyncratic responses to life and its problems, within the confines of a diagnostic system that takes into account only a small number of 'ideal' responses. According to Livesley (2001), no individual can (or will) ever fit the 'ideal' descriptions of personality. This is because many theoretical models of personality, such as the five-factor model of personality, are based on a 'theoretical ideal' of human functioning, which is far removed from the complexity of real-life combinations of personality characteristics, and the pathways and processes of personality development.

In the discussion above, the role of society in the development of personality is emphasised, which brings us to the next dynamic feature of personality. Societies are highly dynamic, and as they change, there will invariably be changes in common practices such as child-rearing. In general, child-rearing practices and expectations for boys differ considerably from those for girls. In the West, between 1900 and 1960, boys were encouraged to learn a trade, to obtain a position in a firm or business, or to aspire to higher learning with the aim of entering a profession such as law, medicine, or scientific research. In Western culture, social, political, and financial contexts supported such learning, in conjunction with the division of labour between women and men; in addition, men were remunerated with higher wages than women for the same tasks.

A number of research findings suggest that a dysfunctional personality style is influenced by authoritarian child-rearing practices and social attitudes. Schlachter and Duckitt (2002) found a link between authoritarian social attitudes and prejudice on the one hand, and a maladjusted personality style, on the other hand. Almajali (2005), in turn, found that an authoritative parenting style, coupled with a child with an internal locus of control, promoted creative thinking in adolescence.

Supporting evidence comes from Langley and Klopper (2005), who found that the establishment of 'trust' was the foundation for therapeutic interventions with patients with Borderline Personality Disorder. This suggests that clients with Borderline Personality Disorder were not able to develop an adequate sense of basic trust with their primary caregiver. Considering the complexity of Borderline Personality Disorder and its associated disorders like alcohol abuse, Dysthymia, Gender Identity Disorder, Schizotypal Personality Disorder, Posttraumatic Stress Disorder, and eating disorders, it becomes clear that the client might not have developed these co-morbid disorders (or Borderline Personality Disorder) if the individual had developed a sense of basic trust. Thus, one could argue that personality disorders could also be considered to be 'socialisation disorders of childhood'.

If changing societies influence the development of personality disorders, one cannot help but wonder what effect the rapid changes in a society like South Africa will have on the prevalence of personality disorders. Since the advent of democracy in South Africa, women rather than men are preferred as employees, and remuneration for men and women is related to the task rather than their gender. This transformation has impacted both negatively and positively on family structures and socialisation processes for boys and girls. Both boys and girls are now encouraged to learn domestic, financial, and academic skills. One could thus expect that the high rate of apparent Dependent Personality Disorder in women will diminish whilst at the same time the rate may increase in the case of men. This would be due to the fact that men might become more financially dependent on their mothers and spouses, as a result of being denied access to the fields of their chosen professions.

The argument for this possible outcome is based on the observed trends in the changes to the classification of personality disorders. When one looks at the history of the classification of these disorders, it is evident how certain personality disorders have 'disappeared' over time, and how others have 'emerged'. The most recent of these changes is the Passive-Aggressive Personality Disorder that has been moved from the main classification to the appendix of DSM-IV-TR, and the possible inclusion of a new personality disorder, the Depressive Personality Disorder. These disorders have, however, not been included in any way in the DSM-5.

According to Lamiell (2007), we will have ongoing difficulties in categorising and diagnosing personality disorders if we do not interrogate our current understanding of personality research. We need to investigate the inconsistency and fundamental incoherence in thinking that has led to the formulation of a 'trait theory of personality'. Lamiell's (2007) historical research regarding the development of thought about what a scientific psychology of personality should be has uncovered a false premise on which our present 'trait theory of personality' has been based. Instead of generating knowledge about a single individual, psychological research practices revolved around generating knowledge about attributes in general. According to Lamiell (2007), the fundamental error is that inter-attribute correlations obtained from studies of individual differences have been used for interpreting single individuals.

Recently, person-centred approaches to studying development in context have uncovered the complex nature of parallel pathways and processes in individual and social development (Estell, Farmer, Pearl, Van Acker, & Rodkin, 2003). This complexity of 'being and becoming' makes it extremely difficult to identify and understand the different contributions of inherent personality traits, wilful responses or reactions to social and/or cultural norms, prescriptions and expectations, and complex inner developmental processes, all in the context of a constantly changing multicultural society.

CONCLUSION

When individual behaviour is classified as abnormal by comparing it to what is customary in the culture in which the individual lives, it is quite possible that perfectly adaptive behaviour can be classified as abnormal. By polarising normal and abnormal behaviour on the grounds of comparing it to the individual's culture, the possibility of finding fault with the cultural norms is automatically excluded when viewed from the linear perspective. This problematic state of using culture as a rule by which individual normality and abnormality are determined has been perpetuated since the inception of the first DSM in 1952. Cultural norms have changed tremendously over the last decades, while the rule of culture as a normative entity has been maintained, even in multicultural societies.

The discussion with regard to the two different diagnostic systems, DSM-5 and ICD-10, demonstrates that the two epistemological systems for communicating knowledge about health and illness differ in their presuppositions about health and illness. The difference between a disease classification (ICD-10) and a psychological disorder classification (DSM-5) constitutes a fundamental difference between a biological aetiology and a psychological and behavioural identification of mental disorders. This chapter provides a window into the psychologically, socially, politically, and environmentally mediated ways in which disorders develop. From this perspective, personality disorders can ultimately be seen as the interacting outcomes of social practices, within the context of the family and the wider social, political, cultural, and environmental field of values and norms, which are themselves situated within the context of a dominant culture.

The implications of these aetiological findings also throw light on the other issues that have plagued the classification of personality disorders for many years, such as the high rate of overlap between different personality disorders. The 'whole individual' within the context of their environment needs to be considered when possible classifications of personality disorders are made.

MULTIPLE-CHOICE QUESTIONS

1. On which axis of the DSM-5 are personality disorders coded?
   a) I
   b) II
   c) III
   d) DSM-5 does not have a multi-axial diagnostic system

2. The DSM-5 divides personality disorders into how many distinct clusters?
   a) one
   b) two
   c) three
   d) four

3. Which set of adjective pairs correctly describes the clusters into which DSM-5 personality disorders are grouped?
   a) odd/eccentric, dangerous/inconsistent, and shy/withdrawn
   b) shy/withdrawn, anxious/fearful, and dangerous/inconsistent
   c) shy/withdrawn, dramatic/emotional, and bizarre/thought-disordered
   d) odd/eccentric, dramatic/emotional, and anxious/fearful

4. The diagnosis of more than one personality disorder in an individual patient is:
   a) common
   b) impossible unless the person suffers from Dissociative Identity Disorder
   c) rare
   d) only possible for personality disorders in the same DSM-5 cluster

5. One of the influences that has been associated with the development of Borderline Personality Disorder is:
   a) child abuse or neglect
   b) head injuries
   c) parental alcoholism
   d) abnormal dopamine levels

PARAGRAPH AND ESSAY QUESTIONS

1. Describe the three clusters of DSM-5 personality disorders and provide an example of at least one personality disorder that belongs to each cluster. How would you characterise each cluster?

2. Compare and contrast the behaviours, thoughts, and motivations of an individual with Avoidant Personality Disorder against someone with Schizoid Personality Disorder. Make sure to note similarities and differences.

3. Explain what differentiates individuals with Schizotypal Personality Disorder from Schizophrenia. What are the similarities observed in individuals diagnosed with Schizotypal Personality Disorder and those diagnosed with Schizophrenia?

13 NEURODEVELOPMENTAL AND OTHER CHILDHOOD DISORDERS

Adri Vorster

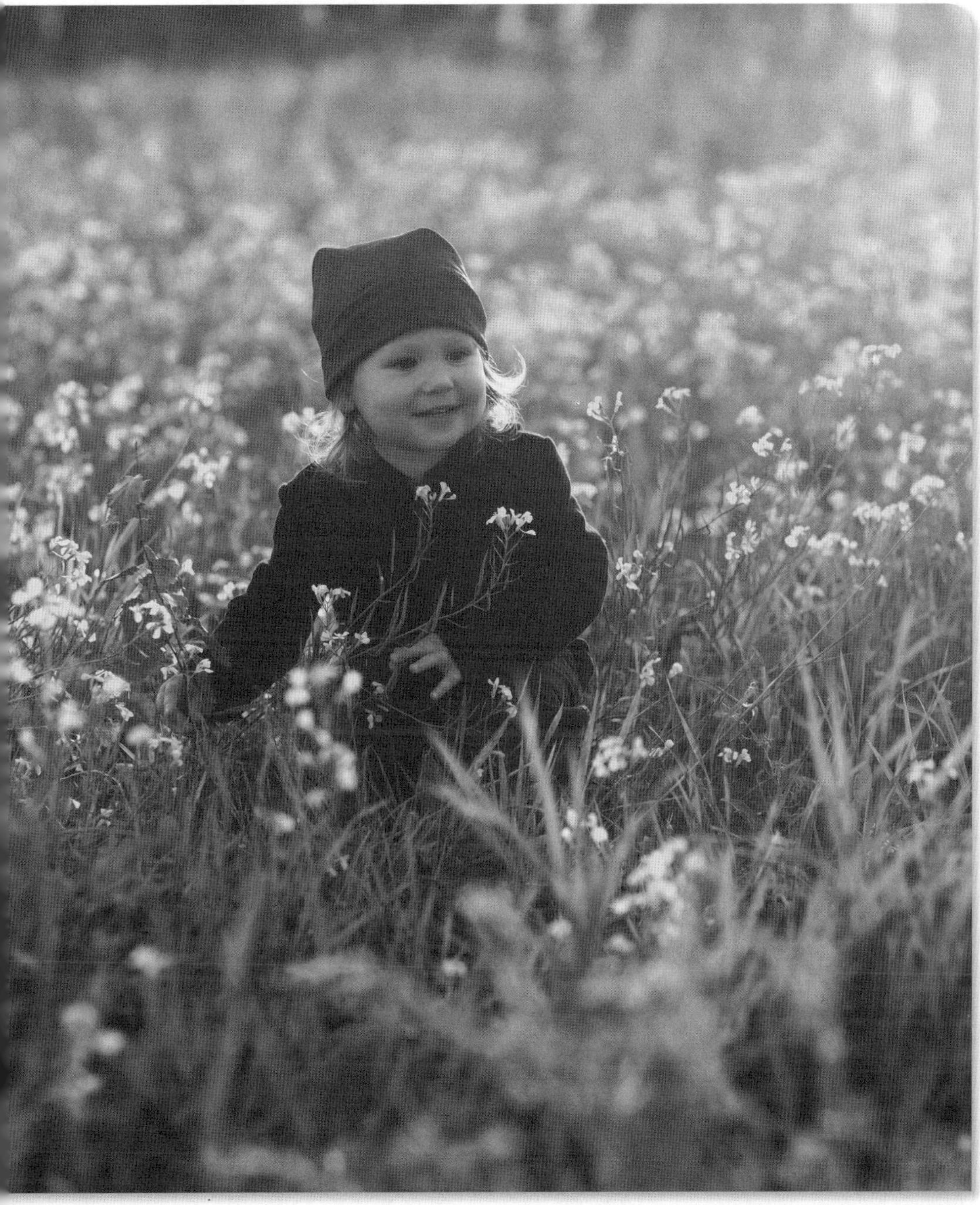

13 CHAPTER OUTLINE

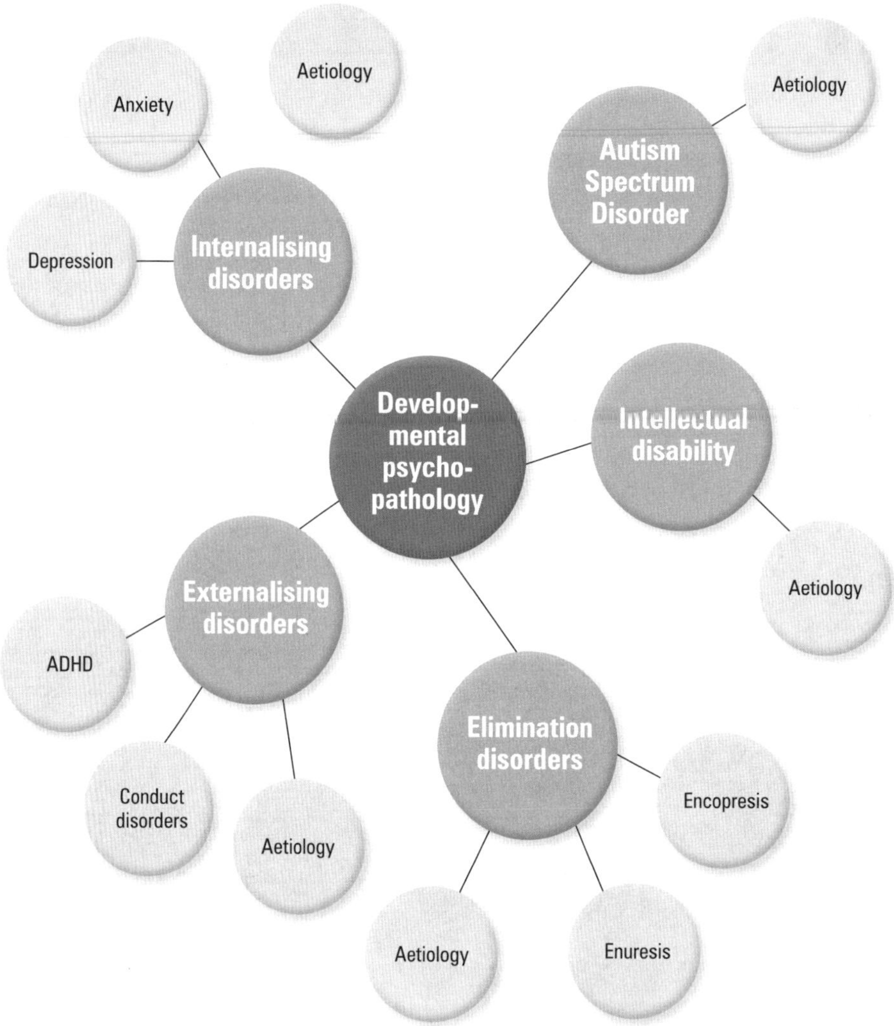

LEARNING OUTCOMES

After studying this chapter you should be able to:

- Demonstrate knowledge of the key concepts, assumptions, and principles associated with developmental psychopathology.
- Employ a broad range of criteria for differentiating between normal and abnormal development in young people.
- Identify multiple factors and processes associated with the cause and course of a range of disorders experienced by young people.
- Identify risk and protective factors and processes associated with a specific disorder.
- Demonstrate knowledge of factors associated with the development and maintenance of internalising, externalising, intellectual, autism spectrum, and elimination disorders in young people.
- Apply a theoretical model of psychopathology to the development of internalising, externalising, intellectual, autism spectrum, and elimination disorders in young people.

INTRODUCTION

Children and adolescents are multifaceted thinking and feeling beings, with a degree of mental complexity that the world has only recently started to truly grasp (World Health Organisation, 2005). For centuries, children were seen as miniature adults. For this reason, they were often, from a very young age, employed as apprentices in professions that required manual labour, including farming, blacksmithing, and carpentry, or as servants in the ancient Greek and Roman societies (Burns, 2007; Mash & Wolfe, 2005). It was also not strange for children to be married at a very young age. However, towards the end of the Middle Ages, with the rise of the Renaissance and the economic, technical, scientific, and philosophical changes that accompanied it, many occupations required stronger academic skills, rather than manual skills (Burns, 2007). In addition, the Renaissance gave rise to humanist thinking. John Locke, an English philosopher and physician, was one of the first men who became famous not only for his humane thinking, but also for his special interest in the right of children to be treated with kindness, understanding, and respect, and to be provided with proper educational opportunities (Mash & Wolfe, 2005). These changes transformed the fate of children and, whereas they had been previously considered to be cost-effective manual labourers, the focus now shifted towards educational instruction and understanding children not as small adults, but as beings in their own right, with their own developmental tasks, abilities, and challenges. Likewise, whereas children's difficulties were previously treated as downward extensions of adult disorders, clinicians now recognise that there are very important differences between adult and childhood disorders (Comer, 1995).

HUMAN DEVELOPMENT

Although the concept of human development can appear relatively simple, one should be careful not to oversimplify it and to take into consideration the essential characteristics that define development:

- Development refers to specific changes that occur over a person's lifespan. These changes are the result of a person's interactions with biological, psychological, and sociocultural variables, which themselves are constantly changing (Wicks-Nelson & Israel, 2009).
- Over the lifespan, people normally change both quantitatively and qualitatively. Whereas children can initially only speak single words, they can later form sentences (quantitative changes) and even later add to the quality of their sentences through appropriate adverbs, correct grammar, etc. (qualitative changes) (Wicks-Nelson & Israel, 2009).
- Children's biological, motor, physical, cognitive, emotional, and social systems follow a common course of development, with early global structures and functions becoming increasingly more differentiated and integrated (Wicks-Nelson & Israel, 2009).
- Added to the above, from a holistic point of view, it is vital to remember that a person's different systems are in continual interaction with one another and through these interactions, a person's structures become increasingly complex and organised, with new structures emerging out of the ones that came before (Wenar & Kerig, 2006).
- A child's development can be compared to a flight of stairs, with one stage building on the next. This implies that not only are the different developmental stages connected and

that a child's current functioning is connected to both past and future functioning, but also that a disturbance in one area, will affect all of the others (Barlow & Durand, 2009).

- Finally, development implies change; however, change is not always positive (Wicks-Nelson & Israel, 2009).

DEVELOPMENTAL PSYCHOPATHOLOGY

In line with our understanding of development, developmental psychopathology refers to understanding how psychopathology emerges over the course of a person's lifespan and how the person's developing systems, in interaction with the noted variables, contribute to the formation of psychopathology or protection against it (Wenar & Kerig, 2006). In addition, developmental psychopathology assumes that psychopathology does not just appear suddenly or unexpectedly. It gradually emerges as a person's systems interact with constantly changing sociocultural, biological, and psychological variables. People differ in their ability to adapt to these changes. If we again consider development as a flight of stairs that follows a specific path, a person's position on the path can at any time be considered either developmentally appropriate or inappropriate. However, one should never think that a person's developmental path is fixed, as new interactions or different reactions to previous circumstances can lead to new directions and either a more appropriate or unfavourable path.

Within the field of developmental psychopathology, developmental disorders are defined as a unique group of disorders that originate in infancy, childhood, or adolescence and that generally impact on specific areas of a person's development. The clinical features of developmental disorders vary with regard to severity and the area of functioning that is affected (Institute of Medicine, 2001). From the different theories of physical, cognitive, language, social, personality, emotional, and moral development, it is evident that childhood is a very important period as far as neurological changes and the completion of certain developmental tasks and competencies are concerned. For this reason, it is important that these disorders are identified and diagnosed as they occur. Not only can this assist parents, caregivers, teachers, and other professionals to assist those whose lives are affected by them, but it could also minimise the impact that they have on the young person's developmental course.

HISTORY OF DEVELOPMENTAL PSYCHOPATHOLOGY

Although the field of psychopathology is not new, the branch of developmental psychopathology as a unique field only emerged about three decades ago from the fields of developmental psychology, clinical psychology, educational psychology, and psychiatry (Wadsworth, 2005). In the 1970s, one of the earliest definitions of developmental disorders was constructed in the United States. This was a result of the forward thinking of some individuals who served with President John F. Kennedy on the president's panel on mental retardation. The goal of this panel was to prevent mental retardation across the globe. This work laid the foundation for the construction of subsequent legislation on developmental disorders. In addition, it also created a structure from which developmental disorders could be defined and treated over the next few decades (Harper, 2008).

From the 1970s to 2000, the definition of developmental disorders changed significantly. While the focus in the 1970 definition fell on defining mental retardation, this was widened in 1975 to incorporate autism and some specific learning disabilities. In 1978, the Developmental Disabilities Act was passed; this provided a detailed explanation of developmental disorders that influenced decision-making, educational interventions, and federal policy for many years to come. The new definitions of developmental disorders became less categorical and placed greater emphasis on the functional limitations that resulted from a specific disorder. In addition, researchers also started to use the word 'impairment' in the place of 'disease' (Harper, 2008).

Together with the significant changes that took place in legislation during the 1970s, the dominant diagnostic system of psychopathology, the *Diagnostic and Statistical Manual of Mental Disorders* (DSM) published by the American Psychiatric Association also went through significant changes as far as developmental psychopathology was concerned. In the early 1970s, the DSM gave almost no attention to developmental psychopathology, mostly because it was assumed that children either did not suffer from psychological disorders or, if they did, they would look much the same as they did in adults (Wadsworth, 2005).

Then, with the publication of Thomas Achenbach's book *Developmental Psychopathology* in 1974, it was proposed that childhood psychopathology should be viewed as a separate and unique branch of psychopathology. In 1983, Rutter and Garmezy took the matter a step further by publishing their chapter on developmental psychopathology in the *Handbook of Child Psychology*. Finally, in 1989 and 1990, the distinction was well cemented as a distinct and unique branch within the broader field of psychopathology when the Rochester Symposium on Developmental Psychopathology brought together a diverse group of students with a specific interest in the field and the *Journal of Development and Psychopathology* was established (Wadsworth, 2005).

CONTEXTUALISING DEVELOPMENTAL PSYCHOPATHOLOGY IN SOUTH AFRICA

It has long been understood that a person's physical health and well-being can be influenced by genetic and environmental factors. However, health care professionals are also acknowledging the adverse impact that these factors can have on a person's mental health and well-being (World Health Organisation, 2005). Taking poverty as an example, Petersen (2010) notes that the social conditions associated with poverty (e.g. poorer education and malnutrition) often lead to physical health difficulties (see Figure 13.1 on the next page). In addition, however, poverty can also lead to helplessness and shame, which are linked to mental health difficulties such as depression and anxiety. On the other hand, when people are stressed or depressed, they often engage in high-risk health behaviours such as excessive alcohol use and unsafe sex, which can in return impact on their physical health. Also, continuous stress, anxiety, and depression can compromise a person's immune system and endocrine functioning, exacerbating the risk of infection. Thus, the interrelationship between environmental risk factors and mental and physical health should not be underestimated.

Environmental factors like poverty that can increase the risk of the developmental of mental health difficulties within a specific context are called risk factors. The World Health

Figure 13.1: The interrelationship between poverty and mental and physical health difficulties

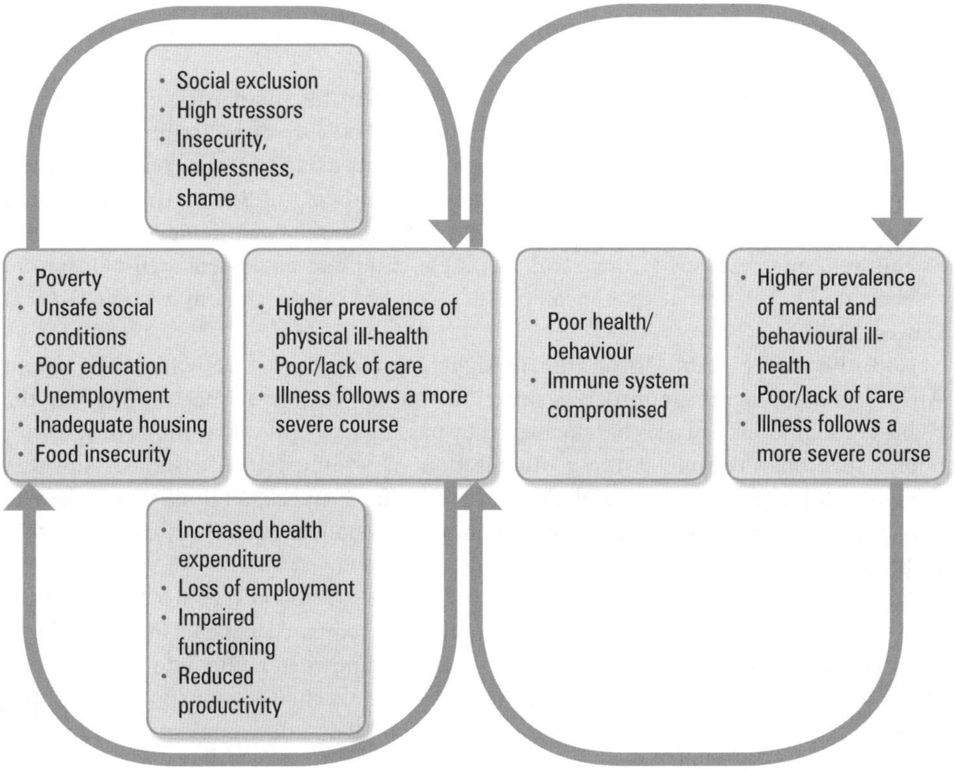

Source: Adapted from Petersen, 2010, p. 8.

Organisation (2005) defines risk factors as those variables that increase the probability of the development and existence of mental health difficulties; protective factors are those variables that moderate the effects of risk exposure and assist in the development of resilience (see Chapter 3). In understanding and treating developmental disorders, it is essential to understand the risk factors within a specific context that can contribute to the development and prolongation of these disorders. Furthermore, in developing a more pro-active approach aimed at preventing developmental disorders, it is important to understand the protective factors within an environment which can enhance mental well-being and resilience in children and adolescents.

From an ecosystemic perspective (see Chapter 2), it is important to understand that risk and protective factors can exist in a child and adolescent's biological, socio-economic, and psychological domains. In the biological domain, the exposure to toxins, genetic influences, and malnutrition are examples of risk factors, whereas age-appropriate physical development and good intellectual stimulation are examples of protective factors. Within the psychological domain, neglect, abuse, and learning disorders are examples of risk factors, whereas good self-esteem and social skills can be considered protective factors. Finally, within the socio-economic domain, family factors such as inconsistent parenting, school factors such as academic failure, and community factors such as discrimination and marginalisation, are all considered examples of risk factors, whereas family attachment and opportunities for involvement in one's school and community are considered protective factors (World Health Organisation, 2005).

In identifying the risk and protective factors within the South African context it is helpful to adopt a rights-based approach as this not only gives us insight into a wide spectrum of risk factors, but also into the developments that have taken place to expand protective factors and hence improve the mental well-being of South African children and adolescents. Furthermore, in linking child and adolescent well-being with the rights of children, one develops a framework to assess child and adolescent well-being from an ecosystemic perspective that encompasses a concern for the child as a whole (Bray & Dawes, 2007).

According to the South African Human Rights Commission and UNICEF (2011), South Africa has made significant progress since the end of apartheid in 1994 in fulfilling the rights of its children. This has been achieved by passing new laws and through progressive public spending, as well as the reorganisation of administrative systems. However, there are still large disparities: a black child is still, for instance, 18 times more likely to live in poverty and only half as likely to complete secondary education, compared to a white child.

Furthermore, as far as household income is concerned, the poorest 20% of South Africa's households house approximately seven million children, compared to the 1.7 million children living in the richest 20% of households. This is significant when taking into consideration that compared to a child growing up in the richest quintile, a child growing up in the poorest quintile is only half as likely to be exposed to early childhood developmental programmes and only a third as likely to complete secondary education.

A large number of the risk factors still faced by South African children and adolescents fall within the psychological domain and violate the rights of children to be protected against all forms of violence, as well as their right to special protection (South African Human Rights Commission & UNICEF, 2011). Some examples are violence and sexual offences against children. In addition, one in three children are exposed to severe corporal punishment and a 1999 survey found that 36% of children above five years of age were engaged in at least one form of work activity.

In the biological domain, several risk factors show how the rights of children to life, to an adequate standard of living, and basic health are still being violated (South African Human Rights Commission & UNICEF, 2011). These include problems with hunger and malnutrition, infection with HIV, and lack of immunisation.

Within the socio-economic domain, there are also still several risk factors that violate the rights of children to social security, housing, water and sanitation, education, and family care (South African Human Rights Commission & UNICEF, 2011). These include that only one in three children live with both their biological parents with many living with a grandparent or other relative.

NEURODEVELOPMENTAL AND OTHER CHILDHOOD DISORDERS

With the publication of the new *Diagnostic and Statistical Manual of Mental Disorders – Fifth Edition* (DSM-5)(American Psychiatric Association, 2013), most of the so-called childhood disorders have been group under the category Neurodevelopmental Disorders. However, others such as Conduct Disorder, Oppositional Defiant Disorder, Enuresis and Encopresis have been grouped elsewhere (See Figure 13.2).

For the purpose of this chapter, the different developmental disorders will be grouped into five categories in the following manner:

- Internalising disorders (including depression and Separation Anxiety Disorder)
- Externalising disorders (including Attention-Deficit/Hyperactivity Disorder, Oppositional Defiant Disorder and Conduct Disorder)
- Intellectual disability (Intellectual Development Disorder)
- Autism Spectrum Disorder
- Elimination disorders (including Enuresis and Encopresis).

By grouping the different disorders in this manner, one develops a better understanding of the interrelationship between the different disorders, as well as the underlying risk and protective factors.

Figure 13.2: DSM-5 classifications of childhood disorders

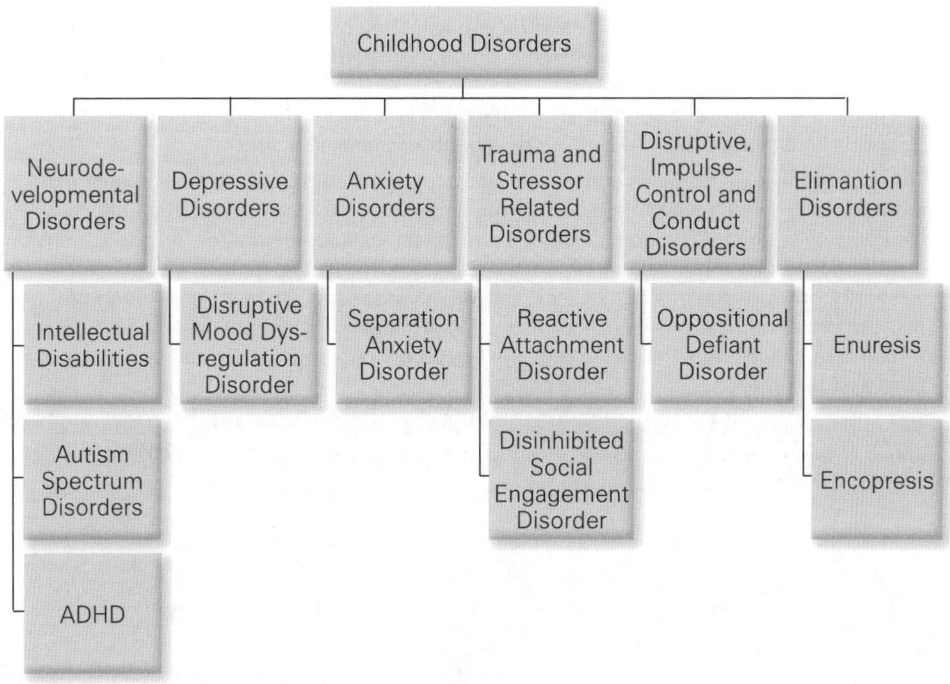

SECTION 1: INTERNALISING DISORDERS

Internalising disorders of childhood and adolescence are best described as disorders that occur within the child. As a result of their difficulties, these children and adolescents often appear shy, withdrawn, and fearful. Unlike externalising disorders, these disorders are usually within the child, rather than being acted out externally in the environment (Helm, 2008). The internalising disorders that will be described in this chapter include depression and anxiety. It is important to note that these disorders should be read in conjunction with the disorders described in Chapter 4 and Chapter 5.

Table 13.1: Diagnostic criteria for emotional disorders with onset specific to childhood, according to the ICD-10

ICD-10
In child psychiatry, a differentiation has traditionally been made between emotional disorders specific to childhood and adolescence and adult-type neurotic disorders. There have been four main justifications for this differentiation. 1. First, research findings have been consistent in showing that the majority of children with emotional disorders go on to become normal adults; only a minority show neurotic disorders in adult life. Conversely, many adult neurotic disorders appear to have an onset in adult life without significant psychopathological precursors in childhood. Hence, there is considerable discontinuity between emotional disorders occurring in these two age periods. 2. Second, many emotional disorders in childhood seem to constitute exaggerations of normal developmental trends rather than phenomena that are qualitatively abnormal in themselves. 3. Third, related to the last consideration, there has often been the theoretical assumption that the mental mechanisms involved in emotional disorders of childhood may not be the same as for adult neuroses. 4. Fourth, the emotional disorders of childhood are less clearly demarcated into supposedly specific entities such as phobic disorders or obsessional disorders. The third of these points lacks empirical validation, and epidemiological data suggest that, if the fourth is correct, it is a matter of degree only (with poorly differentiated emotional disorders quite common in both childhood and adult life). Accordingly, the second feature (i.e. developmental appropriateness) is used as the key diagnostic feature in defining the difference between the emotional disorders with an onset specific to childhood and the neurotic disorders. The validity of this distinction is uncertain, but there is some empirical evidence to suggest that the developmentally appropriate emotional disorders of childhood have a better prognosis.

Source: Reprinted with permission from the ICD-10 Classification of Mental and Behavioural Disorders: Diagnostic Criteria for Research, World Health Organisation, Geneva, 2007.

Depression

CASE STUDY

Lerato was a 16-year-old girl, referred to the adolescent unit of an inpatient psychiatric hospital. Her mother, Lorraine, referred Lerato after discovering her daughter one afternoon after school, bleeding from her wrists. Although the amount of blood was not substantial, Lorraine got quite a fright and immediately took Lerato to the emergency room for treatment. The doctor who attended to Lerato confirmed that she was not seriously injured; but, as he felt concerned as to why the teenager would hurt herself, he referred her to the psychiatric hospital for further assessment and possible inpatient treatment. An interview with a psychiatrist was arranged for the next day.

During this interview, Lerato mentioned that her parents had recently separated after her mother was physically assaulted by her drunken father. Lerato moved with her mother to her maternal grandparents in another province and was hence transferred to a new school. She noted that she did not feel welcome in her new school after some children had made derogatory remarks about her weight. Lerato presented as overweight during the interview with the psychiatrist and when questioned in this regard, noted that she has gained a substantial amount of weight since they moved in with her grandparents.

Lerato also disclosed to the psychiatrist that her parents had been fighting a lot about her father's constant drinking after he had been retrenched the previous year. On the day of the assault, Lerato recalled the feeling of helplessness she felt when she was unable to stop her father from assaulting her mother. As her older brothers decided to stay with their father, Lerato had lost all contact with them and noted that she missed them terribly as they had a very close bond.

It appeared as if Lerato's mood had worsened over the two weeks prior to the incident where she had tried to cut her wrists. She longed for her family to be together and felt increasing concern about her school marks that kept dropping, despite the fact that she had previously been a very diligent student. Lerato constantly felt tired and unable to concentrate on the work in front of her.

Source: Adapted from Kearney, 2010, pp. 25-26.

Depression, currently one of the most common psychiatric diagnoses, impacts on the child or adolescent's cognitive, emotional, and physical functioning. It is of great concern that depression often goes undetected in childhood and adolescence. Thus, instead of being diagnosed as a major disorder with a significant impact on the child's development, it is often interpreted as part of a normal pattern of mood swings. Also, as the externalising disorders often attract more attention, children's internal sufferings often go undetected (Mash & Wolfe,

2005). It is also said that professionals are often reluctant to prematurely diagnose and label a young person with depression (Knox & Lichtenberg, 2005). The danger, however, is that if the disorder goes undiagnosed and hence untreated, it not only has a major impact on the child's current functioning, but also on their future development and functioning.

For a child or adolescent to be diagnosed with a Major Depressive Disorder, they not only need to present with the symptoms of Major Depressive Disorder (see Chapter 5), but other possible disorders also need to be excluded. According to the DSM-5 (American Psychiatric Association, 2013), adults with a Major Depressive Disorder often present with depressed mood; whereas children and adolescents might rather appear irritable, agitated, angry and hostile. Other symptoms noted in children and adolescents who have been diagnosed with depression include, amongst others:

- Persistent sadness and crying or outbursts of shouting and complaining
- Loss of interest in activities that were once enjoyed (e.g. social gatherings, play-dates, and sport)
- Social isolation
- Alcohol and/or substance use/abuse
- An increase or decrease in appetite with subsequent weight loss or gain
- Sleeping difficulties
- Loss of energy, lethargy, and fatigue
- Feelings of worthlessness and guilt without reason
- Extreme sensitivity to rejection or failure
- Talk of running away, or even efforts to run away, from home, or truancy
- Difficulty in sustained attention and concentration, and poor school performance
- Fear of death
- Frequent, non-specific physical complaints such as headaches, stomach pains, and muscle aches
- Boredom and/or reckless behaviour.

These symptoms are expressed in a variety of ways, based on the child or adolescent's developmental level and their ability to express emotions.

Anxiety

Anxiety is typically characterised by two key features – strong negative emotion and a state of fear (see Chapter 4). In addition, it is also accompanied by bodily symptoms of tension. When children and adolescents experience excessive and debilitating anxieties, they are often diagnosed with an anxiety disorder (Mash & Wolfe, 2005). Although there are several types of anxiety disorders, this chapter will focus only on Separation Anxiety Disorder as it is the one most commonly experienced by children and adolescents. However, it is important to note that the different anxiety disorders all share common characteristics, which include (Lopez & Silverman, 2004):

- Maladaptive thoughts or cognitions of harm to self or loved ones
- Physiological arousal or reactions
- Avoidance of, or attempts to avoid, certain situations, objects or events
- The presence of anxiety, fear, and/or worry that is developmentally inappropriate
- Significant distress and impact on the child or adolescent's normal functioning
- Prolonged periods of anxiety, stress, and/or worry.

Anxiety may also manifest through behavioural symptoms that include motor restlessness, difficulty sitting still, and attempts to escape the source of the anxiety (Lowe & Raad, 2007). In addition, children and adolescents who experience anxiety may also present with the following cognitive symptoms: excessive worry, concentration difficulties, attention difficulties, and memory problems. Finally, the physiological symptoms of anxiety include muscle tension, increased perspiration, rapid heartbeat, headaches, and stomach aches.

Although fear and anxiety can be considered normal human responses to danger or threat, they are clinically significant if they are persistent, cause significant functional impairment, or interfere with the child or adolescent's quality of life. In children and adolescents, it is often difficult to diagnose anxiety as it is often considered normal depending on their developmental stage. For instance, children around the age of three years are often afraid of the dark or monsters (Arnold et al., 2003; Lowe & Raad, 2007). However, when the anxiety experienced by a child or adolescent persists past what is expected of a certain developmental stage, causes significant impairment in their daily functioning, and interferes with their quality of life, further diagnosis and intervention are required.

Separation Anxiety Disorder

Separation anxiety often occurs during childhood. It refers to an excessive, age-inappropriate, and unrealistic worry in response to separation from home or a caregiver and is often accompanied by physical symptoms such as headaches, stomach aches, heart palpitations, sweating, shortness of breath, or nausea. Nightmares and sleeping difficulties are also quite common (Lowe & Raad, 2007). As children with this anxiety disorder are scared to separate from home or their caregivers, this disorder has a significant impact on their daily functioning at home and school. In addition, it also has an impact on their social development as they tend to avoid camps, school, or even sleepovers at a friend's house (Lee, 2005b).

Table 13.2: Diagnostic criteria for Separation Anxiety Disorder as adapted from the DSM-5 and ICD-10

DSM-5	ICD-10
A. Developmentally inappropriate and excessive fear or anxiety concerning separation from those to whom the individual is attached, as evidenced by at least three of the following: (1) Recurrent excessive distress when anticipating or expecting separation from home or from major attachment figures. (2) Persistent and excessive worry about losing major attachment figures or about possible harm to them, such as illness, injury, disasters, or death. (3) Persistent and excessive worry about experiencing an untoward event (e.g. getting lost, being kidnapped, having an accident, becoming ill) that causes separation from a major attachment figure.	• The key diagnostic feature is a focused, developmentally inappropriate, excessive anxiety concerning separation from those individuals to whom the child is attached (usually parents or other family members), that is not merely part of a generalised anxiety about multiple situations. The anxiety may take the form of: ‣ An unrealistic, preoccupying worry about possible harm befalling major attachment figures or a fear that they will leave and not return.

DSM-5	ICD-10
(4) Persistent reluctance or refusal to go out, away from home, to school, to work, or elsewhere because of fear of separation. (5) Persistent and excessive fear of or reluctance about being alone or without major attachment figures at home or in other settings. (6) Persistent reluctance or refusal to sleep away from home or to go to sleep without being near a major attachment figure. (7) Repeated nightmares involving the theme of separation. (8) Repeated complaints of physical symptoms (e.g. headaches, stomachaches, nausea, vomiting) when separation from major attachment figures occurs or is anticipated. B. The fear, anxiety or avoidance is persistent, lasting at least 4 weeks in children and adolescents and typically 6 months or more in adults. C. The disturbance causes clinically significant distress or impairment in social, academic, occupational, or other important areas of functioning. D. The disturbance is not better explained by another mental disorder, such as refusing to leave home because of excessive resistance to change in autism spectrum disorder; delusions or hallucinations concerning separation in psychotic disorders; refusal to go outside without a trusted companion in agoraphobia; worries about ill health or other harm befalling significant others in generalized anxiety disorder; or concerns about having an illness in illness anxiety disorder.	‣ An unrealistic, preoccupying worry that some untoward event, such as the child being lost, kidnapped, admitted to hospital, or killed, will separate him or her from a major attachment figure. ‣ Persistent reluctance or refusal to go to school because of fear about separation (rather than for other reasons such as fear about events at school). ‣ Persistent reluctance or refusal to go to sleep without being near or next to a major attachment figure.

Source: Reprinted with permission from the Diagnostic and Statistical Manual of Mental Disorders (DSM), Fifth Edition, American Psychiatric Association (APA), 2013 and ICD-10 Classification of Mental and Behavioural Disorders: Diagnostic Criteria for Research, World Health Organisation (WHO), Geneva, 2007.

Aetiology of internalising disorders

It is said that depression and anxiety are often the result of interdependent physiologically and genetically based causes that can be triggered by certain life events such as familial discord or parental divorce and personal stresses such as academic problems, grief or the end of a significant relationship. Other risk factors include attention difficulties, conduct problems, learning disabilities, chronic illness, abuse or neglect, and trauma (Fried, 2004; Knox & Lichtenberg, 2005).

Genetic and family factors

As far as genetic influences are concerned, children and adolescents who develop symptoms associated with a Major Depressive Disorder and anxiety disorders will most likely have a parent with, or a family history of, depression (Fried, 2004; Knox & Lichtenberg, 2005). Twin and family studies have suggested a genetic vulnerability to the development of affective disorders in childhood and adolescence. However, the influence of familial factors extends far beyond that of genetics. As we have seen in Chapter 5 and will be explained in more detail below, depression and anxiety are often associated with certain negative thinking patterns and it is believed that depressed parents or caregivers may model these to their children and that this, rather than the genetic vulnerability may explain why children with depressed parents also often develop depression (Sander & McCarty, 2005; Wicks-Nelson & Israel, 2006).

In addition, this negative parental cognitive style may also result in children developing lower self-worth, a negative attributional style, and feelings of hopelessness, all of which may contribute to the development of depression and anxiety. Furthermore, research has indicated that parental depression may result in disruption in effective parenting as it can lead to a lower frustration tolerance, hostility, irritation, withdrawal, and/or a lack of nurturance (Jewell & Stark, 2003; Wicks-Nelson & Israel, 2006). Although there thus appears to be a genetic link in the development of emotional disorders, the influence of parental styles should not be underestimated.

Personal and emotional factors

Quite recently, researchers have begun to look at the role that emotional processing plays in the development of internalising developmental disorders and, more specifically, paediatric affective disorders. The results of a study conducted by Ladouceur et al. (2005) suggest that children and adolescents with depression and anxiety, which are often co-morbid, seemed to process emotional information differently from those from their normative sample. For instance, children and adolescents with Major Depressive Disorder and co-morbid anxiety tend to spend more time processing negative emotional information than their peers. In addition, anxiety and depression are also associated with an attentional bias towards negative or even threatening information. Therefore, although further research in this area is required, it would appear that children and adolescents with depression and/or anxiety disorders tend to pay more attention to negative and threatening emotions and linger on these for longer periods than other children and adolescents (Ladouceur et al., 2005).

This idea links to the theory of Aaron Beck (see Chapter 5) which stated that children and adolescents develop depression as a result of the fact that they use negative and biased filters for processing information and interpreting events (Mash & Wolfe, 2005). As far as their biased filters are concerned, Beck stipulated that depressive children and adolescents display negative automatic thoughts that include thoughts of physical and social threat, personal failure, and hostility. As they are biased in the processing of information, they selectively attend to negative information and ignore positive information.

Beck further stipulated that adolescents and children with depression also display a negative cognitive triad (Mash & Wolfe, 2005). This implies that they have negative thoughts and feelings about themselves, the world, and the future. Finally, as far as cognitions are concerned, Beck stipulated that children and adolescents with depression present with negative cognitive schemata. Schemata are stable structures in the child's memory that are used to process information. When these are negative, children and adolescents will tend to filter information in a negative manner. Also, when these are rigid and resistant to change, children and adolescents will be more prone to depression. In addition, these children and adolescents have negative thought patterns about themselves and their environment, which influences their mood. These are called depressogenic cognitions.

A variety of negative attributions, misperceptions, and deficiencies in cognitive problem-solving skills are also related to depression. According to Mash and Wolfe (2005), children and adolescents with depression often display internal, stable, and global attributions to explain the causes of negative events. Thus, when something bad happens, they will often attribute this to something that they have done and hold themselves responsible (internal). Also, the reason that they are to blame will not change over time (stable). Finally, the reason that bad things happen applies to most things they do (global). In contrast to this, they tend to attribute positive things to something outside of themselves (external) and believe that they are not likely to happen again (unstable). Finally, they also tend to think that positive events are unique (specific).

Learning and conditioning

In terms of anxiety disorders, learned behaviour is often considered significant in the development of the disorder. According to the behaviourists, anxiety is a learned behaviour that is both acquired and maintained through operant conditioning, a combination of operant and classical conditioning, and/or modelling. For instance, when a neutral stimulus like a dog is paired repeatedly with an aversive stimulus such as a loud noise (e.g. barking) to produce a conditioned response such as a startled reaction, anxiety problems can develop and the presence of a dog may evoke the startled response. This will result in the avoidance of the dog, which will relieve the anxiety. According to operant conditioning, the avoidance behaviour will be maintained because the reduction of the anxiety is a negative reinforcement. In modelling, a child or adolescent develops an anxiety disorder through the observation and modelling of the behaviour of a significant other. For instance, when a mother avoids snakes for which she has a phobia, a child may develop a similar phobia through simply modelling her mother's behaviour (Lowe & Raad, 2007; Mash & Wolfe, 2005).

As far as depression is concerned, the behaviourists emphasise the importance of learning, environmental consequences, and skills and deficits during the onset and maintenance of depression. Thus, they propose that depression in childhood and adolescence is often related to a lack of response-contingent positive reinforcement (Mash & Wolfe, 2005). According to this theory, a lack of positive reinforcement may occur for three reasons. First, a child may not be able to experience positive reinforcement due to interfering anxiety. Second, changes in the child's environment, such as a divorce or the loss of a significant other, may result in a lack of availability of reward. Finally, a child may not have the skills or ability to have rewarding and satisfying social relationships. When a child continuously experiences a lack of positive reinforcement, they may be vulnerable to the development of depression.

Another theory in the development of anxiety and depression is Bowlby's theory of attachment (Sander & McCarty, 2005). According to this theory, fearfulness in children and adolescents is biologically rooted in the emotional attachment that is needed for survival. For instance, for an infant to survive, it needs to be emotionally and physically attached to its parents. When infants are not near their parents, they tend to display attachment behaviours such as crying, 'clinging', and fear of strangers, in an effort to maintain or restore proximity to their caregivers.

Separation will generally become more tolerable as the child matures. However, when a child is separated from their significant caregivers too early, is treated harshly, is abused, or does not have their primary needs met, they will react differently from their peers to separation and reunion. Also, when children view their environment as unpredictable or hostile, they tend to develop anxieties and fears (Mash & Wolfe, 2005). In addition, children and adolescents who are often confronted with unresponsive and emotionally unavailable caregivers go through a typical set of emotions that include despair, protest, and detachment. In addition, these children will start to feel unworthy and unloved, which places them at a greater risk of developing depression (Mash & Wolfe, 2005).

SECTION 2: EXTERNALISING DISORDERS

Externalising disorders of childhood and adolescence are best described as disorders characterised by behaviours directed outward. The primary difference between these and internalising disorders is in the way in which they are expressed. Unlike internalising disorders, externalising disorders are always expressed outward and become noticeable in the child and adolescent's interpersonal relations and interactions with others. It is here that we often notice behaviours such as disobedience, defiance, aggression, stubbornness, temper tantrums, fidgetiness, and hyperactivity that understandably cause a lot of tension and conflict between the child or adolescent and significant others such as parents and teachers (Helm, 2009).

Figure 13.3: Development of behavioural disorders across developmental stages

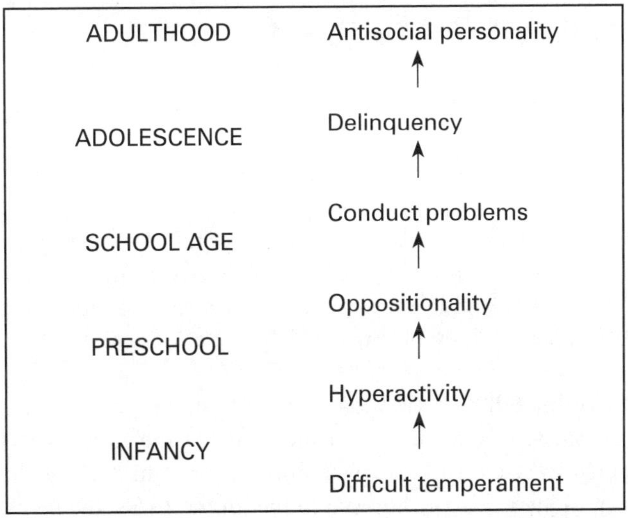

Source: Adapted from Wenar & Kerig, 2000, p. 195.

The externalising disorders that will be discussed in this section include Attention-Deficit/Hyperactivity Disorder (ADHD), which DSM-5 categorised under Neurodevelopmental Disorders, as well as Conduct Disorder and Oppositional Defiant Disorder, which have been listed under the category: Disruptive, Impulse-Control and Conduct Disorders. According to the American Psychiatric Association (2013), there was strong evidence to support the categorisation of ADHD as part of the latter category; however, based on the pattern of its symptoms, the underlying risk factors and the comorbidity of ADHD with a number of other disorders, it was categorised as a Neurodevelopmental Disorder.

Attention-Deficit/Hyperactivity Disorder

CASE STUDY

Eight-year-old Eric lives in a dynamic and ever-changing world; a kaleidoscope where sounds, images, and thoughts are constantly moving, shifting, and altering. As his mind manoeuvres him from one thought and activity to the next, frustration has become his companion. Unimportant sounds and sights distract him and he struggles to keep his thoughts on the task at hand. He gets so wrapped up in a collage of thoughts and pictures that he doesn't even realise when people are talking to him. At times, he is not fully aware of what is going on around him. His parents and teachers describe him as disorganised and constantly caught up in a whirlwind of frenzied activities. The difficulty is that there are some days or situations where he appears fine, which makes others believe that he can control his behaviour. Just to put the proverbial cherry on top of it all, all of the above has an enormous impact on his emotional well-being as it disrupts his life, harms his relationships, and damages his self-esteem.

Source: Adapted from The Colorado Personal Growth and Therapy Resources, 1998, p. 2.

History of ADHD

ADHD was first described in 1902 by an English paediatrician, George Still. He noticed that some of the children in his practice, mostly boys, struggled to inhibit their behaviour and adhere to social rules. According to Still, this problem went beyond simple social etiquette; these children were suffering from a lack of 'moral control' (Barkley, 1995; Green & Chee, 1997).

Over the next few decades following Still's observations, scientists started to study the possible causes of this phenomenon, mostly focussing on the brain. In the early 1960s, the focus shifted to the behaviours associated with the phenomenon (Brochin & Horvath, 1996), which then became known as 'hyperactive child syndrome'. In the 1970s, the focus again shifted, this time to difficulties with impulse control and sustained attention. It was then labeled Attention-Deficit Disorder (with or without Hyperactivity).

Clinical picture

According to Anastopoulos, Guevremont, Shelton, and DuPaul (1992), ADHD is a chronic and pervasive developmental condition characterised by problems with sustained attention, impulse control, and activity regulation. Anastopoulos et al. (1992) add that ADHD can be very disruptive to the person and the people around him or her (e.g. parents, teacher, peers, etc.) and have a significant impact on a person's cognitive, emotional, and social functioning and development.

Anastopoulos (1998) maintains that in diagnosing ADHD, it is always important to consider the child's developmental level. In terms of age of onset, clinicians have started to recognise that ADHD is not only a disorder of childhood, and can also be diagnosed in adulthood (Kieling et al, 2010). Accordingly, the DSM-5 notes that instead of the symptoms being diagnosed before the age of seven years as in the previous DSM-IV-TR, it must now be diagnosed before the age of 12 years.

According to Green and Chee (1997), ADHD contains three essential parts:

- Core behaviours, which include the hyperactive-impulsive and the attention-deficit behaviours
- Secondary behaviours, which include social clumsiness, poor coordination, disorganisation, and poor self-esteem
- Co-morbid conditions, which include specific learning disabilities, Oppositional Defiance Disorder, Conduct Disorder, and depression.

Hyperactive-impulsive behaviours

The DSM-5 describes children who are hyperactive as fidgety and restless. At times, they run or climb excessively in an inappropriate manner given the situation, their age and developmental level. They may have difficulty playing or taking part in leisure activities quietly. They are often on the go or act as if a motor drives them. During their formal school years, they present with many of the behaviours mentioned in the DSM-5. They generally struggle with situations where they have to make transitions from the class to the playground or back again (Brochin & Horvath, 1996).

Anastopoulos (1998) says that hyperactivity is not just displayed through physical restlessness but also verbal restlessness, and parents will regularly describe their children as 'chatterboxes' or 'motor mouths'. Children with ADHD are also hyper-responsive and, compared to other children, they are much more likely to respond to the stimuli in their environments (Barkley, 1995).

ADHD children also tend to be impulsive, behaving 'too quickly' and 'too forcefully'. Thus, they tend to blurt out answers before questions have been completed (American Psychiatric Association, 2013; Green & Chee, 1997). These answers are usually wrong as they have not been well considered. Children with ADHD generally only listen to half of the instructions before they react. They rush through their work, making careless mistakes; they often have difficulty in waiting their turn, interrupting or intruding on others. Children with ADHD seldom set out to get into trouble, but they act without thinking of the repercussions and seldom learn from previous experiences. Although they are able to distinguish between right and wrong, this will usually register only after they have reacted to a certain stimulus and, even when the outcome is negative, they tend to repeat the same mistakes. As a result, they tend to be accident-prone, climbing on roofs or running across busy roads without thinking about the consequences.

Attention-deficit behaviours

According to the DSM-5 (American Psychiatric Association, 2013), children who are inattentive have difficulty with sustaining their attention on tasks or other activities, they fail to pay close attention to details and often make careless mistakes. At times it appears as if they don't listen when spoken to. These children subsequently often fail to follow through on instructions and often fail to finish their schoolwork. They also tend to get bored easily and will leave a task after a few minutes as their mind drifts to something new. Attention-deficit children also display problems with short-term memory and will forget something that was mentioned to them two minutes previously, yet remember something that happened two years before.

Children who are inattentive struggle to organise tasks and activities and often forget or lose things that are necessary to complete tasks. They are easily distracted by sounds and other stimuli in their environments and are forgetful in daily activities. These children tend to avoid tasks, chores, or duties that require a lot of sustained attention and mental effort, but they may give effortless attention to activities that they enjoy. This creates a confusing picture for parents, because on the one hand, their children are easily bored, but on the other, they tend to focus on activities that they enjoy and that are varied. For this reason, one will often hear parents complain that their children cannot finish their schoolwork, but they can sit in front of the television or computer games for hours. Taking this into consideration, Green and Chee (1997) divide attention-deficit into two broad categories, under-attention and over-attention, and say that a child's ability to sustain attention is strongly influenced by situational factors.

Table 13.3: Diagnostic criteria for Attention-Deficit/Hyperactivity Disorder as adapted from the DSM-5 and for Hyperkinetic Disorder as adapted from ICD-10

DSM-5 Attention-Deficit/Hyperactivity Disorder	ICD-10 Hyperkinetic Disorders
A. A persistent pattern of inattention and/or hyperactivity-impulsivity that interferes with functioning or development, as characterized by (1) and/or (2): (1) Inattention: Six (or more) of the following symptoms have persistend for at least 6 months to a degree that is inconsistent with developmental level and that negatively impacts directly on social and academic/occupational activities: **Note:** The symptoms are not solely a manifestation of oppositional behaviour, defiance, hostility, or failure to understand tasks and instructions. For older adolescents or adults (age 17 and older), at least five symptoms are required. a) Often fails to give close attention to details or makes careless mistakes in schoolwork, at work, or during other activities (e.g. overlooks or misses details, work is inaccurate).	• This group of disorders is characterised by: early onset; a combination of overactive, poorly modulated behaviour with marked inattention and lack of persistent task involvement; pervasiveness over situations and persistence over time of these behavioural characteristics. These deficits in persistence and attention should be diagnosed only if they are excessive for the child's age and IQ. • **Diagnostic guidelines:** The cardinal features are impaired attention and overactivity; both are necessary for the diagnosis and should be evident in more than one situation (e.g. home, classroom, clinic).

DSM-5 Attention-Deficit/Hyperactivity Disorder	ICD-10 Hyperkinetic Disorders
b) Often has difficulty sustaining attention in tasks or play activities (e.g. has difficultly remaining focused during lectures, conversations, or lengthy reading). c) Often does not seem to listen when spoken to directly (e.g. mind seems elsewhere, even in the absence of any obvious distraction). d) Often does not follow through on instructions and fails to finish schoolwork, chores, or duties in the workplace (e.g. starts tasks but quickly loses focus and is easily sidetracked). e) Often has difficultly organizing tasks and activities (e.g. difficulty managing sequential tasks; difficulty keeping materials and belongings in order; messy, disorganized work; has poor time management; fails to meet deadlines). f) Often avoids, dislikes, or is reluctant to engage in tasks that require sustained mental effort (e.g. schoolwork or homework; for older adolescents and adults, preparing reports, completing forms, reviewing lengthy papers). g) Often loses things necessary for tasks and activities (e.g. school materials, pencils, books, tools, wallets, keys, paperwork, eyeglasses, mobile telephones). h) Is often easily distracted by extraneous stimuli (for older adolescents and adults, may include unrelated thoughts). i) Is often forgetful in daily activities (e.g. doing chores, running errands; for older adolescents and adults, returning calls, paying bills, keeping appointments). 2. Hyperactivity and impulsivity: Six (or more) of the following symptoms have persisted for at least 6 months to a degree that is inconsistent with developmental level and that negatively impacts directly on social and academic/occupational activities:	‣ Impaired attention is manifested by prematurely breaking off from tasks and leaving activities unfinished. The children change frequently from one activity to another, seemingly losing interest in one task because they become diverted to another (although laboratory studies do not generally show an unusual degree of sensory or perceptual distractibility). ‣ Overactivity implies excessive restlessness, especially in situations requiring relative calm. It may, depending upon the situation, involve the child running and jumping around, getting up from a seat when he or she was supposed to remain seated. • The following associated features are all characteristic of children with this disorder, but they are not sufficient for the diagnosis, or even necessary, but help to sustain it. ‣ Disinhibition in social relationships. ‣ Recklessness in situations involving some danger. ‣ Impulsive flouting of social rules (as shown by intruding on or interrupting others' activities, prematurely answering questions before they have been completed, or difficulty in waiting turns). ‣ Learning disorders and motor clumsiness occur with undue frequency, and should be noted separately when present; they should not, however, be part of the actual diagnosis of hyperkinetic disorder.

DSM-5 Attention-Deficit/Hyperactivity Disorder	ICD-10 Hyperkinetic Disorders
Note: The symptoms are not solely a manifestation of oppositional behaviour, defiance, hostility, or failure to understand tasks and instructions. For older adolescents or adults (age 17 and older), at least five symptoms are required. a) Often fidgets with or taps hands or feet or squirms in seat. b) Often leaves seat in situations when remaining seated is expected (e.g. leaves his or her place in the classroom, in the office or other workplace, or in other situations that require remaining in place). c) Often runs about or climbs in situations where it is inappropriate. (**Note:** In adolescents or adults, may be limited to feeling restless.) d) Often unable to play or engage in leisure activities quietly. e) Is often "on the go", acting as if "driven by a motor" (e.g. is unable to be or uncomfortable being still for extended time, as in restaurants, meetings; may be experienced by others as being restless or difficult to keep up with). f) Often talks excessively. g) Often blurts out an answer before a question has been completed (e.g. completes other people's sentences; cannot wait for turn in conversation). h) Often has difficulty waiting his or her turn (e.g. while waiting in line). i) Often interrupts or intrudes on others (e.g. butts into conversations, games, or activities; may start using other people's things without asking or receiving permission; for adolescents and adults, may intrude into or take over what others are doing). B. Several inattentive or hyperactive-impulsive symptoms were present prior to age 12 years. C. Several inattentive or hyperactive-impulsive symptoms are present in two or more settings (e.g. at home, school, or work; with friends or relatives; in other activities).	

DSM-5 Attention-Deficit/Hyperactivity Disorder	ICD-10 Hyperkinetic Disorders
D. There is clear evidence that the symptoms interfere with, or reduce the quality of, social, academic, or occupational functioning. E. The symptoms do not occur exclusively during the course of schizophrenia or another psychotic disorder and are not better explained by another mental disorder (e.g. mood disorder, anxiety disorder, dissociative disorder, personality disorder, substance intoxication or withdrawal).	

Source: Reprinted with permission from the Diagnostic and Statistical Manual of Mental Disorders (DSM), Fifth Edition, American Psychiatric Association (APA), 2013 and ICD-10 Classification of Mental and Behavioural Disorders: Diagnostic Criteria for Research, World Health Organisation (WHO), Geneva, 2007.

Secondary symptoms

In addition to the core symptoms that are associated with ADHD, there are also some secondary symptoms that we frequently find in children diagnosed with ADHD. Among these are difficulties with regards to social and motor development, as well as emotional worries (APA, 2013):

- ***Social clumsiness:*** Many children with ADHD are socially 'clumsy' despite the fact that they can be very sensitive and caring. According to Brochin and Horvath (1996), children with ADHD are often rejected by their peers, because they tend to misinterpret social cues and will say and do things that are quite inappropriate within a specific situation. They also tend to be bossy (Green & Chee, 1997).
- ***Poor coordination:*** Children with ADHD tend to experience problems with fine and gross motor skills. They have particular problems with their handwriting and some of them are very clumsy and have difficulty coordinating a sequence of movements or doing two things at once, for example, simultaneously moving their arms and their legs. However, this does not apply to all children with ADHD, as some of them turn out to be exceptional athletes (Green & Chee, 1997).
- ***Disorganisation:*** Often, children with ADHD are highly disorganised. A school bag will be left somewhere and books are forgotten at school. They also have difficulty getting started on a particular project and can be very untidy (Green & Chee, 1997).
- ***Poor self-esteem:*** Children who are diagnosed with ADHD often present with low self-esteem (Johnson & Bunce, 2008). They are constantly faced with failure and rejection at school and at home; they may feel as if they can never do anything right, no matter how hard they try.

Co-morbid conditions

According to Green and Chee (1997) and Brochin and Horvath (1996), more than half of the children who are diagnosed with ADHD also display symptoms of one or more co-morbid conditions. This has important implications for the treatment of the conditions.

The following are the most common conditions that co-exist with ADHD:

- ***Specific learning disability:*** Approximately half the children with ADHD will also have some kind of learning disability, which differs from the academic problems directly related to the ADHD. When a child has a specific learning disability, they present with a significant discrepancy between their intellectual potential and their academic performance. This may be due to, for instance, a specific reading disability (Green & Chee, 1997).
- ***Oppositional Defiant Disorder (ODD):*** Between 40% and 60% of the children who display ADHD symptoms will also display symptoms of ODD, which creates quite a volatile mixture. Children with ADHD may act before they think, but they are still remorseful and caring towards others. This will not be the case with children who have ODD, who think that their behaviour is totally justified (Green & Chee, 1997).
- ***Conduct Disorder (CD):*** Children with ADHD and CD are also more likely to use alcohol and other illegal recreational drugs than children with just ADHD (Brochin & Horvath, 1996).
- ***Depression:*** Many children with ADHD feel inadequate as they are unable to behave or perform well or be accepted by others. This can lead to a low self-esteem and co-morbid depression and anxiety. Children with a co-morbid depressive disorder will often appear moody, sad, socially withdrawn, and preoccupied (The Colorado Personal Growth and Therapy Resources, 1998; Green & Chee, 1997). It is important to determine the source of the depression as this will have very important implications for treatment.

Conduct disorders

Most children and adolescents are occasionally non-compliant in that they defy their parents or refuse to comply with their parents' requests (Erickson, 1998). However, when there is continuous defiance or non-compliance, this has a significant impact on the child's and family's well-being. The more serious forms of this behaviour are classified in the DSM-5 as Oppositional Defiant Disorder (ODD) and Conduct Disorder (CD) (APA, 2013).

Oppositional Defiant Disorder

Children and adolescents with ODD display a recurrent and repetitive pattern of negative and antagonistic behaviour that significantly impacts on their academic and family functioning, as well as their social and emotional well-being (Halgin & Whitbourne, 2003; Masse & McNeil, 2008). Although some children and adolescents occasionally display rebellious and non-compliant tendencies, the behaviour of children and adolescents with ODD is more extreme. This behaviour differs from the behaviour of others of the same developmental age such that they are considered to be much more than 'just in a phase' that will pass in time (Erickson, 1998). However, although their behaviour can be verbally aggressive and hurtful towards others, children and adolescents with ODD are generally not physically aggressive and they do not become involved in serious criminal acts (Joyce, 2007).

Children and adolescents with ODD often lose their temper, are generally angry, irritable and argumentative, tend to be resentful, actively defy or refuse to comply with adults' requests or social rules and norms, and are easily annoyed. They will also purposefully and deliberately annoy others, blame others for their wrongdoings and mistakes, and often swear and use obscene language, and are often self-righteous, spiteful, or vindictive (APA, 2013; Erickson, 1998; Halgin & Whitbourne, 2003). What often starts as ODD may develop into the more serious pattern of non-compliance typical of Conduct Disorder (CD) (Barrett, 2004).

In considering possible changes for the diagnostic criteria of Oppositional Defiant Disorder in the DSM-5, the workgroup felt that the DSM-IV-TR criteria were fairly successful in describing a group of children who were impaired and at risk for future problems in adjustment. Based on this, no major changes were recommended (American Psychiatric Association, 2012). However, a severity index was developed, based on the cross-situation pervasiveness of the symptoms. Consequently, the DSM-5 distinguishes between mild, moderate and severe ODD. Children with mild ODD display challenging behaviour in only one setting, whereas children with moderate ODD do so in at least two settings, and children with severe ODD in three or more settings. The DSM-5 also removed the exclusionary criteria for Conduct Disorder, but added that children cannot be diagnosed with ODD if they have been diagnosed with Disruptive Mood Dysregulation Disorder (Chapter 5). In addition, the DSM-5 organises the symptoms of ODD so that one can distinguish between emotional and behavioural symptoms; hence the division of symptoms as part of one of the following three categories: angry/irritable mood, argumentative/defiant behaviour, and vindictiveness. The latter category describes children who are considered to be spiteful and vindictive. Finally, the DSM-5 also provides standard and objective definitions for the frequency of ODD symptoms (American Psychiatric Association, 2013) (see Table 13.4).

Table 13.4: Diagnostic criteria for Oppositional Defiant Disorder as adapted from the DSM-5 and ICD-10

DSM-5	ICD-10
A. A pattern of angry/irritable mood, argumentative/defiant behaviour, or vindictiveness lasting at least 6 months as evidenced by at least four sympotms from any of the following categories, and exhibited during interaction with at least one individual who is not a sibling. Angry/Irritable Mood (1) Often loses temper. (2) Is often touchy or easily annoyed. (3) Is often angry and resentful. Argumentative/Defiant Behaviour (4) Often argues with authority figures or, for children and adolescents, with adults. (5) Often actively defies or refuses to comply with requests from authority figures or with rules. (6) Often deliberately annoys others. (7) Often blames others for his or her mistakes or misbehavior.	• This type of conduct disorder is characteristically seen in children below the age of nine or ten years. • It is defined by the presence of markedly defiant, disobedient, provocative behaviour and by the absence of more severe dissocial or aggressive acts that violate the law or the rights of others. • The disorder requires that the overall criteria be met; even severely mischievous or naughty behaviour is not in itself sufficient for diagnosis. • The essential feature of this disorder is a pattern of: ‣ Persistently negativistic, hostile, defiant, provocative, and disruptive behaviour, which is clearly outside the normal range of behaviour for a child of the same age in the same sociocultural context, and which does not include the more serious violations of the rights of others as reflected in the aggressive and dissocial behaviour specified for categories.

DSM-5	ICD-10
Vindictiveness (8) Has been spiteful or vindictive at least twice within the past 6 months. **Note:** The persistence and frequency of these behaviours should be used to distinguish a behaviour that is within normal limits from a behaviour that is symptomatic. For children younger than 5 years, the behaviour should occur on most days for a period of at least 6 months unless otherwise noted (Criterion A8). For individuals 5 years and older, the behaviour should occur at least once a week for at least 6 months, unless otherwise noted (Criterion A8). While these frequency criteria provide guidance on a minimal level of frequency to define symptoms, other factors should also be considered, such as whether the frequency and intensity of the behaviours are outside a range that is normal for the individual's developmental level, gender, and culture. B. The disturbance in behaviour is associated with distress in the individual or others in his or her immediate social context (e.g. family, peer group, work colleagues), or it impacts negatively on social, educational, occupational, or other important areas of functioning. C. The behaviours do not occur exclusively during the course of a psychotic, substance use, depressive, or bipolar disorder. Also, the criteria are not met for disruptive mood dysregulation disorder.	‣ Frequently and actively defy adult requests or rules and deliberately act to annoy other people. ‣ Usually they tend to be angry, resentful, and easily annoyed by other people whom they blame for their own mistakes or difficulties. ‣ Low frustration tolerance and readily lose their temper. ‣ Typically, their defiance has a provocative quality, so that they initiate confrontations and generally exhibit excessive levels of rudeness, uncooperativeness, and resistance to authority. ‣ Frequently, this behaviour is most evident in interactions with adults or peers whom the child knows well, and signs of the disorder may not be evident during a clinical interview. • The key distinction from other types of conduct disorder is the absence of behaviour that violates the law and the basic rights of others, such as theft, cruelty, bullying, assault, and destructiveness. The definite presence of any of the above would exclude the diagnosis. However, oppositional defiant behaviour, as outlined in the paragraph above, is often found in other types of conduct disorder. • *Excludes:* Conduct disorders including overtly dissocial or aggressive behaviour.

Source: Reprinted with permission from the Diagnostic and Statistical Manual of Mental Disorders (DSM), Fifth Edition, American Psychiatric Association (APA), 2013 and ICD-10 Classification of Mental and Behavioural Disorders: Diagnostic Criteria for Research, World Health Organisation (WHO), Geneva, 2007.

Conduct Disorder

Juvenile delinquency is a legal term that is used to describe antisocial and criminal behaviours that are committed by persons younger than a specified statutory age and that are in direct violation of a country's laws and cultural norms (Erickson, 1998). Upon investigation, most juvenile delinquents present with symptoms associated with Conduct Disorder (CD).

The most common characteristic of CD is a repetitive and persistent violation of the rights of others. In addition, adolescents with CD also tend to defy societal norms and rules, and they often perform illegal acts against others (Erickson, 1998). The typical behaviours associated with CD are mentioned below. Many adolescents with CD are also addicted to alcohol or other recreational drugs. As is the case with ODD, adolescents with CD tend to blame others for their misbehaviour, refuse to accept responsibility, and display a lack of remorse for their behaviours and the consequences thereof (Halgin & Whitbourne, 2003).

Although CD is often diagnosed in adolescents, a differentiation is often made between CD with childhood onset (at least one symptom characteristic of CD before the age of ten years); CD with adolescent onset (no symptoms characteristic of CD before the age of 10 years); and unspecified onset (not enough information available on the presentation of symptoms before or after the age of 10 years) (American Psychiatric Association, 2013). One should also differentiate between more severe cases, that usually result in arrest and include a pattern of delinquent behaviour, where the symptoms are in excess of those required to make the diagnosis and the child's difficulties cause major harm to others; mild cases that include pranks, insignificant lying, and/or group mischief which cause only mild harm to others; and moderate cases where the individual's symptoms and the harm it causes to others are somewhere in-between the mild and severe categories (American Psychiatric Association, 2013; Halgin & Whitbourne, 2003).

According to Erickson (1998), there are four types of conduct disorders, varying in terms of degree of socialisation and aggression. The four types are:

- Undersocialised aggressive
- Undersocialised non-aggressive
- Socialised aggressive
- Socialised non-aggressive.

Those adolescents with CD who are undersocialised generally have superficial, one-sided relationships. They do not have normal patterns of affection and are generally considered to be egocentric. They will manipulate others for their own advantage without feeling guilt or remorse. Although people with the socialised types are generally more attached to others, they are also manipulative and they show little remorse in their interactions with people to whom they are not attached. These adolescents are often part of gangs where they join others in performing illegal acts. People with the aggressive types often violate the rights of others and tend to become involved in physical acts of violence outside of the home. These include assault, physical harm to animals, sexual violence, and direct confrontation with their victims, during hijackings, for instance. Non-aggressive adolescents with Conduct Disorder tend to avoid violence, but constantly violate rules and become involved in activities such as truancy and running away from home, constant lying both in and out of home, vandalism, fire-setting, property damage or loss, deceitfulness, and theft (Erickson, 1998).

As far as Conduct Disorder in the DSM-5 is concerned, no major revisions were recommended. However, an additional specifier for 'with limited prosocial emotions' in Conduct Disorder has been included (APA, 2013). Included in this are individuals who show a lack of remorse or guilt, a callous lack of empathy, a lack of concern about performance, and/or a shallow or deficient affect (American Psychiatric Association, 2013).

Table 13.5: Diagnostic criteria for Conduct Disorder as adapted from the DSM-5 and ICD-10

DSM-5	ICD-10
A. A repetitive and persistent pattern of behaviour in which the basic rights of others or major age-appropriate societal norms or rules are violated, as manifested by the presence of at least three of the following 15 criteria in the past 12 months from any of the categories below, with at least one criterion present in the past 6 months: Aggression to People or Animals (1) Often bullies, threatens, or intimidates others. (2) Often initiates physical fights. (3) Has used a weapon that can cause serious physical harm to others (e.g. a bat, brick, broken bottle, knife, gun). (4) Has been physically cruel to people. (5) Has been physically cruel to animals. (6) Has stolen while confronting a victim (e.g. mugging, purse snatching, extortion, armed robbery). (7) Has forced someone into sexual activity. Destruction of property (8) Has deliberately engaged in fire setting with the intention of causing serious damage. (9) Has deliberately destroyed others' property (other than by fire setting). Deceitfulness or Theft (10)Has broken into someone else's house, building, or car. (11)Often lies to obtain goods or favours or to avoid obligations (i.e. "cons" others). (12)Has stolen items of nontrivial value without confronting a victim (e.g. shoplifting, but without breaking and entering; forgery).	• **Diagnostic guidelines:** Judgements concerning the presence of Conduct Disorder should take into account the child's developmental level. ‣ Temper tantrums, for example, are a normal part of a three-year-old's development and their mere presence would not be grounds for diagnosis. ‣ Equally, the violation of other people's civic rights (as by violent crime) is not within the capacity of most seven-year-olds and so is not a necessary diagnostic criterion for that age group. • Examples of the behaviours on which the diagnosis is based include the following: ‣ Excessive levels of fighting or bullying. ‣ Cruelty to animals or other people. ‣ Severe destructiveness to property. ‣ Fire-setting. ‣ Stealing. ‣ Repeated lying. ‣ Truancy from school and running away from home. ‣ Unusually frequent and severe temper tantrums. ‣ Defiant provocative behaviour. ‣ Persistent severe disobedience. • *Exclusion criteria* include uncommon but serious underlying conditions such as Schizophrenia, Mania, Pervasive Developmental Disorder, Hyperkinetic Disorder, and depression. • This diagnosis is not recommended unless the duration of the behaviour described above has been six months or longer.

DSM-5	ICD-10
Serious Violations of Rules (13)Often stays out at night despite parental prohibitions, beginning before age 13 years. (14)Has run away from home overnight at least twice while living in the parental or parental surrogate home, or once without returning for a lengthy period. (15)Is often truant from school, beginning before age 13 years. B. The disturbance in behaviour causes clinically significant impairment in social, academic, or occupational functioning. C. If the individual is age 18 or older, criteria are not met for antisocial personality disorder.	

Source: Reprinted with permission from the Diagnostic and Statistical Manual of Mental Disorders (DSM), Fifth Edition, American Psychiatric Association (APA), 2013 and ICD-10 Classification of Mental and Behavioural Disorders: Diagnostic Criteria for Research, World Health Organisation (WHO), Geneva, 2007.

Co-morbid disorders

The most common disorders that occur in conjunction with the conduct disorders include ADHD, substance abuse disorders, mood disorders such as depression, anxiety, poor self-esteem, adjustment disorders, and learning difficulties or academic underachievement (Masse & McNeil, 2008). It is very difficult to establish whether these disorders led to the development of the conduct disorder, or whether they exist as a result of the child or adolescent's severe behavioural difficulties (Acosta & Rosen, 2008). However, it is important to remember that when a conduct disorder co-exists with another disorder, it is important that both are identified and treated.

Aetiology of externalising disorders

When considering the aetiology of all of the externalising disorders, clinicians will find it valuable to take a multidimensional approach and take cognizance of the fact that externalising disorders are not caused by a single identifiable factor. It is through the interaction of several factors that externalising disorders are developed and maintained.

Genetic factors

Twin and adoption studies confirm the presence of a genetic influence in the development of ADHD (Johnson & Bunce, 2008; Whitman, 1991). A 1989 twin study found a 51% concordance for ADHD between monozygotic twins and a 31% concordance between dizygotic twins (Bennett, 2003). More recent studies found a higher concordance between monozygotic twins, ranging between 58% and 83% (Bennett, 2003). As far as dizygotic twins are concerned, Bennett (2003) describes recent research indicating concordance ranges between 31% and 47%.

As is the case with ADHD, research conducted through twin and adoption studies has shown that a child's risk of developing a conduct disorder increases significantly if a parent has been diagnosed with a substance use disorder, a mood disorder, Schizophrenia, ADHD, Antisocial Personality Disorder or Conduct Disorder (Joyce, 2007).

Neurological factors

According to Green and Chee (1997), children with ADHD display an unusual imbalance in their neurotransmitters. Dopamine and noradrenalin are the two chemicals involved (Bennett, 2003). These neurotransmitters are either produced in lower volumes by the pre-synaptic cell, or picked up less efficiently by the post-synaptic cell. These neurotransmitters have different functions. Amongst other effects, dopamine prevents our own thoughts or outside activities from distracting us. Low levels of dopamine explain why children with ADHD are easily distracted. Noradrenalin helps us to focus on what is important and to act appropriately. Children whose noradrenalin levels are low tend to become withdrawn. When these levels are too high, these children are hyperactive and impulsive (Green & Chee, 1997).

An imbalance in the functioning of certain neurotransmitters is not the only neurological factor contributing to ADHD. Although the central nervous system is, out of necessity and for survival purposes, equipped to deal with all external stimuli (e.g. visual, auditory, kinaesthetic, etc.), it is impossible for the brain to attend to all stimuli. In order to deal effectively with external stimuli, the central nervous system prioritises stimuli and, in order to formulate a coordinated response, filters out less important stimuli before these stimuli are relayed to the cortex (Green & Chee, 1997). It is postulated that, in the case of ADHD children, stimuli are not filtered properly, which leads to a stimulus overload and uncoordinated responses to these stimuli.

Family factors

People are always influenced by, and influence, other people, groups, organisations, and the environment (Donald, Lazarus, & Lolwana, 1997). People and groups in a specific context form interdependent, dynamic, and interacting relationships with the people around them and with their physical environment. Given these relationships, Barkley (1995) suggests that ADHD is not caused by poor parenting or other environmental factors. On the contrary, it is usually the children with ADHD who place substantial stress on their parents and others in their environment. Parents may start to see themselves as less skilled and knowledgeable than others and they may start to doubt their own parenting style (Anastopoulos, 1998). However, despite the fact that poor parenting does not cause ADHD, it can make the situation worse (Barkley, 1995; Green & Chee, 1997). According to Johnson and Bunce (2008), the parents of children with ADHD often experience problems with parenting, parent-child relationships, and parental stress. Not only are their relationships with their children marked by conflict, but they also tend to use more harsh and punitive methods of discipline.

Likewise, parents of children and adolescents who have been diagnosed with a conduct disorder are also more likely to make fewer positive and more negative statements towards their children. They are also more likely to fail to supervise or monitor their children on a regular basis, to perceive the behavioural problems of their children to be intentional, to present with poor problem-solving skills, and to abuse or neglect their children. Children and adolescents who have been diagnosed with a conduct disorder also often do not receive adequate support from their parents (Barrett, 2004). In addition to these factors, Acosta and Rosen (2008) have identified that family break-up, single parent homes, and even large family size place the family context under huge pressure and often precede the development of serious behavioural difficulties in some of the family members.

Socio-economic factors

In South Africa, there are many children and adolescents who survive in very poor socio-economic circumstances and, although not all of these children will develop a conduct disorder, it is important to note that low socio-economic status and high rates of crime have been associated with the development of conduct disorders (Acosta & Rosen, 2008; Barrett, 2004).

School and academic factors

According to Barrett (2004), children and adolescents with a conduct disorder often attend schools where there is little emphasis on academic work. In addition, these educators may spend less time on lessons and show little appreciation for good school work. In addition, there is little emphasis placed on individual responsibility and there are very poor working conditions for learners.

Personal and emotional factors

According to Joyce (2007), children and adolescents who are diagnosed with a conduct disorder generally display a lack of self-evaluative insight. For this reason, they struggle to take responsibility for their own behaviour and, as mentioned earlier, will often blame others for their wrongdoings. In addition, they also tend to become impulsively involved in high-risk behaviour without considering the consequences for either themselves or others (Masse & McNeil, 2008). They are also highly reactive to emotional situations or perceived injustices and display a very low tolerance for frustration. Research has found that children and adolescents with serious behavioural difficulties have very poor emotional self-regulation, and it has been hypothesised that their emotional self-control is either delayed or poorly developed (Joyce, 2007).

In addition to poor emotional self-control, researchers such as Kenneth Dodge have noted that these children and adolescents have poor communication patterns and tend to misinterpret ambiguous social cues. This not only leads to poor social relations but also tends to escalate hostility (Acosta & Rosen, 2008; Joyce, 2007).

Another personal and emotional risk factor for developing a conduct disorder is temperament (Joyce, 2007). Temperament involves the relatively consistent and stable personality characteristics that influence a person's behaviour. Carl Jung was the first to explain temperament in terms of opposites, including extraversion and introversion, and sensing and intuition. In the studies of Joyce and Oakland (Joyce, 2007), it has been noted that children and adolescents with conduct disorders generally show a preference for extraversion and sensing functions. The latter implies that in learning new information, individuals with conduct disorders place a lot of emphasis on facts as perceived by them, and not on concepts. This could explain why they tend to be argumentative about rules and struggle to generalise behaviour expectations across different circumstances.

Alexander Thomas and Stella Chess took the concept of temperament further in describing the concept of goodness-of-fit. According to this concept, conflict often arises (and increases) when a parent's and child's temperaments are dramatically different and there is thus less understanding and tolerance for the child's behaviour (Joyce, 2007).

Diet

In 1973, Dr Benjamin Feingold suggested that there might be a relationship between a child's diet and their hyperactive behaviour (Green & Chee, 1997). According to Barkley (1995), a substantial amount of research has been done; however, no support for this claim has been found. According to Green and Chee (1997), aspects of diet never cause ADHD; however, some foods can make some children more active and irritable.

SECTION 3: INTELLECTUAL DISABILITY (INTELLECTUAL DEVELOPMENT DISORDER)

According to the DSM-5 (American Psychiatric Association, 2013) children with an intellectual disability or intellectual developmental disorder, display "deficits in general mental abilities such as According to the DSM-5 (American Psychiatric Association, 2013) children with an intellectual disability or intellectual developmental disorder, display "deficits in general mental abilities such as reasoning, problem solving, planning, abstract thinking, judgement, academic learning, and learning from experience" (p.). The World Health Organisation (2007) adds that these abilities/skills contribute to a person's general level of intelligence; thus, individuals with an intellectual disability display deficits in their cognitive, language, motor and social development. As a result they often struggle to become independent and interact socially at an age appropriate level.

In the former DSM-IV-TR (2000) intellectual disability was termed mental retardation and classified as an Axis II diagnosis. When the multiaxial system fell away in the publication of the new DSM-5, mental retardation was grouped under the neuro-developmental disorders and given a new name; intellectual disability. According to Schalock et al. (2007, as cited in Wicks-Nelson & Israel, 2009) this concept was introduced by the influential American Association of Mental Retardation (AAMR), who later changed their name to the American Association on Intellectual and Developmental Disabilities (AAIDD). The new term was adopted as it appears to better describe the current understanding of intellectual disability, and seems to be in agreement with terms used in other parts of the world, i.e. Europe. It is proposed that the new ICD-11 will use the concept intellectual developmental disorder (American Psychiatric Association, 2013), hence the mention thereof in the new DSM-5. For the purpose of this chapter, the concept intellectual disability will be used as it appears in the DSM-5.

When examining the diagnostic criteria as stipulated in the DSM-5 (American Psychiatric Association, 2013), it is evident that people with an intellectual disability present with difficulties in both their intellectual and adaptive functioning. As far as their intellectual functioning is concerned, these individuals struggle with the skills noted earlier; i.e. reasoning, problem solving, planning, abstract thinking, judgment, academic learning, and learning from experience and instruction. Taking their adaptive functioning into consideration, it is noted that individuals with an intellectual disability display significant restrictions in terms of their adaptive behaviour. They thus struggle to communicate with others, take part in social activities and life independently. These intellectual and adaptive difficulties, which first appear during the developmental period, hinders a person's functioning in a variety of environments and can be classified as mild, moderate, severe or profound; depending on the person's level of adaptive functioning. Whereas the former DSM-IV-TR (American Psychiatric Association, 2000) distinguished a person's level of functioning based on his/her intellectual abilities as measured on a standardised intelligence test, the DSM-5 shifted the focus to a person's adaptive functioning as the this determines the type and level of support required (See Table 13.7) (American Psychiatric Association, 2013).

Regardless of the focus on adaptive functioning, the diagnosis of an intellectual disability still depends on a clinical assessment and standardised tests of intelligence; specifically as far as the person's difficulties with regards to his/her intellectual functioning is concerned (American Psychiatric Association, 2013). However, the DSM-5 adds a note of caution as far as standardised intelligence tests are concerned by advising that the test/s administered should be psychometrically valid and sound, individually administered and culturally appropriate. Given the current concerns about the validity and fairness of intelligence tests in a multicultural and multilingual society such as South Africa, it is felt that the diagnosis of an intellectual disability should be made with great caution and a greater focus on a person's adaptive functioning seems more appropriate. However, there currently do not appear to be any standardised assessments of adaptive functioning in the South African context.

Table 13.6 Diagnostic criteria for Intellectual Disability as adapted from the DSM-5

DSM-5
Intellectual disability (intellectual disability disorder) is a disorder with onset during the developmental period that includes both intellectual and adaptive functioning deficits in conceptual, social, and practical domains. The following three criteria must be met: A. Deficits in intellectual functions, such as reasoning, problem solving, planning, abstract thinking, judgment, academic learning, and learning from experience, confirmed by both clinical assessment and individualized, stardardised intelligence testing. B. Deficits in adaptive functioning that result in failure to meet developmental and sociocultural standards for personal independence and social responsibility. Without ongoing support, the adaptive deficits limit functioning in one or more activities of daily life, such as communication, social participation, and independent living, across multiple environments, such as home, school, work and community. C. Onset of intellectual and adaptive deficits during the developmental period. **Note:** The diagnostic term *intellectual disability* is the equivalent term for the ICD-11 diagnosis of *intellectual developmental disorders*. Although the term *intellectual disability* is used throughout this manual, both terms are used in the title to clarify relationships with other classification systems. Moreover, a federal statue in the United States (Public Law 1110256, Rosa's Law) replaces the term *mental retardation with intellectual disability*, and research journals use the term intellectual disability. Thus, *intellectual disability* is the term in common use by medical, educational, and other professions and by the lay public and advocacy groups.

Table 13.7: Severity Levels for Intellectual Disability (Intellectual Developmental Disorder)

Severity level	Conceptual domain	Social domain	Practical domain
Mild	For preschool children, there may be no obvious conceptual differences. For school-age children and adults, there are difficulties in learning academic skills involving reading, writing, arithmetic, time, or money, with support needed in one or more areas to meet age-related expectations. In adults, abstract thinking, executive function (i.e., planning, strategizing, priority setting, and cognitive flexibility), and short-term memory, as well as functional use of academic skills (e.g., reading, money management), are impaired. There is a somewhat concrete approach to problems and solutions compared with age-mates.	Compared with typically developing age-mates, the individual is immature in social interactions. For example, there may be difficulty in accurately perceiving peers' social cues. Communication, conversation, and language are more concrete or immature than expected for age. There may be difficulties regulating emotion and behavior in age-appropriate fashion; these difficulties are noticed by peers in social situations. There is limited understanding of risk in social situations; social judgment is immature for age, and the person is at risk of being manipulated by others (gullibility).	The individual may function age-appropriately in personal care. Individuals need some support with complex daily living tasks in comparison to peers. In adulthood, supports typically involve grocery shopping, transportation, home and child-care organizing, nutritious food preparation, and banking and money management. Recreational skills resemble those of age-mates, although judgment related to well-being and organization around recreation requires support. In adulthood, competitive employment is often seen in jobs that do not emphasize conceptual skills. Individuals generally need support to make health care decisions and legal decisions, and to learn to perform a skilled vocation competently. Support is typically needed to raise a family.

Moderate	All through development, the individual's conceptual skills lag markedly behind those of peers. For preschoolers, language and pre-academic skills develop slowly. For school-age children, progress in reading, writing, mathematics, and understanding of time and money occurs slowly across the school years and is markedly limited compared with that of peers. For adults, academic skill development is typically at an elementary level, and support is required for all use of academic skills in work and personal life. Ongoing assistance on a daily basis is needed to complete conceptual tasks of day-to-day life, and others may take over these responsibilities fully for the individual.	The individual shows marked differences from peers in social and communicative behaviour across development. Spoken language is typically a primary tool for social communication but is much less complex than that of peers. Capacity for relationships is evident in ties to family and friends, and the individual may have successful friendships across life and sometimes romantic relations in adulthood. However, individuals may not perceive or interpret social cues accurately. Social judgment and decision-making abilities are limited, and caretakers must assist the person with life decisions. Friendships with typically developing peers are often affected by communication or social limitations. Significant social and communicative support is needed in work settings for success.	The individual can care for personal needs involving eating, dressing, elimination, and hygiene as an adult, although an extended period of teaching and time is needed for the individual to become independent in these areas, and reminders may be needed. Similarly, participation in all household tasks can be achieved by adulthood, although an extended period of teaching is needed, and ongoing supports will typically occur for adult-level performance. Independent employment in jobs that require limited conceptual and communication skills can be achieved, but considerable support from co-workers, supervisors, and others is needed to manage social expectations, job complexities, and ancillary responsibilities such as scheduling, transportation, health benefits, and money management. A variety of recreational skills can be developed. These typically require additional supports and learning opportunities over an extended period of time. Maladaptive behaviour is present in a significant minority and causes social problems.
Severe	Attainment of conceptual skills is limited. The individual generally has little understanding of written language or of concepts involving numbers, quantity, time, and money.	Spoken language is quite limited in terms of vocabulary and grammar. Speech may be single words or phrases and may be supplemented through augmentative means. Speech and communication are focused on the here and now within everyday events.	The individual requires support for all activities of daily living, including meals, dressing, bathing, and elimination. The individual requires supervision at all times. The individual cannot make responsible decisions regarding well-being of self or others.

Severe	Caretakers provide extensive supports for problem solving throughout life.	Language is used for social communication more than for explication. Individuals understand simple speech and gestural communication. Relationships with family members and familiar others are a source of pleasure and help.	In adulthood, participation in tasks at home, recreation, and work requires ongoing support and assistance. Skill acquisition in all domains involves long-term teaching and ongoing support. Maladaptive behaviour, including self-injury, is present in a significant minority.
Profound	Conceptual skills generally involve the physical world rather than symbolic processes. The individual may use objects in goal-directed fashion for self-care, work, and recreation. Certain visuospatial skills, such as matching and sorting based on physical characteristics, may be acquired. However, co-occurring motor and sensory impairments may prevent functional use of objects.	The individual has very limited understanding of symbolic communication in speech or gesture. He or she may understand some simple instructions or gestures. The individual expresses his or her own desires and emotions largely through nonverbal, nonsymbolic communication. The individual enjoys relationships with well-known family members, caretakers, and familiar others, and initiates and responds to social interactions through gestural and emotional cues. Co-occurring sensory and physical impairments may prevent many social activities.	The individual is dependent on others for all aspects of daily physical care, health, and safety, although he or she may be able to participate in some of these activities as well. Individuals without severe physical impairments may assist with some daily work tasks at home, like carrying dishes to the table. Simple actions with objects may be the basis of participation in some vocational activities with high levels of ongoing support. Recreational activities may involve, for example, enjoyment in listening to music, watching movies, going out for walks, or participating in water activities, all with the support of others. Co-occurring physical and sensory impairments are frequent barriers to participation (beyond watching) in home, recreational, and vocational activities. Maladaptive behavior is present in a significant minority.

Source: Reprinted with permission from the Diagnostic and Statistical Manual of Mental Disorders (DSM), Fifth Edition, American Psychiatric Association (APA), 2013.

Aetiology of intellectual disability

In discussing the aetiology of intellectual disabilities, Wicks-Nelson and Israel (2009) and Mash and Wolfe (2010) acknowledges a two-group approach. On the one hand one finds individuals whose intellectual difficulties have clear underlying organic causes and are more often than not classified with moderate, severe or profound intellectual disabilities. These individuals also often present with other physical disabilities. In the other group one finds cultural-familial factors, where individuals with intellectual disabilities often have a family member with the same difficulties. These individuals' intellectual difficulties are often mild in nature and can also be attributed to socio-economic factors. They generally display few association medical or psychical difficulties/disabilities (Wicks-Nelson & Israel, 2009). Although the distinction between the two groups is helpful in understanding the aetiology of intellectual disabilities, Wicks-Nelson and Israel (2009) cautions that multiple factors can play a role. Although a person may for instance have a biomedical vulnerability to develop an intellectual disability, cultural and familial factors may play an important role in the severity of the disability.

The DSM-5 (American Psychiatric Association, 2013) identifies several factors in the prenatal, perinatal and postnatal period which can contribute to an individual developing an intellectual disability. In the prenatal period chromosomal disorders, maternal disease, genetic factors and brain malformations are all potential risk factors. In addition, the use and abuse of alcohol and recreational drugs, as well as the ingestion of other teratogens and toxins, can pose a significant risk to an unborn child. In the perinatal period, difficulties during the actual birth process that leads to neurological damage in the infant can form the basis of an intellectual disability. In the postnatal period, various diseases, as well as traumatic brain injuries, intoxications, demyelinating disorders, and seizure disorders are all considered potential risk factors that underlie the development of an intellectual disability. With regards to the latter, the influence of social-economic factors should also not be underestimated as leading causes of an intellectual disability (American Psychiatric Association, 2013).

For the purpose of this discussion, these views are combined in understanding the aetiology of intellectual disabilities (see Table 13.8).

Table 13.8: The Aetiology of Intellectual Disabilities

	Organic	Cultural-Familial
Prenatal	Factors such as: • Chromosomal Disorders • Brain Malformations • Genetic Abnormalities • Multiple Congenital Anomalies • Clear Evidence of Brain Dysfunction • Maternal Disease	Factors such as: • Hereditary Influences • Maternal Recreational Drug and Alcohol Use/Abuse • Ingestion of Teratogens and Toxins

Perinatal	Factors such as: • Birth Difficulties • Prematurity • Neonatal Disorders	Factors such as: • Lack of Access to Birth Care • Parental Abondonment of Child • Lack of Medical Interventions upon Discharge
Postnatal	Factors such as: • Traumatic Brain Injuries • Demyelinating Disorders • Seizure Disorders • Various Diseases • Malnutrition	Factors such as: • Inadequate family support • Social Deprivation • Lack of Stimulation • Poverty

Source: Adapted from Wicks-Nelson & Israel, 2009, p. 308.

Organic factors

In considering the role of organic factors in the development of intellectual difficulties, one acknowledges that biological conditions can pose a significant risk to a person's development (Wicks-Nelson & Israel, 2009). Mash and Wolfe (2010) adds that accidents in utero can have a detrimental effect on a child's intellectual development in the prenatal period. In the perinatal period, prematurity and anoxia are considered significant risks and in the postnatal period; head trauma and diseases such as meningitis (Mash & Wolfe, 2010). According to Haugaard (2008) these include chromosomal and genetic abnormalities such as Down Syndrome, Fragile X Syndrome, Phenylketonuria, Williams Syndrome, Prader-Willi Syndrome, and Angelman Syndrome. This author further acknowledges the detrimental effect of prenatal exposure to alcohol and the comorbidity of intellectual disabilities with foetal alcohol syndrome (Haugaard, 2008).

Cultural-familial factors

According to Wicks-Nelson and Israel (2009) twin and adoption studies have shown that there is evidence to suggest that hereditary factors, in combination with other risks, play some role in the development of intellectual disabilities. Other factors that can come into play include psycho-social risks, i.e. low parental education, lack of access to prenatal care, child abuse and neglect, poverty, social deprivation, etc. (Wicks-Nelson & Israel, 2009). Mash and Wolfe (2010) adds that undetected organic conditions can also pose a significant risk to the development of intellectual difficulties.

AUTISM SPECTRUM DISORDER

Autism Spectrum Disorder (ASD) incorporates a group of unique disorders previously listed separately in the DSM-IV-TR (American Psychiatric Association, 2000); including Autism, Asperger's, Childhood Disintegrative Disorder, and Pervasive Developmental Disorder; Not Otherwise Specified. Although these terms are subsequently not used in the DSM-5, ASD is still characterised by a number of overlapping characteristics that was evident in these disorder; primarily in the areas of communication, social interaction, and other distinctive behavioural characteristics (American Psychiatric Association, 2013; Shriver, 2005).

According to the American Psychiatric Association (2012), the workgroup reviewing the changes that were going to be made for the DSM-5, considered the new name because, although autistic spectrum disorders could be reliably and validly distinguished from typical development, it was often difficult to distinguish between the different disorders. Indeed, it had been found that distinctions amongst the autistic spectrum disorders were often inconsistent and dependent upon time, situational variables, severity, language level, and/or intelligence rather than the features of the disorder. Also, because these disorders were recognised by a common set of behaviours, it could best be represented as a single diagnostic criterion that is adapted to the individual's clinical presentation by inclusion of specific clinical specificiers and associated features (American Psychiatric Association, 2012).

CASE STUDY

Twelve-year-old Fundiswa is the apple of her mother's eye. Although she doesn't say much, she is a lovable and well-behaved child. In comparison to her peers, she does not seem much different as she waits in her school uniform for the taxi which will take her to her special school quite far from her house. Quite recently her school hired a new teacher, who was given the responsibility of supervising the education and training of a small group of children that included Fundiswa. Her first task was to assess the children in the group and formulate special education plans for each.

She started her assessment of Fundiswa by observing her in the classroom and noticed that she rarely made eye contact with anyone. She was also quite non-responsive to others. When left alone, she would often stand, put her hands over her throat, stick out her tongue and make strange, soft noises that did not necessarily disturb anyone else in the classroom. However, every time her teacher noticed her doing this, she would gently take her to her seat, where Funsidwa would sit and rock backwards and forwards.

Although Fundiswa rarely disturbed anyone and was generally a very well-behaved child, she would occasionally become quite aggressive when introduced to something or someone new. As she appeared to struggle to speak and only made soft noises, she expressed her anger by pulling her own hair. As part of her assessment of Fundiswa, the new teacher also studied her history and noted that Fundiswa's mother initially thought her child was deaf as she did not speak until after the age of three years. She also preferred to play alone and did not appear to seek physical contact with others. Fundiswa was enrolled at her current school when her mother realised that she was not developing as fast as her friends and appeared not to understand simple commands such as 'don't touch that.'

Source: Adapted from Kearney, 2010, pp. 124-126.

Table 13.9: Some common autism myths and facts

MYTH	FACT
'Cold' parenting causes autism.	There are no known types of parenting practices that cause autism.
Autism is seen primarily in families of high socio-economic status.	Autism is found across all socio-economic classes, and across all cultures and races.
Individuals with autism often have exceptional specialised abilities such as adding or memorising geography.	Although some individuals with autism may have specific exceptional abilities, this is uncommon and not a distinguishing characteristic of autism.
Individuals with autism typically spend their time alone, spinning objects or engaged in other maladaptive behaviour such as self-injury or having tantrums.	Although there is qualitative impairment in social interaction, this may present itself in many different ways for the individual.
Autism is not treatable.	Effective interventions are available to teach social and communication skills and reduce maladaptive behaviours.
Autism is caused by immunisations (e.g. MMR), gastrointestinal disorders, mercury or lead poisoning, and vitamin deficiencies.	There is not a specific identifiable cause for autism at this time. It is likely that the cause includes both genetic and environmental variables.

Source: Shriver, 2005.

The term 'autism' is derived from the Greek word *autos*, which means self. It was most likely first used by the Swiss psychologist Eugene Blueler, who used it to describe children who had schizophrenic symptomology and difficulties in engaging with others (Simpson & LaCava, 2007). Autism as a disorder was, however, first described by Kanner in 1943, after he had studied the behaviour of eleven children in his practice who all displayed similar symptoms (Shriver, 2005). According to Kanner, these children all started to display these symptoms in infancy or early childhood. Amongst the symptoms he included:

- An inability to relate normally to others
- Delayed speech and language development
- Failure to use developed language for communication purposes
- Speech and language irregularities
- Pronoun reversals and misusage
- Extreme literalness
- Normal physical growth and development
- Obsessive insistence on environmental sameness
- An extreme fascination and preoccupation with objects
- Stereotypic, repetitive, and other self-stimulatory responses (Simpson & LaCava, 2007).

Although these defining characteristics of autism have been refined over the years since Kanner first noticed them, an essential cluster of symptoms has remained. These include difficulties with social interaction and communication, and restrictive behaviours and interests (Shriver, 2005).

In 1944, during the same period that Kanner first described autism, the German physician Hans Asperger published a paper entitled Autistic Psychopathy in Childhood. In doing this, Asperger became the first person to describe the cluster of symptoms that comprised what we knew as Asperger's Disorder (Mayes, Calhoun, & Crites, 2001). However, due to the Second World War and a language barrier, it was not until the 1980s that this paper was translated into English. This allowed it to be read more widely and the disorder to be recognised worldwide (Shriver, 2005; Simpson & LaCava, 2007). As noted earlier the DSM-5 no longer uses the term Asperger's Disorder, most likely because it has always been seen as a milder form of autism (McClaren & Winsler, 2005).

As far as ASD is concerned, the DSM-5 (American Psychiatric Association, 2013), groups a person's difficulties with regards to social interaction and communication into one dimension of symptoms and includes difficulties with regards to social-emotional reciprocity; deficits in non-verbal communicative behaviours used for social interaction; and deficits in developing, maintaining and understanding relationships. This change was recommended as the workgroup (American Psychiatric Association, 2012) felt that a child's impairments with regards to social interaction and communication are inseparable and can more accurately be considered as symptoms with contextual and environmental specifiers. Furthermore, language delays are not unique to autism spectrum disorders and by combining these criteria and requiring both to be completely fulfilled, one is contributing to the detail of the diagnosis, without taking anything away from the sensitivity.

The second dimension of symptoms covers the person's restrictive, repetitive behaviours and interests and include stereotyped or repetitive motor movements; insistence on sameness, an inflexible adherence to routines or ritualised patterns of verbal and non-verbal behaviour; highly restricted, fixated interests; and hypo- or hyperactivity to sensory input (American Psychiatric Association, 2013). These difficulties generally have a significant impact on a person's social, educational and occupational functioning. In addition, DSM-5 has also added severity specifiers; level 1, level 2 or level 3. People with level 1 ASD require some support, people with level 2 require substantial support and people with level 3 require very substantial support (see Table 13.10).

ASD is generally first diagnosed in infancy or childhood; thus in the early developmental period. Although it was previously said that a child's symptoms is noticeable before the age of three years (Nissenbaum, 2005), the DSM-5 makes provision for the fact that the child's symptoms might only become noticeable when social demands exceed his/her limited capacity (American Psychiatric Association, 2103). It was previously noted that most children with autism also display some degree of cognitive impairment (Shriver, 2005; Simpson & LaCava, 2007). Although the DSM-5 (American Psychiatric Association, 2013) makes provision for this, it notes that the difficulties experienced by a person with ASD should not be better accounted for by an intellectual disability or global developmental delay.

Depending on the severity of the disorder, it is still believed that children with ASD generally fail to develop suitable peer relationships; in addition, they struggle to share enjoyment with others, and show an appropriate awareness of others. They also present with poor social reciprocity, display great difficulty in pretend or make-believe play, and struggle to understand social relationships. They generally do not like to be touched. In communicating with others, children with ASD present with language delays, have difficulty in initiating and sustaining conversations, use stereotypical or repetitive language, struggle to maintain eye contact, and present with a poor understanding of non-verbal behaviour (Nissenbaum, 2005; APA, 2013).

Furthermore, whilst observing children with ASD, one will notice that they present with stereotypical and repetitive behavioural patterns that include preoccupations, resistance to change, inflexibility, and repetitive motor movements such as rocking. In addition, they also display a need for sameness, a fascination with parts of objects, sensitivity to certain textures, and hand-flapping (Nissenbaum, 2005). Amongst their unusual responses to the environment, children with ASD also occasionally display insensitivity to pain and an over-reactivity or under-reactivity to noise (Boorstein, Fein, & Wilson, 2005). The extent to wich they require support with these once again depends on the severity of the disorder.

Table 13.10: Diagnostic criteria for Autistic Disorder as adapted from the DSM-5 and ICD-10

DSM-5	ICD-10
A. Persistent deficits in social communication and social interaction across multiple contexts, as manifested by the following, currently or by history (examples are illustrative, not exhaustive; see text): (1) Deficits in social-emotional reciprocity, ranging, for example, from abnormal social approach and failure of normal back-and-forth conversation; to reduced sharing of interests, emotions, or affect; to failure to initiate or respond to social interactions. (2) Deficits in nonverbal communication behaviours used for social interaction, ranging, for example, from poorly integrated verbal and nonverbal communication; to abnormalities in eye contact and body language or deficits in understanding and use of gestures; to total lack of facial expressions and nonverbal communication.	• A pervasive developmental disorder defined by the presence of abnormal and/or impaired development that is manifest before the age of three years, and by the characteristic type of abnormal functioning in all three areas of social interaction, communication, and restricted, repetitive behaviour. • **Diagnostic guidelines:** ‣ Usually there is no prior period of unequivocally normal development but, if there is, abnormalities become apparent before the age of three years. ‣ Qualitative impairments in reciprocal social interaction. These take the form of an inadequate appreciation of socio-emotional cues, as shown by a lack of responses to other people's emotions and/or a lack of modulation of behaviour according to social context. ‣ Poor use of social signals and weak integration of social, emotional, and communicative behaviours, and, especially, a lack of socio-emotional reciprocity.

<table>
<tr><th>DSM-5</th><th>ICD-10</th></tr>
<tr><td>
(3) Deficits in developing, maintaining, and understanding relationships, ranging, for example, from difficulties adjusting behaviour to suit various social contexts; to difficulties in sharing imaginative play or in making friends; to absence of interest in peers.
B. Restricted, repetitive actions of behaviour, interests, or activities, as manifested by at least two of the following, currently or by history (examples are illustrative, not exhaustive; see text):
(1) Stereotyped or repetitive motor movements, use of objects, or speech (e.g. simple motor stereotypies, lining up toys or flipping objects, echolalia, idiosyncrative phrases).
(2) Insistence on sameness, inflexible adherence to routines, or ritualized patterns of verbal or nonverbal behaviour (e.g. extreme distress at small changes, difficulties with transitions, rigid thinking patterns, greeting rituals, need to take same route or eat same food every day).
(3) Highly restricted, fixated interests that are abnormal in intensity or focus (e.g. strong attachment to or preoccupation with unusual objects, excessively circumscribed or perseverative interests).
(4) Hyper- or hypoactivity to sensory input or unusual interests in sensory aspects of the environment (e.g. apparent indifferent to pain/temperature, adverse response to specific sounds or textures, excessive smelling or touching of objects, visual fascination with lights or movement).
C. Symptoms must be present in the early developmental period (but may not become fully manifest until social demands exceed limited capacities, or may be masked by learned strategies in later life).
</td><td>
‣ Qualitative impairments in communications, i.e:
– Lack of social usage of whatever language skills are present.
– Impairment in make-believe and social imitative play.
– Poor synchrony and lack of reciprocity in conversational interchange.
– Poor flexibility in language expression and a relative lack of creativity and fantasy in thought processes.
– Lack of emotional response to other people's verbal and non-verbal overtures.
‣ Impaired use of variations in cadence or emphasis to reflect communicative modulation, and a similar lack of accompanying gesture to provide emphasis or aid meaning in spoken communication.
• The condition is also characterised by:
‣ Restricted, repetitive, and stereotyped patterns of behaviour, interests, and activities.
‣ In early childhood, particularly, there may be specific attachment to unusual, typically non-soft objects.
‣ The children may insist on the performance of particular routines in rituals of a non-functional character; there may be stereotyped preoccupations with interests such as dates, routes, or timetables.
• Often there are:
‣ Motor stereotypes.
‣ Specific interest in non-functional elements of objects (such as their smell or feel) is common.
‣ There may be a resistance to changes in routine or in details of the personal environment (such as the movement of ornaments or furniture in the family home).
</td></tr>
</table>

DSM-5	ICD-10
D. Symptoms cause clinically significant impairment in social, occupational, or other important areas of current functioning. E. These disturbances are not better explained by intellectual disability (intellectual developmental disorder) or global developmental delay. Intellectual disability and autism spectrum disorder frequently co-occur; to make comorbid diagnoses of autism spectrum disorder and intellectual disability, social communication should be below that expected for general developmental level	• A range of other non-specific problems such as fear/phobias, sleeping and eating disturbances, temper tantrums, and aggression. Self-injury (e.g. by wrist-biting) is fairly common, especially when there is associated severe mental retardation. • Lack of spontaneity, initiative, and creativity in the organisation of their leisure time and they have difficulty applying conceptualisations in decision-making in work (even when the tasks themselves are well within their capacity). • The specific manifestation of deficits characteristic of autism change as the children grow older, but the deficits continue into and through adult life with a broadly similar pattern of problems in socialisation, communication, and interest patterns.

Source: Reprinted with permission from the Diagnostic and Statistical Manual of Mental Disorders (DSM), Fifth Edition, American Psychiatric Association (APA), 2013 and ICD-10 Classification of Mental and Behavioural Disorders: Diagnostic Criteria for Research, World Health Organisation (WHO), Geneva, 2007.

Aetiology of Autism Spectrum Disorder

The aetiology of ASD is still very unclear, but it is widely assumed to be caused by a convergence of genetic, biological, and environmental variables (Shriver, 2005). In addition, ASD has also been associated with a number of medical illnesses, including maternal rubella, phenylketonuria, encephalitis, meningitis, fragile X syndrome, seizure disorder, and tuberous sclerosis (Simpson & LaCava, 2007). The previous assumption that certain familial and parental factors play a role has been widely disproved.

However, research does support the suggestion that there is a genetic component in the development of ASD (Rutter, 2000). Studies of families of those diagnosed with ASD have shown that there is a much higher rate of ASD in monozygotic twins, compared with dizygotic twins. In addition, a family member of a person with ASD has a much higher chance of developing an autism spectrum disorder than do the general population (Simpson & LaCava, 2007). Research has further indicated that parents who have one child with ASD have a 3%–5% chance of having another child with the disorder, which is also much higher than the general population (Fritson, 2007).

In the past, there has been speculation that ASD is caused by the MMR (measles-mumps-rubella) vaccination, vitamin deficiencies, and food allergies. This is, however, not supported by scientific research (Nissebaum, 2007).

SECTION 4: ELIMINATION DISORDERS

One of the most important milestones in a child's developmental path is the ability to control bodily functions. As a young child spends the first few years of life, exploring, understanding, and manipulating his or her body, the ability to control bodily functions such as urination is a very important and exciting step. In addition, due partly to social pressure to attain control of one's bodily functions, difficulties in managing to do so can cause major stress and distress in a young child's life (Wenar & Kerig, 2006). Children who have an elimination disorder struggle to exercise control over two very specific bodily functions and will repeatedly and age-inappropriately urinate (Enuresis) or pass faeces (Encopresis) in unacceptable settings (Comer, 1995).

Enuresis

Table 13.11: Diagnostic criteria for Enuresis as adapted from the DSM-5 and ICD-10

DSM-5 Enuresis	ICD 10
A. Repeated voiding of urine into bed or clothes, whether involuntary or intentional. B. The behaviour is clinically significant as manifested by either a frequency of at least twice a week for at least 3 consecutive months or the presence of clinically significant distress or impairment in social, academic (occupational), or other important areas of functioning. C. Chronological age is at least 5 years (or equivalent developmental level). D. The behaviour is not attributable to the physiological effects of a substance (e.g. a diuretic, an antipsychotic medication) or another medical condition (e.g. diabetes, spina bifida, a seizure disorder).	• A disorder characterised by involuntary voiding of urine, by day and/or by night, which is abnormal in relation to the individual's mental age and which is not a consequence of a lack of bladder control due to any neurological disorder, to epileptic attacks, or to any structural abnormality of the urinary tract. The enuresis may have been present from birth (i.e. an abnormal extension of the normal infantile incontinence) or it may have arisen following a period of acquired bladder control. The later onset (or secondary) variety usually begins about the age of five to seven years. The enuresis may constitute a monosymptomatic condition or it may be associated with a more widespread emotional or behavioural disorder.

Source: Reprinted with permission from the Diagnostic and Statistical Manual of Mental Disorders (DSM), Fifth Edition, American Psychiatric Association (APA), 2013 and ICD-10 Classification of Mental and Behavioural Disorders: Diagnostic Criteria for Research, World Health Organisation (WHO), Geneva, 2007.

Enuresis comes from the Greek *ouresis* (urination) and refers to how children repeatedly and mostly involuntarily (in some cases intentionally) urinate in inappropriate places, i.e. their bed and/or clothes (American Psychiatric Association, 2000; Haugaard, 2008). For a child to be diagnosed with Enuresis, the inappropriate urination takes place after the age at which most children are expected to have learned to urinate in an appropriate place such as a toilet. Although this is dependent upon social norms and customs, a child needs to be at least five years of age, or functioning at an equivalent developmental level, to meet the diagnostic criteria for Enuresis (American Psychiatric Association, 2013; Wicks-Nelson & Israel, 2009).

According to the DSM-5 (American Psychiatric Association, 2013), the behaviour becomes clinically significant when it occurs frequently (at least twice weekly for at least three consecutive months) or if it causes significant distress or impairment in social, academic (occupational), or other important areas of functioning.

In addition to the above, the DSM-5 (American Psychiatric Association, 2013) stipulates that the incontinence is not due exclusively to the direct physiological effect of a substance or a general medical condition (such as diabetes, spina bifida, or a seizure disorder).

In order to truly understand Enuresis and the different subtypes, it is important to understand that the ability to withhold urination, until it is appropriate to do so, involves the complex coordination between a child's physical and cognitive abilities. On a physical level, the child's bladder needs to develop to the size that it can hold a meaningful amount of urine (American Academy of Child and Adolescent Psychiatry, 2004). However, there is a difference between the actual amount of urine that a child's bladder can hold and the bladder's functional capacity, which refers to the amount of urine that a child's bladder can hold before he/she feels the urge to urinate. A person's functional bladder capacity is always smaller than the actual bladder capacity, which is one of the reasons why we can withhold urination after experiencing the urge to do so (Haugaard, 2008).

Another physical ability which a child needs to develop is the ability to exercise control over the external urinary sphincter so that urine can be voluntarily retained in the bladder. Once in an appropriate place, the child then needs to be able to relax the external urinary sphincter whilst contracting the muscles of the bladder so that urine can be expelled. In order to do this, the child needs to develop voluntary control of the micturition reflex (American Academy of Child and Adolescent Psychiatry, 2004). On a cognitive level, the child needs to develop the ability to recognise the physical sensations indicating that the bladder is full.

Difficulties with any of the stated abilities can contribute to enuresis (Haugaard, 2008). Wenar and Kerig (2006) add that children also require the necessary communication skills to advise their parents that they need to go to the bathroom and the social and emotional knowledge to understand the importance of adhering to social norms.

Based on the above, Haugaard (2008) quotes Von Gontard (1998) in identifying three different subtypes of enuresis:

- **Urge incontinence** occurs when a child cannot suppress his/her bladder contractions whilst the bladder fills with urine, resulting in frequent and uncontrollable emptying of the bladder.
- On the other hand, **voiding postponement** occurs when a child does not urinate for long periods on purpose. When the child can then no longer hold the urine, there is a sudden, uncontrollable void of urine. There are several reasons why children might purposely refuse to urinate, including fear of the bathroom and a desire to continue playing.
- Finally, there is **detrusor-sphincter dyscoordination** where a child cannot relax the external urinary sphincter whilst contracting the muscles around the bladder, resulting in strained urination and usually only small amounts of urine. Enuresis then occurs when the child's bladder becomes so full that involuntary voiding occurs.

In addition to the noted subtypes, the DSM-5 (American Psychiatric Association, 2013) also distinguishes between Nocturnal (night-time) and Diurnal (day-time) Enuresis. Children may, however, also present with a combination of the two. In addition, Enuresis may either be primary or secondary. Primary Enuresis indicates that the child has never had a period of urinary continence. Secondary Enuresis indicates that the child has had a period of urinary continence, but has returned to wetting incidents (American Academy of Child and Adolescent Psychiatry, 2004).

Encopresis

Encopresis, derived from the Greek word *kopros* (excrement) is described as repeated, often involuntary (in some cases voluntary) passing of faeces in inappropriate places that usually starts after the age of four years (Comer, 1995; Haugaard, 2008). To receive a diagnosis of Encopresis, a child needs to pass faeces in inappropriate places at least once a month, for at least three months. Therefore, a child who has very rare incidents will not qualify for the diagnosis (Haugaard, 2008).

The most common form of Encopresis is the type with constipation and overflow incontinence (Wicks-Nelson & Israel, 2009). In this type, hard faeces blocks the bowel, but liquid faeces leaks past. There are, however, some children who struggle with Encopresis without constipation and overflow incontinence (American Psychiatric Association, 2013).

Table 13.12: Diagnostic criteria for Encopresis as adapted from the DSM-5 and ICD-10

DSM-5	ICD 10
A. Repeated passage of faeces into inappropriate places (e.g. clothing, floor), whether involuntary or intentional. B. At least one such event occurs each month for at least 3 months. C. Chronological age is at least 4 years (or equivalent developmental level). D. The behaviour is not attributable to the physiological effects of a substance (e.g. laxatives) or another medical condition except through a mechanism involving constipation.	Repeated voluntary or involuntary passage of faeces, usually of normal or near-normal consistency, in places not appropriate for that purpose in the individual's own sociocultural setting. The condition may represent an abnormal continuation of normal infantile incontinence, it may involve a loss of continence following the acquisition of bowel control, or it may involve the deliberate deposition of faeces in inappropriate places in spite of normal physiological bowel control. The condition may occur as a monosymptomatic disorder, or it may form part of a wider disorder, especially an emotional disorder or a conduct disorder.

Source: Reprinted with permission from the Diagnostic and Statistical Manual of Mental Disorders (DSM), Fifth Edition, American Psychiatric Association (APA), 2013 and ICD-10 Classification of Mental and Behavioural Disorders: Diagnostic Criteria for Research, World Health Organisation (WHO), Geneva, 2007.

Using the same criteria as those applied to Enuresis, children can either have Diurnal Encopresis or Nocturnal Encopresis or both. Likewise, they can suffer from either primary or secondary Encopresis (Haugaard, 2008). Comer (1995) is of the opinion that Encopresis usually occurs during the day and seldom at night. Ondersma and colleagues (2001, in Haugaard, 2008) have suggested that there are three different subtypes of Encopresis depending on their cause:

- **Retentive Encopresis** is similar to Encopresis with constipation and overflow incontinence.
- **Manipulative Encopresis** where the child purposely expels a stool to achieve some goal (e.g. seeking attention or expressing anger and frustration).
- **Stress-related Encopresis** is related to stressful life experiences.

Aetiology of elimination disorders

Early conceptualisations of elimination disorders stated that they were mainly caused by psychological difficulties; however, more recent research has indicated that most cases of elimination disorders are caused by biological difficulties while the psychological difficulties experienced by children are usually secondary to the elimination difficulties (Haugaard, 2008; Wicks-Nelson & Israel, 2009). According to the ICD-10 criteria (World Health Organisation, 2007), elimination disorders may, however, be associated with a more widespread emotional or behavioural disorder. The American Academy of Child and Adolescent Psychiatry (2004) agrees, but warns that this only accounts for Enuresis in a small subgroup of children who develop secondary enuresis in response to a stressful situation.

It is often difficult to ascertain which is cause and which is effect, as emotional problems may arise as a result of the elimination difficulties and the distress and stigma attached to them. Haugaard (2008) describes these emotional difficulties and notes that children with Enuresis or Encopresis are usually aware that they have not developed the type of physical control that is expected of their developmental level and that this can impact on their self-worth and self-esteem. In addition, these children often experience negative reactions from those around them and are often teased by others.

On the other hand, elimination difficulties may also develop due to some other emotional or behavioural problems and one occasionally sees children who expel faeces as an expression of anger. There is generally no straightforward way to decide which problem occurred first and a clinician also has to take into consideration that Enuresis or Encopresis may have developed together with emotional or behavioural difficulties as a result of related aetiological factors. The most important rule in making a diagnosis is to consider which difficulty (i.e. the Enuresis/Encopresis or the emotional/behavioural difficulty) is the most prominent problem (World Health Organisation, 2007).

Physiological causes

In the case of Enuresis, as noted above, a child's functional bladder capacity is smaller than their actual bladder capacity. Children with Nocturnal Enuresis, tend to urinate automatically when the bladder reaches its functional capacity and the urge to do so arises. As a result, children with a smaller functional capacity may urinate more often during the night than those who have an average capacity (American Academy of Child and Adolescent Psychiatry, 2004). Furthermore, according to research by Kawauchi et al. (2003, in Haugaard, 2008), children with Nocturnal Enuresis have smaller functional bladder capacities during the night than during the day.

Research into children's sleeping patterns and the times at which Nocturnal Enuresis occurs produced conflicting results. Earlier studies showed that Enuresis occurs during all four stages of sleep, whilst a more recent study indicated that no wetting incidents occur during a normal REM cycle (Haugaard, 2008; Wicks-Nelson & Israel, 2009). The research also indicated that children struggled more with Enuresis on nights when they had longer periods of deep sleep, than on nights where they had shorter periods of stages 3 and 4 sleep. In addition, some research has also indicated that children with Enuresis struggle more to wake from sleep than their counterparts who do not experience Enuresis. Although there thus appears to be a link between deep sleep and Enuresis, more research is required (Haugaard, 2008; Wicks-Nelson & Israel, 2009).

Some research on the physiological causes of Nocturnal Enuresis has indicated that some children secrete less anginine vasopressin, an antidiuretic hormone that reduces urine production at night. Whereas most people produce more anginine vasopressin during the night than during the day, it would appear that children with Nocturnal Enuresis secrete less of this hormone and hence produce more urine at night (Haugaard, 2008). According to Wenar and Kerig (2006), evidence in support of the anginine vasopressin hypothesis is questionable as not all the children who struggle with Nocturnal Enuresis produce excessive urine.

As far as Encopresis is concerned, Wicks-Nelson and Israel (2009) state that, as is the case with Enuresis, physiological difficulties, for instance with the normal defaecation reflex, may contribute to the development of Encopresis.

Genetic factors

Most children with Enuresis have a close relative who has experienced the same difficulty, suggesting that there is a genetic link (Comer, 1995). According to Wicks-Nelson and Israel (2009), there are higher concordance rates for Enuresis between monozygotic twins than between dizygotic twins. Wenar and Kerig (2006) note that when both parents have been enuretic as children, there is an estimated 80% risk that their child will also have Enuresis. However, when only one parent had Enuresis, the child only has an estimated 45% risk. If neither parent had it, the estimated risk is 15%.

According to Haugaard (2008), genes on several chromosomes play a role in the development of Enuresis as they influence the child's ability to develop functional bladder capacity. Alternatively, Enuresis may be the result of combinations of different genes which impede the maturation needed for urinary continence.

As far as the genetic link in the development of Encopresis is concerned, constipation, which can cause Encopresis, can be influenced by genetic factors. Genes can either reduce a child's awareness of a full colon and the need for a bowel movement or cause difficulty with normal bowel movements (Haugaard, 2008).

Stool-toilet refusal

One of the causes of constipation can be stool-toilet refusal. This occurs when children refuse to use a toilet for bowel movements despite having learned to urinate in it. As is the case with postponement of urinary voiding, children with stool-toilet refusal withhold bowel movements as long as they can or until they are given a diaper to wear. This delay in passing faeces can then lead to constipation which can result in painful bowel movements, making the child even more reluctant to pass a stool. As for voiding postponement, children may avoid passing faeces because of fear of the bathroom or the toilet training that they have received (Haugaard, 2008).

Family factors

Studies on the familial factors involved in Enuresis have indicated that the way caregivers manage normal bedwetting during the toilet-training process can play a significant role. One common mistake is to wake children several times during the night to urinate. Not only can this be quite stressful for parents and children, children also learn a pattern of urinating when they are only half awake. They can then continue doing this even when they are in bed and only half aroused or woken by the urge to empty their bladders. Also, as children are then taught to empty their bladders when they are not yet full, they do not learn to recognise the physical sensations associated with bladders which have reached their functional capacity (Haugaard, 2008). Consequently, children learn to urinate frequently when there are only small amounts of urine in their bladders (Haugaard, 2008).

Some caregivers also tend to limit the amount of fluids that their children take during the evening. However, this might also impede the development of the child's functional bladder capacity as well as their awareness of the physical sensations associated with it.

Certain caregivers believe that it is helpful to punish children for elimination difficulties. When Enuresis or Encopresis are involuntary, however, punishment will not resolve the problem. Also, punishment can create stress and fear which can actually worsen the situation; this can lead to resentment and result in children who intentionally urinate or pass faeces out of anger and frustration (Comer, 1995; Haugaard, 2008).

CONCLUSION

One of the biggest challenges facing most developing countries is not only the extent of the developmental disorders experienced by their children and adolescents, and the constant increase in prevalence, but also the treatment of such disorders. It is extremely costly to manage developmental disorders effectively, as this involves intervention on many different levels of the social context. Not only does this require individual intervention and/or therapy but also teacher training and support, community education, school-based interventions, parental training and support, and hospital-based interventions.

In addition, it urgently requires a national strategy to assist children in dealing with the challenges that they face every day, including broader socio-economic and political problems. Indeed, should we ever succeed in effectively addressing these, the benefits of reduced dependency and improved productivity and quality of life will be immense (Institute of Medicine, 2001).

MULTIPLE-CHOICE QUESTIONS

1. The main reason that it is so important to identify children with developmental disorders as early as possible is that:
   a) medications are most effective when administered at an early stage of the disorder
   b) skill deficits can be identified and addressed before they impact on later development
   c) family functioning often declines as the developmental disorder progresses
   d) children are more receptive to therapy when they are young

2. An individual diagnosed with Attention-Deficit/Hyperactivity Disorder will always present with:
   a) hyperactive behaviour that alternates with periods of distraction
   b) patterns of inattention OR hyperactivity/impulsivity
   c) both patterns of inattention AND hyperactivity/impulsivity
   d) periods of distraction that lead to hyperactive/impulsive behaviour

3. The inattention cluster of Attention-Deficit/Hyperactivity Disorder symptoms is characterised by:
   a) careless mistakes
   b) fidgeting
   c) not waiting one's turn to answer questions
   d) all of these

4. One of the most characteristic patterns for children with ASD is that they are generally:
   a) uninterested in people
   b) very intelligent
   c) extremely talkative
   d) hyperactive

5. The two-group approach to the development of intellectual disabilities, state that the following factors are possible causes of these disabilities:
   a) organic/genetic-familial factors
   b) MMR and tuberculosis vaccinations
   c) German measles and mumps
   d) authoritarian parenting

6. Which one of the following is not considered a subtype of enuresis:
   a) urge incontinence
   b) voiding postponement
   c) voiding obstruction
   d) detrusor-sphincter dyscoordination

7. Which one of the following is not considered a subtype of encopresis:
   a) voiding encopresis
   b) manipulative encopresis
   c) retentive encopresis
   d) stress-related encopresis

PARAGRAPH AND ESSAY QUESTIONS

1. Most models of developmental psychology suggest that normal childhood development progresses as a series of steps, with each new achievement building on prior development. Given this model, select any childhood developmental disorder and describe how it can influence current and future deficits for the individual.

2. Explain the statement: 'We are not sure whether academic difficulties of children with Attention-Deficit/Hyperactivity disorder are a result of the disorder or a result of the symptoms of the disorder'.

3. Describe the causes of Intellectual Abilities using the two-group approach as explained by Wicks-Nelson and Israel (2009).

4. Describe the different subtypes of enuresis and encopresis and how they differ from one another given their underlying causes.

14 LEGAL AND ETHICAL ISSUES IN MENTAL DISORDERS

Christiaan Bezuidenhout

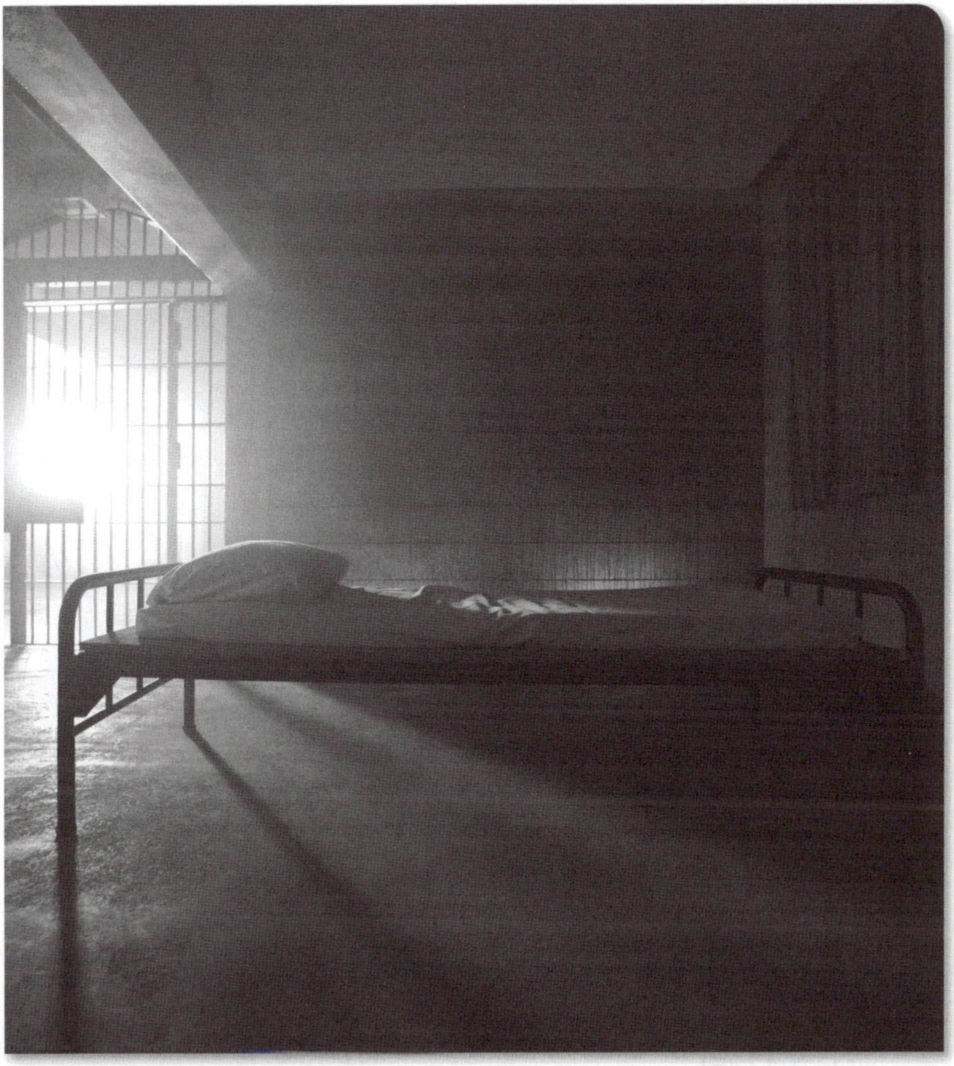

14 CHAPTER OUTLINE

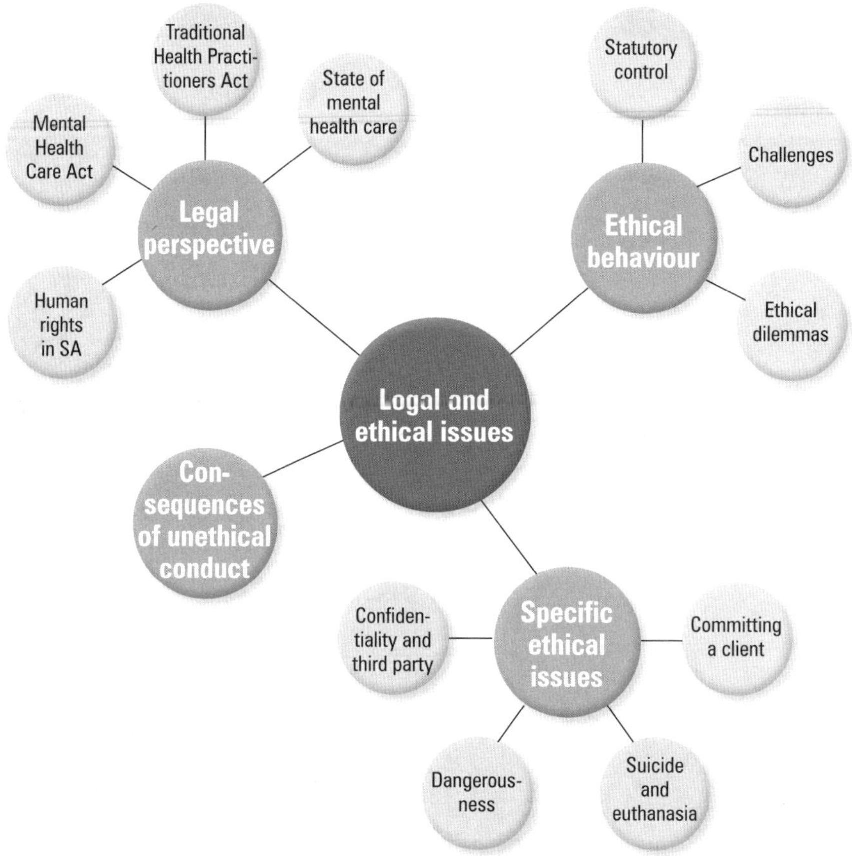

LEARNING OUTCOMES

After studying this chapter you should be able to:

- Critically highlight the prerequisites for ethical conduct.
- Outline the concept 'ethical behaviour'.
- Explain the role of the Health Professions Council of South Africa in ensuring ethical conduct in the health and behavioural medicine disciplines.
- Critically debate the different circumstances under which a therapist can divulge client information to a third party.
- Explain what possible consequences unethical conduct can have for a practitioner.
- Explain in your own words certain unique factors to consider in the South African context, to ensure ethical conduct at all times.

INTRODUCTION

After studying the preceding chapters, you should see very clearly that most people who suffer from a mental disorder are extremely vulnerable. Especially when one deals with a vulnerable population, one must always make sure that their rights, dignity, and safety are addressed. As the incidence of certain mental disorders changes, for example, the projected impact of depression, mental health practitioners will increasingly be confronted with different challenges in the future. It is estimated that by the year 2020, depression will be the second leading cause of disability worldwide (SADAG Conference, 2011). Projections like this emphasise the likelihood that, in the future, practitioners will consult with an increasing number of clients/patients with mental problems. This increases the challenges regarding consistent ethical behaviour by the practitioner.

In addition, now more than ever, have human rights for all become a key aspect on the global agenda. In many historical texts it is evident that individuals with odd behaviour were often treated inhumanely and had no human rights. In many cases abnormal and/or criminal behaviour was treated as evil. Before the eighteenth century, eccentric or unacceptable behaviour was attributed to supernatural powers such as demons, evil spirits, and witches (see Chapter 1). Since no scientific explanations existed for this type of behaviour, the 'mad' and the 'bad' were tortured and often executed by being burnt at the stake. Sometimes a hole was drilled or chipped into the skull to release the evil spirits (Brown, Esbensen, & Geis, 2007).

Amongst different ethnic groups of South Africa, similar executions for 'odd' behaviour are still taking place and many people (usually older women) have been killed after being accused of witchcraft. The human rights dogma of South Africa is particularly important here because these individuals are not tried by a court of law but by so-called 'kangaroo courts' mostly set up in rural areas, informal settlements, or townships. The killing of witches and other accused people thus serves to remove from society individuals who are undesirable according to societal and cultural beliefs.

The purpose of this chapter is to provide the reader with an understanding of the legal rights of people who have been diagnosed with a mental disorder, the new legal framework to accommodate indigenous beliefs, recognise traditional healers' role in psychology, as well as the ethical standards health professionals such as psychologists and social workers should adhere to when they interact with their clients.

CORE ETHICAL VALUES AND STANDARDS

The core ethical values and standards required of health care practitioners include the following (Health Professions Council of South Africa [HPCSA], 2008, p. 2):

1. ***Respect for persons:*** Practitioners should respect patients as persons, and acknowledge their intrinsic worth, dignity, and sense of value.
2. ***Best interests or well-being* (non-maleficence):** Practitioners should not harm or act against the best interests of patients, even when the interests of the latter conflict with their own self-interest.
3. ***Best interests or well-being* (beneficence)**: Practitioners should act in the best interests of patients even when the interests of the latter conflict with their own personal self-interest.
4. ***Human rights:*** Practitioners should recognise the human rights of all individuals.
5. ***Autonomy:*** Practitioners should honour the right of patients to self-determination to make their own informed choices and to live their lives by their own beliefs, values, and preferences.
6. ***Integrity:*** Practitioners should incorporate these core ethical values and standards as the foundation for their character and practice as responsible health care professionals.
7. ***Truthfulness:*** Practitioners should regard the truth and truthfulness as the basis of trust in their professional relationships with patients.
8. ***Confidentiality:*** Practitioners should treat personal or private information as confidential in professional relationships with patients – unless over-riding reasons confer a moral or legal right to disclosure.
9. ***Compassion:*** Practitioners should be sensitive to, and empathise with, the individual and social needs of their patients and seek to create mechanisms for providing comfort and support where appropriate and possible.
10. ***Tolerance:*** Practitioners should respect the rights of people to have different ethical beliefs as these may arise from deeply held personal, religious, or cultural convictions.
11. ***Justice:*** Practitioners should treat all individuals and groups in an impartial, fair, and just manner.
12. ***Professional competence and self-improvement:*** Practitioners should continually endeavour to attain the highest level of knowledge and skills required within their area of practice.
13. ***Community:*** Practitioners should strive to contribute to the betterment of society in accordance with their professional abilities and standing in the community.

LEGAL PERSPECTIVE

The Universal Declaration of Human Rights was adopted by the United Nations General Assembly (10 December 1948, at Palais de Chaillot, Paris). This declaration emerged following the atrocities that took place before and during the Second World War. Its aim was to ensure that all humans on earth should have the same basic rights purely because they are human. In this Universal Declaration it is stated that 'all human beings are inherently entitled' to basic rights. In Article 1 of the Declaration it is declared that: 'All human beings are born free and equal in dignity and rights. They are endowed with reason and conscience and should act towards one another in a spirit of brotherhood.'

Similarly, basic human rights became a very important aspect in South Africa after apartheid was toppled. The new Constitution was promulgated to ensure human rights for all human beings in South Africa.

Human rights in South Africa

When dealing with people with mental disorders, it is important to remember that no matter how severe their disorder, one is first and foremost dealing with another human being, and as such, this person has certain human rights. This person is protected by the Constitution of the Republic of South Africa, and practitioners should be acutely aware of the constitutional rights of their clients (see Table 14.1).

Table 14.1: Relevant excerpts from the Constitution of the Republic of South Africa, 1996

The Republic of South Africa is one, sovereign, democratic State founded on the following values:

(a) Human dignity, the achievement of equality and the advancement of human rights and freedoms.
(b) Non-racialism and non-sexism.
(c) Supremacy of the constitution and the rule of law.

Rights

7. (1) This Bill of Rights is a cornerstone of democracy in South Africa. It enshrines the rights of all people in our country and affirms the democratic values of human dignity, equality, and freedom.

Equality

9. (1) Everyone is equal before the law and has the right to equal protection and benefit of the law.
(2) Equality includes the full and equal enjoyment of all rights and freedoms. To promote the achievement of equality, legislative, and other measures designed to protect or advance persons, or categories of persons, disadvantaged by unfair discrimination may be taken.
(3) The state may not unfairly discriminate directly or indirectly against anyone on one or more grounds, including race, gender, sex, pregnancy, marital status, ethnic or social origin, colour, sexual orientation, age, disability, religion, conscience, belief, culture, language, and birth.

(4) No person may unfairly discriminate directly or indirectly against anyone on one or more grounds in terms of subsection (3). National legislation must be enacted to prevent or prohibit unfair discrimination.
(5) Discrimination on one or more of the grounds listed in subsection (3) is unfair unless it is established that the discrimination is fair.

Human dignity
10. Everyone has inherent dignity and the right to have their dignity respected and protected.

Life
11. Everyone has the right to life.

Freedom and security of the person
12. (1) Everyone has the right to freedom and security of the person, which includes the right:
(a) not to be deprived of freedom arbitrarily or without just cause;
(b) not to be detained without trial;
(c) to be free from all forms of violence from either public or private sources;
(d) not to be tortured in any way; and
(e) not to be treated or punished in a cruel, inhuman, or degrading way.
(2) Everyone has the right to bodily and psychological integrity, which includes the right
(a) to make decisions concerning reproduction;
(b) to security in and control over their body; and
(c) not to be subjected to medical or scientific experiments without their informed consent.

Privacy
14. Everyone has the right to privacy, which includes the right not to have:
(d) the privacy of their communications infringed.

Health care, food, water, and social security
27. (1) Everyone has the right to have access to:
(a) health care services, including reproductive health care;
(3) No one may be refused emergency medical treatment.

Access to information
32. (1) Everyone has the right of access to:
(b) any information that is held by another person and that is required for the exercise or protection of any rights.

Source: Adapted from an excerpt from Act No. 108 of 1996 (adapted from www.hpcsa.co.za).

Despite the increased focus on a rights-based approach, mistreatment of people with mental disorders continues. In recent years, there have been many media reports of abuse of patients by the State, institutions, or individuals. The South African Constitution states very clearly that all people must be treated with dignity and respect. Further pertinent issues, for the purposes of this chapter, include the right to privacy and the right to information. This implies that all mental health care practitioners must respect the privacy of their clients and also that they may not withhold any information from their clients.

Further aspects of importance are those of forced detention and treatment of psychiatric patients. Previously, it was relatively easy to have a patient certified and admitted to a psychiatric hospital without their consent and against their will. However, in order to protect the legal rights of patients in this regard, the Mental Health Care Act (No. 17 of 2002) has stipulated the exact procedures that need to be complied with, with regard to admitting patients to psychiatric and rehabilitation institutions. Furthermore, any treatment and research has to comply with the Constitution. Finally, all laws, acts, and professional codes of conduct must adhere to the Constitution.

The Mental Health Care Act (No. 17 of 2002)

It was envisaged that many past ethical abuses against individuals with mental disorders would be corrected by the new Mental Health Care Act (No. 17 of 2002) (MHCA) (implemented in 2004). The act sought to bring mental health care practices in line with those of the World Health Organisation (WHO) and to promote the human rights of people with mental disorders in South Africa.

The purpose of the Mental Health Care Act (No 17 of 2002) is:

> *To provide for the care, treatment, and rehabilitation of persons who are mentally ill; to set out different procedures to be followed in the admission of such persons; to establish Review Boards in respect of every health establishment; to determine their powers and functions; to provide for the care and administration of the property of mentally ill persons; to repeal certain laws; and to provide for matters connected therewith.*

The Act covers, inter alia, the following:

- Designation of health establishments administered under the auspices of the State as psychiatric hospitals or as care and rehabilitation centres
- Provision of mental health care, treatment, and rehabilitation services at health establishments
- Respect, human dignity, and privacy
- Consent
- Determinations concerning mental health status
- Disclosure of information
- Knowledge of rights
- Appointment of an administrator for care and administration of property of the mentally ill person or person with severe or profound intellectual disability.

One way of viewing this act is that it operationalises the terms of the Constitution as they apply to patients with a mental disorder. The act also clearly defines different mental health professionals and their roles and responsibilities (see Table 14.2). Any person who acts outside these makes him- or herself guilty of a crime.

Table 14.2: Relevant definitions from the Mental Health Care Act (No. 17 of 2002)

Term	Definition
Assisted care, treatment, and rehabilitation	The provision of health interventions to people incapable of making informed decisions due to their mental health status and who do not refuse the health interventions.
Assisted mental health care user	A person receiving assisted care, treatment, and rehabilitation.
Care and rehabilitation centres	Health establishments for the care, treatment, and rehabilitation of people with intellectual disabilities.
Health establishment	Institutions, facilities, buildings, or places where people receive care, treatment, rehabilitative assistance, diagnostic or therapeutic interventions, or other health services. Includes facilities such as community health and rehabilitation centres, clinics, hospitals, and psychiatric hospitals.
Involuntary care, treatment, and rehabilitation	The provision of health interventions to people incapable of making informed decisions due to their mental health status and who refuse health intervention but require such services for their own protection or for the protection of others.
Involuntary mental health care user	A person receiving involuntary care, treatment, and rehabilitation.
Medical practitioner	A person registered as such in terms of the Health Professions Act (No. 56 of 1974).
Mental health care practitioner	A psychiatrist or registered medical practitioner or a nurse, occupational therapist, psychologist, or social worker who has been trained to provide prescribed mental health care, treatment, and rehabilitation services.
Mental health care provider	A person providing mental health care services to mental health care users and includes mental health care practitioners.
Mental health care user	A person receiving care, treatment, and rehabilitation services or using a health service at a health establishment aimed at enhancing the mental health status of a user, State patient, or mentally ill prisoner, or where the person concerned is below the age of 18 years or is incapable of taking decisions, and in certain circumstances may include: (i) prospective user; (ii) the person's next of kin; (iii) a person authorised by any other law or court order to act on that person's behalf; (iv) an administrator appointed in terms of this act; and (v) an executor of that deceased person's estate.

Term	Definition
Mental illness	A positive diagnosis of a mental health-related illness in terms of accepted diagnostic criteria made by a mental health care practitioner authorised to make such diagnosis.
Psychiatric hospital	A health establishment that provides care, treatment, and rehabilitation services only for users with mental illness.
Psychiatrist	A person registered as such in terms of the Health Professions Act (No. 56 of 1974).
Psychologist	A person registered as such in terms of the Health Professions Act (No. 56 of 1974).
Social worker	A person registered as such in terms of the Social Services Professions Act (No. 110 of 1978).
Voluntary care, treatment, and rehabilitation	A provision of health interventions to a person who gives consent to such interventions.

Source: Adapted from www.hpcsa.co.za

Moosa and Jeenah (2010) state that the act was intended to 'remove distinctions between health professionals, in that any registered medical practitioner or psychiatrically trained nurse/occupational therapist/psychologist/social worker (defined as a 'mental health care practitioner') is allowed to provide mental health care, treatment, and rehabilitation (CTR) services'.

In addition, The National Health Act (No. 61 of 2003) (NHA) refers to categories of workers in more general terms as 'health care providers', where a 'health practitioner or provider' is a person providing health services in terms of any law such as the Allied Professions, Health Professions, Nursing, Pharmacy, and Dental Technicians Acts. The NHA is meant to be one of the legislative measures that will facilitate the progressive realisation of the right to health. This act also refers to the fact that everyone in South Africa should have access to health care services.

Traditional Health Practitioners Act (No. 35 of 2004)

South Africa is a diverse country where the majority of people are black and a significant proportion of this majority believes in indigenous medicines and practices to heal emotional problems. It is therefore not uncommon for the majority of black South Africans to consult with a traditional healer when they feel emotionally disturbed in some way. Traditional healers are an important source of psychiatric support in South Africa. Two types of traditional healers exist, namely a *sangoma* and an *inyanga*. A *sangoma* uses traditional medicines, but relies primarily on divination and communication with the ancestors for healing powers/purposes (see Chapter 2). The *inyanga* is a herbalist who is concerned with medicines made from plants and animals; *izinyanga* pass their knowledge of traditional medicines on through the generations usually from parent to child.

It is has been discussed in several previous chapters how some indigenous diagnoses (e.g. *amafufunyana* and *ukuthwasa*) have symptoms that may be seen as evidence of Schizophrenia (Bezuidenhout & Klopper, 2011; Zabow, 2007). Based on this, it has become evident that the human rights of the client and the traditional healer need to be protected through a legal mandate. In this context, the purpose of the Traditional Health Practitioners Act (No. 35 of 2004) is to:

- Establish the Interim Traditional Healers Council of South Africa.
- Provide for the registration, training, and practice of traditional healers.
- Serve and protect the interest of the public who use the services of traditional health practitioners.
- The need for this act was precipitated by the significant political and social changes that have occurred in South Africa since 1994 (Janse van Rensburg, 2009). Since democratisation, a very high premium is placed on human rights which entail the equal, just, and fair treatment of all people. Cross-cultural diagnosis and treatment present serious challenges in this context; thus, mental health professionals need to be trained to recognise and accommodate diverse customs and practices, and to support people with a variety of needs.

Figure 14.1: A traditional healer

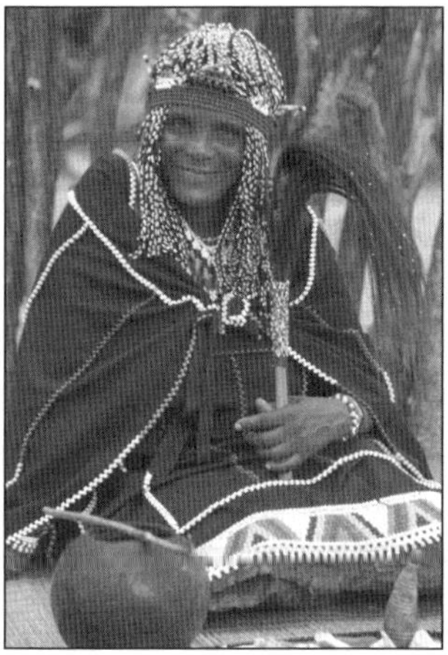

Table 14.3: Psychologists actively registered with the HPCSA per ethnic group as of February 2012

Ethnicity of psychologist	Number	% of registered psychologists
African	685	9.70
Chinese	1	0.01
Coloured	240	3.40
Indian	412	5.83
White	4,062	57.51
No information	1,663	23.55
TOTAL	7,063	100

Source: Adapted from www.hpcsa.co.za

In addition, as a result of historically privileged access to training, most psychologists practising in South Africa are white and from a Western background (see Table 14.3). Burke, Harper, Rudnick and Kruger (2007, p. 114) suggest that 'the importation of Western pathology texts into Africa, the racist legacy of apartheid, an African cosmology at odds with Western values, and the realities of language barriers in a country with 11 official languages are undeniable challenges facing the psychological profession in South Africa'.

The challenge lies in the ability to understand other cultures and ethnic groups. In professional practice, when a client from a different ethnic background approaches a psychologist in need of assistance, the psychologist is obliged to serve the client with a high level of professionalism and ethical standards. In some cases, this may be difficult because of language problems and differences in belief systems. Some African cultures or ethnicities, for example, lack separate words for manifestations of depression or panic attacks (SADAG Conference, 2011). In many cases, depression or panic attacks will be seen as 'madness' because the behaviour is out of context and most often not understood. If no indigenous concepts exist for a symptom or condition, how can Western definition and interpretation of it make sense?

If necessary, the professional should acknowledge their incapacity to treat someone and, in this case, they should refer a client to a suitable therapist, colleague, or traditional healer. Incompetence or the inability to understand the genuine need of the client can make the client vulnerable to many varieties of unethical actions of the practitioner. The act and a dialogue about different disorders should contribute to more ethical actions and an increased culture of understanding.

The state of mental health care in South Africa

Despite South Africa's progressive mental health legislation, ongoing barriers to the financing and development of mental health services exist, which result in: (*i*) psychiatric hospitals remaining outdated, falling into disrepair, and often unfit for human use; (*ii*) serious shortages of mental health professionals; (*iii*) inability to develop vitally important tertiary level psychiatric services (such as child and adolescent services, psychogeriatric services, neuropsychiatric services, etc.); and (*iv*) community mental health and psychosocial rehabilitation services remaining undeveloped, so that patients end up institutionalised, without hope of rehabilitation back into their communities. This state of affairs remains unchanged despite the legislated commitments to reform mental health care in the MHCA (2002).

However, the MHCA has not yet brought about the envisaged changes to ensure fair, just, and ethical treatment of all patients. Many facilities and psychiatric hospitals are still delivering substandard services. Patients are still being housed in dilapidated buildings with poor infrastructure. Ramlall, Chipps, and Mars, (2010, p. 669) state in this regard that 'in such conditions, the shortage of specialist facilities, admission beds, and staff trained in psychiatry is of concern'.

HISTORY OF THE SOUTH AFRICAN ETHICAL CODE FOR PSYCHOLOGISTS

According to Pettifor and Sawchuk (2006), codes of ethics for psychologists were established about 50 years ago. In 1953, the American Psychological Association set the tone when it published a provisional code of ethics for acceptable professional conduct. The main aims of the code were to ensure respect, confidentiality, and doing no harm to a patient.

The global professionalisation of psychology escalated rapidly after the Second World War. In 1948, the first professional association in South Africa was formed, namely the South African Psychological Association (SAPA). This was the first body in South Africa that discussed a possible list of regulations or ethics for psychologists. In 1955, SAPA eventually accepted a set of ethical standards that was largely based on the ethical standards that the

American Psychological Association proposed in 1953. This was called Ethical Standards of Psychologists, Summary of Ethical Principles. Prior to this, no action could be taken when a complaint was lodged against a member of SAPA. Although membership of SAPA was voluntary, this code allowed for the termination of membership in cases of misconduct.

Although SAPA ceased to exist in 1982, and a new body, the Psychological Association of South Africa (PASA), was established in 1983, the ethical standards set by SAPA were adhered to until 1985. PASA then set new ethical standards until this association was replaced by the Psychological Society of South Africa (PsySSA) in 1994. It must be noted that although SAPA, PASA, and PsySSA were or are all professional bodies, they do not have any statutory powers. In South Africa, the statutory power over health professionals is held by the Health Professions Council of South Africa (HPCSA), which was established in 1999, having previously been known as the South African Medical and Dental Council (SAMDC) (Scherrer, Louw, & Möller, 2002). Guided by the Medical, Dental, and Supplementary Service Professions Act (No. 56 of 1974), the name of this statutory body was changed to acknowledge psychology and other supplementary health professions.

In an endeavour to make psychology more formalised and structured in South Africa, a Professional Board for Psychology was set up in 1974. This was done in terms of the Medical, Dental, and Supplementary Service Professions Act (No. 56 of 1974). The Professional Board for Psychology is currently one of the 12 professional boards under the auspices of the HPCSA. Since 1974, the HPCSA has been charged 'by statute to register those persons wishing to use the title 'psychologist' and to practise as such' (Louw, 1997a, pp. 183–185). The Professional Board for Psychology ensures that psychologists register with the Council before they can enter professional practice. The Board also ensures that people who request official registration as psychologists have sufficient professional training (Scherrer et al., 2002).

The Professional Board for Psychology developed a set of rules during 1977 that can be seen as the first official code of conduct for psychologists in South Africa. Although the professional bodies or associations (e.g. SAPA, PASA, & PsySSA) had voluntary membership, and each association had its own set of rules and regulations, registration as a practising psychologist could (and can) only take place through the Professional Board for Psychology. Thus, practising psychologists (and psychometrists) do not have to be members of professional associations as long as they are officially registered with the Professional Board for Psychology. The Professional Board for Psychology is furthermore responsible for disciplinary actions if a registered psychologist is accused of unprofessional behaviour (Louw, 1997b).

The American Psychological Association has been the global leader with regard to ethical standards for psychologists and is required to update the code of ethics regularly to adhere to social changes and demands internationally. In this regard, Canter, Bennett, Jones, and Nagy (1994, p. xv) reported that 'to address the many changes that have occurred in recent years as the profession of psychology has evolved, the APA, ... developed a new code of ethics, titled Ethical Principles of Psychologists and Code of Conduct (1992)'. However, more recently, suggestions have been forthcoming from the global psychology community to develop an international code of ethical principles for psychologists. These suggestions were answered when the International Union of Psychological Science passed a resolution in 2002 that urged member societies to enact codes of ethics and to take action against members who were guilty of human rights abuses. This endeavour 'denounced all practices that were inconsistent with the high moral standards required for psychologists to conduct scientific and professional activities' (Pettifor & Sawchuk, 2006, p. 217).

Gobodo-Madikizela and Foster (2005, p. 344) assert that 'every person should be accorded a sense of value, worth, and dignity, and that every person should be protected from infringements and abuses of these fundamental rights'. The aim of the following section is to address the complex and sometimes poorly understood phenomenon of ethical conduct in the behavioural sciences. Apart from being a human rights abuse, unacceptable conduct with a client or research participant during any interaction has the potential to result in disciplinary action or a legal encounter. Knowledge gained from this section should enable learners and practitioners to understand clearly the complex challenges to maintaining acceptable professional conduct.

ETHICAL BEHAVIOUR

Ethics are 'moral principles' that a mental health practitioner should uphold at all times. According to Burke et al. (2007), the word ethics is derived from the Greek word *ethos* (character). It refers to a set of moral principles which define what is acceptable and unacceptable and which appeal to a person's moral responsibility to act within the acceptable boundaries of humanity. Zabow and Kalsiki (2006, p. 357) assert that 'ethical principles and the law frequently interact'. According to Pope and Vasques (2007), it is important that practitioners are aware of the ethical code that applies to their profession; however, this awareness alone is not sufficient. According to these authors, a code of ethics cannot be followed in a thoughtless, rote manner, as ethical codes merely prompt, guide, and inform a practitioner's ethical deliberations. Professional conduct requires an ethical character first and foremost, and also requires an active, thoughtful, and creative approach, for the following reasons (Pope & Vasques, 2007):

- Each client or patient is unique; therefore, one cannot make ethical judgements based only on similarities with other clients. In each new case, the practitioner must apply his or her mind anew to the ethical considerations.
- Related to the above, each situation is unique, and ethical codes, no matter how thorough they are, cannot prescribe for all situations that a practitioner may encounter.
- Ethical codes may, in different situations and with different clients, provide us more or less clarity regarding the types of ethical considerations that may be significant, but often the code provides only broad guidelines that are open to interpretation by practitioners.

In the context of professional practice, ethical behaviour refers to a set of behavioural expectations that need to be adhered to by psychologists when they interact with clients so as to avoid causing harm to these clients. They should respect and honour the emotions and opinions of others and they should never exploit or abuse these (Alvesson & Sköldberg, 2000; Becker, 1992).

The essence of ethical behaviour is to act in a way that is always in the best interest of the client (principle of beneficence), for example, by making sure that the client always receives the best possible treatment. In addition, the professional should not take any action that can be damaging to the client (principle of non-maleficence). Ethical behaviour is nested in a set of values that every behavioural and health care professional should internalise.

Statutory control over ethical behaviour

One of the distinctions between a profession and an occupation is that all professions have codes of ethics, and there is always a statutory body that takes the responsibility for setting up and implementing an ethical code of behaviour for a particular profession. As described earlier, in South Africa, the Health Professions Council of South Africa (HPCSA) is the statutory body that performs this function for all health and allied professions. The HPCSA is the overarching body that is made up of professional boards of all the professions that fall under its auspices.

The Professional Board for Psychology is responsible for setting up and implementing the ethical code for psychologists. The ethical code for psychologists is an extensive document that covers a wide array of professional conduct (see Table 14.4). It must be remembered, however, that the field of ethics and ethical conduct is complicated, and given the fact that this book focuses mainly on abnormal behaviour, this section cannot cover the ethical code in its entirety. The most recent ethical rules for psychologists were promulgated by the Professional Board for Psychology in August 2006, and are available on the HPCSA website.

The code of conduct for psychologists was guided and developed from a generic set of ethical and professional standards of the HPCSA. This is because each discipline is confronted with unique ethical challenges that differ in intricacy and relevance (Zabow & Kaliski, 2006). However, codes of conduct all have one thing in common, namely, to ensure that a set of standards or rules is established and that the members or individuals who are associated with the body or organisation that prescribes these codes or rules should adhere to them. If an individual breaches the prescribed code of behaviour or expectations, sanctions of some kind should be forthcoming.

Table 14.4: Excerpts from the ethical code for psychologists as it relates to abnormal behaviour

Broad area	Examples of sub-areas
Professional competence	Competency limits Maintaining competence Adding new competencies
Professional relations	Respect for human rights and for others Informed consent Unfair discrimination Sexual and other harassment Avoiding harm Conflict of interest Multiple relationships Exploitative relationships Cooperation with other professionals
Privacy, confidentiality, and records	Rights to confidentiality Limits on intrusions on privacy Legally dependent clients Release of confidential information

Broad area	Examples of sub-areas
Assessment activities	Appropriate use of assessment methods Informed consent in assessments Communication of results Scoring, interpreting, and explaining assessment results
Therapeutic activities	Informed consent to therapy Interruption of therapy Terminating therapy

With regard to the formulation of board-specific ethical codes, Burke et al. (2007, p. 113) maintain that 'the South African context poses the additional challenge of multiple levels of practitioner registration (e.g. psychological counsellors and psychologists)'. According to these authors, an ethics manual will probably be more useful than a specific code of ethics. As more and more practitioners with different levels of training are being allowed to do therapeutic work, for example, debriefing and play therapy, different levels of registration should guide the future development of the proposed manual. The following psychological professions are currently registered under the auspices of the Professional Board for Psychology: Psychologists, Intern Psychologists, Student Psychologists, Registered Counsellors, Psychometrists, and Psychotechnicians. There are also five specific categories of registration for psychologists: Clinical, Counselling, Educational, Industrial, and Research Psychology.

In concluding this section, it is clear that the appropriate governing or administrative body with the legal mandate to represent its registered members should ensure that a code of conduct is developed and that its members adhere to it. The Professional Board for Psychology used these guidelines to develop a board-specific code of conduct. The relevant code of conduct must always incorporate the core values of integrity, trust, and honesty. After a proper investigation, a confirmed breach of the code of conduct by the members should be punished in accordance with the level of unethical behaviour.

Challenges to ethical behaviour

Regardless of the current dilemmas and standing of a professional or statutory body, its 'watchdog' presence over practitioners in the mental health and medical sciences cannot be overemphasised as, annually, a number of practitioners are found guilty of misconduct. HPCSA statistics show that between 2007 and 2010, penalties were applied in 562 finalised matters. In terms of psychologists, 21 cases were finalised by the Professional Board for Psychology between 1 April 2009 and 31 March 2012.

However, the full extent of unethical conduct is unknown and inadequately understood. Although many complaints are lodged against psychologists, 'organised statistics on the exact scope of these complaints are not readily available. This is both odd and regrettable since complaints against psychologists in South Africa are not uncommon' (Scherrer et al., 2002, p. 55). The most common issues that can lead to a complaint are as follows (Louw, 1997b; PsySSA, 1994):

- ***Professional disrespect:*** Derogatory statements between psychologists about each other's training and skills.
- ***Breaches of confidentiality:*** A breach of confidentiality occurs when the psychologist tells someone the content of therapy sessions or divulges the diagnosis of a client without the client's permission.
- ***Confidentiality and forensic reports:*** When a psychologist is doing an interview for court work (forensic) purposes, the interviewee should be informed at the outset that confidentiality is not possible as the psychologist is going to write a report of their findings for the court and is most probably going to testify in court about the findings. The interviewee cannot complain about the contents of the report if the information was given voluntarily and if the psychologist explained to them that confidentiality was not possible.
- ***Inappropriate relationships with clients:*** A therapist should not enter non-professional relationships with their clients and they should refrain from socialising with clients where possible. This includes any sexual relationships with clients.
- ***Selection assessments:*** A psychologist who evaluates a person for selection procedures for employment placement should obtain written consent from the candidate to divulge information to the employer.
- ***Fees:*** Overcharging and inflated fees can be seen as fraud. The psychologist should charge a patient strictly according to the actual duration of the therapy session and according to the agreed fees.
- ***Advertising:*** There are strict guidelines about appropriate advertising for professional services. For example, it would be inappropriate for a psychologist to announce their name and contact details during a school assembly.
- ***Competence:*** Professionals should be careful not to act outside their level of competence as this may lead to harm to the client. In particular, psychologists may misuse psychological tests, or use inappropriate tests, which can contribute to an incorrect diagnosis of a client's problem.

CASE STUDY

Crystal, a 20-year-old female client, has been consulting with Dr B, a male psychologist, for six months. During the consultations, the client has disclosed her feelings of incompetence and her low self-esteem to her therapist. This has become a discussion point during every consultation. She also disclosed to the therapist that she stays at home over weekends as she does not have any male friends and she feels too shy to go out on her own. Eventually, she tells Dr B that she feels safe with him and that she does not feel incompetent when she interacts with him. During a consultation, Dr B suggests that she go out with her female friends, as group socialisation may help her to feel more confident to go out over weekends. Crystal then suggests to Dr B that he should take her out one weekend, as she feels safe with him.

DISCUSSION

In this context, an appropriate and ethical response would be to treat the suggestion in a professional manner without hurting the client's feelings. Clearly, Dr B should not accept the invitation to take Crystal out. It would be inappropriate and unethical behaviour for Dr B to enter into a social relationship with his client. Dr B should always act in such a way that he will help the client with her problem but he should refrain from getting involved with her on a personal level.

As is indicated above, practitioners may be guilty of a wide range of misbehaviours that include unacceptable marketing practices, harmful interventions, inappropriate relationships with clients (see the case study of Dr. B), professional sabotage or malicious gossip, sexual harassment, overcharging of medical schemes and patients, and breaking confidentiality through careless discussions about clients in public settings (see the case study of Dr C). 'Interesting' clients are sometimes mentioned in social discussions. Practitioners may mask the individual's name and gender but provide enough information in the conversation to allow an educated guess to be made about who the person may be. The casual sharing of the client's information to make conversation or to sound informed and astute is a serious breach of client–therapist confidentiality.

In the human sciences, a scrupulous respect for human dignity is required; however, it is often difficult to adhere to the code of conduct relevant to the discipline because it is human nature to inquire, to experiment, and to bend the rules. Thus, as previously mentioned, some professionals do act outside the prescribed boundaries of the code of conduct. However, all professionals who are bound by their relevant code of conduct should always act ethically and strive towards a shared commitment to their profession's vision, principles, and ethical standards of behaviour.

Ethical dilemmas

Sometimes, practitioners are faced with two or more ethical principles from the code of conduct that are in direct conflict with one another. Practitioners then have to use their personal discretion to decide which principle to prioritise and abide by. According to Burke et al. (2007, p. 111), 'few ethical codes provide criteria to decide the relative importance of such principles. However, the practitioner is required to make the judgement'. This supports the suggestion that a manual for practitioners should be developed, with best-practice examples and real-life dilemmas, and added discussions around the issues involved.

SPECIFIC ETHICAL ISSUES FOR MENTAL HEALTH CARE PROFESSIONALS

A basic premise of mental health care is confidentiality. This means that the professional commits to keeping what the client tells them confidential. However, there are some exceptions to this in that information can be divulged in certain situations. For example, a practitioner may be confronted by a visibly aggressive client who clearly does not want to calm down even if asked politely to do so, or a person who divulges information about their terrorist cell which plans to blow up the Union Buildings, or a person who describes his fantasies about killing his estranged girlfriend or a person who has given up hope and threatens to commit suicide. Is there merit in all these cases to divulge information? It is not within the scope of this chapter to explore all these debates. However, in the following sections, four aspects will be addressed to answer some of these difficult questions in mental health intervention. These include breaches of confidentiality and reporting to third parties, dangerous clients, suicidal clients, as well as committing of a client.

CASE STUDY

During a soccer game Dr C bumped into a female client at the cold-drink stand. After he greeted the client, Dr C and his friend made their way to their seats. Dr C's friend asked him about the woman he had greeted at the cold-drink stand. His friend was very inquisitive and asked Dr C several questions about the woman. Dr C replied 'professionally' by saying, 'She is a client and unfortunately I cannot tell you anything about her'. However, after the game, Dr C and his friend went to a pub to have a few drinks and to celebrate their team's victory. The friend once again enquired about the woman they saw earlier at the soccer. Dr C, now under the influence of alcohol, told his friend that her previous boyfriend had drugged and raped her and had taken intimate photographs of her and posted them on the World Wide Web.

DISCUSSION

There are several ethical issues here. Firstly, Dr C should not have revealed that the woman in question was a client (principle of privacy). Secondly, this kind of discussion with friends is forbidden according to the code of conduct, as it betrays the client's confidentiality. If the client or another professional learn about this, they can report Dr C to the HPCSA and the Professional Board for Psychology. The HPCSA will then investigate the matter and will deal with Dr C according to its prescribed mandate.

Confidentiality and reporting to third parties

Athough the HPCSA prescribes certain guidelines, the onus still lies on the professional to decide whether or not to break confidentiality by divulging the information to a third party. The premise of ethical conduct is based on the professional's respect for, and dedication to, the client. This means that they do not tell anyone else what the client has said or done (see the case study of Dr C). However, the HPCSA allows a registered practitioner to break confidentiality in the following instances (HPCSA, 2007):

1. A practitioner shall divulge verbally or in writing information regarding a patient which he or she ought to divulge only:
   a. In terms of a statutory provision;
   b. At the instruction of a court of law; or
   c. Where justified in the public interest.
2. Any information other than the information referred to in subrule (1) shall only be divulged by a practitioner:
   a. With the express consent of the patient;
   b. In the case of a minor under the age of 14 years, with the written consent of his or her parent or guardian; or
   c. In the case of a deceased patient, with the written consent of his or her next-of-kin or the executor of such deceased patient's estate

In Rule 30 of the Professional Board for Psychology regarding 'Rules of Conduct Pertaining Specifically to Psychology', it is stated in Chapter 2 that a psychologist may release confidential information 'upon court order or to conform to legal imperatives or upon the written authorisation of the client, parent of a minor client, or legal guardian'.

Dangerousness

To complicate the challenges of ethical conduct and keeping confidentiality, therapists sometimes consult with dangerous or high-risk individuals who may talk about their intense anger and frequent violent thoughts. A question that arises from this is whether a therapist is obligated to warn others (authorities or a third party, e.g. the intended victim) that the client has indicated to them that they have fantasies of acting dangerously, or they intend to, or have already, acted dangerously (see discussion of the Tarasoff case in Box 14.1).

BOX 14.1: THE TATIANA TARASOFF CASE

The 'Tarasoff Case' has been highly publicised since the early 1970s and is regularly used to support discussions on dangerousness, the assessment of risk, and the divulging of patient information. Prosenjit Poddar, who was an outpatient at the University of California's Berkeley campus clinic, revealed to his psychiatrist his desires to harm or kill a girl he had met at a dance. Poddar had dated this young woman (Tatiana Tarasoff) for a short time after he met her. After their brief relationship ended, Poddar became highly distressed and paranoid. After Poddar threatened to blow up Ms Tarasoff's house, a friend persuaded Poddar to seek therapy at the campus clinic. However, after eight sessions, Poddar discontinued his therapy after the psychiatrist warned that he would restrain Poddar if he continued to make threats against his ex-girlfriend. The psychiatrist consulted his supervisor and together they decided to inform the university campus police about Poddar's threats and to ask for their assistance in admitting Poddar to hospital.

The campus police investigated the case and subsequently questioned Poddar; they reported that he appeared quite rational during the interview and that he had promised to stay away from his ex-girlfriend. He also promised that he would never harm Tatiana. The clinic director instructed his staff not to pursue efforts to hospitalise Poddar. Poddar kept a low profile after the arrest and, for some time, complied with his promise not to contact or hurt Tatiana. However, two months after this event, he went to Tatiana's home and stabbed her to death.

Although the clinic initiated the contact with the campus police, they never contacted Tatiana Tarasoff to warn her of any potential danger. Her parents subsequently sued the Berkeley Clinic on the grounds of negligence. They were of the opinion that the psychiatrist who treated Poddar had been negligent in not warning Tarasoff (or them) of the danger she was in. The case was dismissed by the lower courts, but when the Tarasoff parents took the case to the Supreme Court of California, it confirmed that therapists have a duty to break confidentiality to warn of potential harm. This decision has been controversial and was later amended to say that therapists need to take measures to protect intended victims.

DISCUSSION

It is good practice for psychologists to warn clients at the beginning of their therapy that there may be circumstances under which confidentiality could be broken. These would include the threat of harm to themselves (suicide) or to others (assault or homicide).

Source: Herbert & Young, 2002.

In view of the rules (described in the previous section) that regulate the instances when a counsellor can breach the confidentiality clause, the following questions arise: How does one determine which cases should be shared with the authorities because this is justified as acting in the public interest? If a client reveals information that indicates possible aggressive or dangerous behaviour in the future, should the therapist inform the authorities, considering that a 'false alarm' would constitute a breach of confidentiality?

In this situation, the professional has to balance the risk of harm to others against adhering to the ethical code of conduct by maintaining confidentiality. However, it is very difficult to make an accurate prediction of dangerousness and violence. To illustrate some of the problems with the prediction of dangerousness, the potential physical and/or emotional harm caused by a client, and the role of the practitioner in this context, read the case study of Sipho.

CASE STUDY

During a visit to his lecturer, who is also a clinical psychologist, Sipho shares the following information with his lecturer. He explains to her that his academic performance is suffering because his girlfriend has recently ended their three-year relationship and she immediately started seeing someone new. The lecturer convinces Sipho to come and see her in her capacity as a clinical psychologist to address his emotional distress. After four counselling sessions, Sipho shares enough detail of his post-relationship behaviour with the lecturer for her to make the following conclusions: Sipho is obsessed with his ex-girlfriend, he shows self-mutilating behaviour, stalks his ex-girlfriend, photographs her against her wishes, telephones her repeatedly, and makes threats to commit suicide after he has killed her. This type of behaviour can clearly be categorised as potentially harmful to others. Depending on the personality of the ex-girlfriend and her knowledge of Sipho, she may see his behaviour either as childish and a nuisance or as posing a serious threat to her and other community members. If she is distressed by his behaviour and feels that it has a negative effect on her well-being, she may believe that she is being harmed emotionally.

Sipho is diagnosed as suffering from a Borderline Personality Disorder. However, this diagnosis and the ex-girlfriend's distress do not enable a professional to predict accurately the level of dangerousness the behaviour poses. Thus, the lecturer has a dilemma. Should Sipho be referred for further therapy or should he be admitted to a mental hospital for both his own and for his ex-girlfriend's protection? Many individuals (male and female) show 'dangerous tendencies' follow the break-up of a love relationship or something similarly traumatic. What should the lecturer do?

DISCUSSION

Firstly, the lecturer should have referred Sipho to another professional, as, by seeing him as a client, she entered into a dual relationship with him (as lecturer and counsellor). Secondly, the practitioner's present dilemma is whether she should inform the authorities of Sipho's behaviour before something destructive takes place. The counsellor is bound by a code of ethical conduct to keep the client's information to herself. However, there seems to be a real risk of harm to her client and his ex-girlfriend. In cases like these, counsellors are guided by their own discretion, but they are also guided by the Tatiana Tarasoff case (see Box 14.1).

The case study of Sipho clearly illustrates an ethical dilemma that some practitioners face from time to time. According to the HPCSA criteria (see Table 14.4), a client has the right to confidentiality; however, in this case, the client's fantasies had a direct impact on the safety of another person. These kinds of situations force practitioners to make a judgement as to the seriousness of the matter and to what extent it is anticipated that clients will act on their fantasies, delusions, or hallucinations. In the Tarasoff case, it is quite clear that the practitioner judged that there was a real threat, otherwise the campus police would not have been notified. Notifying the police was clearly a breach of confidentiality; the question is, was this justified? In addition, the question needs to be asked as to why the victim was not notified.

It is usually agreed that behaviour that causes physical injury and/or damage to property can be deemed dangerous. However, not only physical actions may be regarded as dangerous or destructive. In some cases, the court accepts that actions causing psychological or emotional damage are also characteristic of dangerous behaviour. The legal definition is, however, largely focused on physical or tangible harm and does not really accommodate psychological or emotional damage (Bartol, 2002; Bartol & Bartol, 2005; Bartol & Bartol, 2011; Blackburn, 1993).

One of the difficulties illustrated by the Tarasoff Case is that some people who seem to pose no threat to society may indeed be dangerous, while others regarded as dangerous may show no such behaviour following release from care. The MacArthur Risk Assessment Study in the United States (see Table 14.5), which is hailed as one of the most prominent studies in connection with dangerousness, showed that in a significant number of cases, people were incorrectly judged to be dangerous.

Clinicians are not able to predict with accuracy the probability of harm occurring, nor can they accurately specify the type of violence or severity of harm an individual may cause. The tendency amongst clinicians is to over-predict a person's level of dangerousness. Some studies suggest that two out of every three (66%) predictions are 'false positives' (Bartlett & Sandland, 2003; Bartol & Bartol, 2011; Walker, 1996). A false positive refers to the situation when a person is labelled dangerous but does not exhibit dangerous behaviour after the prediction. However, Ashworth (2000) refers to other prediction studies which found 50% accuracy in prediction of dangerousness. Ashworth (2000, p. 180) also states that no 'significant improvements [in prediction] have been reported in recent years'. Prediction thus remains unreliable in the determination of dangerousness. In support of this, Kaliski (2006, p. 117) claims that 'the sad reality is that few experts, regardless of their professional backgrounds, can provide reliable predictions of future violence'.

Table 14.5: Factors that can contribute to risk of violent behaviour

Factor	Contribution to risk of violent behaviour
Gender	Slight difference in terms of gender, with men being slightly more prone to violence than women.
Prior violence	A history of violent behaviour seems to be strongly related to future violence.
Childhood experiences	A history of serious and frequent physical abuse and a father with a criminal record or with a history of substance abuse predict subsequent violent behaviour.
Neighbourhood and race	Race is not a factor as different race groups from the same disadvantaged neighbourhoods had the same rates of violence.
Diagnosis of mental disorder	A diagnosis of Schizophrenia is associated with a lower rate of violence than a diagnosis of certain personality or adjustment disorders. A co-occurring diagnosis of substance abuse is strongly predictive of violence.
Delusions	The presence of delusions is not associated with violence; however, a generally 'suspicious' attitude toward others seems to be related to later violence.
Hallucinations	Hallucinations in general do not seem to be related to violence with the exception of where voices specifically commanded a violent act.
Violent thoughts	Thinking or daydreaming about harming others was associated with violence, particularly if the thoughts or daydreams were persistent.

Source: Adapted from http://www.macarthur.virginia.edu/risk.html

Whether or not one has a statutory or ethical duty to warn or protect, many practitioners regard the Tarasoff ruling as the 'standard of practice' with regard to potentially dangerous clients (Bartol & Bartol, 2008). However, others do not agree with the Tarasoff ruling in therapeutic situations where an individual divulges their intention to hurt another person. For example, Bersoff (2002, p. 570) is of the opinion that the Tarasoff case should be seen as 'bad law, bad social science, and bad social policy'. Bersoff insists that Poddar was an outpatient and not under the control of a mental hospital and therefore not eligible for involuntary commitment. This means that there was no legal duty on the psychiatrist to protect private third parties from harm.

Suicide and euthanasia

Mental health practitioners are often confronted by someone who expresses their intent to take their own life because of some form of distress. Two of the most common underlying disorders that are related to suicide are Schizophrenia and depression. The suicide incidence among people suffering from Schizophrenia is at least 20 times higher than the incidence amongst the general population. Alcoholism and substance addiction also often correlate with suicidal behaviour. Suicide is common in most cultures of the world and it occurs at all social levels and amongst all races in South Africa.

Due partly to the fact that there are so many myths about suicide, it can be very difficult to predict whether a client or patient who expresses their will to die will actually go through with their intention. The mental health practitioner should always consider a suicide threat to be serious and should treat a suicidal person ethically and with dignity. Anyone expressing suicidal feelings needs immediate attention. However, it is often difficult to intervene and to prevent suicide because of the level of distress suicidal clients manifest with. The client usually does not realise the limitations and irrationality of their thought processes. Many insist that it would be better if they take their own life.

This opens up the question whether any person has the right to intervene if another human being decides to take their own life. The Constitution states that we have a right to life but the same argument can be put forward for death. We have a right to die and probably a right to die as we wish to die. For example, one might ask whether an aged person with a terminal illness has the right to insist on suicide or assisted suicide (euthanasia). This becomes a very controversial issue since health care practitioners are trained to save lives and to help humans. This issue continues to be the subject of fierce legal and moral debate.

Although euthanasia has been legalised in a few countries, in South Africa it is illegal to assist a person to take their own life, even on request. It is also vital for mental health practitioners to act according to the current legal guidelines; otherwise, they could face serious criminal charges such as accessory to murder or murder. In addition, should a practitioner treat a suicidal client inappropriately or neglect to take reasonable steps to assist a suicidal person, they could be charged with unethical behaviour by the HPCSA. Neglecting this duty can have very serious mental health implications for clients (Bhamjee, 2010; Egan, 2008; Hoffmann, Myburgh, & Poggenpoel, 2010; Lippi, Smit, Jordaan, & Roos, 2009; Prinsloo & Louw, 1989; Sneiderman & McQuoid-Mason, 2000).

The two underlying principles of the ethical code, namely beneficence (acting in the best interest of the client) and non-maleficence (minimising harm) are relevant here. On the one hand, one could argue that the decision to break confidentiality 'on behalf of the client' could be deemed by the client to be an act of maleficence; clients could argue that the practitioner is not treating them with the necessary respect and dignity. However, suicidal clients may be very vulnerable and unable to make a rational decision for themselves. In this situation, it may be in the client's best interest (beneficence) to make a decision to protect him or her from harm. In this case, the beneficence outweighs any potential maleficence. Allan (1997, p. 80) states that 'where a client is in immediate and real danger of serious harm but is incapable of giving consent, or refuses, and where there is no reasonable alternative to the course of action considered ... contacting the person's relatives or the police may be justified'. Others would say that this action is not only justified but an obligation of professional ethical behaviour.

In addition, family murders are increasing in South Africa amongst all cultural and ethnic groups (known as murder-suicide or extended suicide). Extended suicide occurs when the parent carefully plans the murder and tries to prevent the victims from experiencing any pain. Murder-suicide is likely to be preceded by a pathological possessiveness of the husband in respect of his wife and children, especially his wife. Males who view their family members as property are more likely to commit an impulsive family murder or murder-suicide. It is difficult for the practitioner to decide whether the client who raises a possible family murder during therapy will commit either one of these types of family murder. The question arises whether this intention provides enough grounds to inform the other members of the family and the authorities.

In addition to all the factors discussed above, in the case of psychologists, their decision about possibly breaking confidentiality about these matters is often influenced by their own values as well as their therapeutic modality.

Committing a client

Committing or referring a client for observation has considerable implications for both parties. The mere committal to a psychiatric institution is stigmatising and potentially degrading. Referral for observation is a commonly used mental health intervention whereby the referred individual is monitored or treated for specific behaviour. It is essential to adhere to guidelines for good medical practice during the referral process, as incomplete assessments and poor quality of referral could have detrimental consequences for both the health professional referring the person as well as for the practitioner receiving the patient in the facility. Poor quality of referrals to mental health service providers should be seen as a serious infringement of human rights. Typical infringements include unclear referrals and breaches of patient confidentiality (Struwig & Pretorius, 2009).

Should it become evident that a client needs to be committed, a health professional is obliged to discuss with the client the possibilities of treatment and the possible effects of non-treatment (e.g. distress, injury and, in extreme cases, death). Other options such as medication should also be discussed. This is important especially if the person has the capacity to make informed decisions about his or her care. In cases where a person poses a risk, the person should be informed that a risk assessment is needed and that it should be considered as an attempt to reduce harm.

Some individuals with a severe mental illness may lack the capacity to recognise the presence of a disorder, to consider advice regarding the risks and benefits of treatment, or to make an informed choice about their condition and the best option for treatment. Swanepoel (2010) proposes that three factors should be considered when confronted with the ethics of decision-making regarding a client/patient:

- Psychologists always have choices they can select from as they make decisions.
- The consequences of each of the different choices should be taken into account.
- The context of the specific ethical dilemma must be considered as it will have an effect on the eventual decision.

The health care professional could, where possible, obtain a second opinion if uncertain about aspects of the person's condition. Although the legal capacity of a person can be assessed quite accurately, we should stay mindful of our limitations in terms of predicting dangerousness. Should a person lack the capacity to make a decision on their commitment, the health care professional should discuss the person's condition with other relevant role-players such as a spouse or other direct family members, and take immediate action. This swift action could reduce risks in cases where a person has a severe mental condition or poses a safety risk to others. In this case, the patient should be committed to ensure immediate proper care and to reduce any form of risk (Ryan, Nielssen, Paton, & Large 2010). However, Zabow (2008. p. 62) warns practitioners not to be over-enthusiastic with committing of clients. He summarises the pitfalls of committing as follows:

> *'It is important that all clinicians remain aware of recent developments, the extent of the current legislation, and any ongoing changes. In the current situation a 'dangerousness' alert due to publicised incidents has become a determinant for involuntary hospitalisation, but should be specifically reserved for those cases in which restoring mental health is the reason for use of legislation to detain the patient. Beneficence requires the provision of care for those patients incapable of caring for themselves. Arguments opposing the above also relate to autonomy and the infringement of the person's liberty'.*

CONSEQUENCES OF UNETHICAL CONDUCT

The HPCSA will investigate any written allegations submitted to it regarding the violation of the code of ethical behaviour by a mental health care practitioner. If a client wishes to lodge a complaint of unethical behaviour against a psychologist, they should direct a letter describing the complaint to the HPCSA. The complainant could also be a colleague or an ordinary member of society.

Following receipt of a complaint, the Professional Board will notify the accused that a complaint has been lodged and request him or her to submit an explanation in defence of the alleged malpractice. The defence or explanation is put before the Committee for Preliminary Inquiry. This committee deals with all matters, within current policy parameters, relating to preliminary enquiries regarding complaints, determination of accounts, and fines, in terms of the Medical, Dental, and Supplementary Health Service Professions Act (No. 56 of 1974) and reports to the Board about these.

The Committee for Preliminary Inquiry will decide whether the complaint warrants further investigation. If a satisfactory explanation is given by the practitioner, it is usually accepted and no further action is taken. However, the accused can be called to meet with the committee if it is not satisfied with the justification. If the explanation is not accepted, an inquiry by the Disciplinary Committee will follow.

Corrective actions for confirmed breaches of ethical conduct by members of the HPCSA are described in the disciplinary policies. The legal implications that can be expected when a member breaches the Code of Conduct or behaves unethically are stipulated on the official website of the HPCSA (www.hpcsa.co.za). If the transgression is minor, for example advertising services inappropriately, the practitioner will be warned or fined. If the transgression is of a more serious nature, the practitioner can be put on probation, suspended for a specified time, or struck off the roll. In very serious cases, where criminal charges are laid against the professional, a prison sentence may be imposed. The complainant can also lodge a civil case against the practitioner.

Even if psychologists are successful with their defence of the complaint, they are likely to suffer as the complaint itself may damage their reputation. In addition, the process may have severe financial implications, both directly in terms of legal costs and indirectly in terms of loss of income (Scherrer et al., 2002).

In addition to the process described above, from September 2005, the HPCSA appointed an ombudsman to assist in investigating and settling complaints referred by the legal services department of the Committee for Preliminary Inquiry. The ombudsman addresses complaints against registered practitioners and determines their nature and validity in terms of the Medical, Dental, and Supplementary Health Service Professions Act (No. 56 of 1974). The Office of the Ombudsman also renders a mediation service and endeavours to resolve matters amicably, if at all possible (www.hpcsa.co.za).

This regulatory framework therefore governs the disciplinary processes when a complaint is lodged against a practitioner. The HPCSA also follows a policy of transparency by posting on their website all the cases that they investigate, the names of the offending parties, and their punishment, to ensure that the public is protected from similar malpractice in the future.

CASE STUDY

Dr A is a well-known psychiatrist who falsely claims from medical schemes for 'consultations with patients' he sees on a weekly basis. He also overcharges some patients and claims for chronic depression medicines that he 'prescribes and provides' for them on a monthly basis. Through these actions, Dr A is fraudulently claiming thousands of rand from medical schemes for fictitious 'patients' with behavioural disorders.

In a severe case of unethical behaviour like this the following needs to be considered: Dr A's actions are premeditated and harmful, but he did not hurt his patients directly (either physically or psychologically). However, his actions run the risk of exhausting the patients' medical funds. The primary victims in this context are the medical schemes. The secondary victims are the patients because their capacity to get treatment when they indeed need it is damaged.

DISCUSSION

Should Dr A get a warning with the requirement that he pay the medical schemes back what he owes them or should Dr A get a fine? OR Should he be suspended from practice for some period of time? In a case like this, Dr A would probably be required to pay back the fees to the medical schemes, he would probably have to pay a fine, and he would most likely be removed from the register for a period of time. In addition, depending on the extent of the fraud, he may face criminal charges.

CONCLUSION

When dealing with people with a mental disorder we must always remind ourselves that we are dealing with vulnerable people. Swanepoel (2010. p. 853) feels that 'making ethical or moral decisions, like any other decision in health care, is not a precise art but a learned skill'. Furthermore, in this context it is evident that mental health professionals are in a position of power in relation to their clients; therefore, they should be very careful not to abuse this position or to harm the client in a therapeutic environment. Professional behaviour is expected at all times, partly 'because of the essentially private, highly personal, and sometimes intensely emotional nature of the relationship' (Zabow & Kaliski, 2006, p. 360). The practitioner should always ensure that they act professionally in a clinical or therapeutic situation and they should guard against any situation or action that can be deemed as unprofessional or unethical. It goes without saying that the practitioner should never fuel or encourage a situation that could lead to unethical behaviour.

This chapter has provided a brief overview of important elements regarding legal and ethical issues concerning the management of people with a mental disorder. Any mental health professional must have a working knowledge of the relevant legal acts and ethical codes to ensure that their conduct is above reproach at all times. This chapter should, however, have made it abundantly clear that ethical decisions are not always as clearcut as they may seem at first glance. Practitioners, relying on their own ethical character, their knowledge of relevant laws, and their knowledge of the ethical code, need to navigate themselves through any difficult situations they may encounter. Failure to do this successfully makes them vulnerable to litigation and disciplinary action.

PARAGRAPH AND ESSAY QUESTIONS

1. Critically discuss the prerequisites for ethical conduct in a therapeutic context.
2. Define ethical behaviour in your own words.
3. Examine the role of the Health Professions Council of South Africa in ensuring ethical conduct in the health and behavioural disciplines.
4. Explain why it is important to accommodate indigenous belief systems in modern psychology.
5. Critically explain the different circumstances under which a therapist can divulge client information to a third party. Illustrate your answer with a case study.
6. Debate the possible consequences which unethical conduct can have for a practitioner.
7. Explain what legal implications unethical conduct can have for a practitioner.
8. Explain in your own words what unique factors need to be considered in the South African context in order to ensure ethical conduct at all times.

Appendix A

PSYCHOLOGICAL MANIFESTATIONS OF MEDICAL DISEASE

Conrad Visser

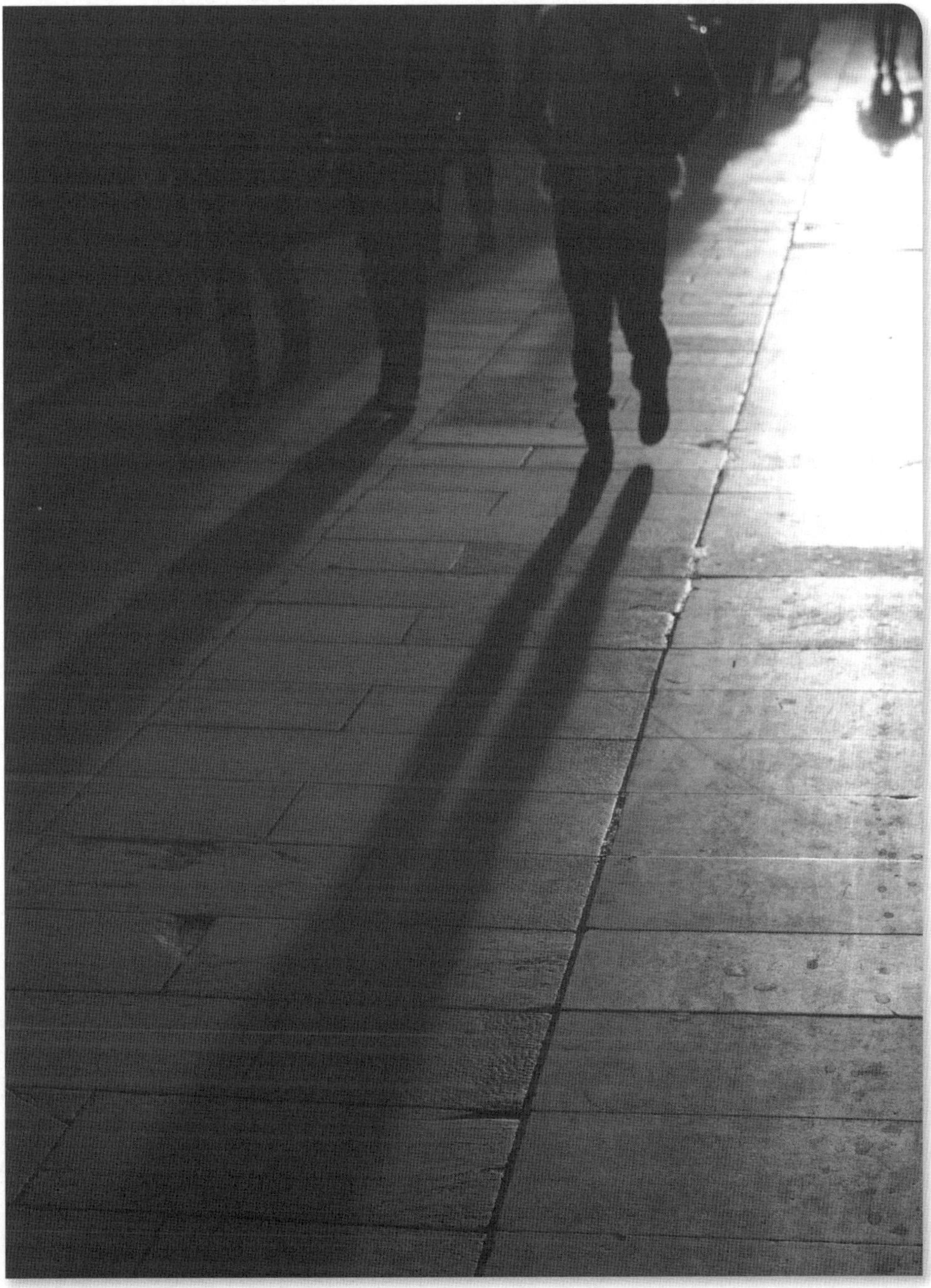

A APPENDIX OUTLINE

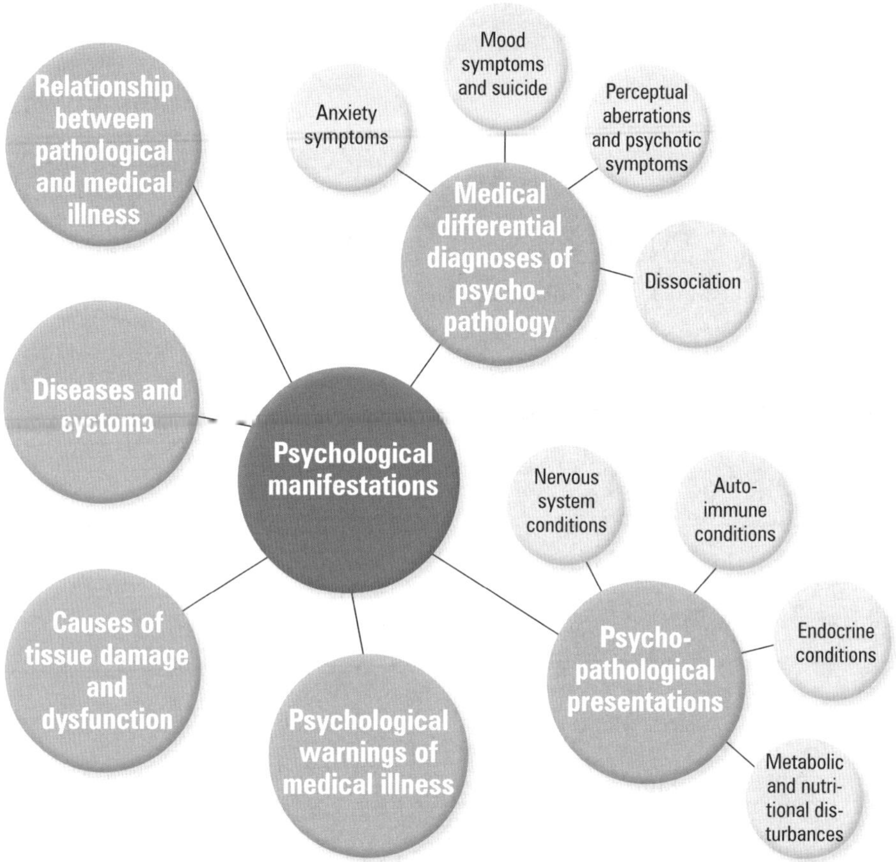

- Introduction
- Causes of tissue damage and dysfunction
- Disease and systems
- Relationship between psychopathology and medical illness
- Medical differential diagnoses of psychopathology
  - **Anxiety symptoms**
  - **Mood symptoms and suicide**
  - **Perceptual aberrations and psychotic symptoms**
  - **Dissociation**
- Psychopathological presentations of selected medical conditions
  - **Nervous system conditions**
    - Epilepsy
    - Neurodegenerative disorders
    - Central nervous system infections
    - Head trauma
    - Cerebral neoplasm
    - Demyelinating disorders
  - **Auto-immune conditions**
  - **Endocrine conditions**
  - **Metabolic and nutritional disturbances, toxins, and organ failure**
- Psychological warnings of medical illness
- Conclusion

LEARNING OUTCOMES

After studying this section, students should be able to:

- List causes of cellular and tissue damage and provide a classification for medical illness according to bodily systems.
- Describe the relationships between psychological symptoms and syndromes and medical illness.
- List medical differential diagnoses of psychopathological presentations.
- Describe the psychological manifestations of a selection of common medical conditions: epilepsy, neurodegenerative disorders, central nervous system infection, head trauma, cerebral neoplasm, demyelinating disorders, autoimmune disorders, endocrine conditions, and metabolic and nutritional disturbances, toxins, and organ failure.
- Describe psychopathological manifestations pointing towards medical causation.
- Recognise warning signs of medical causation in psychopathological case material.

INTRODUCTION

We know that the experience of disease always has psychological elements: it cannot be any other way. The presence of so-called bodily illness is universally accompanied by subjective phenomena like pain and malaise. When are sick, we feel down, we are listless, have little appetite, and we worry. Whilst mindful of this ever-important aspect of caring for the sick, the aim of this section is to draw attention to another phenomenon: psychological symptoms *caused* by medical illness.

While the brain is responsible for mental functions like thoughts and behaviour, it is also a bodily entity just like the lungs, gall bladder, and bone marrow. Like any other organ, normal brain function requires intact bodily systems to ensure adequate energy, maintenance of structure and biochemical environment, and protection from injury. The brain is therefore susceptible to the same injuries and harm that affect other bodily systems. In its broadest sense, pathology refers to abnormal functioning and structure at the systemic, organ-specific, tissue, cellular, and molecular levels the body. This section hopes to help students understand the many injuries and other aberrations that can give rise to pathology anywhere in the body. We will look at a practical way to classify disease and consider the medical causation of psychological symptoms. We will also explore differential diagnoses of common psychological symptoms and the psychological signature of a selection of medical conditions. Finally, we will show how psychological symptoms can draw our attention to their probable medical causation.

CAUSES OF TISSUE DAMAGE AND DYSFUNCTION

The cells that make up most of the body's tissues have many characteristics in common: they metabolise nutrients to meet their energy requirements; they have ways of maintaining their biochemistry; they interact with neighbouring cells as well as the extracellular environment; and can refashion their structure or function in response to change. Many cells can even multiply and seed new populations.

Causes of cellular injury could be classified as:

- ***Vascular*** (e.g. stroke, myocardial infarction, etc.)
- ***Infective*** (e.g. brain abscesses, malaria, etc.)
- ***Toxic*** (e.g. mercury, lead, etc.)
- ***Traumatic*** (e.g. burns, lacerations, etc.)
- ***Auto-immune*** (e.g. rheumatic fever, systemic lupus erythematosis, etc)
- ***Allergic*** (e.g. asthma, eczema, etc.)
- ***Metabolic*** (e.g. diabetes, myxoedema, etc.)
- ***Inherited*** (e.g. Down's syndrome)
- ***Neoplastic*** (e.g. carcinoma, leukaemia, etc.)
- ***Nutritional*** (e.g. anaemia, beriberi, etc.)
- ***Degenerative*** (e.g. Parkinson's disease, osteoarthritis, etc.)

Insults can be acquired (e.g. infection or trauma) or inherited. Often, as we have seen with the diathesis-stress model, interplay between an inherited vulnerability and exposure to environmental factors precipitates pathology. Autoimmune conditions are examples of this stress-vulnerability interplay. For example, a person may inherit a vulnerability to eczema which 'flares up' when they experience life stress.

DISEASES AND SYSTEMS

Tissue damage of any kind can affect isolated tissues or organs or involve the whole body. For the purposes of this section, it is easiest to grasp the varied nature of bodily pathology by considering its occurrence across organ systems (see Table 1). Such a classification is based on artificial boundaries whereas there is considerable overlap between organ systems for example, a stroke be classified as neurological or cardiovascular disease. Practically, three factors determine the allocation of diseases to different systems within a system-based classification:

- The primary mode of presentation
- The speciality traditionally regarded to possess the expertise in management
- Knowledge of aetiology and pathogenesis.

Table 1: Disease types by system

System	Description	Example of illnesses
Cardiovascular	heart, arteries, and veins	cardiac ischaemia, valvular lesions, cardiac failure, vasculitis, arteriosclerosis, aneurysm, varicose veins, deep vein thrombosis
Gastrointestinal	oesophagus, stomach, small and large bowel, anus; liver, biliary tree, pancreas, and spleen	oesophageal carcinoma, gastro-oesophageal reflux disease, duodenal ulcer, cholelithiasis, acute pancreatitis, colonic carcinoma
Genito-urinary	kidneys, ureters, urinary bladder, urethra, and male and female reproductive organs	polycycystic kidney disease, acute glomerulonephritis, renal failure, ectopic pregnancy, acute cystitis, cervical carcinoma, gonorrhoea
Musculoskeletal	bony and cartilaginous skeleton, joints, ligaments, fascias, muscles, and tendons	compound fracture of the humerus, osteoarthritis, septic arthritis, tennis elbow, compartment syndrome
Neurological	central and peripheral nervous system	stroke, epilepsy, Alzheimer's, Parkinson's, transverse myelitis, diabetic neuropathy, myasthenia gravis, polymyositis, muscular dystrophy
Cutaneous	skin and its appendages – hair and nails	acne vulgaris, porphyria, squamous cell carcinoma, malignant melanoma, eczema, alopecia, onychomycosis
Otorhino-laryngological	ear, nose, and throat (ENT)	vestibulitis, hearing loss, otitis media, tonsillitis, pharyngeal carcinoma, nasal polyps, fractured nasal septum
Orodental	teeth, gums, palate, tongue, and salivary glands	dental caries, dental abscess, periodontal disease, dental loss, malocclusion, haemangioma of the tongue, Sjögren's syndrome
Ophthalmologic	eyes and adnexa	laceration of the lid, conjunctivitis, trachoma, keratitis, acute glaucoma, retinal tear, macular degeneration
Lympho-haematological	formed elements, other blood products, bone marrow, and lymphoid tissue	iron-deficiency anaemia, neutropaenia, acute myeloblastic leukaemia, polycythemia rubra vera, Hodgkin's disease

System	Description	Example of illnesses
Endocrine	hormone-releasing organs; regulation and functioning of hormones across the body	Cushing's syndrome, diabetes mellitus, hypothyroidism, hyperparathyroidism, polycystic ovaries

RELATIONSHIP BETWEEN PSYCHOPATHOLOGY AND MEDICAL ILLNESS

The relationship between psychopathology and medical illness assumes one of six patterns:

1 ***Incidental*** (i.e. a chance relationship)
2 ***Psychological reaction to medical illness*** (e.g. anger, depression, hopelessness, and guilt *following* diagnosis of breast cancer)
3 ***Modification of expression of medical illness with antecedent psychiatric disorder*** (e.g. treatment-resistant Major Depressive Episode with atypical features, established Major Depressive Disorder *and* chronic hepatitis; induction of rapid cycling, established Bipolar II Disorder *and* hyperthyroidism)
4 ***Precipitation of new episode of medical illness with antecedent psychiatric disorder*** (e.g. new Major Depressive Episode, established Bipolar II Disorder *and* co-morbid osteoarthritis)
5 ***First expression of psychiatric disorder with antecedent medical vulnerability*** (e.g. first ever Manic Episode, family history of Bipolar I Disorder *and* co-morbid diabetes mellitus)
6 ***Psychological symptoms with medical causation*** (e.g. delirium *due to* renal failure; panic-like syndrome *due to* complex partial epilepsy; depersonalisation *due to* migraine).

It is important to note that factors 3, 4, and 5 are closely related to factor 6 and probably share a neural substrate in symptom genesis. Factor 2 concerns adjustment reactions and subthreshold anxiety or mood syndromes. By implication, symptoms could not have arisen without some awareness of the medical condition. The focus of this section is on Factor 6 – psychological symptoms with medical causation.

There are various ways that these can present. The psychopathological presentation can define or dominate the clinical picture, it can exist in isolation, or there can be a combination of physical symptoms and various types and combinations of psychological symptoms: cognitive, perceptual, thought. To simplify discussion and conform to DSM-IV-TR constructs, this section will group the psychopathological presentation according to whether or not it is dominated by cognitive impairments.

When the clinical picture is dominated by the acute onset or rapid progression of cognitive impairments, notably in terms of consciousness, with possible impairments in attention, memory, language, praxis, and gnosis, the presenting pattern suggests delirium. Although non-specific, delirium announces the presence of a very sick brain with gross functional disruption. Brain and systemic infection, gross metabolic disturbances, poisoning, trauma, and seizures may all cause delirium.

A clinical presentation dominated by cognitive impairments but without disturbed consciousness suggests dementia or one of the specific neuropsychiatric syndromes like

Korsakoff's Amnesic Syndrome. Dementia can emerge from the remnants of a delirium or arise independently. Whilst delirium, dementia, and the specific neuropsychiatric syndromes may demonstrate prominent emotional disturbances, aberrant perceptions, disturbed reality testing, and personality changes, these are not their defining features. (Delirium, dementia, and related conditions are considered in Chapter 7.)

Psychopathological symptoms not dominated by cognitive impairment but often affected by medical illness include anxiety, depression, mania, psychosis, and dissociation. Even if cognitive symptoms accompany a mood or psychotic presentation, they never dominate the clinical picture. Examples of non-cognitive conditions are: Psychotic Disorder due to Hypothyroidism and phobic behaviour due to Parkinson's disease.

MEDICAL DIFFERENTIAL DIAGNOSES OF PSYCHOPATHOLOGICAL PRESENTATIONS

Anxiety systems

Nowhere is the intertwining of mind and body as obvious as in our experience of anxiety. We 'go pale', our mouths go dry, and we talk of 'butterflies in our stomach'. The Panic Attack can be part of normal human experience where it serves as an intense, but non-specific alarm.

With panic being the archetypal response to smothering, it is unsurprising to find it closely associated with lung and heart disease. Hypoventilation with acute carbon dioxide retention in the lungs precipitates panic. Hypoxia, cardiac ischaemia, arrhythmia, hypoglycaemia, electrolyte, acid-base, and mineral disturbances, and direct brain lesions can all cause panic. In addition, it is interesting that connective tissue laxity with double-jointedness and a 'floppy' mitral valve relate to Panic Disorder.

Over and above the examples mentioned above, various illnesses of the different body systems may present as panic. Examples of these include:

- ***Cardiovascular:*** Myocardial ischaemia, myocarditis, and pericarditis
- ***Pulmonary:*** Pneumonia, pulmonary embolism and oedema, pneumothorax, and bronchospasm
- ***Systemic:*** anaemia, poisoning, sepsis, or neoplasm
- ***Neurological:*** Epilepsy, strokes, neoplasms, multiple sclerosis, and neurodegenerative disorders.

Differential diagnoses for generalised anxiety are similar to those for panic but they favour chronic states. Phobic behaviours are seen most often in ischaemic heart disease and chronic lung disease, as well as ulcerative colitis, extensive surgical resection of bowel, epilepsy, movement disorders, concussion, and infection with the human immunodeficiency virus (HIV). The strong association between phobic behaviour and Parkinson's disease may relate to shared brain networks involving the basal ganglia.

Obsessive-Compulsive Disorder (OCD) and the OCD spectrum are among the most 'neurological' of psychiatric conditions. Functional imaging, pharmacological and neuropsychological insights, and lesion studies have implicated orbito-fronto-striatal networks in obsessive ideas, compulsive behaviours, and accompanying anxiety. Not surprisingly, obsessive-compulsive phenomena are found in neurological disorders, particularly the movement disorders.

Mood symptoms and suicide

Primary to the presentation of many medical conditions, notably infections and cancer, is a sense of malaise. Malaise involves poor sleep, decreased appetite, fatigue, and apathy, and thus its presentation is difficult to distinguish from Major Depression. In medical conditions, emotional changes are probably due to a combination of a patient's adjustment and the direct pathological impacts on the neural substrate subserving emotion, motivation, and vegetative functions. As was the case with panic disorders, there are various illnesses that could present as depression. Examples of these include:

- ***Cardiovascular:*** Ischaemic heart disease and cardiac failure.
- ***Pulmonary:*** Chronic lung diease.
- ***Organ:*** Kidney and liver failure.
- ***Systemic:*** Viral infections and neoplasms.
- ***Neurological:*** Epilepsy, strokes, neoplasms, multiple sclerosis, and neurodegenerative disorders.

A permissive association between cytokines and depression exists. Cytokines are messenger molecules involved in the marshalling of immune responses in infection and cancer. Viral infections like influenza, infectious mononucleosis and hepatitis A have a reputation for causing depression. Serum levels of cytokines Interleukin 1, 2, and 6, and Tumour Necrosis Factor α are raised in Major Depression and Somatisation Disorder (see Chapter 8). Cytokines' behavioural impact is adaptive: reduced physical activity and social withdrawal aid convalescence and limit complications like further infection.

Cortisol and catecholamines are implicated in depressive symptoms. Cognitive disturbances, notably to short-term memory, can accompany depression in medical conditions and are believed to be related to a cascade of limbic events initiated by cortisol's binding to glucocorticoid III-receptors on hippocampal cells. The strong correlation between Cushing's syndrome, where cortisol is released in excess, and depression underscores this pathogenic mechanism.

Nutritional deficiencies, hypoxia, electrolyte and mineral disturbances, and acid-base imbalance must also be considered, particularly if symptoms are of abrupt onset. Hypothyroidism, or myxoedema, involves insufficient release and activity of thyroid hormones with reduced metabolism throughout the body. Patients with hypothyroidism are tired, lack motivation, sluggish, overweight despite little appetite, cold intolerant, and depressed. Hyperthyroidism also produces depression with a testy mood.

Table 2: Medical differential diagnoses for manic symptoms

- Use of exogenous corticosteroids
- Endocrinopathies:
  - Hyperparathyroidism and hyperthyroidism
- Other metabolic conditions (e.g. porphyria variegata)
- Organ failure: kidneys and liver
- Neurological disorder:
  - Multiple sclerosis
  - Infections (syphilis, HIV/AIDS, herpes simplex encephalitis)
  - Stroke (fronto-polar)
  - Cerebritis with systemic lupus erythematosis
  - Epilepsy
  - Neoplasm
  - Degenerative conditions

Excessive serum calcium, or hypercalcaemia, is another cause of depression. Damage to the brain networks which subserve depression may be causal in certain epilepsies, neurodegenerative conditions, brain abscess, tumours, stroke, and mechanical trauma. Lately, a particularly tight neural correlation between unipolar depression and epilepsy has been proposed. Chronic pain, as encountered in rheumatoid arthritis, cancerous infiltrations, and neuralgias, goes hand in hand with depression (see Chapter 5). Manic reactions are encountered in multiple sclerosis, neurosyphilis, focal epilepsies, and exposure to exogenous corticosteroids (i.e. cortisone given medicinally). The reason why exogenous cortisol should precipitate mania whilst endogenous cortisol precipitates depression is unknown. Hyperthyroidism may cause manic symptoms, but not as often as depression. Even in the absence of clinical thyroid disease, thyroid hormone disturbances and thyroid auto-antibodies have been shown in major depression, Dysthymic Disorder and bipolar disorders. See Table 2 for the medical differential diagnoses for manic symptoms.

Suicide is not uncommon in medical settings. There are many theories about this, but a satisfactory universal explanation has not been established. Suffering, impairment, loss of opportunity, and social embarrassment all contribute to the helplessness felt in the face of serious, chronic, debilitating, and life-threatening illness. However, direct involvement of neural circuits active in suicidal behaviour also appears likely. Conditions like epilepsy, Huntington's disease, renal and hepatic failure, cancer, and HIV/AIDS have suicide rates substantially higher than expected for their severity and chronicity alone.

Perceptual aberrations and psychotic symptoms

In medical conditions with psychological disturbances, perceptual aberrations far outnumber delusions and disorganisation. Hallucinations are typically simpler than in primary psychoses with noises, flashes, or shadows, rather than voices or formed images. While undoubtedly hallucinated, the squiggles and lines typical of the aura of migraine can hardly be regarded as psychotic and the sufferer recognises them as abnormal. Insight into their unreality is preserved because the brain aberration is restricted to the primary visual cortex, a part of brain quite unconcerned with establishing meaning.

Medical conditions sometimes feature complex or 'formed' hallucinations and, if visual, classically involve 'animules' or little animals. Hallucinated objects that appear smaller than expected are highly suggestive of medical causation. Often, they are called Lilliputian hallucinations, after Lilliput, the magical island of miniscule people where Gulliver had washed ashore. An acrid smell, like that of burning rubber, classically presages a convulsion in grand mal epilepsy and is an example of an olfactory (smell) hallucination. Gustatory (taste) and tactile hallucinations also suggest medical causation, as do hallucinated sounds like buzzing, ticking, and recurrent musical phrases. Formication, or feeling ants crawling under or on the skin, is a tactile hallucination found in organ failure, epilepsy, and cocaine intoxication. Hallucinations in medical illness often worsen with nightfall. Passivity phenomena (i.e. where a person feels that some aspect of themselves is under the external control of others, e.g. feeling that arms or legs are moved by somebody else) and dissociation may accompany hallucinations. If present, delusions typically involve simple themes, often persecution, but neurosyphilis, HIV/AIDS, and multiple sclerosis can involve grandeur. Schizophrenic-like psychoses are found in hypothyroidism and temporal lobe epilepsy. Medical differential diagnoses of psychotic symptoms are described in Table 3.

Dissociation

Although the dissociative symptom dimension permeates most of psychiatry – Schizophrenia, Panic Disorder, Acute Stress Disorder, Borderline Personality Disorder, and the dissociative and somatoform disorders – it is also common in medical illness. Epilepsy is regarded as the prototypical dissociative condition; it also accompanies metabolic disturbances, nutritional deficits, and migraine. Particular forms of dissociation, like alienation, suggest medical causes (see Chapter 8 and Tables 8.1.and 8.14).

Table 3: Medical differential diagnoses of psychotic symptoms

- Any condition causing decreased brain perfusion and/or oxygen delivery
- Endocrinopathies:
  - Hyperthyroidism and hypothyroidism, hyperparathyroidism, Cushing's syndrome, and Addison's disease
- Metabolic disturbances (acidosis, hyponatraemia, hypocalcaemia, hypercalcaemia, polytrauma
- Infection (urinary tract infection, particularly in elderly patients, pneumonia, e.g. Legionella, overwhelming sepsis)
- Organ failure: kidneys and liver
- Neurological disorder:
  - Infections (neurosyphilis, HIV/AIDS, herpes encephalitis, tuberculosis, brain abscess)
  - Nutritional deficiency (vitamin B_{12} – cobalamine – and B_1 – thiamine)
  - Neoplasm (primary and secondary tumours, infiltrates, and para-neoplastic effects like limbic encephalitis)
  - Stroke
  - Epilepsy
  - Migraine
  - Multiple sclerosis and other demyelinating conditions
  - Heavy metals and other toxins
  - Systemic lupus erythematosus
  - Degenerative conditions (Lewy-body dementia, Alzheimer's disease, multisystem atrophy)
  - Trauma
  - Sensory loss (blindness – with Charles Bonnet syndrome – and deafness)

PSYCHOPATHOLOGICAL PRESENTATIONS OF SELECTED MEDICAL CONDITIONS

Nervous system conditions

Epilepsy

Epilepsy has a prevalence of about 1% of the population worldwide and even higher in developing countries. Epilepsy is *not* a disease, but a symptom complex and is defined as the occurrence of two or more unprovoked seizures. Seizures have many causes: electrolyte disturbances, hypoglycaemia, infections, fever, organ failure, and malignant hypertension. A seizure is a period of abnormal brain electrical activity. A generalised seizure involves the entire brain and the person always loses consciousness. In contrast, a focal or partial seizure involves only part of the brain. When consciousness is preserved, the seizure is called a simple focal seizure. If consciousness is disturbed, the focal or partial seizure is called a complex partial seizure. This kind of seizure usually occurs in the temporal or frontal lobes. Temporal-lobe epilepsy is the commonest form of adult epilepsy.

Epileptic psychopathology is best considered in terms of the four phases that characterise epilepsy: prodromal, ictal, post-ictal, and inter-ictal. (Ictal refers to the actual seizure or ictus.) Although epilepsy commonly proceeds through all four phases, it does not always. Epileptic psychopathology can also involve any psychological domain: cognition, emotion, thought, perception, and motor behaviour. The prodromal phase usually sets in quietly, emerging gradually from the preceding inter-ictal period. Prodromal symptoms are mostly subtle and lack specificity. For up to some days before the seizure, the patient may feel different and 'out of sorts', experiencing lethargy, irritability, sullenness, and apprehension. Seldom does he or she feel elated. Thinking may become clouded and the person may experience an increase in twitches and jerks.

The ictus strikes suddenly. If seizure onset is focal, emanating from the motor strip (primary motor cortex), rhythmical muscle twitching may grip a limb, with progressively greater involvement, as if marching from thumb, along the arm, to the face. A similarly progressive sensory march involves tactile sensation.

Psychological ictal symptoms occur in simple partial epilepsies but are more suggestive of complex ones. Patients may feel terrified, panicky, depressed, or burdened with intense guilt. Much rarer is rapture. The person may also experience déjà vu, a sense of having already experienced a situation. Obsessive thoughts, forced thinking, and thought alienation are other typical cognitive symptoms.

HELPFUL HINT

Common causes of epilepsy

- Perinatal trauma
- Infectious processes (CNS and systemic)
- Head trauma
- Brain tumours (primary or secondary)
- Drug intoxication and withdrawal
- Toxins
- Hypoxic brain damage
- Recurrent febrile convulsions
- Congenital neurocutaneous syndromes
- Neurodegenerative conditions
- Vascular anomalies
- Unknown: e.g. cortical dysgenesis.

Patients also report so-called 'gaze attraction' where, compelled by the seizure to stare at something in the environment, they experience intense dysphoria. They may smell something offensive like burning rubber, experience a sudden taste, feel sensations on the skin, and hallucinate sounds or voices. Objects may look much larger (macropsia) or smaller (micropsia) than their expected size or they may appear to change shape (metamorphosia). Dissociative experiences, like depersonalisation, are commonplace. Autonomic symptoms like flushing, shallow breathing, a racing heart, and stomach churning or belching occur.

As patients with complex partial epilepsy experience disturbances of consciousness of variable intensity, they have variable impairment in recollection of experiences during the seizure. Anxiety, terror, depression, déjà vu-like phenomena, forced thinking (repetitive, intrusive thoughts experienced at the onset of a seizure), hallucinations, and autonomic symptoms dominate the person's experience. Patients are frequently seen to perform stereotypical, repetitive behaviours called epileptic automatisms (e.g. lip smacking, fluttering of the eyes, etc.).

The complex ictus often merges imperceptibly with the post-ictal delirium. Impaired consciousness may be evident for hours and even days. During this protracted disturbance, also called a twilight state, the patient lies still and unresponsive to the environment.

Generalised seizures lack psychic experiences and the ictus may be an absence (petit mal) seizure or generalised convulsion. Convulsive seizures manifest first with tonic muscle contraction, followed by rhythmic jerking that eventually dies down. It is during the tonic phase that person may utter a scream, fall to the ground often with injury, stop breathing and turn blue, bite his or her tongue, or lose bladder control. In the clonic phase, as breathing resumes, pooled secretions of saliva froth up out of the mouth. In generalised epilepsy, the post-ictal phase is typically a delirium of variable severity and duration. Usually, the patient enters a deep sleep, scowls when disturbed, and has a severe headache and muscle pain.

In the inter-ictal phase, psychosis and depression are the most common psychopathology. Suicide is strikingly over-represented among epileptic patients. Mania is not common. Temporal lobe epilepsy, frequent seizures, and poor psychosocial adaptation are positively correlated with severity of inter-ictal psychopathology. Psychosis encountered in temporal lobe epilepsy resembles Schizophrenia except for a few subtle differences (e.g. patients' affects tend to be warmer and more congruent than Schizophrenics' and formal thought disorder is less pronounced).

Seizures per se do not cause cognitive deterioration except in patients with repeated or prolonged status epilepticus (repeated seizures without regaining consciousness in between) and subsequent hypoxic brain damage. Cognitive impairments encountered in epileptic patients relate to an underlying pathology responsible for both seizures and cognitive impairments. Thus, patients with neurological disorders often also have epilepsy. The observed discrepancy between epileptic and non-epileptic persons on standard intelligence measures is attributable to factors like missing school, restrictions on activities, lack of career advancement, social embarrassment, stigmatisation, and the deleterious effects of anti-epileptic medications, particularly older ones like phenobarbitone.

The idea of a uniquely epileptic personality is controversial. The personality is characterised by a tendency to imbue even neutral things with emotion, excessive writing (hypergraphia), religious preoccupations, reduced sexuality, a serious, sullen, and sometimes officious disposition, and a 'viscous' or 'sticky' style of interacting. This 'stickiness' is striking in conversation and it is difficult to make a polite exit from this engagement.

Neurodegenerative disorders

Involvement of the basal ganglia in neurodegenerative disorders is associated with psychopathological manifestations. Parkinson's disease, Huntington's disease, Lewy body dementia, and other multisystem atrophic conditions can present with depression, psychosis, and anxiety even before movement disorder signs have become obvious. Parkinson's disease correlates particularly with depression and phobias. Huntington's disease demonstrates one of the strongest correlates with suicide of all medical conditions.

Central nervous system infections

In a patient with normal immunity, bacterial meningitis and viral encephalitis present in a clinically suggestive manner: headache, photophobia, nausea and vomiting, fever, stiff neck, lethargy, sleepiness, confusion, and seizures. More challenging are infections characterised by their atypical symptoms or where they occur in the immune-compromised patient. At first presentation, herpes simplex encephalitis is not infrequently misinterpreted as a psychiatric condition. The infection tends to occur in the frontal and temporal lobes, tends to be asymmetrical, and to produce bloody lesions where grey matter and white matter meet. It often presents with agitation, irritability, and psychosis, including gustatory hallucinations. Patients often display bizarre behaviour and marked motor agitation. Seizures are not uncommon, notably partial seizures referable to the temporal lobe. Localising neurological signs may be absent. A high index of suspicion, laboratory examination of cerebrospinal fluid, neuro-imaging with contrast-enhancement, and electroencephalography assist with correct diagnosis and treatment.

Over the past two decades, chronic meningitis has been on the rise, mirroring the explosion of HIV/AIDS-related infections. Tuberculous and cryptococcal meningitis are the two main types in this context. Psychological signs such as cognitive impairment, lethargy, emotional dullness, or lability warn of their presence. Positive HIV serology and other signs of HIV/AIDS-related infection add to the suspicion.

With the rise of HIV/AIDS, neurosyphilisis is also making an unwelcome comeback. It can present with few physical signs. Mental state changes like cognitive impairments, irritability, impulsivity, and paranoid psychoses serve as warning signs. Serological evidence in the cerebrospinal fluid of the presence of treponema pallidum confirms the diagnosis.

The human immunodeficiency virus (HIV) is a cause of substantial psychological morbidity. Although the mechanism has not been clearly identified, HIV directly infects the nervous system. Opportunistic infections and malignancies associated with HIV can further add to the emergence of psychological abnormalities. The initial seroconversion illness can present with non-specific malaise, while subtle cognitive impairments and personality changes become evident from early in the infection. The so-called HIV encephalopathy presents as a subcortical dementia with slowed cognitions, memory deficits, and depression. Delirium can supervene at any stage of the infection. Up to 40% of patients infected with HIV are depressed. A characteristic maniform psychosis is recognised to occur in a proportion of patients. A maniform psychosis indicates an elevated mood without other vegetative or cognitive symptoms. Suicide is more common in HIV-infected patients than in patients with other chronic multisystem illnesses.

Head trauma

What concerns us in this section is closed head trauma, where its presence is signalled by psychopathological symptoms. The most frequent brain trauma in this category is chronic subdural haematoma. This usually arises in elderly persons, often with a history of alcohol abuse and dementia, where cerebral atrophy has set in. Cerebral atrophy increases risk of a subdural bleed because veins have to stretch across the shrunken brain. Even a minor blow to the head can cause rupture of these veins, which is followed by a slow venous bleed into the space between the brain and its outer membranous covering the dura mater. Blood slowly accumulates in the subdural space and, for a while, the brain accommodates this expanding mass. As a consequence, symptoms develop slowly and may not be noticed for a while. Usually, patients initially show subtle cognitive deterioration, depression, and lethargy. Not infrequently, a history of head trauma is absent. Bilateral subdural haematomata are even more of a diagnostic challenge because unilateral localising neurological signs are absent. Early surgical evacuation of the subdural clot can result in spectacular recovery. Where there is no history of trauma and where there are aggression, catatonia, impaired consciousness, apparent disorganised communication, or suspected focal cognitive deficits, cerebral trauma must be actively ruled out, or in.

CASE STUDY 1: Desmond

Late one night, an unidentified young male was brought to casualty by security guards who had found him walking aimlessly near the stock exchange in Sandton. He was unable to give a history and was noted to be incoherent. A cursory physical examination revealed no abnormalities. His chest and skull X-rays were normal. He was admitted and a psychiatric assessment requested. A junior medical officer on the psychiatric unit assessed him to be psychotic with pronounced formal thought disorder. No localising neurological signs were noted. He was started on neuroleptic treatment, but no improvement was noted after two weeks on the psychiatric ward. When the patient had a seizure, the medical officer organised an emergency brain scan that revealed a subdural blood clot overlying his left parieto-temporal junction. After review by the consultant psychiatrist, the formal thought disorder turned out to have been receptive aphasia. While fluent, he spoke gibberish and was unable to carry out instructions. Surgical drainage of the clot proceeded and he made an uneventful recovery. He identified himself as Desmond, a newspaper seller. Although amnesic to events that led to hospitalisation, it later became known that he had been mugged and robbed of his mobile phone, cash, and identity book.

Cerebral neoplasm

Cerebral neoplasms or brain tumours produce psychological symptoms in about half of cases. Tumours can be primary (e.g. atrocytoma and meningioma), when they arise in or around the brain. Secondary tumours are metastases, or seedlings of cancers from a site elsewhere in the body, typically lung, breast, or colon. Primary brain tumours are usually histologically not cancer, but are dangerous because of their situation inside the confines of the skull.

Fast-growing tumours announce themselves early with features of raised intracranial pressure and other predictable signs: headaches made worse when reclining, visual blurring, focal cognitive abnormalities, and seizures. Slow-growing tumours, particularly if located in the frontal lobes, can reach a substantial size before they are noticed. They are the ones most likely to present with psychological symptoms. Frontal meningioma, a tumour of the membranous lining of the brain, is the most common. Psychological features include subtle personality changes, depression, lability, and impulsivity. Depending on location, tumours can present in any conceivable way – hallucinations, dissociation, panic, obsessions, and cognitive impairments.

Demyelinating disorders

Multiple sclerosis is the prototypical demyelinating disorder and suspected to be of autoimmune pathogenesis. It involves the destruction of the fatty myelin sheath surrounding nerve fibres in the central nervous system, thereby slowing nerve conduction. Multiple sclerosis mostly affects people of northern-European extraction. In South Africa, patients are overwhelmingly first-generation European immigrants. Of considerable epidemiological interest, white South Africans born in South Africa appear mostly protected from multiple sclerosis. Similar demyelinating conditions are found among black Africans but their association with multiple sclerosis remains unsettled.

About half of all these patients have cognitive impairment, particularly affecting memory. General intellectual decline is also noted. About 25% of patients display a low-grade, chronic euphoria; a frankly manic syndrome can also develop. Depression is very common, affecting up to 50% of patients and the suicide rate is substantially elevated. Otherwise, personality changes can set in with irritability, apathy, and histrionic outbursts. Neurologically, multiple sclerosis features visual loss, ataxia, cerebellar involvement, and spasticity. Different patterns of symptom expression are recognised.

Autoimmune conditions

Systemic lupus erythematosus involves multiple organs, notably skin, kidneys, and brain. Half of all lupus patients present with mainly psychological symptoms like depression, lability, anxiety, sleep problems, and cognitive impairments. Focal epilepsy is not uncommon. Frank mania and psychosis can also develop. Psychological symptoms are caused by the combined effect of cerebritis (autoimmune inflammation of brain cells) and vasculitis (inflamed blood vessels causing brain ischaemia).

Rheumatic fever is an autoimmune condition triggered by infection with streptococcus group A. It produces cardiac valve lesions, glomerulonephritis, and attacks neural cells in the basal ganglia of the brain. Basal ganglia involvement causes jolting, jerky, 'dance-like' movements known as Sydenham's chorea or St. Vitus' dance. A subgroup of patients with Obsessive-Compulsive Disorder show immunological evidence of streptococcus group A infection and autoimmune neural damage is believed to release obsessive and compulsive symptoms.

Endocrine conditions

Hypo- and hyperthyroidism respectively refer to under- and overactivity of thyroid hormone. Thyroid hormone modulates cellular metabolism across the body. Hyperthyroidism has several causes. Typically it is the result of an autoimmune process, Grave's disease. Grave's has other very recognisable clinical signs, like protruding eyes (exophthalmos) caused by autoimmune inflammation and swelling of the fatty tissue that surrounds the eyeballs. A close relationship exists between thyroid hormone regulation and mood. Not surprisingly, psychological symptoms are often the first to appear in hyperthyroidism and involve anxiety, irritability, and depression. Maniform disturbances and psychosis can occur. Memory impairments are common. Physically, patients lose weight despite excessive hunger and food intake, they feel excessively tired, have tremors, racy pulse rates, and are sweaty and heat intolerant. Invariably, Grave's evolves into hypothyroidism.

Often referred to by the old term myxoedema, hypothyroidism is also caused by dietary iodine deficiency, lithium use, surgical ablation of the thyroid, and destruction by radioactive iodine. Depression, apathy, delusions, manic-like states, and psychosis are associated with hypothyroidism. 'Myxoedema madness' is a slightly pejorative term for a severe psychotic state resembling Schizophrenia. Pronounced cognitive impairments make hypothyroidism an exemplar of reversible dementia. Physically, patients are overweight (despite little food intake), sluggish, and cold-intolerant.

Hyperparathyroidism is surprisingly common in the elderly and is related to calcium metabolism. The excessive serum calcium causes personality changes, moodiness, and cognitive impairments. Rapid changes in calcium concentration may precipitate delirium. Patients also have weakness, lose bone density, and can develop kidney stones. Hypoparathyroidism, in contrast, causes hypocalcaemia with neural excitability, muscle twitchiness, and cramps or tetany. If serum calcium drops rapidly, delirium and seizures result. If change is slow, psychopathology may be present without physical signs like tetany. Dissociative phenomena are not uncommon and personality changes occur.

Despite its rarity, phaechromocytoma must remain on the list of differential diagnoses for panic and other anxiety states. Phaeochromocytoma is an adrenal medullary tumour, although it can occur elsewhere. The tumour secretes excessive catecholamines (adrenaline and noradrenaline) intermittently and in bursts. As a result, physical signs are confined to an attack and may even go unnoticed by patients. However, the intense psychological symptoms are a different story and unlikely to be missed.

Metabolic and nutritional disturbances, toxins, and organ failure

Electrolytes like sodium and potassium are essential for normal cell function and play a major role in nerve conduction. Likewise, the acid-base balance directly impacts basic cellular function. Disturbances in electrolyte and acid-base status produce significant disruption of normal neural function. If electrolyte and acid-base changes are rapid, delirium results, with seizures, coma, and death. Besides the acute attentional, memory, and other cognitive impairments, patients may look agitated, feel apprehensive, and become restless. Chronic electrolyte and acid-base changes produce less spectacular effects and may go unnoticed for quite some time. Low blood glucose caused by excessive or inappropriate administration of insulin, liver failure, or insulinoma (insulin-secreting tumour) all cause a psychic syndrome indistinguishable from a Panic Attack. If hypoglycaemia persists, global cognitive deficits, impaired consciousness, seizures, coma, and death may follow.

Deficiencies of B-group vitamins, notably thiamine (B_1), niacin (B_3), and cobalamine (B_{12}) may present with psychological and neurological symptoms. Thiamine deficiency causes Wernicke-Korsakoff's syndrome. It is more common in alcoholics and is occasionally encountered in patients receiving total intravenous feeding. The initial acute stage is characterised by a delirium and characteristic neurological abnormalities involving gait and eye movements. Patients who survive this phase may be left with a permanent deficit involving short-term memory, the so-called Korsakoff's amnesic syndrome.

Beriberi, also caused by thiamine deficiency, may present with lassitude, irritability, and depression. However, its physical signs are far more spectacular than the psychological ones. Niacin deficiency causes pellagra and can present with a delirium. Predictable skin lesions and diarrhoea accompany it. If untreated, pellagra is deadly. Cobalamine deficiency can present with a wide range of psychological manifestations including dementia, depression, and psychosis. Cobalamine deficiency causes loss of integrity of white matter in the central nervous system.

Heavy metals or divalent cationic metals are particularly neurotoxic. With increased public, industrial, and regulatory awareness, lead poisoning is much less of a public health problem than it was fifty years ago. High blood concentration of lead causes encephalopathy with irritability, agitation, and difficulty sleeping. A delirium sets in characterised by hallucinations and motor excitability. Convulsions, depressed consciousness, and death may follow. Predictable physical signs are noted, including clumsiness, unsteady gait, vomiting, and a distinctive purplish discoloration of gums – in past eras, this was a hallmark of plumbism or lead poisoning.

Thankfully, the former scourge of mercury poisoning has also receded. The last major mercury scare was on the Japanese island Okinawa in the late 1960s where entire communities reliant on fish as their staple food were affected following contamination of offshore fishing areas by mercury containing industrial waste. Psychologically, mercury poisoning presents with depression and pronounced psychosis with formal thought disorder. Cognitive impairments, tremors, cerebellar signs, and involvement of peripheral nerves with loss of sensation also develop. Manganese is notorious for causing a movement disorder reminiscent of Parkinson's disease. 'Manganese madness' is characterised by emotional lability, hallucinations, obsessive-compulsive behaviour, nightmares, and spells of uncontrolled laughter.

Renal failure, also called uraemia, causes substantial electrolyte and acid-base disturbances. In the uraemic state, patients may feel euphoric. Sometimes they are restless. They demonstrate global cognitive impairments, predominantly affecting attention and memory. Delirium may supervene. Tactile hallucinations are experienced. Myoclonus (a sudden violent jerk) and seizures may occur. In chronic renal failure, cognitive deficits may be irreversible. In the past, dialysis caused a state of dementia, believed to have been related to aluminium atoms in the dialysate.

Table 4: Factors suggestive of the presence of medical illness with psychological symptoms

A ATYPICAL AGE OF ONSET

- The prevalence of physical illness increases with increasing age. Most mental disorders emerge in adolescence or early adulthood. It is rare for a first psychotic experience at 60; OCD is unusual in an octogenarian; new or isolated cognitive impairments are unusual in a young person.

B ATYPICAL PRIMARY COMPLAINTS AND MODE OF ONSET

- **Atypical and suggestive symptoms** (symptoms that are unusual for presentation specific for each syndrome)
  - e.g. bias towards visual/tactile/olfactory/gustatory hallucinations; hallucinations are poorly formed; if visual, zoological and Lilliputian varieties are common.
- **Incongruous and inconsistent symptoms** (deviation from predictable syndromal nature of disease)
  - e.g. occurrence of hallucinations without predictable delusional interpretation
- **Atypical mode of onset and course**
  - e.g. precipitous onset, rapid deterioration without prodromal warning or presence of an identifiable stressor

C OCCURRENCE OF COGNITIVE, NEUROLOGICAL, AND PHYSICAL COMPLAINTS

- **Occurrence of cognitive symptoms** (any new or unexplained symptoms, when prominent or dominant)
  - e.g. gross memory lapses, experienced and reported disorientation, periods experienced as 'confusion'
- **Occurrence of physical symptoms** (any new or unexplained symptoms)
  - e.g. in panic, crushing central chest pain with typical ulnar radiation, nausea, and sweating, particularly on exertion suggest cardiac ischaemia; night sweats, loss of weight with apathy, tiredness, and depression suggests TB; any neurological symptoms

D SUGGESTIVE PATTERN OF RISK FACTORS

- **Absence of significant personal or family psychiatric or substance-use history**
- **No significant identifiable psychosocial stressors**
- **Positive personal and family medical history**
  - e.g. cardiovascular disease

E MENTAL STATE BIASES

- **Cognitive abnormalities** (any new or unexplained, when prominent or dominant)
  - e.g. impairment in consciousness, attention, learning, memory, and executive deficits; any aphasia, apraxia, and agnosia
- **Incongruity of symptoms and internal inconsistencies:**
  - **Affect** e.g. unexpected affective warmth and responsivity, distress shown at symptoms (particularly if 'psychotic')
  - **Thought content** e.g. poorly developed delusional themes if presentation is psychotic
  - **Thought form** e.g. absent or slight formal thought disorder if psychotic presentation is expected

F	PHYSICAL AND NEUROLOGICAL ABNORMALITIES
	• **Abnormal physical signs on general examination, demonstrable abnormalities with special investigations** • **Neurological signs** (any new or unexplained) ‣ e.g. localising signs, pronounced 'soft' signs, adventitious movements, abnormal gait and sphincter tone, raised intracranial pressure
G	POOR OR ATYPICAL TREATMENT RESPONSE

Liver failure produces a classical encephalopathy, probably on the basis of GABA-like neurotransmitters bypassing the liver and entering the systemic circulation from the gut. This happens as a consequence of portal hypertension, obstruction to blood flow in the liver's portal circulation because of the disrupted, chaotic hepatic structure typical of cirrhosis. Hypoglycaemia found in late stages of liver failure adds to deranged neural function. Drowsiness is common, cognitive functions are globally impaired, and patients are unable to keep their wrists extended for long, resulting in the so-called 'liver flap'. Earlier in the disease process, personality changes become evident: patients are less inhibited, show poor judgement, and progressive cognitive impairments. Psychiatric medications must be used with great caution as they are no longer metabolised by the liver, leading to toxicity and unexpected responses and adverse effects.

Heart failure results in decreased oxygen delivery to tissues. A host of electrolyte and acid-base disturbances may also emerge. If acute, delirium usually sets in. If chronic, subtler but progressive cognitive decline, depression, and tiredness become noticeable. Acute respiratory failure produces panic and restlessness and later delirium and coma. Chronic respiratory failure presents more subtly.

Limited to a few Afrikaans families, porphyria variegata, so-called South African porphyria, is characterised by skin and neurological involvement. Porphyria is a disorder of haeme-synthesis (haeme is a constituent of haemoglobin). An enzyme deficiency in the synthetic pathway causes accumulation of toxic metabolites that deposit in skin and nervous tissue. Blistering skin lesions result. Severe abdominal pain is caused through abdominal visceral innervation. Porphyria causes many psychological symptoms like anxiety, depression, mania, and psychosis. Porphyric attacks occur upon exposure to substances that induce haeme-synthesis. As a result, most psychiatric medications are contraindicated in patients with porphyria, as are many antibiotics and anaesthetic agents.

PSYCHOLOGICAL WARNINGS OF MEDICAL ILLNESS

Failure to recognise medical illness in a patient presenting primarily with psychopathology may result in fruitless treatment, needless suffering, and preventable death. The process of diagnosis entails securing and integrating clinical information so as to form a workable concept of the patient's presenting problem. Clinical information is evaluated against known pathology. Undoubtedly, the accurate diagnosis of medical illness requires knowledge of *all* of pathology. So, armed only with knowledge of psychopathology, what would lead the student reading this text to suspect a medical causation of psychic symptoms?

Fortunately, common themes are recognisable. Recognition relies on a firm grasp of psychopathology and a degree of suspicion that physical or neurological problems are present. The approach revolves about the recognition of what is atypical in a presentation and considers the following:

- Age at onset.
- Nature of primary complaint and its mode of onset.
- Occurrence of physical, neurological and cognitive complaints.
- Suggestive pattern of risk factors.
- Biases noted on mental state examination.
- The presence of abnormalities on general and neurological examination.
- Poor or atypical response to conventional treatment.

Table 4 lists these factors with examples. The two case studies are illustrative of medical illness masquerading as a psychological syndrome or presenting with psychological symptoms. After each case, factors suggestive of medical causation are highlighted using the terminology of Table 4.

CASE STUDY 2: Iqbal

Iqbal is a highly intelligent and driven 18-year-old law student. He comes from a high-achieving family, has been top of his class all year, and his parents expect him to pass his end-of-year examinations with a 90% average. After the exams, he is due to represent South Africa at a law Olympiad in Dubai. On the eve of the exams, he presented to a local casualty with shortness of breath, crushing central chest pain radiating down his left arm, and a feeling of unbearable foreboding. He complained of feeling dizzy, having pins and needles, and being nauseous. When the episode had started some two hours earlier, he felt alienated from his body and experienced the world as 'far away and detached'. Besides chicken pox and mumps, he had been a healthy boy. He never underwent psychological treatment and has no family history of any significant medical or psychiatric illness. As a devout Muslim, he has never used drugs. Initial examination revealed marked pallor, clamminess, prominent arcus lipidis,* and general puffiness. A cursory entry dotted in his clinical file read 'Panic Attack – stressed individual, refer to psychiatry'.

As protocol dictates the recording of an ECG on all patients presenting with chest pain, this was done. The ECG suggested a massive anterior infarction of his heart muscle. With renewed urgency, Iqbal was rushed to high care and appropriate treatment initiated. He made an uneventful recovery. Extensive investigations were embarked upon to pinpoint the cause of his heart attack. It transpired that he had

*** arcus lipidis is a white ring around the edge of the clear part of the eye, formed by cholesterol deposition.**

severe hypercholesterolaemia, his LDL cholesterol being more than five times the upper limit of normal. Soon, it was discovered that he suffered from nephrotic syndrome, a kidney condition where protein is wasted in the urine. The liver produces excessive LDL in response to the protein loss, accounting for his high serum-cholestrol that resulted in significant arterial disease and his untimely heart attack.

Case study 2 contains the following themes (see Table 4) that alert us to the presence of a medical condition:

- ***Factor B:*** Symptoms are suggestive of a panic attack, although the pain's radiation, and sweatiness and nausea are more ominous (see Factors C and F below). The duration of two hours far outstrips a panic attack's customary duration of ten to fifteen minutes, pointing to something very different.
- ***Factor C:*** The radiation of Iqbal's chest pain is not typical of a Panic Attack and suggests pain of cardiac origin. Similarly, nausea is not common in Panic Attacks and suggests cardiac pathology.
- ***Factor D:*** Though compatible with a first Panic Attack or first manifestation of an anxiety or other psychiatric disorder, the absence of a psychiatric history favours medical causation.
- ***Factor F:*** Abnormal findings are present on physical examination. The patient was noted to be markedly pale, clammy, and puffy with a prominent arcus. Whereas pallor is associated with panic, puffiness is altogether foreign and warns of something very different – fluid in tissues. The abnormal ECG and blood work cement the medical causation of psychic symptoms.

Both the puffiness and arcus can be explained by nephrotic syndrome: renal protein wasting and low serum protein concentration causes fluid leakage into tissue; in compensating for protein loss, the liver produces excessive LDL. LDL cholesterol deposits in the eyes causing arcus lipidis. LDL cholesterol contributed to forming of atherosclerotic plaque in his coronary arteries causing the infarction.

CASE STUDY 3: Themba

A familiar face on late-night television, where he hosts an arts magazine show, Themba, now 60, was originally trained as a teacher. He left South Africa during the struggle to live in London. Upon returning just over ten years ago, he adapted slowly to his new life. Things improved when he landed a position as lecturer in African Art History at a local university, where he also met his wife – a Scottish woman. They were divorced recently – an ugly and very public affair because of his celebrity status in the art world. This experience left him reeling, vulnerable, and angry: 'She had always assured me of her devotion, yet cheated on me for all our ten years of marriage.' Miserable, he planned a return to London.

Recently, his family doctor referred him to a psychiatrist for 'psychosis with paranoia and hallucinations'. The doctor had started Risperidone, an antipsychotic agent, but noted no improvement. Themba related how he would hear his ex's voice castigating and belittling him for harbouring thoughts on London. 'But I cannot control it, I feel compelled to think of London, I don't want to; it's always the same repetitive thought, over and over; then she starts shouting in that metallic-sounding voice, saying she wants to kill me, over and over', he grumbled. When he hears her voice, Themba feels 'spaced out'. At once, he halts whatever he is busy doing and cannot even move. After 20 minutes, it is all over. Feeling better, he wonders how he could ever have had 'these silly thoughts', reassuring himself that 'she wouldn't actually kill me', but he worried that 'something serious must be wrong with my brain.'

More pointed questioning revealed that he experiences tingling in his right arm when he hears the voice and jumbles his words when trying to speak. He also described a tendency to dissociate with marked depersonalisation experiences, occurring unexpectedly once or twice a month. Except for the tumultuous divorce and initial struggle settling down in South Africa, his history was unremarkable. He stopped smoking dagga 'years ago' and does not drink alcohol. As a preschooler, he had frequent febrile convulsions. He has no other medical history. Mental state examination revealed an intelligent, intense, and worried man, with an appropriate and warm affect and no formal thought disorder.

The general and neurological examinations were unremarkable. Worried about a neurological problem, the psychiatrist requested an electroencephalogram (EEG) and magnetic resonance imaging (MRI) of his brain. Both proved significant: the EEG demonstrated left temporal abnormal activity and the MRI mesial temporal sclerosis,* also on the left. The psychiatrist stopped Themba's antipsychotic medication and introduced antiepileptic treatment. Symptoms resolved completely. Themba settled down, ready to face the future, thankful for relatively benign positive diagnosis of temporal lobe epilepsy.

* Mesial temporal sclerosis is scarring of the hippocampus, part of the limbic cortex on the inner aspect of the temporal lobe and it strongly correlates with temporal lobe epilepsy. It is a likely consequence of repeated febrile convulsions in childhood.

In case study 3 we can highlight the following:

- ***Factor A:*** Themba is 60, an unusually advanced age of onset for a first psychotic episode or for the emergence of gross psychopathology in the absence of medical causation. In general, mental illness typically shows its hand in the late teens or early adulthood.
- ***Factor B:*** Although Themba experienced hallucinations, their phenomenology was atypical. They occurred in stereotyped relation to an obsessive thought. The patient retained insight into their abnormal nature (he felt there was 'something seriously wrong with my brain') and never elaborated a delusional belief around them (he reassured himself that she would not kill him). The disturbances were also brief and episodic – atypical for

a psychotic state, but suggestive of a brain disturbances like a seizure. Symptoms were also experienced as attacks, paroxysmal or of precipitous onset – again less suggestive of psychosis or other primary psychological disturbance and more supportive of seizures. Feeling 'spaced out' may indicate an alteration in consciousness or dissociation.

- ***Factor C:*** During an episode, Themba experienced cognitive and neurological symptoms: his inability to move, jumbled speech, tingling in one arm, and possibly alteration in consciousness. He also describes frequent depersonalisation experiences.
- ***Factor D:*** Themba's history is not out of keeping with the final diagnosis – it shows no risk of mental illness, but reveals childhood febrile convulsions – a recognised risk factor for developing temporal lobe epilepsy.
- ***Factor E:*** Themba displayed a normal mental state with no formal thought disorder as might be expected of psychosis. While highly suggestive of cerebral pathology, lasting cognitive abnormalities are neither necessary for, nor typical of, a diagnosis of temporal lobe epilepsy.
- ***Factor F:*** The demonstration of a brain abnormality on two independent tests – EEG and MRI - supports our suspicions and confirms the presence of neurological illness.
- ***Factor G:*** Lastly, Themba's condition did not respond as expected to conventional treatment. Risperidone, an antipsychotic agent, may even aggravate epilepsy. Resolution of symptoms followed introduction of appropriate antiepileptic treatment and cessation of the antipsychotic.

CONCLUSION

When sick, we *experience* being sick. We *behave* as if we are sick. Mind and body are not separate. Yet, the relationship between medical illness and psychopathological symptoms is a complex one. Over and above our psychological reactions to medical conditions, medical illness also has a direct hand in the causation of psychological symptoms. Sometimes, medical conditions manifest primarily with psychopathological phenomena. Psychological symptoms may in fact announce the presence of a medical condition, for example, in neurological and endocrine conditions. At other times, medical conditions produce only vague psychological syndromes which lack specificity, for example, in infections and in electrolyte, metabolic, and nutritional abnormalities. Medical conditions that evolve rapidly also tend to produce non-specific psychological manifestations such that physical signs and symptoms dominate the clinical picture. Psychological symptom expression is graded on a continuum: at its one extreme it has general malaise, delirium, and dementia; at the other extreme are syndromes quite indistinguishable from mental disorders like Schizophrenia, mania, and major depression. Being mindful of those factors warning of medical causation of psychological symptoms would stand the psychologist in good stead when faced with real-world patients.

ANSWERS TO MCQs

Chapter	Question	Answer
1	1	a
	2	b
	3	c
	4	c
	5	d
	6	a
	7	d
	8	d
	9	a
	10	a
2	1	c
	2	a
	3	d
	4	d
	5	c
	6	c
	7	a
	8	c
	9	b
	10	a
3	1	c
	2	b
	3	c
	4	b
	5	a
4	1	b
	2	a
	3	c
	4	b
	5	c
5	1	d
	2	c
	3	d
	4	a
	5	c
	6	d
6	1	e
	2	c
	3	d
	4	c
	5	b
	6	c
	7	a
	8	c
	9	c
7	1	a
	2	c
	3	c
	4	d
	5	c
8	1	b
	2	c
	3	b
	4	d
	5	c
9	1	a
	2	b
	3	a
10	1	c
	2	d
	3	d
11	1	a
	2	a
	3	d
	4	c
	5	a
	6	a
	7	c
	8	c
12	1	b
	2	b
	3	d
	4	a
	5	d
	6	c
	7	a
13	1	a
	2	d
	3	b
	4	b
	5	c
	6	d
	7	d

REFERENCES

Abdussalam-Bali, W. (2004). *Sword against black magic and evil magicians.* London: Al-Firdous Books.

Acosta, S. J., & Rosen, L. A. (2008). *Conduct disorder.* Encyclopedia of counseling. http://www.sage-ereference.com/counseling/Abstract_n30.html. Retrieved on 20 March 2009.

Adams, G. L. (1984). *Normative adaptive behavior checklist.* San Antonio, TX: The Psychological Corporation.

Adams, W. J. (2004). Promoting environmentally responsible behaviour: An evaluation of the global learning and observations to benefit the environment (globe) programme. Unpublished master's dissertation, University of South Africa, Pretoria.

Adebimpe, V. (1981). Overview: White norms and psychiatric diagnosis of black patients. *American Journal of Psychiatry*, 138(3), 279–285.

Affleck, G., & Tennen, H. (1996). Constructing benefits from adversity: Adaptational significance and dispositional underpinnings. *Journal of Personality*, 64, 899–902.

Agras, W. S. (1987). *Eating disorders: Management of obesity, bulimia, and anorexia nervosa.* New York: Elmsford.

Ahmed, R., & Pretorius-Heuchert, J. W. (2001). Notions of social community psychology: Issues and challenges. In M. Seedat, N. Duncan & S. Lazarus (Eds.), *Community psychology: Theory, method and practice.* South African and other perspectives (pp. 67–85). Cape Town: Oxford University Press.

Ahmer, S., Faruqui, R. A., & Aijaz, A. (2007). Psychiatric rating scales in Urdu: a systematic review. *BioMed Central Psychiatry*, 7(1),59.

Akbarian, S., Kim, J. J., Potkin, S. G., Hagman, J. O., Tafazzoli, A., Potkin, S. G., Bunney, W. E., & Jones, E. G. (1995). Gene expression for glutamic acid decarboxylase is reduced without loss of neurons in prefrontal cortex of schizophrenics. *Archives of General Psychiatry*, 52, 258–266.

Akiskal, H. S. (1979). *Affective disorders: Special clinical forms.* Philadelphia: Saunders.

Akst, D. (2011). *Procrastination, problematic internet addiction and resilience.* The Resilience Institute Newsletter. Retrieved March 10, 2012, from http://www.resiliencei.com

Akyüz, G. D. (1999). Frequency of dissociative identity disorder in the general population in Turkey. *Comprehensive Psychiatry*, 40(2), 151–159.

Alcoholics Anonymous World Services, Inc. (2012). *Welcome to Alcoholics Anonymous.* Retrieved March 10, 2012, from www.aa.org/

Allan, A. (1997). *The law for psychotherapists and counsellors.* Somerset West: Inter-Ed Publishers.

Allen, D. F., Postel, J., Berrios, G. E. (2000). The Ganser Syndrome. In G. H. Berrios. *Memory disorders in psychiatric practice.* Cambridge University Press, 443–454.

Almajali, H. K. (2005). The influence of family upbringing style and locus of control on the creative thinking of preparatory school learners in the United Arab Emirates. Unpublished doctoral thesis, University of South Africa, Pretoria.

Alvesson, M. & Sköldberg, K. (2000). *Reflexive methodology: New vistas for qualitative research.* London: Sage Publications Inc.

American Academy of Child and Adolescent Psychiatry. (2004). Practice parameter for the assessment and treatment of children and adolescents with enuresis. *American Academy of Child and Adolescent Psychiatry*, 43(12), 1540–1550.

American Psychiatric Association. (1980). *Diagnostic and statistical manual of mental disorders* (3rd Ed.). Washington DC: APA.

American Psychiatric Association. (1987). *Diagnostic and statistical manual of mental disorders* (3rd Ed. – revised). (DSM–III–R). Washington DC: APA.

American Psychiatric Association. (1994). *Diagnostic and statistical manual of mental disorders* (4th Ed.). Washington DC: APA.

American Psychiatric Association. (2000). *Diagnostic and statistical manual of mental disorders.* (4th Ed. – Text Revision). Washington DC: APA.

American Psychiatric Association. (2012). *DSM-5 development.* Retrieved February 10, 2012 from, http://www.dsm5.org/Pages/Default.aspx

American Psychiatric Association. (2013). Diagnostic and statistical manual of mental disorders (5th Ed.). Washington DC: APA.

American Psychological Association. (2002). *Personality disorders and the five-factor model of personality.* Washington DC: APA.

American Society of Addiction Medicine. (2011). *Public Policy Statement: Definition of Addiction.* Adopted by the ASAM Board of Directors April 12, 2011. Retrieved March 10, 2012 from http://www.asam.org

Anastasi, A. (1988). *Psychological testing* (6th Ed.). New York: Oxford University Press.

Anastasi, A., & Urbina, S. (1997). *Psychological testing* (7th ed.). Chicago: Prentice Hall.

Anastopoulos, A. D. (1998). A training program for parents of children with Attention Deficit Hyperactivity Disorder. In J. M. Briesmeister & C. E. Schaefer (Eds). *Handbook of parent training* (2nd Ed.). New York: John Wiley & Sons, Inc.

Anastopoulos, A. D., Guevremont, D. C., Shelton, T. L., & DuPaul, G. J. (1992). Parenting stress among families of children with Attention Deficit Hyperactivity disorder. *Journal of Abnormal Child Psychology*, 20(5), 503–520.

Andersen, B. L., Cyranowski, J. C., & Espindle, D. (1999). Men's sexual self-schema. *Journal of Personality and Social Psychology*, 76, 645–661.

Andersen, B., & Cyranowski, J. (1994). Women's sexual self-schema. *Journal of Personality and Social Psychology*, 67, 1079–1100.

Andrasik, F. (2000). Biofeedback. In D. I. Motofsky & D. H. Barlow (Eds). *The management of stress and anxiety in medical disorders*. Needham Heights: Allyn & Bacon, 66–83.

Andreasen, N. (1999) Understanding the causes of schizophrenia. *New England Journal of Medicine*, 340, 645–647.

Andreasen, N. C. & Swaze, V. W. (1993). Neuroimaging. In J. A. Costa, E. Silva, & C. C. Nadelson (Eds). *International review of psychiatry*, 1. Washington: American Psychiatric Press.

Andreasen, N. C., Olsen, S. A., Dennert, J. W., & Smith, M. R. (1982). Ventricular enlargement in Schizophrenia: Relationship to positive and negative symptoms. *American Journal of Psychiatry*, 139, 297–302.

Andreasen, N. C., Rezai, K., Alliger, R., Swayze, V. W, Flaum, M., Kirchner, P., Cohen, G., & O'Leary, D. S. (1992). Hypofrontality in neuroleptic-naive patients and in patients with chronic Schizophrenia: Assessment with xenon 133 single-photon emission computed tomography with the Tower of London. *Archives of General Psychiatry*, 49, 943–958.

Andreasen, N. C., Swayze, V. W., Flaum, M., Yates, W. R., Arndt, S., & McChesney, C. (1990). Ventricular enlargement in Schizophrenia evaluated with computed tomographic scanning: Effects of gender, age, and stage of illness. *Archives of General Psychiatry*, 47, 1008–1015.

Andrèasson, S., Engström, A., Allebeck, P., & Rydberg, U. (1987). Cannabis and Schizophrenia: A longitudinal study of Swedish conscripts. *The Lancet*, 330(8574), 1483–1486.

Andrist, L. (2003). Media images, body dissatisfaction, and disordered eating in adolescent women. *American Journal of Maternal Child Nursing*, 28, 119–123.

Angleitner, A. & Ostendorf, F. (1994). Temperament and the Big Five factors of personality. In C. F. Halverson, Jr., G. A. Kohnstamm, & R. P. Martin (Eds). *The developing structure of temperament from infancy to adulthood.* Hillsdale, NJ: Lawrence Erlbaum.

Arnold, P., Bhandan, S. P., Lorch, E., Ivey, J., Rose, M., & Rosenberg, D. R. (2003). Childhood anxiety disorders and developmental issues in anxiety. *Current Psychiatry Reports*, 5, 252–265.

Arnone, D., McIntosh, A. M., Ebmeier, K. P., Munafò, M. R., & Anderson, I. M. (2011). Magnetic resonance imaging studies in unipolar depression: Systematic review and meta-regression analyses. *Neuropsychopharmacology,* Jul 2. [Epub ahead of print].

Ashworth, A. (2000). *Sentencing and criminal justice* (3rd Ed.). Oxford: Oxford University Press.

Asuni, T., Schoenberg, F., & Swift, C. (1994). *Mental health and disease in Africa.* Ibadan: Spectrum Books.

Austin, E. J., Saklofske, D. H., & Egan, V. (2005). Personality, well-being and health correlates of trait emotional intelligence. *Personality and Individual Differences*, 38, 547–558.

Balaban, C. D. & Jacob, R. G. (2001). Background and history of the interface between anxiety and vertigo. *Journal of Anxiety Disorders*, 15(1–2), 27–51.

Bandura, A. (1969). *Principles of behavior modification.* New York: Holt, Rinehart & Winston.

Barkley, R. A. (1995). *Taking charge of ADHD: The complete authoritative guide for parents.* London: Guilford Press.

Barlow, D. H. & Durand, V. M. (2004). *Abnormal psychology: An integrative approach* (4th Ed.). Pacific Grove, CA: Wadsworth.

Barlow, D. H. & Durand, V. M. (2005). *Abnormal Psychology: An integrative approach*. Belmont: Thomson.
Barlow, D. H. & Durand, V. M. (2009). *Abnormal psychology: An integrative approach* (5th Ed.). Belmont: Wadsworth Cengage Learning.
Barlow, D. H. & Durand, V. M. (2011). *Abnormal psychology: An integrative approach*. Belmont, C.A.: Wadsworth.
Barlow, D. H. (2000). Unraveling the mysteries of anxiety and its disorders from the perspective of emotion theory. *American Psychologist*, 55(11), 1245–1263.
Barlow, D. H. (2002). *Anxiety and its disorders: The nature and treatment of anxiety and panic* (2nd Ed.). New York: Guilford Press.
Barlow, D. H. (2003). Anxiety and its disorders: The nature and treatment of anxiety and panic (2nd Ed.). *Journal of Clinical Psychiatry*, 64, 345–346.
Barlow, D. H. (2004). Covert sensitization for paraphilia. In D. Wedding & R. J. Corsini (Eds). *Case studies in psychotherapy* (4th Ed.). Belmont, CA: Thomson, 105–113.
Barlow, D. H. (2005). What's new about evidence-based assessment? *Psychological Assessment*, 17, 308–311.
Barlow, D. H. (2006). Psychotherapy and psychological treatments: The future. *Clinical Psychology: Science and Practice*, 13, 216–220.
Barlow, D. H. (2007). *Clinical handbook of psychological disorders: A step-by-step treatment manual* (4th Ed.). New York: Guilford Press.
Barlow, D. H., & Allen, L. B. (2004). The scientific basis of psychological treatments for anxiety disorders: Past, present and future. In J. M. Gorman (Ed.). *Fears and anxiety: Benefits of translational research*. Washington, DC: American Psychiatric Press.
Barlow, D. H., & Durand, V. M. (2005). *Abnormal psychology: An integrative approach* (4th ed.). London: Cengage.
Barrett, J. G. (2004). *Conduct Disorders*. Encyclopedia of Applied Developmental Science. http://www.sage–ereference.com/applieddevscience/Article_n111.html. Retrieved on 20 March 2009.
Bartlett, P. & Sandland, R. (2003). *Mental health law: Policy and practice*. Oxford: Oxford University Press.
Bartol, C. R. & Bartol, A. M. (2005). *Current perspectives in forensic psychology and criminal justice*. New York: Sage.
Bartol, C. R. & Bartol, A. M. (2008). *Current perspectives in forensic psychology and criminal behavior*. New York: Sage.
Bartol, C. R. (2002). *Criminal behavior: A psychosocial approach* (6th ed.). Upper Saddle River, NJ: Prentice Hall.
Bartol, C. R., & Bartol, A. M. (2005). *Criminal behavior: A psychosocial approach* (7th ed.). Upper Saddle River, NJ: Pearson
Bartol, C. R., & Bartol, A. M. (2008). *Criminal behavior: A psychosocial approach* (8th ed.). Upper Saddle River, NJ: Pearson
Bartol, C. R., & Bartol, A. M. (2011). *Criminal behavior: A psychosocial approach* (9th ed.). Upper Saddle River, NJ: Pearson
Bateson, G. (1959). Cultural problems posed by a study of schizophrenic process. In A. Auerback (Ed.), *Schizophrenia: An integrated approach*, (pp. 125–149). New York: Ronald Press.
Batson, C. D., Ahmad, N., Lishner, D. A., & Tsang, J. (2005). Empathy and altruism. In C. R. Snyder & S. J. Lopez (Eds.), *Handbook of positive psychology* (pp. 485–498). Oxford: Oxford University Press.
Baumeister, R. F., Vohs, K. D., & Tice, D. M. (2007). The strength model of self-control. *Current Directions in Psychological Science*, 16(6), 351–355.
Baumeister, R., & Vohs, K. D. (2002). The pursuit of meaningfulness in life. In C. R. Snyder & S. J. Lopez (Eds.), *Handbook of positive psychology* (pp. 608–617). New York: Oxford University Press.
Baumgardner, S. R., & Crothers, M. K. (2009). *Positive psychology*. Upper Saddle River, NJ: Pearson.
Beck, A. T. (1967). *Depression: Clinical, experimental, and theoretical aspects*. New York: Hoeber.
Beck, A. T. (1972). *Depression: Causes and treatment*. Philadelphia: University of Pennsylvania Press.
Beck, A. T. (1976). *Cognitive therapy and the emotional disorders*. New York: International Universities Press.
Beck, A. T. (2005). The current state of cognitive therapy – A 40-year retrospective. *Archives Of General Psychiatry*, 62(9), 953–959.

Beck, A. T., Brown, G., Berchick, R. J., Stewart, B. L. & Steer, R. A. (1990). Relationship between hopelessness and ultimate suicide: A replication with psychiatric outpatients. *American Journal of Psychiatry*, 147, 190–195.

Beck, J. G., McNiff, J., Clapp, J. D., Olsen, S. A., Avery, M. L., & Hagewood, J. H. (2011). Exploring negative emotion in women experiencing intimate partner violence: Shame, guilt, and PTSD. *Behaviour Therapy*, 42, 740–750. doi 10.1016/j.beth.2011.04.001

Beck, J. S. (2005a). *Cognitive Behavior Therapy: Basics and Beyond.* New York, NY: The Guilford Press.

Beck, J. S. (2005b). *Cognitive Therapy for Challenging Problems.* New York, NY: The Guilford Press.

Becker, L. C. (1992). Places for Pluralism. *Ethics*, 102(4), 707–719.

Becker, L. C. (Ed.). (1992). *Encyclopaedia of ethics*, 1, 329–330.

Becvar, D. S. & Becvar, R. J. (2009). *Family therapy: A systemic integration* (7th ed.). Boston: Allyn and Bacon/ Pearson.

Beekman, A. T., Geerlings, S. W., Deeg, D. J., et al. (2002). The natural history of late-life depression: A 6-year prospective study in the community. *Archives of General Psychiatry*, 59, 605–611.

Bell, C. J. & Nutt, D. J. (1998). Serotonin and panic. *British Journal of Psychiatry*, 172, 465–471.

Bell, V. (2007). Online information, extreme communities and internet therapy: Is the internet good for our mental health? *Journal of Mental Health*, 16(1), 115–157.

Bellak, L. (1979). Introduction: An idiosyncratic overview. In L. Bellak (Ed.). *Disorders of the schizophrenic syndrome* (pp. 3–24). New York: Basic Books.

Bemporad, J. R. (1997). Cultural and historical aspects of eating disorders. *Theoretical Medicine*, 18, 401–420.

Bennett, P. (2003). *Abnormal and clinical psychology: An introductory textbook.* Maidenhead: Open University Press.

Bernstein, D. P., Useda, D., & Siever, L. J. (1995). Paranoid personality disorder. In W. J. Livesley (Ed.). *The DSM-IV personality disorders.* New York: Guilford Press, 45–57.

Berrios, G. E., Luque, R., & Villagrán, J. M. (2003). Schizophrenia: A conceptual history. *International Journal of Psychology and Psychological Theory*, 3 (2), 111–140.

Berry, J. W., Poortinga, Y. H., Segall, M. H., & Dasen, P. R. (2002). *Cross-cultural psychology: Research and applications* (2nd ed.). Cambridge: Cambridge University Press.

Bersoff, D. N. (2002). Some contrarian concerns about law, psychology, and public policy. *Law and Human Behavior*, 26(5), 565–574.

Bertelsen, A. (2002). Schizophrenia and related disorders: Experience with current diagnostic systems. *Psychopathology*, 35(2–3), 89–93.

Bessenhof, G. R. (2006). Can media affect us? Social comparison, self-discrepancy, and the thin ideal. *Psychology of Women Quarterly*, 30, 239–251.

Bevilacqua, L., & Goldman, D. (2009). Genes and Addictions. *Clinical Pharmacology & Therapeutics.* 85, 359–361.

Bezuidenhout, C., & Klopper, H. (2011). Crimes of a violent nature. In C. Bezuidenhout (Ed.). *A Southern African perspective on fundamental criminology.* Cape Town: Pearson.

Bhamjee, S. (2010). Is the right to die with dignity constitutionally guaranteed? Baxter v Montana* and other developments in patient autonomy and physician assisted suicide. *Obiter*, 31(2), 333–352.

Bhana, D. (2008). Beyond stigma? Young children's responses to HIV and AIDS. *Culture, Health & Sexuality*, 10(7), 725–738.

Bielski, R. J. & Friedel, R. O. (1977). Subtypes of depression—Diagnosis and medical management. *Western Journal of Medicine*, 126(5), 347–352.

Billings, A. G., Cronkite, R. C., & Moos, R. H. (1983). Social–environmental factors in unipolar depression: Comparisons of depressed patients and nondepressed controls. *Journal of Abnormal Psychology*, 92(2), 119–133.

Binitie, A. (1975). A factor–analytical study of depression across cultures (African and European). *British Journal of Psychiatry*, 127, 559–563.

Birley, J., & Brown, G. W. (1970). Crisis and life changes preceding the onset or relapse of acute Schizophrenia: Clinical aspects. *British Journal of Psychiatry*, 16, 327–333.

Bjorck, J. P. & Thurman, J. W. (2007). Negative life events, patterns of positive and negative religious coping, and psychological functioning. *Journal for the Scientific Study of Religion*, 46(2), 159–167.

Black, D. S. (2004). Conversion hysteria: Lessons from functional imaging. *Journal of Neuropsychiatry and Clinical Neurosciences*, 16(3), 245–251.

Blackburn, R. (1993). *The psychology of criminal conduct: Theory, research and practice.* New York: Wiley & Sons.

Blashfield, R. K. (1984). *The classification of psychopathology. Neo-Kraepelinian and quantitative approaches.* New York: Plenum.

Bleueler, E. (1911/1950) *Dementia praecox or the group of schizophrenias.* New York: International Universities Press.

Board, B. J., & Fritzon, K. (2005). Disordered personalities at work. *Psychology, Crime and Law*, 11(1), 17–32.

Bojuwoye, O. & Sodi, T. (2010). Challenges and opportunities to integrating traditional healing into counselling and psychotherapy. *Counselling Psychology Quarterly*, 23(3), 283–296. doi: 10.1080/09515070.2010.505750

Bojuwoye, O. (2003). Mental health care delivery practices among traditional African cultures – nature, process and virtues. In N. S. Madu (Ed.). *Contributions to psychotherapy conference in Africa* (pp. 188–206). Turfloop: University to the North.

Boll, T. J. (1985). Developing issues in clinical neuropsychology. *Journal of Clinical and Experimental Neuropsychology*, 7(5), 473–485.

Boog, G. (2004). Obstetrical complications and subsequent Schizophrenia in adolescent and young adult offspring: Is there a relationship? *European Journal of Obstetrics & Gynaecology and Reproductive Biology*, 114(2), 130–136.

Boorstein, H. C., Fein, D. A., & Wilson, L. B. (2005). *Pervasive developmental disorders. Encyclopedia of Human Development.* http://www.sage-ereference.com/humandevelopment/Article_n477.html. Retrieved on 20 March 2009.

Boss, L. (1997). Epidemic hysteria: A review of the published literature. *Epidemiologic Reviews*, 19(2), 233–243.

Botha, U. A., Koen, L., Joska, J. ., Parker, J. S., Horn, N., Hering, L. M., & Oosthuizen, P. P. (2010). The revolving door phenomenon in psychiatry: Comparing low-frequency and high-frequency users of psychiatric inpatient services in a developing country. *Social Psychiatry, Psychiatric Epidemiology*, 45(4), 461–468.

Botta, R. A. (2003). For your health? The relationship between magazine reading and adolescents' body image and eating disturbances. *Sex Roles*, 48, 389–399.

Botta, R. A. (2006). Television images and adolescent girls' body image disturbance. *Journal of Communication*, 49, 22–41.

Bowlby, J. (1980). *Attachment and Loss (3): Loss, sadness and depression.* New York: Basic.

Boyle, M. (1990). *Schizophrenia: A scientific delusion?* London: Routledge.

Brandtstädter, J., & Rothermund, K. (2002). The life-course dynamics of goal pursuit and goal adjustment: A two-process framework. *Developmental Review*, 22, 117–150.

Bray, R., & Dawes, A. (2007). A rights-based approach to monitoring the well-being of children in South Africa. In A. Dawes, R. Bray, & A. van der Merwe (Eds.), *Monitoring child well-being: A South Africa rights-based approach* (pp. 29–52). Cape Town: Human Science Research Council.

Brett-Jones, J., Garety, P., & Hemsley, D. (1987). Measuring delusional experiences: A method and its application. *British Journal of Clinical Psychology*, 26, 257–265.

Briggs, H. (2012). *Web addicts have brain changes, research suggests.* Retrieved January 15, 2012 from BBC News website.

Brochin, H. A., & Horvath, J. A. (1996). Attention Deficit Hyperactivity Disorder. In G. M. Blau, & T. P. Gullotta (Eds). *Adolescent dysfunctional behaviour: Causes, interventions and prevention.* Thousand Oaks: Sage.

Brodrick, K. (2002). Correlation between scores on two screening tools for dementia in Xhosa women. *SA Journal of Occupational Therapy*, 32(3), 8–13.

Brotto L. A. & Klein, C. (2007). Sexual and gender-identity disorders. In M. Hersen, S. M. Turner & D. Beidel (Eds). *Adult psychopathology and diagnosis* (5th ed.) Hoboken: John Wiley & Sons, 504–570.

Brown, G. W, Birley, J. L. T., & Wing, J. K. (1972). The influence of family life on the course of schizophrenic disorders: A replication. *British Journal of Psychiatry*, 121, 241–58.

Brown, G. W. & Harris, T. O. (1989). *Life events and illness.* New York: Guilford Press.

Brown, G. W., Harris, T. O., & Hepworth, C. (1994). Life events and endogenous depression. A puzzle reexamined. *Archives of General Psychiatry*, 51, 525–534.

Brown, R. S. (2005). Dissociation, childhood interpersonal trauma, and family functioning in patients with Somatization Disorder. *American Journal of Psychiatry*, 162, 899–905.

Brown, R. T. & McMillan, K. (2005). *Rett syndrome*. Encyclopedia of human development. http://www.sage-ereference.com/humandevelopment/Article_n525.html. retrieved on 20 March 2009.

Brown, S. (1997). Excess mortality of Schizophrenia: A meta-analysis. *The British Journal of Psychiatry*, 171, 502–508.

Brown, S. E., Esbensen, F. A., & Geis, G. (2007). *Criminology: Explaining crime and its context* (6th ed.). Cincinnati, OH: Anderson.

Brownell, K. D. & Fairburn, C. G. (Eds). (1995). *Eating disorders and obesity: A comprehensive handbook*. New York: Guilford Press.

Brownell, K. D. & Rodin, J. (1994).The dieting maelstrom: Is it possible and advisable to lose weight? *American Psychologist*, 49(9), 781–791.

Brownell, K. D. (1991). Dieting and the search for the perfect body: Where physiology and culture collide. *Behavior Therapy*, 22, 1–12.

Brownell, K. D. (2003). *Food fight: The inside story of the food industry, Americas obesity crisis and what we can do about it*. New York: McGraw-Hill.

Bruch, H. (1985). Four decades of eating disorders. In D. M. Garner & P. E. Garfmkel (Eds.). *Handbook of psychotherapy for anorexia nervosa and bulimia*. New York: Guilford Press, 7–18.

Bruch, H. (1986). Anorexia nervosa: The therapeutic task. In K. D. Brownell & J. P. Foreyt (Eds) . *Handbook of eating disorders*. New York: Basic, 328–332.

Bryant, R. (2007). Does dissociation further our understanding of PTSD? *Journal of Anxiety Disorders*, 21(2), 183–191.

Buhrman, M. V. (1984). *Living in two worlds: Communication between a white healer and her black counterparts*. Cape Town: Human & Rosseau.

Bulhan, H. A. (1985). *Franz Fanon and the psychology of oppression*. New York: Plenum.

Bureau of Census (1983). *Statistical abstract of the United States*. Washington DC: US Government Printing Office.

Burke, A. (2010). The abuse of social science research results for political gain: The apartheid system as case study. *Journal of Public Administration*, 45(3), 403–419.

Burke, A., Harper, M., Rudnick, H. & Kruger, G. (2007). Moving beyond statutory ethical codes: Practitioner ethics as a contextual, character-based enterprise. *South African Journal of Psychology*, 37(1), 107–120.

Burnam, M. A., Stein, J. A., Golding, J. M., & Siegel, J. M. (1988). Sexual assault and mental disorders in a community population. *Journal of Consulting and Clinical Psychology*, 56, 843–850.

Burns, J. K. (2009). Dispelling a myth: Developing world poverty, inequality, violence and social fragmentation are not good for outcome in Schizophrenia. *African Journal of Psychiatry*, 12, 200–205.

Burns, J. K., Jhazbhay, K., Esterhuizen, T., & Emsley, R. (2010). Exposure to trauma and the clinical presentation of first-episode psychosis in South Africa. *Journal of Psychiatric Research*, 45(2), 179–184.

Burns, S. R. (2007). *Childhood and Adolescence*. 21st century psychology: A reference handbook. Encyclopedia of Counseling. http://www.sage-ereference.com/psychology/Article_n54.html. retrieved on 20 March 2009.

Butcher, J. N. (2000). Revising psychological tests: Lessons learned from the revision of the MMPI. *Psychological Assessment*, 12, 263–271.

Butcher, J. N., Graham, J. R., Williams, C. L., & Ben-Porath, Y. S. (1990). *Development and use of the MMPI–2 content scales*. Minneapolis: University of Minnesota Press.

Butcher, J. N., Mineka, S., & Hooley, J. M. (2010). *Abnormal psychology* (14th ed.). Boston: Allyn & Bacon.

Byres, A. L., Yaffe, K., Covinsky, K. E., Friedman, M. B., Bruce, M. L. (2010). High Occurrence of mood and anxiety disorders among older adults. *Archives of General Psychiatry*, 67(5), 489–496.

Callard, F. (2006). Understanding agoraphobia: Women, men, and the historical geography of urban anxiety. In C. Berkin, J. Pinch & C. Appel (Eds.), *Exploring Women's Studies: Looking Forward, Looking Back*. New York: Prentice Hall, 201–217.

Campbell, J. (1999). Schizophrenia, the space of reasons and thinking as a motor process. *The Monist*, 82(4), 609–625.

Cannon, T. D., Barr, C. E., & Mednick, S. A. (1991). Genetic and perinatal factors in the etiology of Schizophrenia. In E. F. Walker (Ed.), *Schizophrenia: A life-course developmental perspective*. New York: Academic Press, 9–31.

Canter, M. B., Bennett, B. E., Jones, S. E. & Nagy, T. F. (1994). *Ethics for psychologists: A commentary on the APA ethics code*. Washington, DC: American Psychological Association.

Caradas, A. A., Lambert, E. V., & Charlton, E. (2001). An ethnic comparison of eating attitudes and associated body image concerns in adolescent South African schoolgirls. *Journal of Human Nutrition and Dietetics*, 14, 111–120.

Cardeña, E. (1994). The domain of dissociation. In S. J. Rhue. *Dissociation, Clinical and Theoretical Perspectives*. New York: Guilford Press, 15–31.

Carothers, J. C. (1959). Culture, psychiatry, and the written word. *Psychiatry*, 22, 307–320.

Carpenter, W. T. (1994).The negative symptom challenge. *Archives of General Psychiatry*, 49, 236–237.

Carrey, N., & Ungar, M. (2007). Resilience theory and the diagnostic and statistical manual: Incompatible bed fellows? *Child and Psychiatric Clinics of North America*, 16, 497–513.

Carson, R. C. (1985). The schizophrenias. In H. E. Adams & P. B. Sutker (Eds.), *Comprehensive Textbook of Psychopathology*. New York: Plenum, 411–434.

Carson, R. C., Butcher, J. N., & Coleman, J. C. (1988). *Abnormal psychology and modern life*. Glenview: Scott, Foresman.

Carson, T. P. & Carson, R. C. (1984). The affective disorders. In H. E. Adams & P. B. Sutker (Eds). *Comprehensive handbook of psychopathology*. New York: Plenum Press, 349–381.

Carter, M. M., Hollon, S. D., Carson, R. S., & Shelton, R. C. (1995). Effects of a safe person on induced distress following a biological challenge in panic disorder with agoraphobia. *Journal of Abnormal Psychology*, 104, 156–163.

Cartwright, D. (2008). Psychopathology. In L. Swartz, C. de la Rey, N. Duncan, & L. Townsend (Eds). *Psychology: An introduction*. Cape Town: Oxford University Press.

Carver, C. S. (2004). Self-regulation of action and affect. In R. F., Baumeister & K. D. Vohs (Eds.), *Handbook of self-regulation: Research, theory, and applications*. London: Guilford Press, 13–39.

Carver, C. S., & Scheier, M. F. (2005). Optimism. In C. R. Snyder & S. J. Lopez (Eds.) *Handbook of positive psychology*. Oxford: Oxford University Press, 231–243.

Cash T. E., Morrow, J. A., Hrabosky, J. I., & Perry, A. A. (2004). How has body image changed? A cross sectional investigation of college women and men from 1983 to 2001. *Journal of Consulting and Clinical Psychology*, 72, 1081–1089.

Casino Association of South Africa. (2011). *Problem gambling and responsible gambling*. Retrieved December 15, 2011, from www.casasa.org.za

Caspi, A., Sugden, K., Moffitt, T. E. (2003). Influence of life stress on depression: Moderation by a polymorphism in the 5-HTT gene. *Science*, 301(5631), 386–89.

Castillo, R. J. (Ed.). (1998). *Meanings of Madness*. Pacific Grove, CA: Brooks/Cole.

Castro, M. (2006). *The world's most dangerous drug*. National Geographic,

Cauce, A. M. (2011). Is multicultural psychology a-scientific? Diverse methods for diversity research. *Cultural Diversity and Ethnic Minority Psychology*, 17(3), 228–233.

Cervilla, J. A., Molina, E., Rivera, M., Torres-González, F., Bellón, J. A., Moreno, B., et al. (2007). The risk for depression conferred by stressful life events is modified by variation at the serotonin transporter 5HTTLPR genotype: Evidence from the Spanish PREDICT–Gene cohort. *Molecular Psychiatry*, 12 (8), 748–55.

Chamorro-Premuzic, T., Bennett, E., Furnham, A. (2007). The happy personality: Meditational role of trait emotional intelligence. *Personality and Individual Differences*, 42, 1633–1639.

Charney, D. A., Paraherakis, A. M. & Gill, K. J. (2000). The treatment of sedative–hypnotic dependence: Evaluating clinical predictors of outcome. *Journal of Clinical Psychiatry*, 61, 190–195.

Charney, D. S., Deutsch, A. V., Krystal, J. H., Southwick, A. M., & Davis, M. (1993). Psychobiologic mechanisms of post-traumatic stress disorder. *Archives of General Psychiatry*, 50, 295–305.

Charney, D.S. (2004). Psychobiological mechanisms of resilience and vulnerability: implications for successful adaptation to extreme stress. *American Journal of Psychiatry*, 161, 195–216.

Chelminski, I. & Zimmerman, M. (2003). Pathological worry in depressed and anxious patients. *Journal of Anxiety Disorders*, 17(5), 533–546.

Chen, J., Nakano, Y., Ietzugu, T., Ogawa, S., Junayama, T., & Watanabe, N. (2007). Group cognitive behavior therapy for Japanese students with social anxiety disorder: Preliminary outcomes and their predictors. *BioMed Central Psychiatry*, 7(69), 1–10.

Child and adolescent mental health policies and plans. Geneva: World Health Organisation.

Chua, S. E., & McKenna, P. J. (1995). Schizophrenia – a brain disease? A critical review of structural and functional cerebral abnormality in the disorder. *British Journal of Psychiatry*, 166, 563–82.

Clausen, J. A. (1957). Social and psychological factors in narcotics addiction. *Law and Contemporary Problems*, 22, 34–51.

Cleghorn, J. M., Franco, S., Szechtman, B., Kaplan, R. D, Szechtman, H., Brown, G. M., Nahmias, G. M., & Garnett, E. S. (1992). Toward a brain map of auditory hallucinations. *American Journal of Psychiatry*, 149, 1062–1069.

Cloninger, C. R., & Gottesman, I. I. (1987). Genetic and environmental factors in antisocial behavior disorders. In S. A. Mednick, T. E. Moffitt, & S. A. Stack (Eds). *The cause of crime: New biological approaches*. New York: Cambridge University Press, 92–109.

Cloninger, C., & Yutzy, S. (1993). Somatoform and dissociative disorders: A summary of changes for DSM–IV. In D. Dunner (Ed.). *In current psychiatric therapy*. Philadelphia: W.B. Saunders, 310–313.

Cohn, L. D., Adler, N. E., Irwin, C. E., Millstein, S. G., Kegeles, S. G., & Stone, G. (1987). Body-figure preferences in male and female adolescents. *Journal of Abnormal Psychology*, 96, 276–279.

Coleman, R., Morison, L., Paine, K., Powell, R. A., & Walvaren, G. (2006). Women's reproductive health and depression: A community survey in Gambia, West Africa. *Social Psychiatry and Psychiatric Epidemiology*, 41, 720–727.

Comer, R. J. (1995). *Abnormal psychology* (2nd ed.). New York: W.H. Freeman and Company.

Compton, W. C. (2005). *An introduction to positive psychology*. Belmont, CA: Wadsworth/Cengage Learning.

Compulsive gambling. (2012). Retrieved March 10, 2012 from http://www.miph.org/projects/gambling-problems-resource-center

Connors, M. E., & Morse, W. (1993). Sexual abuse and eating disorders: A review. *International Journal of Eating Disorders*, 13, 1–11.

Conway, K. P., Compton, W., Stinson, F. S., & Grant, B. F. (2006). Lifetime comorbidity of DSM-IV mood and anxiety disorders and specific drug use disorders: Results from the National Epidemiologic Survey on Alcohol and Related Conditions. *Journal of Clinical Psychiatry*, 67(2), 247–257.

Cooper, D. (1967). *Psychiatry and anti-psychiatry*. London: Tavistock Publications.

Cooper, R. (2005). *Classifying madness: A philosophical examination of the Diagnostic and Statistical Manual of Mental Disorders*. Berlin: Springer.

Corin, E., & Murphy, H. B. M. (1979). Psychiatric perspectives in Africa Part I: The Western viewpoint. *Transcultural Psychiatric Research Review*, 16, 147–169.

Cornblatt, B., & Erlenmeyer-Kimling, L. E. (1985).Global attention deviance in children at risk for Schizophrenia: Specificity and predictive validity. *Journal of Abnormal Psychology*, 94, 470–486.

Corsini, R. & Wedding, D. (2005). *Current psychotherapies* (7th Ed.). Toronto: Thomson/Brooks Cole Publishers.

Cox, B. J. (1994). Alexithymia in somatoform disorder patients with chronic pain. *Journal of Psychosomatic Research*, 38(6), 523–527.

Coyne, R. (2005). Strategic therapy with depressed married persons: Initial agenda, themes and interventions. *Journal of Marital and Family Therapy*, 10, 53–62.

Cranco, R., & Lehman, H. E. (2000). Schizophrenia: Clinical features. In B. J. Sadock & V. A. Sadock (Eds.), *Kaplan & Sadock's comprehensive textbook of psychiatry* (Vol. 7). Philadelphia: Williams & Wilkins, 1663–1676.

Craske, M. G. & Barlow, D. H. (2001). Panic disorder and agoraphobia. In D. H. Barlow (Ed.). *Clinical handbook of psychological disorders: A step-by-step treatment manual* (3rd Ed). New York: The Guilford Press, 1–59.

Craske, M. G. & Barlow, D. H. (2007). Panic disorder and agoraphobia. In D. H. Barlow (Ed.). *Clinical handbook of psychological disorders: A step-by-step treatment manual* (4th Ed). New York: The Guilford Press.

Craske, M. G. (2003). *Origins of phobias and anxiety disorders: Why more women than men?* New York: Pergamon Publishers.

Critser, G. (2003). *Fat land: How Americans became the fattest people in the world*. Boston: Houghton Mifflin.

Crosson, B. & Warren, R. L. (1982). Use of the Luria-Nebraska Neuropsychological Battery in aphasia: A conceptual critique. *Journal of Consulting and Clinical Psychology*, 50, 22–31.

Crow, T. J. (1985). The two-syndrome concept: Origins and current status. *Schizophrenia Bulletin*, 11, 471–486.

Csikszentmihalyi, M. (1990). *Flow: The psychology of optimal experience*. New York: Harper Row.

Cunnien, A. J. (1997). Psychiatric and medical syndromes associated with deception. In R. Rogers, *Clinical Assessment of Malingering and Deception*. New York: Guilford, 23–46.

Cutter, W. J., Norbury, R., & Murphy D. G. (2003).Oestrogen, brain function, and neuropsychiatric disorders. *Journal of Neurology, Neurosurgery and Psychiatry*, 74(7), 837–840.

Dahl, A. A. (1993). The personality disorders: A critical review of family, twin, and adoption studies. *Journal of Personality Disorders*, Suppl. 1, 86–99.

Dana, R. H. (2000). *Handbook of cross-cultural personality assessment*. Mahwah, NJ: Lawrence Erlbaum Associates Publishers.

Daubenton, F., & Van Rensburg, P. (2001). Schizophrenia and other psychotic disorders. In B. Robertson, C. W. Allwood, & C. Gagiano (Eds.), *Textbook of Psychiatry for Southern Africa*. Cape Town: Oxford University Press, 92–110.

Davidson, L. L., & Heinrichs, R. W. (2003). Quantification of frontal and temporal lobe brain imaging findings in Schizophrenia: a meta-analysis. *Psychiatry Research*, 122(2), 69–87.

Davidson, M., Keefe, R. S. E., Mohs, R. C., Siever, L. J., Losonczy, M. E, Horvath.T. B., & Davis, K. L. (1987). L-Dopa challenge and relapse in Schizophrenia. *American Journal of Psychiatry*, 144, 934–938.

Davis, C. (1996). The interdependence of obsessive-compulsiveness, physical activity, and starvation: A model for anorexia nervosa. In W. F. Epling & W. D. Pierce (Eds). *Activity nervosa: Theory, research, and treatment*. Mahwah, NJ: Erlbaum, 209–218.

Davis, C. (1997). Normal and neurotic perfectionism in eating disorders: An interactive model. *International Journal of Eating Disorders*, 22, 421–426.

Davis, K. L., Kahn, R. S., Ko, G., & Davidson, M. (1991). Dopamine and Schizophrenia: A review and reconceptualization. *American Journal of Psychiatry*, 148, 1474–1486.

Davison, G. & Neale, J. (2001). *Abnormal psychology* (8th Ed.). New York: John Wiley & Sons Inc.

Day, M. (1998) Mostly in the mind. *New Scientist*, July, 2142, 159.

Day, R., Nielsen, J. A., Korten, A., Ernberg, G., Dube, K. C., Gebhart. J., Jablensky, A., Leon, C., Marsella, A., Olatawatura, M., Sartorius, N., Stromgren, E., Takahashi, R., Wig, N., & Wynne, L. C. (1987). Stressful life events preceding the acute onset of Schizophrenia: A cross-national study from the World Health Organization. *Cultural Medicine and Psychiatry*, 11, 123–205.

De Bruin, G. P., Swartz, L., Tomlinson, M., Cooper, P. J., & Molteno, C. (2004). The factor structure of the Edinburgh Postnatal Depression scale in a South African peri-urban settlement. *South African Journal of Psychology*, 34(1), 113–121.

De la Rey, C. & Eagle, G. (1997). Gender and mental health policy development. In D. Foster, M. Freeman, & Y. Pillay (Eds). *Mental health policy issues for South Africa*. Cape Town: MASA Multimedia, 143–165.

De Leon, J., Diaz, F. J., Rogers, T., Browne, D., & Dinsmore, L. (2002). Initiation of daily smoking and nicotine dependence in Schizophrenia and mood disorders. *Schizophrenia Research*, 56(1), 47–54.

De Shazer, S., & Berg, I. K. (1997). What works? Remarks on research aspects of solution-focused brief therapy. *Journal of Family therapy*, 19, 121–124.

DeFronzo-Dobkin, R. D., Panzarella, C., Alloy, L. B., Cascardi, M., Truesdell, K. & Gara, M. (2007). Assessing an interpersonal–cognitive risk factor for depression: Preliminary validation of the Social Feedback Questionnaire. *Journal of Social and Personal Relationships*, 24(5), 675–680.

DeGrandpre, 2006

Dell'Osso, L., Shear, M. K., Carmassi, C., Rucci, P., Maser, J. D., Frank, E., Endicott, J., Lorettu, L., Altamura, C. A., Carpiniello, B., Perris, F., Conversano, C., Ciaparelli, A., Carlina, M., Sarno, N., & Cassano, G. B. (2008). Validity and reliability of the Structured Clinical Interview for the Trauma and Loss Spectrum (SCI-TALS). *Clinical Practice & Epidemiology in Mental Health*, 4, 2.

Delport, I. & Szabo, C. P. (2008). Eating disorders in South Africa: an inter-ethnic comparison of admission data. *South African Medical Journal*. Retrieved December 1, 2011 from http://findarticles.com/p/articles/mi_6869/is_4_98/ai_n28539690/pg_2/?tag=content;co l1

Dennis, C. L. E., Janssen, P.A., & Singer, J. (2004). Identifying women at risk for postpartum depression in the immediate postpartum period. *Acta Psychiatrica Scandinavica*, 110, 338–346.
Diener, E. (2000). Subjective well-being: The science of happiness and a proposal for a national index. *American Psychologist*, 55, 34–44.
Dirks, B. (2001). Eating disorders. In B. Robertson, C. W. Allwood & C. Gagiano (Eds.). *Textbook of Psychiatry for Southern Africa*. Cape Town: Oxford.
Dishion, T. J., & Patterson, G. R. (1997). The timing and severity of antisocial behavior: Three hypotheses within an ecological framework. In D. M. Stoff, J. Breiling, & J. D. Maser (Eds.). *Handbook of Antisocial Personality Disorder*. New York: Wiley, 205–217.
Doer, P., Fichter, M., Pirke, K. M., & Lund, R. (1980). Relationship between weight gain and hypothalamic–pituitary–adrenal function in patients with anorexia nervosa. *Journal of Steroid Biochemistry*, 13, 529–537.
Dolan, B. (1991). Cross-cultural aspects of anorexia and bulimia: A review. *International Journal of Eating Disorders*, 10, 67–78.
Dommisse, J. (1987). The state of psychiatry in South Africa today. *Social Science and Medicine*, 24(9), 749–761.
Donald, D., Lazarus, S., & Lolwana, P. (1997). *Educational psychology in social context: Challenges of development, social issues and special need in southern Africa*. Cape Town: Oxford University Press.
Double, D. B. (1992). Understanding schizophrenia. *British Medical Journal*, 305, 775–776.
Douma, S. L., Husband, C., O'Donnell, M. E., Barwin, B. N., & Woodend A. K. (2005). Estrogen-related mood disorders: Reproductive life cycle factors. *Advances in Nursing Science*, 28(4), 364–375.
Dreger, A. D. (2006). Intersex and human rights: The long view. In S. Sytsma (Ed.). *Ethics and Intersex*. New York: Springer, 73–86.
Drewnowski, A., Yee, D. K., & Krahn, D. D. (1988). Bulimia in college women: Incidence and recovery rates. *American Journal of Psychiatry*, 145, 753–755.
Dreyer, N. (Ed.) (2006). *A century of Sundays*. Cape Town: Struik.
Du Plessis, J. (1999). *Oor gaywees [On being gay]*. Cape Town: Tafelberg.
Du Plessis, L. (2003). An Investigation into models for the assessment of malingering in criminal forensic evaluations: A focus on malingering of mental illness. Unpublished dissertation submitted in part fulfilment of the requirements for the degree of Master of Arts in Clinical Psychology, Unisa.
Duman, R. S., Heninger, G. R., & Nestler, E. J. (1997). A molecular and cellular theory of depression. *Archives of General Psychiatry*, 54(7), 597–606.
Dwork, A. J. (1997). Postmortem studies of the hippocampal formation in Schizophrenia. *Schizophrenia Bulletin*, 23, 385–402.
Dworkin, R. H., Lenzenwenger, M. F., & Moldin, S. O. (1987). Genetics and the phenomenology of Schizophrenia. In P. D. Harvey & E. F. Walker (Eds.), *Positive and negative symptoms of psychosis*. Hillsdale, NJ: Erlbaum, 258–288
Dworkin, S. F., & Wilson, L. (1993). Somatoform Pain Disorder and its Treatment. In D. D. Dunner, *Current Psychiatric Therapy*. Philadelphia: WB Saunders Company, 321–237.
Eagle, G. T. (2005). Grasping the thorn: The impact and supervision of traumatic stress therapy in the South African context. *Journal of Psychology in Africa*, 15(2), 197–207.
Eagles, J. M., (1991).The relationship between Schizophrenia and immigration. Are there alternatives to psychosocial hypothesis? *The British Journal of Psychiatry*, 159, 783–789.
Earl-Taylor, M., & Thomas, L. (2003). *The long term neurological and developmental effects of sexual abuse on infant children*. Retrieved on March 13, 2012 from http://www.scienceinafrica.co.za/2003/march/abuse.htm
Ebata, A. T., Peterson, A. C., & Conger, J. J. (1990). The development of psychopathology in adolescence. In J. Rolf, A. S. Masten, D. Cicchetti, K. H. Nuechterlein, & S. Weintraub (Eds.). *Risk and protective factors in the development of psychopathology*. Cambridge, England: Cambridge University Press, 308–333.
Ebmeier, K. P., Donaghey, C., & Steele, J. D. (2006). Recent developments and current controversies in depression. *Lancet*, 367, 153–167.
Edwards, D. (2005). Critical perspectives on research on Posttraumatic Stress Disorder and implications for the South African context. *Journal of Psychology in Africa*, 15(2), 117–124.

Edwards, D. (2005). Posttraumatic stress disorder as a public health concern in South Africa. *Journal of Psychology in Africa*, 15(2), 125–134.

Edwards, D. (2005). Treating PTSD in South African contexts: A theoretical framework and a model for developing evidence-based practice. *Journal of Psychology in Africa*, 15(2), 209–220.

Edwards, D., Sakasa, P., & Van Wyk, G. (2005). Trauma, resilience and vulnerability to PTSD: A review and clinical case analysis. *Journal of Psychology in Africa*, 15(2), 143–153.

Edwards, S. D. (2010). A Rogerian perspective on empathic patterns in Southern African Healing. *Journal of Psychology in Africa*, 20(2), 321–326.

Egan, A. (2008). Should the state support the 'right to die'? *South African Journal of Bioethics and Law*, 1(2), 47–52.

Eggers, C., & Bunk, D. (1997). The long-term course of childhood onset Schizophrenia: A 42-year follow up. *Schizophrenia Bulletin*, 23, 105–116.

Eisenberg, L. (1995). The social construction of the human brain. *American Journal of Psychiatry*, 152, 1563–1575.

Eisenberg, L. A. (1959). A Clinical study of Gilles de la Tourette's Disease (Maladie des Tics) in children. *American Journal of Psychiatry*, 115, 715–723.

Eisenberg, N., & Ota Wang, V. (2003). Toward a positive psychology: Social development and cultural contributions. In L.G Aspinwall & U.M. Staudinger (Eds.), *A psychology of human strengths. Fundamental questions and future directions for a positive psychology*. Washington, DC: American Psychological Association, 117–129.

Ekman, P. (1993). Facial expression and emotion. *American psychologist*, 48, 384–392.

Ekman, P. (1999). Basic emotions. In T. Dalgleish & M. Power (Eds.). *Handbook of cognition and emotion*. Sussex: John Wiley & Sons Ltd.

Elhai, J. D., Carvalho, L. F., Miguel, F. K., Palmieri, P. A., Primi, R., & Frueh, B. C. (2011). Testing whether Posttraumatic Stress Disorder and Major Depressive Disorder are similar or unique constructs. *Journal of Anxiety Disorders*, 25(3), 404–410.

Eliason, M. J. (1996). *Who cares? Institutional barriers to health care for lesbian, gay, and bisexual people*. New York: National League for Nursing Press.

Ellis, A. (1995). Changing rational-emotive therapy (RET) to rational emotive behavior therapy (REBT). *Journal of Rational-Emotive and Cognitive-Behavior Therapy*, 13, 85–89.

Ellis, A. (2004). How my theory and practice of psychotherapy has influenced and changed other psychotherapies. *Journal of Rational-Emotive & Cognitive-Behavior Therapy*, 22 (2), 79–83.

Elovainio, M., Jokela, M., Kivimäki, M., Pulkki-Råback, M., Lehtimäki, T., Airla, N., et al. (2007). Genetic variants in the DRD2 gene moderate the relationship between stressful life events and depressive symptoms in adults: Cardiovascular risk in young Finns study. *Psychosomatic Medicine*, 69(5), 391–395.

Emsley, R. A., Niehaus, D. J. H., Mbanga, N. I., Oosthuizen, P. P., Stein, D. J., Maritz, J. S., Pimstone, S. N., Hayden, M. R., Laurent, C., Deleuze, J., & Mallet, J. (2001). The factor structure for positive and negative symptoms in South African Xhosa patients with Schizophrenia. *Schizophrenia Research*, 47, 149–157.

Emsley, R. A., Oosthuizen, P. P., Joubert, A. F., Hawkridge, S. M., & Stein, D. J. (1999). Treatment of Schizophrenia in low-income countries. *International Journal of Neuropharmacology*, 2, 321–325.

Ensink, K. R. (1996). Indigenous categories of distress and dysfunction in South African Xhosa children and adolescents as described by indigenous healers. *Transcultural Psychiatry*, 33(2), 137–172.

Ensink, K. R. (1999). Patient and family experiences of psychiatric services and African indigenous healers. *Transcultural Psychiatry*, 36(1), 23–43.

Erickson, M. T. (1998). *Behaviour disorders of children and adolescents: Assessment, etiology and intervention*. Upper Saddle River: Prentice Hall.

Escobar, J. (2004). Transcultural aspects of dissociative and somatoform disorders. *Psychiatric Times*, 21(5).

Escobar, J. I., Gara, M., Silver, R. C., Waitzkin, H., Holman, A., & Compton, W. (1998). Somatisation disorder in primary care. *British Journal of Psychiatry*, 173, 262–266.

Esplen, E. & Jolly, S. (2006). *Gender and sex: A sample of definitions*. Brighton: Bridge Development-Gender.

Estell, D. B., Farmer, T. W., Pearl, R., Van Acker, R., & Rodkin, P. C. (2003). Heterogeneity in the relationship between popularity and aggression: Individual, group, and classroom influences. In S. C. Peck & R. W. Roeser (Eds). *Person-centered approaches to studying development in context*. San Francisco: Jossey-Bass.

Evans, C., & Street, E. (1995). Possible differences in family patterns in anorexia nervosa and bulimia nervosa. *Journal of Family Therapy*, 17, 115–131.

Everill, J. T., & Waller, G. (1995). Reported sexual abuse and eating psychopathology: A review of the evidence for a causal link. *International Journal of Eating Disorders*, 18, 1–11.

Exner, J. E. (2002). *The Rorschach: Basic Foundations and Principles of Interpretation* (1). Hoboken, NJ: Wiley.

Fairburn, C. G., Agras, W. S., & Wilson, G. T. (1992). The research on the treatment of bulimia nervosa: Practical and theoretical implications. In G. H. Anderson & S. H. Kennedy (Eds). *The biology of fast and famine: Relevance to eating disorders*. New York: Academic Press, 317–340.

Fairburn, C. G., Cooper, Z., Bohn, K., O'Connor, M. E., Doll, H. A., & Palmer, R. L. (2007). The severity and states of Eating Disorder NOS: Implications for DSM-V. *Behaviour Research and Therapy*, 45(8), 1705–1715.

Fairburn, C. G., Shafran, R., & Cooper, Z. (1999). A cognitive behavioural theory of anorexia nervosa. *Behaviour Research and Therapy*, 37, 1–13.

Fallon, A. E., & Rozin, P. (1985). Sex differences in perception of ideal body shape. *Journal of Abnormal Psychology*, 94, 102–105.

Fava, M., Copeland, P. M., Schweiger, U., & Herzog, D. B. (1989). Neurochemical abnormalities of anorexia and bulimia nervosa. *American Journal of Psychiatry*, 146, 963–971.

Feighner, J. P., Robins, E., Guze, S. B., Woodruff, R. A., Winokur, G., & Munoz, R. (1972). Diagnostic criteria for use in psychiatric research. *Archives of General Psychiatry*, 26, 57–63.

Ferracuti, S. S. (1996). Dissociative Trance Disorder: Clinical and Rorschach findings in ten persons reporting demon possession and treated by exorcism. *Journal of Personality Assessment*, 66, 525–539

Ferster, C. B. (1973). A functional analysis of depression. *American Psychologist*, 28, 857–870.

Feusner, J. D., Townsend, J., Bystritsky, A., & Bookheimer, S. (2007). Visual information processing of faces in Body Dysmorphic Disorder. *Archives of General Psychiatry*, 64(12), 1417–1425.

Fichter, M. M. & Quadflieg, N. (1997). Six-year course of Bulimia Nervosa. *International Journal of Eating Disorders*, 22(4), 361–384.

Fichter, M. M. & Quadflieg, N. (1999). Six-year course and outcome of Anorexia Nervosa. *International Journal of Eating Disorders*, 26(4), 359–385.

Fichter, M. M., & Naegel, R. (1990). Concordance for bulimia nervosa in twins. *International Journal of Eating Disorders*, 9, 425–436.

Flor-Henry cited in Black, D. N., Seritan, A. L., Taber, K. H., & Hurley, R. A. (2004). Conversion hysteria: Lessons from functional imaging. *Journal of Neuropsychiatry and Clinical Neurosciences*, 16(3), 245–251.

Folkman, S. (1984). Personal control and stress and coping processes: A theoretical analysis. *Journal of Personality and Social Psychology*, 46, 839–852.

Ford, C. V. (1985). Conversion Disorders: An overview. *Psychosomatics*, 26, 371–385.

Forgus, R. H., & DeWolfe, A. S. (1974).Coding of cognitive input in delusional patients. *Journal of Abnormal Psychology*, 83, 278–284.

Foster, D. (1993). On racism: Virulent mythologies and fragile threads. In L. Nicholas (Ed.), *Psychology and oppression: Critiques and proposals*. Johannesburg: Skotaville, pp. 55–80

Foster, D., Freeman, M., & Pillay, Y. (1997). *Mental health policy issues for South Africa*. Medical Association of South Africa, Pinelands.

Fowler, J. S., Volkow, N. D., Kassed, C. A., & Chang, L. (2007). Imaging the addicted human brain. *NIDA Science & Practice Perspectives*, 3(2), 4–15.

Frank, E., Anderson, B., Reynolds, C. F., Ritenour, A., & Kupfer, D. J. (1994). Life events and the research diagnostic criteria endogenous subtype. A confirmation of the distinction using the Bedford College methods. *Archives of General Psychiatry*, 51, 519–524.

Frankl, V. (1959). *The will to meaning: foundations and applications of logotherapy*. New York: World Publishing House.

Frankl, V. E. (1976). *Man's search for meaning. An introduction to Logotherapy* (3rd ed.). New York: Pocket.

Frederiksen, N. (1986). Toward a broader conception of human intelligence. *American Psychologist*, 41(4), 445–452.

Fredrickson, B. L. (2005). Positive emotions. In C. R. Snyder & S. J. Lopez (Eds.), *Handbook of Positive Psychology*. Oxford: Oxford University Press, 120–134.

Freeman, A. & Reinecke, M. A. (Eds). (2007). *Personality disorders in childhood and adolescence.* Hoboken, NJ: John Wiley & Sons.

Freeman, M. (1992). *Providing mental health care for all in South Africa – structure and strategy.* Johannesburg: Centre for Health Policy.

Freeston, M. H., Dugas, M. J., Letarte, H., Rheaume, J., Blais, F., & Ladouceur, R. (1996). Physical symptoms associated with worry in a non-clinical population. *Journal of Anxiety Disorders*, 10(5), 365–377.

Fresco, D. M., Rytwinski, N. K., & Craighead, L. W. (2007). Explanatory flexibility and negative life events interact to predict depression symptoms. *Journal of Social and Clinical Psychology*, 26, 595–608.

Freud, S. (1895). Project for a scientific psychology. In *Standard edition of the complete works of Sigmund Freud.* London: Hogarth Press.

Freud, S. (1900). *The interpretation of dreams.* London: Penguin Books.

Freud, S. (1905). *Three essays on the theory of sexuality.* London: Penguin Books.

Freud, S. (1914). *On narcissism: An introduction.* London: Penguin Books.

Freud, S. (1915). *Thoughts for the times on war & death.* London: Penguin Books.

Freud, S. (1917). *Mourning & melancholia.* London: Penguin Books.

Freud, S. (1920). *Beyond the pleasure principle.* London: Penguin Books.

Freud, S. (1926). *Inhibitions, symptoms & anxiety.* London: Penguin Books.

Freud, S. (1950). *The interpretation of dreams.* New York: Random House.

Freund, B. (1992). The poor whites: A social force and a social problem in South African history. In R. Morell (Ed.), *White but poor: Essays on the history of poor whites in Southern Africa* 1880–1994. Pretoria: University of South Africa, xiii–xxiii.

Fried, A. (2004). Adolescents at risk. *Encyclopedia of Applied Developmental Science.* http://www.sage-ereference.com/applied devscience/Article_n15.html. Retrieved on 20 March 2009.

Fried, A. (2004). Depression in adolescence. *Encyclopedia of Applied Developmental Science.* SAGE Publications. http://www.sage–ereference.com/applied devscience/Article_n15.html. Retrieved on 20 March 2009.

Fritson, K.K. (2007). *Autism.* 21st century psychology: A reference handbook. Encyclopedia of counseling. http://www.sage–ereference.com/psychology/Article_n57.html. Retrieved on 20 March 2009.

Fromm-Reichmann, F. (1948). Notes on the development of treatment of schizophrenics by psychoanalytic psychotherapy. *Psychiatry*, 11, 263–273.

Frude, N. (1998). *Understanding abnormal psychology.* Oxford: Blackwell.

Frydenburg, E. (1997). *Adolescent coping: Theoretical and research perspectives.* London: Routledge.

Frydenburg, E. (2008). *Adolescent coping: Advances in theory, research and practice.* London: Routledge.

Furnham, A., & Baguma, P. (1994). Cross-cultural differences in the evaluation of male and female body shapes. *International Journal of Eating Disorders*, 15, 81–89.

Furukawa, T.A., Watanabe, N., Omori, I.M., & Churchill, R. (2007). Can pill placebo augment cognitive-behavior therapy for panic disorder? *BMC Psychiatry*, 7, 73.

Ganasen, K. A., Finchama, D., Smit, J., Seedat, S. & Stein, D. (2007). Utility of the HIV Dementia Scale (HDS) in identifying HIV dementia in a South African sample. *Journal of the Neurological Sciences*, 269(1–2):62–64.

Garcia-Soriano, G., Belloch, A., Morillo, C., & Clark, D. A. (2011). Symptom dimensions in Obsessive-Compulsive Disorder: From normal cognitive intrusions to clinical obsessions. *Journal of Anxiety Disorders*, 25(4), 474–482.

Garety, P. (1991). Reasoning and delusions. *British Journal of Psychiatry*, 159, 14–18.

Garner, D. M., Olmsted, M. P., & Polivy, J. (1983). Development and validation of a multi-dimensional eating disorder inventory for anorexia nervosa and bulimia. *International Journal of Eating Disorders*, 2, 15–34.

Garner, D. M., Vitousek, K. M., & Pike, K. M. (1997). Cognitive-behavioral therapy for anorexia nervosa. In D. M. Garner & P. E. Garfinkel (Eds). *Handbook of treatment for eating disorders.* New York: Guilford Press, 94–144.

GenderdynamiX. (n.d.). Retrieved March 6, 2012 from http://www.genderdynamix.org.za

George, A. A. (2009). Risk and resilience in adolescent suicidal ideation. Unpublished doctoral dissertation, University of the Free State, Bloemfontein, South Africa.

German, G. A. (1972). Aspects of clinical psychiatry in sub-Saharan Africa. *British Journal of Psychiatry*, 115, 1323–1329.

German, G. A. (1987). Mental health in Africa (II). The nature of mental disorder in Africa today. Some clinical observations. *British Journal of Psychiatry*, 151, 440–446.

Gibson, K., & Swartz, L. (2008). Putting the 'heart' into community psychology: Some South African examples. *Psychodynamic practice,* 14(1), 59–75.

Gillies, L. S. (1992). Depression in newly urbanized elderly South Africans. *Southern African Journal of Gerontology,* 1, 20–24.

Glasser, W. (1984). *Control theory.* New York: Harper & Row.

Gobodo-Madikizela, P. & Foster, D. (2005). Psychology and human rights abuses. In C. Tredoux, D. Foster, A. Allan, A. Cohen, & D. Wassenaar (Eds). *Psychology and Law* (343-383). Pretoria: Juta Legal and Academic Publishers.

Goff, D. C., Cather, C., Evins, A. E., Henderson, D. C., Freudenreich, O., Copeland, P. M., Bierer, M., Duckworth, K., Sacks, F. M. (2005). Medical Morbidity and Mortality in Schizophrenia: Guidelines for Psychiatrists. *Journal of Clinical Psychiatry*, 66(2), 183–194.

Goldfried, M. R. (2001). Integrating gay, lesbian, and bisexual issues into mainstream psychology. *American Psychologist*, 56, 975–988.

Goldman, D., Orozi, G., & Ducci, F. (2006). The genetics of addictions: Uncovering the genes. *Focus*, 4, 401–415.

Goldney, R. D. (2006). The utility of the DSM nosology of mood disorders. *Canadian Journal of Psychiatry*, 51(14), 874–878.

Goldsmith, S. K., Shapiro, R. N., & Joyce, J. N. (1997). Disrupted pattern of D2 dopamine receptors in the temporal lobe in Schizophrenia. A postmortem study. *Archives of General Psychiatry*, 54, 649–58.

Goldstein, S. B. (2000). *Cross-cultural explorations: Activities in culture and psychology.* Boston: Allyn & Bacon.

Golub, D. (1995). Cultural variations in multiple personality disorder. In L. Cohen, J. Berzoff, & M. Elin (Eds.), *Dissociative Identity Disorder*. Northvale: Jason Aronson, 285–326.

Gone, J. P. (2011). Is psychological science a-cultural? *Cultural Diversity and Ethnic Minority Psychology*, 17(3), 234–242.

Gonsiorek, J. C. & Weinrich, J. D. (1991). *Homosexuality: Research implications for public policy.* Newbury Park CA: Sage Publications.

Gonsiorek, J. C. (1988). Mental health issues of gay and lesbian adolescents. *Journal of Adolescent Health Care*, 9, 114–122.

Goodsitt, A. (1997). Eating disorders: A self-psychological perspective. In D. M. Garner & P. E. Garfinkel (Eds.). *Handbook of treatment for eating disorders*. New York: Guilford Press, 205–228.

Goodwach, R. (2005). Sex therapy: Historical evolution, current practice. Part 1. *Anzjft*, 26(3), 155–164.

Goodwin, F. K., & Jamison, K. R. (1990). *Manic-depressive illness*. New York: Oxford University Press.

Gorman, J. M., Papp, L. A., & Coplan, J. D. (1995). Neuroanatomy and neurotransmitter function in panic disorder. In S. P. Roose & R. A. Glick (Eds). *Anxiety as Symptom and Signal*. Hillsdale: Erlbaum, 39–56.

Gotlib, I. H. (1982). Self-reinforcement and depression in interpersonal interaction: The role of performance level. *Journal of Abnormal Psychology*, 91(1), 3–13.

Gottesman, I. I. (1991). *Schizophrenia genesis: The origins of madness*. New York: Freeman.

Gould, S.J. (1981). *The mismeasure of man*. New York: W.W. Norton.

Grabe, H. R. (2000). The relationship between dimensions of alexithymia and dissociation. *Psychotherapy and Psychosomatics*, 69, 128–131.

Grant, B. F., Hasin, D. S., Stinson, F. S., Dawson, D. A., Chou, P. S, June, R. W., & Huang, B. (2005). Co-occurrence of 12-month mood and anxiety disorders and personality disorders in the US: Results from the national epidemiologic survey on alcohol and related conditions. *Journal of Psychiatric Research*, 39(1), 1–9.

Grant, I., Patterson, T. L., & Yager, J. (1988). Social supports in relation to physical health and symptoms of depression in the elderly. *American Journal of Psychiatry*, 145(10), 1254–1258.

Green, C. & Chee, K. (1997). *Understanding ADHD* (2nd Ed.). London: Vermilion.

Greene, R. W., & Ollendick, T. H. (2000). Behavioral assessment of children. In G. Goldstein & M. Hersen (Eds). *Handbook of psychological assessment* (3rd Ed.). Oxford: Elsevier Science (Pergamon), 453–470.

Gross, R. (2010). *Psychology: The science of mind and behaviour* (6th ed). London: Hodder Education.

Gross, S. (n.d.). *Legislative work for intersex rights*. Retrieved March 6, 2012 from http://www.intersex.org.za/publications/judicialmatters.html

Groth-Marnat, G. (1999). *Handbook of psychological assessment* (3rd Ed. – revised). New York: John Wiley & Sons.

Gruenberg, A. M., Goldstein, R. D., & Pincus, H. A. (2005). Classification of depression: Research and diagnostic criteria: DSM-IV and ICD-10. In J. Licinio & M. L. Wong (Eds.) *Biology of Depression*. New York: Wiley.

Gumbiner, J. (2010). *What causes addiction? Psychoanalytic theories of addiction*. Retrieved 2011, from http://www.psychologytoday.com

Gunderson, J. G. (2009). Borderline personality disorder: Ontogeny of a diagnosis. *American Journal of Psychiatry*, 166(5), 530–539.

Gurvits, I. G., Koenigsberg, H. W., & Siever, L. J. (2000). Neurotransmitter dysfunction in patients with borderline personality disorder. *Psychiatric Clinics of North America*, 23, 27–40.

Haeffel, G. J., Getchell, M., Koposov R. A., Yrigollen, C. M., DeYoung, C. G., Klinteberg, B., Oreland, L., Ruchkin, V. V., Pakstis, A., & Grigorenko, E. L. (2008). Association between polymorphisms in the dopamine transporter gene and depression: Evidence for a gene–environment interaction in a sample of juvenile detainees. *Psychological Science*, 19(1), 62–69.

Hales, R. Y. (2008). *American Psychiatric Publishing textbook of psychiatry* (8th Ed.). Washington, DC: American Psychiatric Publishing.

Halgin, R. P. & Whitbourne, S. K. (2003). *Abnormal psychology: Clinical perspectives on psychological disorders*. New York: McGraw-Hill.

Halmi, K. A. (2000). Eating disorders. In B. J. Sadock & V. A. Sadock (Eds). *Kaplan & Sadock's comprehensive textbook of psychiatry* (7th Ed.). Philadelphia: Williams & Wilkins, 1663–1676.

Harper, D. C. (2008). *Developmental disorders*. Encyclopedia of counseling. http://www.sage–ereference.com/counseling/Article_n50.html. Retrieved on 20 March 2009.

Harrison, G. (1990). Searching for the causes of Schizophrenia: The role of migrant studies. *Schizophrenia Bulletin*, 16(4), 663–671.

Harshbarger, J. L., Ahlers-Schmidt, C. R., Mayans, L., Mayans, D., & Hawkins, J. H. (2009). Pro-anorexia websites: What a clinician should know. *International Journal of Eating Disorders*, 42, 367–370.

Harvey, J. A. & Robinson, J. D. (2003). Eating Disorders in Men: Current Considerations. *Journal of Clinical Psychology in Medical Settings*, 10(4), 297–306.

Hashim, I. H. (2003). Cultural and gender differences in perceptions of stressors and coping skills: A study of Western and African college students in China. *School Psychology International*, 24(2), 182–203.

Hattingh, C. (1994). The experience of gays and lesbians who are covert at work. Unpublished Honours Dissertation. Grahamstown: Rhodes University.

Haugaard, J. J. (2008). *Child Psychopathology*. New York: McGraw-Hill.

Hause, J. S. (1984). Barriers to work stress. In W. D. Gentry, H. Benson, & C. de Wolff (Eds.). *Behavioral medicine: Work, stress and health*. The Hague: Nijhoff.

Hay, P. J., & Hall, A. (1991). The prevalence of eating disorders in recently admitted psychiatric in-patients. *British Journal of Psychiatry*, 159, 562–565.

Haynes, S. N. (2000). Behavioural assessment of adults. In G. Goldstein & M. Hersen (Eds). *Handbook of psychological assessment*. New York: Pergamon Press, 471–502.

Heap, M. R. (1991). The quest for wholeness: Health care strategies among the residents of council-built hostels in Cape Town. *Social Science and Medicine*, 32, 117–126.

Heckers, S. (1997). Neuropathology of Schizophrenia: Cortex, basal ganglia, and neurotransmitter-specific projection systems. *Schizophrenia Bulletin*, 23, 403–421.

Hefferon, K., & Boniwell, I. (2011). *Positive psychology: Theory, research and applications*. Berkshire: Open University Press.

Heinrichs, N., Hofmann, S. G., & Barlow, D. H. (2004). Non-specific encoding of threat in social phobia and panic disorder. *Cognitive Behaviour Therapy*, 33(4), 199–207.

Hekma, G. (2009). *ABC van perversies*. Amsterdam: J.M Meulenhoff.

Helm, H. M. (2008). *Externalizing problems of childhood*. Encyclopedia of counseling. http://www.sage-ereference.com/counseling/Article_n64.html. Retrieved on 20 March 2009.

Henquet, C., Murray, R., Linszen, D., & Van Os, J. (2005). The environment and Schizophrenia: The role of cannabis use. *Schizophrenia Bulletin*, 31(3), 608–612.

Herbert, P. B., & Young, K. A. (2002). Tarasoff at twenty-five. *Journal of the American Academy of Psychiatry and Law*, 30, 275–81.

Herkov, M. (2006). *What is sexual addiction*. Retrieved January 15, 2012, from http://psychcentral.com/lib/2006/what-is-sexual-addiction

Herman, A. A., Stein, D. J. Seedat, S., Heeringa, S. G., Moomal, H., & Williams, D. R. (2009). The South African Stress and Health (SASH) study: 12-month and lifetime prevalence of common mental disorders. *South African Medical Journal*, 99(5), 339–344.

Herrmann, L. L., Le Masurier, M., Ebmeier, K. P. (2008). White matter hyperintensities in late life depression: a systematic review. *Journal of Neurology, Neurosurgery, and Psychiatry*, 79(6), 619–24.

Hersen, M., Turner, S. M., & Beidel, D. (2007). *Adult psychopathology and diagnosis* (5th Ed.). Hoboken: John Wiley & Sons.

Hettema, J. M., Neale, M. C., & Kendler, K. S. (2001). A review and meta-analysis of the genetic epidemiology of anxiety disorders. *American Journal of Psychiatry*, 158, 1568–1578.

Hinton, D., Nathan, M., Bird, B., & Park, L. (2002). Panic probes and the identification of panic: A historical and cross-cultural perspective. *Culture, Medicine and Psychiatry*, 26(2), 137–153.

Hirsch, J. K., Wolford, K., Lalonde, S. M., Brunk, L., Morris, A. P. (2007). Dispositional optimism as a moderator of the relationship between negative life events and suicide ideation and attempts. *Cognitive Therapy and Research*, 31(4), 533–546.

Hirschfeld, R. & Shea, T. (1992). Personality. In E. Paykel (Ed.). *Handbook of affective disorders*. New York: Guilford Press, 185–194.

Hoebel, B. G., & Teitelbaum, P. (1966). Weight regulation in normal and hypothalamic hyperphagic rats. *Journal of Comparative and Physiological Psychology*, 61, 189–193.

Hoffmann, W. A., Myburgh, C. & Poggenpoel, M. (2010). The lived experiences of late-adolescent female suicide survivors: 'A part of me died'. *Journal of Interdisciplinary Health Sciences*, 15(1), 1–9.

Hofmann, A. (1980). *LSD: My problem child*. New York: McGraw Hill.

Holdstock, T. L. (1981). Psychology in South Africa belongs to the colonial era: Arrogance or ignorance. *South African Journal of Psychology*, 11, 123–129.

Holland, A. J., Hall, A., Murray, R., Russell, G. F. M., & Crisp, A. H. (1984). Anorexia nervosa: A study of 34 twin pairs and one set of triplets. *British Journal of Psychiatry*, 145, 414–419.

Holtzman, N. A. & Marteau, T. M. (2000). Will genetics revolutionize medicine? *New England Journal of Medicine*, 342, 141–4.

Hook, D. & Eagle, G. (2002). *Psychopathology and social prejudice*. Lansdowne: UCT Press.

Hook, D. (2002). The other side of language: The body and the limits of signification. *Psychoanalytic Review*, 89(5), 681–713.

Hor, K. & Taylor, M. (2010). Review of 'Suicide and Schizophrenia: a systematic review of rates and risk factors'. *Journal of Psychopharmachology*, 24(4), 81–90.

Hoste, R. R. & le Grange, D. (2008). Expressed emotion among white and ethnic minority families of adolescents with Bulimia Nervosa. *European Eating Disorders Review*, 16(5), 395–400.

Howard, R. (1992). Folie a deux involving a dog. *American Journal of Psychiatry*, 149, 414.

HPCSA (Health Professions Council of South Africa). (2007). *Guidelines for good practice in the health care professions*. Ethical and professional rules of the health professions council of South Africa as promulgated in Government Gazette r717/2006. (2nd ed.). Booklet 2 (29th May 2007). Pretoria: HPCSA.

Hsu, L. K. G. (1987). Are eating disorders becoming more common in blacks. *International Journal of Eating Disorders*, 6, 113–124.

Hsu, L. K. G. (1990). *Eating disorders*. New York: Guilford Press.

Hsu, L. K. G., Chesler, B. E., & Santhouse, R. (1990). Bulimia nervosa in eleven sets of twins: A clinical report. *International Journal of Eating Disorders*, 9, 275–282.

Hudson, J. I., Lalonde, J. K., Berry, J. M., Pindych, L. J., Bulik, C. M., Crow, S. J. et al. (2006). Binge-eating disorder as a distinct familial phenotype in obese individuals. *Archives of General Psychiatry*, 63, 313–319.

Hugo, C. J., Boshoff, D. E. L., Traut, A., Zungu-Dirwayi, N., & Stein, D. J. (2003). Community attitudes toward and knowledge of mental illness in South Africa. *Social Psychiatry and Psychiatric Epidemiology*, 38, 715–719.

Hussain, A. F., & Cochrane, R. (2002). Depression in South Asian women: Asian women's beliefs on causes and cures. *Mental Health, Religion & Culture*, 5(3), 285–311.

Husserl, E.G.A. (1952/1989). Ideas pertaining to a pure phenomenology and to a phenomenological philosophy – Second book: Studies in the phenomenology of constitution (R. Rojcewicz, & A. Schuwer, Trans.). *Collected works*, Vol. 3. The Hague, Netherlands: Kluwer.

Husserl, E.G.A. (1971/1980). Ideas pertaining to a pure phenomenology and to a phenomenological philosophy – Third book: Phenomenology and the foundation of the sciences (T. E. Klein & W.E. Pohl, Trans). *Collected works*, Vol. 1. The Hague, Netherlands: Kluwer.

ICD10 Chapter V: Mood (affective) disorders. *Mental and behavioural disorders.* http://en.wikipedia.org/wiki/ICD-10_Chapter_V:_Mental_and_behavioural_disorders. Retrieved 6 November 2007.

Ineichen, B. (2000). The epidemiology of dementia in Africa: A review. *Social Science & Medicine*, 50(11), 1673–1677.

Institute of Medicine: Committee on Nervous System Disorders in Developing Countries, Board on Global Health (2001). *Neurological, psychiatric and developmental disorders: Meeting the challenge in the developing world.* Washington: National Academy Press. http://books.nap.edu/openbook/0309071925/gifmid/112.gif. Retrieved 23 March 2009.

Isaacs, G. & McKendrick, B. (1992). *Male homosexuality in South Africa: Identity formation, culture and crisis.* New York: Oxford University Press.

Janoff-Bulman, R. (1992). *Shattered assumptions.* New York: Free Press.

Janse van Rensburg, A. B. R. (2009). A changed climate for mental health care delivery in South Africa. *Psychiatry*, 12, 157–16

Jarvis, E. (1998). Schizophrenia in British immigrants: Recent findings, issues and implications. *Transcultaral Psychiatry*, 35(1), 39–74.

Jaspers, K. (1962). *General psychopathology.* Manchester: Manchester University Press.

Jewell, J. D., & Stark, K. D. (2003). Comparing the family environments of adolescents with conduct disorder or depression. *Journal of Child and Family Studies*, 12(1), 77–89.

Jimerson, D. C., Wolfe, B. E., Metzger, E. D., Finkelstein, D. M., Cooper, T. B., et al. (1997). Decreased serotonin function in bulimia nervosa. *Archives of General Psychiatry*, 54, 529–536.

Jinabhai, C. C., Taylor, M., Rangongo, M. F., Mkhize, N., Anderson, S., Pillay, B. J., & Sullivan, K. R. (2004). Investigating the mental abilities of rural Zulu primary school children in South Africa. *Ethnicity and Health*, 9, 1, 17–36.

Johnson, B. D., & Bunce, R. (2008). *Attention Deficit/Hyperactivity Disorder.* Encyclopedia of counseling. http://www.sage-ereference.com/counseling/Article_n11.html. Retrieved on 20 March 2009.

Johnson, D. M., Zlotnick, C. & Perez, S. (2011). Cognitive-behavioral treatment of PTSD in residents of battered women's shelters: Results of a randomised clinical trial. *Journal of Consulting and Clinical Psychology*, 79(4), 542–551.

Johnson, J. C. (2006). Dissociative disorders among adults in the community, impaired functioning, and axis I and II comorbidity. *Journal of Psychiatric Research*, 40(2), 131–140.

Johnstone, L. (2000). *Users and abusers of psychiatry: A critical look at psychiatric practice* (2nd Ed.). London: Routledge.

Jones, B. E., & Gray, B. A. (1986). Problems in diagnosing Schizophrenia and affective disorders in Blacks. *Hospital and Community Psychiatry*, 37, 61–65.

Jones, D. J., Fox, M. M., Babigan, H. M., & Hutton, H. E. (1980). Epidemiology of anorexia nervosa in Monroe County, New York: 1960–1976. *Psychosomatic Medicine*, 42, 551–558.

Joseph, S. & Linley, P. A. (2004). Positive therapy: A positive psychological theory of therapeutic practice. In P. A. Linley & S. Joseph (Eds.), *Positive psychology in practice.* Hoboken, NJ: John Wiley, 354–368.

Joyce, D. (2007). *Conduct Disorders Encyclopedia of School Psychology.* Sage Publications. http://www.sage-ereference.com/educationalpsychology/Article_n47.html. Retrieved 9 March 2009.

Junginger, J., Barker, S., & Coe, D. (1992). Mood theme and bizarreness of delusions in Schizophrenia and mood psychosis. *Journal of Abnormal Psychology*, 101, 287–292.

Kabat-Zinn, J. (1990). *Full catastrophe living: Using the wisdom of your body and mind to face stress, pain and illness.* New York: Delacourt.

Kahn, M. S., & Kelly, K. (2001). Cultural tensions in psychiatric nursing: Managing the interface between Western mental health care and Xhosa traditional healing in South Africa. *Transcultural Psychiatry*, 38, 35–50.

Kahn, R. S., Davidson, M., Knott, P., Stern, R. G., Apter, S., & Davis, K. L. (1993). Effect of neuroleptic medication on cerebrospinal fluid monoamine metabolite concentrations in Schizophrenia: Serotonin-dopamine inter-actions as a target for treatment. *Archives of General Psychiatry*, 50, 599–605.

Kale, R. (1995). New South-Africa's mental health. *British Medical Journal*, 310, 1254.

Kaliski, S. Z. (2006). The criminal defendant. In S. Z. Kaliski (Ed.). *Psycholegal assessment in South Africa*. Cape Town: Oxford University Press, 93–112.

Kaminer, D., Grimsrud, A., Myer, L., Stein, D. J., & Williams, D. R. (2008). Risk for post-traumatic stress disorder associated with different forms of interpersonal violence in South Africa. *Social Science & Medicine*, 67, 1589–1595.

Kanacki, L. S., Jones, P. S., & Galbraith, M. E. (1996). Social support and depression in widows and widowers. *Journal of Gerontological Nursing*, 22(2), 39–45.

Kaplan, E. (1989). Thyroid and parathyroid. In S. I. Schwartz, G. Shiars, & F. E. Spencer. *Principles of surgery* (5th Ed.). New York: McGraw-Hill, 1613–1685.

Kaplan, H. I., Sadock, B. J., & Grebb, J. A. (1994). *Kaplan & Sadock's synopsis of psychiatry: Behavioral sciences clinical psychiatry* (7th Ed.). Baltimore: Lippincott Williams & Wilkins.

Kaplan, H. I., Sadock, B. J., & Grebb, J. A. (1996). *Synopsis of psychiatry: Behavioral sciences, clinical psychiatry*. Baltimore: Williams & Wilkins.

Kaplan, H. I., & Sadock, B.J. (2007). *Kaplan & Sadock's synopsis of psychiatry: Behavioral sciences clinical psychiatry* (10th Ed.). Baltimore: Lippincott Williams & Wilkins.

Kaplan, H. S. (1979). *Disorders of sexual desire*. New York: Brunner/Mazel.

Karayiorgou, M., & Gogos, J.A. (2011). *Human genetic approaches*. Retrieved November 30, 2011 from http://schizophreniaresearch.columbia.edu/content/research-program-0

Karim, S., Saeed, K., Rana, M. H., Mubbashar, M., Jenkins, R. (2004). Pakistan mental health country profile. *International Review of Psychiatry*, 16, 83–92.

Karpelowsky, B., & Edwards, D. J. A. (2005). Trauma, imagery and the therapeutic relationship: Langu's story. *Journal of Psychology in Africa*, 15(2), 185–195.

Kasayira, J. M., & Chireshe, R. (2010). Poverty and HIV/AIDS in Sub-Saharan Africa: Implications for psychological well-being. *Journal of Psychology in Africa*, 20(2), 203–208.

Kasset, J. A., Gwirtsman, H. E., Kaye, W. H., Brandt, H. A., & Jimerson, D. C. (1992). Pattern of onset of bulimic symptoms in anorexia nervosa. *Archives of General Psychiatry*, 49, 132–138.

Kavanagh, D. J. (1992). Recent developments in expressed emotion in Schizophrenia. *British Journal of Psychiatry*, 160, 601–620.

Kay, S.R. (1991). *Positive and negative syndromes in Schizophrenia: assessment and research*. New York: Bruner/Mazel.

Kaye, W. H., Barbarich, B. S., Putnam, B. S., Gendall, K. A., Fernstrom, J., Fernstrom, M. et al. (2003). Anxiolytic effects of acute tryptophan depletion in anorexia nervosa. *International Journal of Eating Disorders*, 33, 825–838.

Kaye, W. H., Weltzin, T. E., Hsu, L. K. G., Mcconaha, C. W., & Bolton, B. (1993). Amount of calories retained after binge eating and vomiting. *American Journal of Psychiatry*, 150(6), 969–971.

Kazadi, N. J. B., Moosa, M. Y. H., & Jeenah, F. Y. (2008). Factors associated with relapse in Schizophrenia. *South African Journal of Psychiatry*, 14(2), 52–62.

Kearney, C. A. (2010). *Casebook in childhood behaviour disorders* (4th ed.). Belmont: Wadsworth Cengage Learning.

Keel, P. K., Doer, D. J., Eddy, K. T., Franko, D., Charatan, D. L., & Herzog, D. B. (2003). Predictors of mortality in eating disorders. *Archives of General Psychiatry*, 60, 179–183.

Keeney, B. P. (1983). *Aesthetics of change*. New York: Guilford.

Keith, S. J., Regier, D. A., & Rae, D. S. (1991).Schizophrenic disorders. In L. N. Robins & D. A. Regier (Eds.), *Psychiatric Disorders in America* (pp. 33–52). New York: Free Press.

Kekae-Moletsane, M. (2004). The efficacy of the Rorshach among black learners in South Africa. Unpublished PhD Thesis. Pretoria: University of Pretoria.

Keller, M. C., Neale, M. C., & Kendler, K. S. (2007). Different negative life events are associated with different patterns of depressive symptoms. *American Journal of Psychiatry*, 164, 1521–1529.

Kendler, K. S., & Gardner, C. O. (1998). Boundaries of major depression: An evaluation of DSM–IV criteria. *American Journal of Psychiatry*, 155, 172.

Kendler, K. S., Karkowski-Shuman, L., & Walsh, D. (1996). Age of onset in Schizophrenia and risk of illness in relatives. *British Journal of Psychiatry*, 169, 213–218.

Kendler, K. S., Kessler, R. C., Walters, E. E., MacLean, C., Neale, M. C., Heath, A. C., et al. (1995). Stressful life events, genetic liability, and onset of an episode of major depression in women. *American Journal of Psychiatry*, 152, 833–842.

Kendler, K. S., MacLean, C., Neale, M., Kessler, R., Heath, A., & Eaves, L. (1991). The genetic epidemiology of bulimia nervosa. *American Journal of Psychiatry*, 148, 1627–1637.

Kendler, K. S., Neale, M. C., Kessler, R. C., Heath, A. C., & Eaves, L. J. (1993). A test of the equal–environment assumption in twin studies of psychiatric illness. *Archives of General Psychiatry*, 49, 257–266.

Kernberg, O. F. & Michels, R. (2009). Borderline personality disorder. *American Journal of Psychiatry*, 166, 505–508.

Kessler, R. C., Angermeyer, M., Anthony, J. C., et al. (2007). Lifetime prevalence and age-of-onset distributions of mental disorders in the World Health Organization's World Mental Health Survey Initiative. *World Psychiatry*, 6(3), 168–176.

Kessler, R. C., Keller, M. B., Wittchen, H. U. (2001). The epidemiology of generalized anxiety disorder. *Psychiatric Clinics of North America*, 24, 19–40.

Kessler, R. C., McGonagle, K. A., Zhao, S., et al (1994). Lifetime and 12-month prevalence of DSM-III-R major depressive disorder in the general population: Results from the US national comorbidity survey. *British Journal of Psychiatry*, 168(30), 17–30.

Kessler, R.C., & Wittchen, H.U. (2002). Patterns and correlates of generalized anxiety disorder in community samples. *Journal of Clinical Psychiatry*, 63(Suppl 8), 4–10.

Kety, S. S., Wender, P. H., Jacobsen, B., Ingraham, L. T., Jansson, L., Faber, B., & Kinney, D.K. (1994). Mental illness in the biological and adoptive relatives of schizophrenic adoptees: Replication of the Copenhagen study in the rest of Denmark. *American Journal of Psychiatry*, 144, 934–938.

Keyes, C. L. M., & Lopez, S. J. (2005). Toward a science of mental health: Positive directions in diagnosis and interventions. In C. R. Snyder & S. J. Lopez (Eds.), *Handbook of positive psychology*. Oxford: Oxford University Press, 45–62.

Keyes, C.L.M. (1998). Social well-being. *Social Psychology Quarterly*, 61, 121–140.

Keyes, C.L.M. (2002). The mental health continuum: from languishing to flourishing in life. *Journal of Health and Social Behavior*, 43, 207–222.

Keys, A., Brozek, J., Hsu, L. K. G., McConoha, C. E., & Bolton, B. (1950). *The biology of human starvation*. Minneapolis: University of Minnesota Press.

Khumalo, I. P., Wissing, M. P., & Temane, Q. M. (2008). Exploring the validity of the VIA-Inventory of Strengths in an African Context. *Journal of Psychology in Africa*, 18(1), 133–142.

Kieling, C., Kieling, R. R., Rohde, L. A., Frick, P. J., Moffitt. T., Nigg, J. T., Tannock, R., & Castellanos, F. X. (2010). The age at onset of Attention-deficit/Hyperactivity Disorder. *The American Journal of Psychiatry*, 167, 14–16.

Killen, J. D., Taylor, C. B., Telch, M. J., Saylor, K. E., Maron, D. J., & Robinson, T. N. (1986). Self-induced vomiting and laxative and diuretic use among teenagers: Precursors of the binge–purge syndrome. *Journal of the American Medical Association*, 255, 1447–1449.

Kim, D. (2008). Blues from the neighborhood? Neighborhood characteristics and depression. *Epidemiologic reviews*, 30, 101–117.

Kim, J. H. & Lennon, S. J. (2007). Mass Media and Self-Esteem, Body Image, and Eating Disorder Tendencies. *Clothing and Textiles Research Journal*, 25(1), 3–23.

Kimmel, M. (2000). *The gendered society*. New York: Oxford University Press.

King, M. B. (1993). Cultural aspects of eating disorders. *International Review of Psychiatry*, 5, 205–216.

Kirsten, D. K. & Du Plessis, W. F. (2008). Lived experiences of subclinical eating disorder: Female students' perceptions. *Journal of Psychology in Africa*, 18(4), 561–572.

Klein, D. N., Shankman, S. A., & McFarland, B. R. (2006). Classification of mood disorders. In D. J. Stein, D. Kupfer, & A. Schatzberg (Eds.). *The American Psychiatric Publishing textbook of mood disorders*. New York: American Psychiatric Publishing, 17–32.

Klimidis, S., & Tokgoz, A. (n.d.). *A transcultural perspective on the Mini Mental State Examination*. Victorian Transcultural Psychiatry Unit. Retrieved October 27, 2008 from http://www.tpu.org.au/docs/mmse/mini_mental_document.pdf

Knox, P. L., & Lichtenberg, J. W. (2005). *Depression*. Encyclopedia of school psychology. http://www.sage-ereference.com/schoolpsychology/Article_n76.html. Retrieved on 20 March 2009.

Koen, L., Niehaus, D. J. H., De Jong, G., Muller, J. E., & Jordaan, E. (2006). Morphological features in a Xhosa Schizophrenia population. *Biomed Central Psychiatry*, 6(1), 47.

Kope, T. & Sack, W. (1987). Anorexia nervosa in South-East Asian refugees: A report on three cases. *Journal of the American Academy of Child and Adolescent Psychiatry*, 26, 795–7.

Krahn, L. B. (2008). Looking Toward DSM-V: Should Factitious Disorder become a subtype of Somatoform Disorder? *Psychosomatics*, 49, 277–282.

Krassoievitch, M., Perez-Rincon, H., & Suarez, P. (1982). Correlation entre les hallucinations visuelles et auditives dans une population de schophrenes Mexicains. *Confrontations Psychiatriques*, 15, 149–162.

Kruger, C. S. (2007). Dissociation – a preliminary contextual model. *South African Journal of Psychiatry*, 13(1), 13–17, 20–21.

Kruger, H. S., Puoane, T., Senekal, M., & Van der Merwe, T. (2005). Obesity in South Africa: challenges for government and health professionals. *Public Health Nutrition*, 8, 491–500.

Kruger, H. S., Venter, C. S., & Vorster, H. H. (2001). Obesity in African women in the North West Province, South Africa is associated with an increased risk of non-communicable diseases: The THUSA study. *British Journal of Nutrition*, 86, 733–740.

Kruger, H. S., Venter, C. S., Vorster, H. H., & Margetts, B. M. (2002). Physical inactivity is the major determinant of obesity in black women in the North West province, South Africa: The THUSA study. *Nutrition*, 18, 422–427.

Kua, E. S. (1986). A cross-cultural study of the possession-trance in Singapore. *Australian NZ Journal of Psychiatry*, 20(3), 361–364.

Kuepper, R., Van Os, J., Lieb, R., Wittchen, H. U., Höfler, M., & Henquet, C. (2011). Continued cannabis use and risk of incidence and persistence of psychotic symptoms: 10-year follow-up cohort study. *British Medical Journal Research*, 342, d738.

Kuhl, J., Kazén, M., & Koole, S.L. (2006). Putting self-regulation into practice: A user's manual. *Applied psychology: An international review*, 55(3), 408-418.

Kwom, J. S., Kim, Y. M., Chang , C. G., Park, B. K., & Yoon, D. J. (2000). Three-year follow-up of women with the sole diagnosis of depressive personality disorder: subsequent development of dysthymia and major depression. *American Journal of Psychiatry,* 157(12), 1966–1972.

Labe, D. (2005). Psychotherapy for Posttraumatic Stress Disorder in a young rape survivor: A case study. *Journal of Psychology in Africa*, 15(2), 177–184.

Labre, M. P. (2002). Adolescent boys and the Muscular Male Body ideal. *Journal of Adolescent Health*, 30(4), 233–242.

Lacey, J. H. (1992). The treatment demand for bulimia: A catchment area report of referral rates and demography. *Psychiatric Bulletin*, 16, 203–205.

Ladouceur, C. D., Dahl, R. E., Williamson, D. E., Birmaher, B., Ryan, N. D., & Casey, B. J. (2005). Altered emotional processing in pediatric anxiety, depression and comorbid anxiety–depression. *Journal of Abnormal Child Psychology*, 33 (2), 165–177.

Laing, R. D. (1969). *The divided self*. New York: Pantheon.

Laing, R. D. (1976). A critique of Kallmann's and Slater's henetic theory of Schizophrenia. In R. I. Evans & R. D. Laing (Eds.). *The man and his ideas*. New York: Dutton.

Laing, R. D., & Esterson, A. (1964). *Sanity, madness, and the family*. London: Tavistock.

Lake, A., Staiger, P., & Glowinski, H. (2000). Effect of Western culture on women's attitudes to eating and perceptions of body shape. *International Journal of Eating Disorders*, 27, 83–89.

Lambley, P. (1980). *The psychology of apartheid*. London: Secker & Warburg.

Lamiell, J. T. (2007). On sustaining critical discourse with mainstream personality investigators: Problems and prospects. *Theory & Psychology*, 17(2), 169–185.

Landon, T. M., & Barlow, D. H. (2004). Cognitive-behavioral treatment for panic disorder: Current status. *Journal of Psychiatric Practice*, 10(4), 211–226.

Langer, E. (2005). Well-being: Mindfulness versus positive evaluation. In C. R. Snyder & S. J. Lopez (Eds.), *Handbook of positive psychology*. Oxford: Oxford University Press, 214–230.

Langley, G. C., & Klopper, H. (2005). Trust as a foundation for the therapeutic intervention for patients with borderline personality disorder. *Journal of Psychiatric and Mental Health Nursing*, 12(1), 23–32.

Larsen, R. J. & Buss, D. M. (2002). *Personality psychology*. Boston: McGraw-Hill.

Lasiuk, G. C. & Hegadoren, K. M. (2007). The effects of estradiol on central serotonergic systems and its relationship to mood in women. *Biological Research for Nursing*, 9(2),147–160.

Lauman, E. O., Paik, A., Glasser, D. B., Kang, J. H., Wang, T. & Levinson, B. (2006). A cross-national study of subjective sexual well-being among older women and men: Findings from the global study of sexual attitudes and behaviors. *Archives of Sexual Behavior*, 35(2), 145–161.

Lazarus, R. S. & Folkman, S. (1984). *Stress, appraisal and coping*. New York: Springer.

Lazarus, S. (1988). The role of the psychologist in South African society: In search of an appropriate community psychology. Unpublished doctoral thesis, University of Cape Town, Cape Town.

Le Grange, D., Louw, J., Breen A., & Katzman, M. A. (2004). The meaning of 'self-starvation' in impoverished black adolescents in South Africa. *Culture, Medicine and Psychiatry*, 28, 439–461.

Le Grange, D., Telch, C.F., & Tibbs, J. (1998). Eating attitudes and behaviours in 1435 South African Caucasian and non–Caucasian college students. *American Journal of Psychiatry*, 155, 250–254.

Lechner, S. (2009). Benefit finding. In S. Lopez (Ed.), *The encyclopedia of positive psychology*. Chichester: Blackwell, 99–102.

Lee, S. W. (2005a). *Generalized Anxiety Disorder*. Encyclopedia of school psychology. http://www.sage-ereference.com/schoolpsychology/Article_n123.html. Retrieved on 20 March 2009.

Lee, S. W. (2005b). *Separation Anxiety Disorder*. Encyclopedia of School Psychology. Sage Publications. http://www.sage-ereference.com/schoolpsychology/Article_n123.html. Retrieved 20 March 2009.

Leff, J. (1981). *Psychiatry around the globe: A transcultural view*. New York: Marcel Dekker.

Leff, J., Wig, N. N., Bedi, H., Menon, D. K., Kuipers, L., Korten, A., Ernberg, G., Day, R., Sartorius, N., & Jablenski, A. (1990). Relatives' expressed emotion and the course of Schizophrenia in Chandigarh. *British Journal of Psychiatry*, 156, 351–356.

Leibowitz-Levy, S. (2005). The role of brief-term interventions with South African child trauma survivors. *Journal of Psychology in Africa*, 15(2), 155–163.

Lemonick, M. D., & Alice, P. (2007). The science of addiction. *Time*.

Lenger, V., De Villiers, C., & Louw, S. J. (1996). Informant questionnaires as screening measures to detect dementia. A pilot study in the South African context. *South African Medical Journal*, 86(6), 737–741.

Leon, G. R., Fulkerson, J. A., Perry, C. L., & Early-Zald, M. B. (1995). Prospective analysis of personality and behavioural vulnerabilities and gender influences in the later development of disordered eating. *Journal of Abnormal Psychology*, 104, 140–149.

Lerner, R. M. (2006). Resilience as an attribute of the developmental system: Comments on the papers of Professors Masten & Wachs. *Annals of the New York Academy of Sciences*, 1094, 40–51.

Lesolang-Pitje, N. (2003). African traditional healing and psychotherapy. In N. S. Madu (Ed.), *Contributions to psychotherapy conference in Africa* (pp. 207–213). Turfloop: University of the North.

Lester, D., & Akande, A. (1997). Patterns of depression in Xhosa and Yoruba students. *The Journal of Social Psychology*, 137 (6), 782–783.

Leutscher, P. D., Lagging, M., Buhl, M. R., Pedersen, C., Norkrans, G., Langeland, N., Mørch, K., Färkkilä, M., Hjerrild, S., Hellstrand, K., Bech, P. (2010). Evaluation of depression as a risk factor for treatment failure in chronic hepatitis C. *Hepatology*, 52(2), 430–435.

Levine, M. P., & Troiden, R. R. (1988). The myth of sexual compulsivity. *The Journal of Sex Research*, 25, 347–363.

Levy, L. H. & Derby, J. F. (1992). Bereavement support groups: Who joins; who does not; and why. *American Journal of Community Psychology*, 20, 649–662.

Lewinsohn, P. M. (1974). A behavioral approach to depression. In R. M. Friedman, & M. M. Katz (Eds). *The psychology of depression: Contemporary theory and research*. New York: Wiley.

Lewinsohn, P. M., & Hoberman, H. M. (1982). Depression. In A. S. Bellack, M. Hersen, & A. E. Kazdin (Eds). *International handbook of behavior modification and therapy*. New York: Plenum, 126–148.

Lewis, C. M., Levinson, D. F., Wise, L. H., DeLisi, L. E., Straub, R. E., Hovatta, I , et al. (2003). Genome scan meta-analysis of Schizophrenia and Bipolar Disorder, Part II: Schizophrenia. *U.S. National Library of Medicine National Institutes of Health*, 73(1), 34–48.

Lewis, D. A. & Levitt, P. (2002). Review of Schizophrenia as a disorder of Neurodevelopment. *Annual Review of Neuroscience*, 25, 409–432.

Lewis, R. & Frydenburg, E. (2002). Concomitants of failure to cope: What we should teach adolescents about coping. *British Journal of Educational Psychology*, 72, 419–431.

Lewis-Fernández, R., & Kleinman, A. (1995). Cultural psychiatry: Theoretical, clinical, and research issues. *The Psychiatric Clinics of North America*, 18,3, 433–48.

Lezak, M. D. (1995). *Neuropsychological assessment* (3rd ed.). New York: Oxford University Press.

Lidz, T., Fleck, S., & Cornelison, A. R. (1965). *Schizophrenia and the family*. New York: International Universities Press.

Liebowitz, S. F. (1985). Brain neurotransmitters and appetite regulation. *Psychopharmacology Bulletin*, 21, 415.

Lilienfeld, L. R., Kaye, W. H., Greenco, C. G., Merikangas, K. R., Plotnicov, K., et al. (1998). A controlled family study of anorexia nervosa and bulimia nervosa: Psychiatric disorders in first-degree relatives and effects of proband comorbidity. *Archives of General Psychiatry*, 55, 603–610.

Lim, L., Tze, P. N., Hong, C. C., Peak, C. C., Won, V., Lee, T., Fones, C., & Ee, H. K. (2005). Generalised Anxiety Disorder in Singapore: Prevalence, co-morbidity and risk factors in a multi-ethnic population. *Social Psychiatry and Psychiatric Epidemiology*, 40(12), 972–979.

Lindquist, P., & Allebeck, P. (1990). Schizophrenia and crime: A longitudinal follow-up of 644 schizophrenics in Stockholm. *British Journal of Psychiatry*, 157, 345–350

Lindsey, K. P., & Paul, G. L. (1989). Involuntary commitments to public mental institutions: Issues involving the overrepresentation of blacks and assessment of relevant functioning. *Psychological Bulletin*, 106, 171–183.

Linley, P. A., Joseph, S., Harrington, S., & Wood, A. M. (2006). Positive psychology: Past, present, and (possible) future. *The Journal of Positive Psychology*, 1(1), 3–16.

Lippi, G., Smit, D. J., Jordaan, J.C. & Roos, J. L. (2009). Suicide risk in Schizophrenia – a follow-up study after 20 years Part 1: Outcome and associated social factors. *South African Journal of Psychology*, 15(3), 56–62.

Lipsitz, J. D., Barlow, D. H., Mannuzza, S., Hofmann, S. G., & Fyer, A. J. (2002). Clinical features for four DSM-IV specific phobia subtypes. *Journal of Nervous and Mental Disease*, 190, 471–478.

Littlewood, R., & Lipsedge, M. (1997). *Aliens and alienists: Ethnic minorities and psychiatry* (3rd ed.). London: Routledge.

Livesley, J. W. (2001). Conceptual and taxonomic issues. In W. J. Livesley (Ed.). *Handbook of personality disorders*. New York: Guilford, 3–38.

Livesley, J. W. (2001). *Handbook of personality disorders: Theory, research, and treatment*. New York: Guilford.

Lochner, C. (2003). Exploring the genetics of anxiety disorders. *Science in Africa*. http://www.scienceinafrica.co.za/2003/june/genetics.htm. Retrieved on 28 March 2009.

London, 1999.

Lopata, H. Z. (1993). The support systems of American urban widows. In W. Stroebe, M. S. Stroebe, & R. O. Hanson. *Handbook of bereavement, theory, research and intervention*. New York: Cambridge University Press.

Lopez, B., & Silverman, W. K. (2004). *Anxiety disorders in children*. Encyclopedia of applied developmental science. http://www.sage-ereference.com/applieddevscience/Article_n35.html. retrieved on 20 March 2009.

Lopez, S. J., Floyd, R. K., Ulven, J. C., & Snyder, C. R. (2000). Hope therapy: Helping clients build a house of hope. In C. R. Snyder (Ed.), *Handbook of hope: Theory, measures, and applications*. San Diego, CA: Academic Press, 123–150.

Lopez, S. R., Nelson, K. A., Snyder, K. S., & Mintz, J. (1999). Attributions and affective reactions of family members and course of Schizophrenia. *Journal of Abnormal Psychology*, 108, 307–317.

Louw, D. A. & Allan, A. (1996). Forensic psychology in South Africa. *American Journal of Forensic Psychology*, 14, 1–13.

Louw, D. A. & Edwards, D. J. A. (1993). *Psychology: An introduction for students in Southern Africa*. Johannesburg: Lexicon.

Louw, J. (1997a). Regulating professional conduct. Part I: Codes of ethics of national psychology associations in South Africa. *South African Journal of Psychology*, 27(3), 183–188.

Louw, J. (1997b). Regulating professional conduct. Part II: The professional board for psychology in South Africa. *South African Journal of Psychology*, 27(3), 189–195.

Love, B. (1995). *Encyclopedia of unusual sex practices*. Fort Lee NJ: Barricade Books.

Lowe, P. A. & Raad, J. M. (2007). *Anxiety. Encyclopedia of Educational Psychology*. Sage Publications. http://www.sage-ereference.com/educationalpsychology/Article_n12.html. Retrieved 20 March 2009.

Lucas, A. R., Beard, C. M., O'Fallon, W. M., & Kurlan, L. T. (1990). 50-year trends in the incidence of anorexia nervosa in Rochester Minn.: A population-based study. *American Journal of Psychiatry*, 148, 917–922.

Ludwig, A. (1972). Hysteria: A neurobiological theory. *Archives of General Psychiatry*, 27, 771–777.

Lund, C., Kleintjes, S., Kakuma, R., Flisher, A. J., & the MHaPP Research Programme Consortium. (2010). Public sector mental health systems in South Africa: Interprovincial comparisons and policy implications. *Social Psychiatry and Psychiatric Epidemiology*, 45(3), 393–404.

Luria, A. R. (1966). *Higher cortical functions in man*. New York: Basic Books.

Lyketsos, C. G., & Olin, J. (2002). Depression in Alzheimer's disease: Overview and treatment. *Biological Psychiatry*, 52, 243–252.

Maatz, K. R. (2005). The alcoholic offender – significance for determination of guilt. A legal view. *Nervenarzt*, 76(11), 1389–1401.

MacDonald, A. W., & Schulz, S. C. (2009). What we know: Findings that every theory of Schizophrenia should explain. *Schizophrenia Bulletin*, 35(3): 493–508. First published online: March 27, 2009.

Maddux, J. E. (2008). Positive psychology and the illness ideology: Toward a positive clinical psychology. *Applied Psychology: An International Review*, 57, 54–70. doi: 10.1111/j.1464-0597.2008.00354.x

Maddux, J.E. (2005). Stopping the 'Madness'. Positive psychology and the deconstruction of the illness ideology and the DSM. In C. R. Snyder & S. J. Lopez (Eds.), *Handbook of positive psychology*. Oxford: Oxford University Press, 13–25.

Madu, N. S. (2003). Is psychotherapy a basic need for human? With special reference to Africa. In N. S. Madu (Ed.), *Contributions to psychotherapy conference in Africa*. Turfloop: University of the North, 136–142.

Madu, S. N., & Roos, J. J. (2006). Depression among mothers with preterm infants and their stress-coping strategies. *Social Behavior and Personality*, 34(7), 877–890.

Maes, S., & Karoly, P. (2005). Self-regulation and intervention in physical health and illness: A review. *Applied Psychology: An International Review*, 54(2), 267–299.

Mailis-Gagnon, A., & Israelson, D. (2003). *Beyond pain: Making the mind-body connection*. Toronto: Viking Canada/Penguin Books.

Makkar, S. & Grisham, J. (2011). The predictors and contents of post-event processing in Social Anxiety. *Cognitive Therapy and Research*, 35(2), 118–133.

Malik, K. (2000). Culture and emotions: Depression among Pakistanis. In C. Squire (Ed.), *Culture in psychology*. New York: Routledge, 147–162.

Malindi, J.M., & Theron, L.C. (2010). The hidden resilience of street youth. *South African Journal of Psychology*, 40(3), 318–326.

Manderscheid R. W., Ryff C. D., Freeman E. J., McKnight-Eily L. R., Dhingra S., Strine T. W. (2010). Evolving definitions of mental illness and wellness. *Prev Chronic Dis*, 7(1):A19.

Mann, L., Radford, M., Burnett, P., Ford, S., Bond, M., Leung, K., Nakamura, H., Vaughan, G., & Yang, K. (1998). Cross-cultural differences in self-reported decision-making style and confidence. *International Journal of Psychology*, 33(5), 325–335.

Manson, S., Beals, J., O'Nell, T., Piasecki, J., Bechtold, D., Keane, E., & Jones, M. (1996). Wounded spirits, ailing hearts: PTSD and related disorders among American Indians. In A. J. Marsella, M. J. Friedman, E. T. Gerrity, & R. M. Scurfield (Eds). *Ethnocultural aspects of posttraumatic stress disorder*. Washington: American Psychiatric Press, 255 - 283.

Marcus, J., Hans, S. L., Nagier, S. Auerbach, J. G., Mirsky, A., & Aubrey, A. (1987). Review of the NIMH Israeli Kibbutz-City and the Jerusalem infant development study. *Schizophrenia Bulletin*, 13, 425–438.

Maree, D. J. F., Maree, M., & Collins, C. (2008). The relationship between hope and goal achievement. *Journal of Psychology in Africa*, 18(1), 65–74.

Markov, I. S. & Berrios, G. E. (1992).The meaning of insight in clinical psychiatry. *The British Journal of Psychiatry*, 160, 850–860.

Marrazzi, M. A., & Luby, E. D. (1986). An auto-addiction model of chronic anorexia nervosa. *International Journal of Eating Disorders*, 5, 191–208.

Martinez, J. (2010). *Tiger Woods sex scandal: Golfer being treated for sex addiction at Missisipi rehab, says author*. Retrieved 2011, from NYDailyNews.com.

Mash, E. J. & Wolfe, D.A. (2005). *Abnormal child psychology*. Belmont: Thomson Wadsworth.

Mash, E.J. & Wolfe, D.A. (2010). *Abnormal child psychology* (4th ed.). Belmont, CA: Wadsworth Cengage Learning.

Masse, J. J. & McNeil, C. B. (2008). *Oppositional Defiant Disorder*. Encyclopedia of counseling. http://www.sage-ereference.com/counseling/Article_n105.html. Retrieved on 20 March 2009.

Masten, A. S. (2001). Ordinary magic: Resilience processes in development. *American Psychologist*, 56, 227–238.

Masten, A. S., & Obradovic, J. (2006). Competence and resilience in development. *Annals of the New York Academy of Sciences*, 1094, 13–27.

Masters, W. H., & Johnson, V. E. (1976). Principles of the new sex therapy. *American Journal of Psychiatry*, 133(5), 548–554.

Matthews, A. & MacLeod, C. (1994). Cognitive approaches to emotion and emotional disorders. *Annual Review of Clinical Psychology*, 1, 197–225.

May, J. (1998). *Poverty and inequality in South Africa*. Report prepared for the Office of the Executive Deputy President and the Inter-Ministerial Committee for Poverty and Inequality. Durban: Praxis Publishing Ltd.

Mayberg, H. S. (2007). Brain pathway may underlie depression. *Scientific American*, 17(4), 26–31.

Mayer, J. D., Caruso, D., & Salovey, P. (1999). Emotional intelligence meets traditional standards for an intelligence. *Intelligence*, 27, 267–298.

Mayes, S. D., Calhoun, S. L., & Crites, D. L. (2001). Does DSM-IV Asperger's disorder exist? *Journal of Abnormal Child Psychology*, 29(3), 263–271.

Mbanga, N. I., Niehaus, D. J., Mzamo, N. C., Wessels, C. J., Allen, A., Emsley, R. A., & Stein, D. J. (2002). Attitudes towards and beliefs about Schizophrenia in Xhosa families with affected probands. *Curationis*, 25, 69–73.

McCann, U. D., Rossiter, E. M., King, R. J., & Agras, W. S. (1991). Nonpurging bulimia: A distinct subtype of bulimia nervosa. *International Journal of Eating Disorders*, 10, 679–687.

McClaren, E. & Winsler, A. (2005). *Asperger syndrome*. Encyclopedia of Human Development. http://www.sage-ereference.com/humandevelopment/Article_n53.html. retrieved on 20 March 2009.

McConaghy N. (2005). Time to abandon the gay/heterosexual dichotomy? *Archives of Sexual Behavior*, 34(1),1–2.

McCullough, M. E., & Van Oyen Witvliet, C. (2005). The psychology of forgiveness. In C. R. Snyder & S. J. Lopez (Eds.), *Handbook of positive psychology*. Oxford: Oxford University Press, 446–458.

McDermott, R. (2005). The great arch of unimagined bridges: Integrative play therapy with an abused child. *Journal of Psychology in Africa*, 15(2), 165–175.

McGlashan, T. H., & Fenton, W. S. (1991). Classical subtypes for Schizophrenia: Literature review for DSM-III. *Schizophrenia Bulletin*, 17, 609–622.

McGrath, J., Saha, S., Welham, J., Saadi, O. E., MacCauley, C., & Chant, D. (2004). A systematic review of the incidence of Schizophrenia: The distribution of rates and the influence of sex, urbanicity, migrant status and methodology. *BMC Medicine*, 2, 13.

McGue, M. (1993). From proteins to cognitions: The behavioral genetics of alcoholism. In R. Plomin & G. E. McClearn (Eds). *Nature, nurture, and psychology*. Washington: American Psychological Association Press.

McGuffin, P. & Katz, R. (1993). Genes, adversity and depression. In R. Plomin & G. E. McClearn (Eds). *Nature, nurture and psychology*. Washington DC: American Psychology Association, 217–230.

McGuffin, P. & Martin, N. (1999). Behaviour and genes. *British Medical Journal*, 3(19), 37–40.

Mcguire, P. K., Shah, G. M. S., & Murray, R. M. (1993). Increased blood flow in Broca's area during auditory hallucinations in Schizophrenia. *Lancet*, 342, 703–706.

Medical Research Council. (2006). Alcohol and drug abuse module. In *Healthinfo*, SA, editor.

Mednick, S. A., & Schulsinger, F. (1968). Some premorbid characteristics related to breakdown in children with schizophrenic mothers. *Journal of Psychiatric Research*, 6, 267–291.

Mednick, S. A., Huttonen, M. O., & Machon, R. A. (1994). Prenatal influenza infections and adult Schizophrenia. *Schizophrenia Bulletin*, 20, 263–268.

Meehl, P. E. (1962). Schizotaxia, schizotypia, schizophrenia. *American Psychologist*, 17, 827–838.

Menezes, N. M., Georgiades, K., & Boyle, M. H. (2011). The influence of immigrant status and concentration on psychiatric disorder in Canada: A multi-level analysis. *Psychological Medicine*, Cambridge University, 41, 2221–2231.

Mental State Examination. Victorian Transcultural Psychiatry Unit & Centre for International Mental Health. http://www.vtpu.org.au/docs/mmse/mini_mental_document.pdf. Retrieved on 28 August 2008.

Merskey, H. & Bogduk, N. (Eds). (1986). Pain terms, a current list with definitions and notes on usage. International Association for the Study of Pain. *Classification of chronic pain* (2nd Ed.), 209–214.

Meyer, A. (1951/2). *Collected Papers*. Winters E. Baltimore (Ed.). Baltimore: Johns Hopkins Press.

Meyer, C., Blisset, J., & Oldfield, C. (2001). Sexual orientation and eating psychopathology: The role of masculinity and femininity. *International Journal of Eating Disorders*, 29, 413–318.

Meyer, W. F., Moore, C., & Viljoen, H. G. (1993). *Personality theories – from Freud to Frankl*. Johannesburg: Lexicon.

Meyer, W., Moore, C., & Viljoen, H. (2002). *Personology. From individual to ecosystem*. Cape Town: Heinemann Publishers.

Miller, C. A. & Golden, N. H. (2010). An Introduction to Eating Disorders: Clinical Presentation, Epidemiology, and Prognosis. *Nutrition in Clinical Practice*, 25, 110–115.

Miller, M. N. & Pumarierga, A. J. (2001). Culture and eating disorders: A historical and cross-cultural review. *Psychiatry*, 64, 93–110.

Millon, T. & Davis, R. D. (1996). *Disorders of personality: DSM-IV and beyond*. New York: Wiley.

Millon, T. & Everly, G. S., Jr. (1985). *Personality and its disorders*. New York: Wiley.

Millon, T. (1969). *Modern psychopathology: A biosocial approach to maladaptive learning and functioning*. Philadelphia: W.B. Saunders.

Millon, T. (2004). *Personality disorders in modern life* (2nd ed.). New York: Wiley.

Millon, T., Davis, R., Millon, C., Escovar, L., & Meagher, S. (2000). *Personality disorders in modern life*. New York: Wiley.

Minde, M. (1974). The history of mental health services in South Africa: Part I. In the days of the Dutch East India Company. *South African Medical Journal*, 48, 1270–1272.

Mineka, S. (1985). Animal models of anxiety based disorders: Their usefulness and limitations. In A. H. Tuma & J. Maser (Eds.). *Anxiety and the anxiety disorders*. Hillsdale: Erlbaum, 199–244.

Minuchin, S., Baker, L., Rosman, B., Milman, L., & Todd, T. (1975). A conceptual model of psychosomatic illness in children. *Archives of General Psychiatry*, 32, 1031–1038.

Minuchin, S., Rosman, B. L., & Baker, L. (1978). *Psychosomatic families: Anorexia nervosa in context*. Cambridge, MA: Harvard University Press.

Moldin, S. O. (1997). The maddening hunt for madness genes. *Nature Genetics*, 17, 127–129.

Moletsane, M. (2011). Indigenous African personality and health theories. Paper presented at a seminar, at the University of Western Cape, Department of Psychology.

Money, J. (1984). Paraphilias: Phenomenology and classification. *American Journal of Psychotherapy*, 38(2), 164–179.

Money, J. (1988). *Venuses penuses: Sexology, sexosophy, and exigency theory*. New York: Prometheus Books.

Monteleone, P. (2001). Endocrine disturbances and psychiatric disorders. *Current Opinion in Psychiatry*, 14(6), 605–10.

Moodley, R., & Sutherland, P. (2010). Psychic retreats in other places: Clients who seek healing with traditional healers and psychotherapists. *Counselling Psychology Quarterly*, 23(3), 267–282. doi: 10.1080/09515070.2010.505748

Moore, S. C. & Oaksford, M. (2002). *Emotional cognition: From brain to behaviour*. Amsterdam: John Benjamin's Publishing Company.

Moosa, M. Y. H., Jeenah, F. Y. A. (2010). A review of the applications for involuntary admissions made to the Mental Health Review Boards by institutions in Gauteng in 2008. *South African Journal of Psychology*, 16(4), 125–130.

Moreno, F. A., Rowe D. C., Kaiser, B., Chase, D., Michaels, T., Gelernter, J., Delgado, P. L. (2002). Association between a serotonin transporter promoter region polymorphism and mood response during tryptophan depletion. *Molecular Psychiatry*, 7(2), 213–216.

Morgan, W. G. (1995). Origin and history of the Thematic Apperception Test images. *Journal of Personality Assessment*, 65, 237–252.

Moser, P. W. (1998). Double vision: Why do we never match up to our mind's ideal? *Self Magazine*, January, 51–52.

Mosotho, L., Louw, D., & Calitz, F. J. W. (2011).Schizophrenia among Sesotho speakers in South Africa. *African Journal of Psychiatry*, 14, 50–55.

Mould, J., Grobler, A. A., Odendaal, D. C., & De Jager, L. (2011). Ethnic differences in age of onset and prevalence of disordered eating attitudes and behaviours: A school-based South African study. *South African Journal of Clinical Nutrition*, 24(3), 137–141.

Mowrer, O. H. (1939). A stimulus–response analysis of anxiety and its role as reinforcing agent. *Psychological Review*, 46, 553–566.

Murphy, A., & Janeke, H. C. (2009). The relationship between thinking styles and emotional intelligence: An exploratory study. *South African Journal of Psychology*, 39(3), 357–375.

Murstein, B. I. (1972). A thematic test and the Rorschach in predicting marital choice. *Journal of Personality Assessment*, 36(3), 213–217.

Myer, L., Ehrlich, R. I., & Susser, E. S. (2004). Social epidemiology in South Africa. *Epidemiological Review*, 26(1), 112–123.

Naidoo, A. V. (1996). Challenging the hegemony of Eurocentric Psychology. *Journal of Community and Health Sciences*, 2(2), 9–16.

Narcotics Anonymous, Inc. (2012). *Narcotics anonymous world services*. Retrieved 2012, from www.NA.org/

National Institute on Drug Abuse (NIDA). (1999). *Principles of drug addiction treatment: A research-based guide*.

National Institute on Drug Abuse (NIDA). (2007). *Drugs, brains and behaviour: The science of addiction*.

Ndetei, D. M., & Singh, A. (1983). Hallucinations in Kenyan schizophrenic patients. *Acta Psychiatrica Scandinavica*, 67, 144–147.

Ndetei, D. M., & Vadher, A. (1984). A cross-cultural study of the frequencies of Schneider's first-rank symptoms of Schizophrenia. *Acta Psychiatrica Scandinavica*, 70, 540–544.

Ndetei, D. M., Khasakhala, L., Kuria, M., Mutiso, V., Ongecha, F. A., & Kokonya, D. (2009). The prevalence of mental disorders in adults in different level general medical facilities in Kenya: A cross-sectional study. *Annals of General Psychiatry*, 8(1). Available online at http://www.annals-general-psychiatry.com/content/8/1/1

Nel, J. A. (1999). Sexual and gender identity disorders. In A. Novello (Ed.), *Abnormal psychology: An integrative approach: A workbook for South African Students*. Johannesburg: Thomson, 117–125.

Nel, J. A. (2005). Moving from rhetoric to creating the reality: Empowering South Africa's lesbian and gay community. In M. van Zyl & M. Steyn (Eds). *Performing queer: Shaping sexualities 1994–2004*, (1). Cape Town: Kwela Books, 281–300.

Nel, J. A. (2005a). Hate crimes: A new category of vulnerable victims for a new South Africa. In L. Davis & R. Snyman (Eds.). *Victimology in South Africa*. Pretoria: Van Schaik, 240–256.

Nel, J.A. (2007). *Counteracting heterosexism and introducing LGBTI-affirmative stance in the psychology curriculum: A roundtable discussion*. http://uovs.ac.za/faculties/documents/01/163/conference2007. Retrieved 25 February 2008.

Nemeroff, C. B. (1998). Psychopharmacology of affective disorders in the 21st century. *Biological Psychiatry*, 44, 517–525.

Neumark-Stainer, D., & Haines, J. (2004). Psychological and behavioural consequences of obesity. In J. K. Thompson (Ed.). *Handbook of eating disorders and obesity*. New York: John Wiley, 349–371.

Ngcobo, M., & Pillay, B. J. (2008). Depression in African women presenting for psychological services at a general hospital. *African Journal of Psychiatry*, 11, 2, 133–137.

Nicholas, L., Daniels, P., & Hurwitz, M. (2001). Part 1: A perspective on the people of color. In R. T. Francoeur (Ed.). *International Encyclopedia of Sexuality* (4), London: Continuum International.

Niehaus, D. J. H., Kinnear, C. J., Corfield, V. A., Du Toit, P. L., Van Kradenburg, J., Moolman-Smook, C. M., Weyers, J. B., Potgieter, A., Seedat, S., Emsley, R. A., Knowles, J. A., Brink, P. A., & Stein, D. J. (2001). Association between a catechol-o-methyltransferase polymorphism and Obsessive-Compulsive Disorder in the Afrikaner population. *Journal of Affective Disorders*, 65, 61–65.

Niehaus, D. O. (2004). A culture-bound syndrome 'amafufunyana' and a culture-specific event 'ukuthwasa': Differentiated by a family history of Schizophrenia and other psychiatric disorders. *Psychopathology*, 37(2), 59–63.

Nielsen, E.B., Lyon M., & Ellison, G. (1983). Apparent hallucinations in monkeys during around-the-clock amphetamine for seven to fourteen days. *Journal of Nervous Mental Disorder*, 171, 222–233.

Nissenbaum, M. S. (2005). Autism. *Encyclopedia of human development.* http://www.sage-ereference.com/humandevelopment/Article_n67.html. Retrieved on 20 March 2009.

Noda, Y., Nakano, Y., Lee, K., Ogawa, S., Kinoshita, Y., Funayama, T., Watanabe, N., Chen, J., Noguchi, Y., Kataoka, M., Suzuki, M. & Furukawa, T. A. (2007). Sensitization of catastrophic cognition in cognitive-behavioral therapy for panic disorder. *BMC Psychiatry*, 7, 70.

Nolen-Hoeksema, S. (2007). *Abnormal Psychology* (3rd Ed.). Boston: McGraw-Hill.

Nolen-Hoeksema, S., & Davis, C. G. (2002). Positive responses to loss: Perceiving benefits and growth. In C. R. Snyder & S. J. Lopez (Eds.), *Handbook of positive psychology*. New York: Oxford University Press 598–607.

Nopoulos, P., Flaum, M., & Andreasen, N.C. (1997). Sex differences in brain morphology in Schizophrenia. *American Journal of Psychiatry*, 154 (12), 1648–1654.

Norris, D. L. (1979). Clinical diagnostic criteria for primary anorexia nervosa. *South African Medical Journal*, 56, 987–993.

Norris, M. L., Boydell, K. M., Pinhas, L., & Katzman, D. K. (2006). Ana and the Internet: A review of pro-anorexia websites. *International Journal of Eating Disorders*, 39, 443–447.

Nortje, C., Posthumus, T., & Moller, A. T. (2008). Comparison of integrated cognitive restructuring plus exposure with exposure alone in group treatment of generalised Social Anxiety Disorder. *South African Journal of Psychology*, 38(4), 647–658.

Nzimande, B. (1986). Industrial psychology and the study of black workers in South Africa: A review and critique. *Psychology in Society*, 2, 54–91.

O'Shaughnessy, R. & Dallos, R. (2009). Review of Attachment Research and Eating Disorders: A Review of the Literature. *Clinical Child Psychology and Psychiatry*, 14(4), 559–574.

Obesity and food addiction summit. (2011). Retrieved 2012, from http://www.foodaddictionsummit.org.

Ogden, C. L., Carroll, M. D., Curtin, L. R., McDowell, M. A., Tabak, C. J., & Flegal, K. M. (2006). Prevalence of overweight and obesity in the United States, 1999–2004. *JAMA*, 295, 1549–1555.

Ohaeri, J. U., & Otote, D. I. (2002). Family history, life events and the factorial structure of depression in a Nigerian sample of inpatients. *Psychopathology*, 35(4), 210–219.

Olatunji, B. O., Wolitzky-Taylor, K. B., Sawchuk, C. N., & Ciesielski, B. G. (2011). Worry and the anxiety disorders: A meta-analytic synthesis of specificity to GAD. *Applied and Preventive Psychology* doi:10.1016/j.appsy.2011.03.001.

Oldham, J. M. (2009). Borderline Personality Disorder comes of age. *American Journal of Psychiatry*, 166(5), 509–511.

Orley, J. H. & Wing, J. K. (1979). Psychiatric disorders in two African villages. *Archives of General Psychiatry*, 36, 513–520.

Overbeke, G. (2008). Pro-Anorexia Websites: Content, Impact, and Explanations of Popularity. *Mind Matters: The Wesleyan Journal of Psychology*, 3, 49–62.

Ovuga, E., Boardman, J., & Wasserman, D. (2005). The prevalence of depression in two districts of Uganda. *Social Psychiatry and Psychiatric Epidemiology*, 40, 439–445.

Paquette, M. C., & Raine, K. (2004). Sociocultural context of women's' body image. *Social Science and Medicine*, 59, 1047–1058.

Park, N., Peterson, C., & Seligman, M. E. P. (2004). Strengths of character and well-being. *Journal of Social and Clinical Psychology*, 23(5), 603–619.

Parker, G. (2001). Depression in the planet's largest ethnic group: The Chinese. *American Journal of Psychiatry*, 158(6), 857–864.

Parker, I. (2006). Working out anxiety. Notes on Freud's early case. *Psychodynamic Practice*, 12, 281–329.

Parker, I., Georgaca, E., Harper, D., McLaughlin, T., & Stowell-Smith, M. (1995). *Deconstructing psychopathology*. London: Sage.

Parker, J. D. A., Summerfeldt, L. J., Hogan, M. J., & Majeski, S. A. (2004). Emotional intelligence and academic success: Examining the transition from high school to university. *Personality and Individual Differences*, 36, 163–172.

Parle, J. (2003). Witchcraft or madness? The Amandiki of Zululand, 1894–1914. *Journal of Southern African Studies*, 29(1), 105–132.

Parry, C. D. H., & Swartz, L. (1997). Psychiatric epidemiology. In J. Katzenellenbogen, G. Joubert, & S. S. Abdool-Karim (Eds.), *Epidemiology: A manual for Southern Africa*. Cape Town: Oxford University Press, 230–242.

Patel, V., De Souza, N., & Rodrigues, M. (2003). Postnatal depression and infant growth and development in low-income countries: A cohort study from Goa, India. *Archives of Diseases in Childhood*, 88, 34–37.

Paxton, S. J., Schutz, H. K., Wertheim, E. H., & Muir, S. L. (1999). Friendship clique and peer influences on body image concerns, dietary restraint, extreme weight-loss behaviors, and binge eating in adolescent girls. *Journal of Abnormal Psychology*, 108, 255–264.

Paykel, E. S. (1974). Life stress and psychiatric disorder: Applications of the clinical approach. In B.S. Dohrenwend & B. P. Dohrenwend (Eds.). *Stressful life events: Their nature effects*. New York: Wiley.

Paykel, E. S. (2002). Mood disorders: Review of current diagnostic systems. *Psychopathology*, 35(2–3), 94–99.

Perkins, D. O., Gu, H., Boteva, K., & Lieberman, J. A. (2005). Relationship between duration of untreated psychosis and outcome in first-episode Schizophrenia: A critical review and meta-analysis. *American Journal of Psychiatry*, 162(10), 1785–1804.

Perry, J. C. (1993). Longitudinal studies of personality disorders. *Journal of Personality Disorders*, Suppl. 1, 63–85.

Petchesky, R. (2008). In R. Parker, R, Petchesky, & R. Sembler (Eds). *SexPolitics. Reports from the front lines*. Sexuality Policy Watch. Retrieved February 9, 2012 from http://www.siyanda.org/docs/sexpolitics.pdf

Petersen, I. (2010). At the heart of development: An introduction to mental health promotion and the prevention of mental health disorders in scarce-resource contexts. In I. Petersen, A. Bhana, A. J. Flisher, L. Swartz, & L. Richter (eds.). *Promoting mental health in scare-resource contexts*. Cape Town: Human Science Research Council, 3–36.

Pettifor, J. L. & Sawchuk, T. R. (2006). Psychologists' perceptions of ethically troubling incidents across international borders. *International Journal of Psychology*, 41(3), 216–225.

Phan, T. (2006). Resilience as coping mechanism: A common story of Vietnamese refugee women. In P. Wong & L. Wong (Eds.), *Handbook of multicultural perspectives on stress and coping*. New York: Springer, 427–437.

Phend, C. (2009). APA: Borderline Personality Disorder often missed first time around. *MedPage Today*, 22, 1–3.

Philen, R.M., Kilbourne, E.M., McKinley, T.W., & Parrish, R.G. (1989). Mass sociogenic illness by proxy: parentally reported epidemic in an elementary school. *Lancet*, 9(2), 1372–1376.

Phillips, K. A., Yen, S., & Gunderson, J. G. (2003). Personality disorders. In R. E. Hales & S. C. Yudofsky (Eds). *Textbook of clinical psychiatry* (4th Ed.). Washington: American Psychatric Publishing, 804–832.

Phillips, K., McElroy, S. J., Keck, P., Pope, H. J., & Hudson, J. (1993). Body dysmorphic disorder: 30 cases of imagined ugliness. *American Journal of Psychiatry*, 150, 302–308.

Picchioni, M. M., & Murray, R. (2008). Schizophrenia. *Scholarpedia*, 3(4), 4132.

Pietrzak, R. H., Goldstein, M. B., Malley, J. C., Rivers, A. J., Johnson, D. C., Morgan III, C. A., & Southwick, S. M. (2010). Posttraumatic growth in 'Veterans on Operation Enduring Freedom and Iraqi Freedom'. *Journal of Affective Disorders*, 126(1–2), 230–235.

Pigg, S. L. & Adams, V. (2005). Introduction: The moral object of sex. In V. Adams, & S. L. Pigg (Eds.). *Development science, sexuality and morality in global perspective*. Durham: Duke University Press, 1–38.

Pike, K. M., & Rodin, J. (1991). Mothers, daughters, and disordered eating. *Journal of Abnormal Psychology*, 100(2), 198–204.

Pillay B. J. (2000). Providing mental health services to survivors: A KwaZulu-Natal perspective. *Ethnicity and Health*, 5(3), 269–272.

Pillay, B. J. (1996). A model of help-seeking behaviour for urban Africans. *South African Journal of Psychology*, 1, 4–9.

Pillay, J. (2003). "Community psychology is all theory and no practice": Training educational psychologists in community practice within the South African context. *South African Journal of Psychology*, 33(4), 261–268.

Pinel, P. (1801/1962). *A Treatise of Insanity*. New York: Hafner.

Pliner, P. & Haddock, G. (1996). Perfectionism in weight-concerned and unconcerned women: An experimental approach. *International Journal of Eating Disorders*, 19, 381–389.

Pogue-Geile, M. F., & Keshavan, M. S. (1991). Negative symptomatology in Schizophrenia: Syndrome and subtype status. In J. F. Greden & R. Tandon (Eds.), *Negative schizophrenic symptoms: Pathophysiology and clinical implications*. Washington, DC: American Psychiatric Press, 41–59.

Polders L. A. (2006). Factors affecting vulnerability to depression among gay men and lesbian women. Unpublished master's dissertation, University of South Africa, Pretoria.

Pope, H. G., Jr., & Hudson, J. I. (1992). Is childhood sexual abuse a risk factor for bulimia nervosa? *American Journal of Psychiatry*, 149, 455–463.

Pope, K. S. & Vasques, M. (2007). *Ethics in psychotherapy and counseling: A practical guide* (3rd ed.). San Francisco: Jossey-Bass.

Popkin, B. M. & Doak, C. M. (1998). The obesity epidemic is a worldwide phenomenon. *Nutrition Reviews*, 56, 106–114.

Porter, R. (2002). *Madness: A brief history*. Oxford: Oxford University Press.

Posner, M., & Raichle, M. E. (Eds.). (2007). *Images of Mind*. New York: W.H. Freeman.

Potgieter, C. (1997). From apartheid to Mandela's constitution: Black South African lesbians in the nineties. In B. Greene (Ed.). *Ethnic and cultural diversity among lesbians and gay men*. Thousand Oaks: Sage, 88–116.

Pretorius-Heuchert, J. W., & Ahmed, R. (2001). Community psychology: Past, present and future. In M. Seedat, N. Duncan, & S. Lazarus. *Community Psychology: Theory, Method and Practice – South African and other perspectives*. Cape Town: Oxford University Press.

Prince, R. (1968). The changing picture of depressive syndromes in Africa. Is it fact or diagnostic fashion? *Canadian Journal of African Studies*, 1, 177–192.

Prinsloo, J. F. & Louw, D. A. (1989). Selfmoord. In D. A. Louw. *Suid-Afrikaanse handboek van abnormale gedrag*.

Pro ana tips & tricks (n.d.). Retrieved January 13, 2012 from http://day-by-day87tips.tumblr.com/post/3466665015/you-dont-want-food-food-is-disgusting-and-if-you-eat

Professional Board for Psychology. (1998). *Policy on the classification of psychometric measuring devices, instruments, methods and techniques*. Pretoria: Interim Medical & Dental Council of South Africa.

Psychological Society of South Africa (PsySSA.). (1994). A new-look psychological society for South Africa. *Newsletter of the Psychological Society for South Africa* (PsySSA), 1(1), 1.

Psychological Society of South Africa (PsySSA). (2011). *Annual Report: 2011*. Houghton: PsySSA.

Puaone, T., Steyn, K., Bradshaw, D., Laubscher, R., Lambert, V., & Mbananga, N. (2002). Obesity in South Africa: The South African demographic and health survey. *Obesity Research*, 10, 1038–1048.

Rachman, S. (1997). A cognitive theory of obsessions. *Behaviour Research and Therapy*, 35, 667–682.

Rachman, S. (2000). Obituaries: Joseph Wolpe (1915–1997). *American Psychologist*, 55(4), 441–442.

Rado, T. (1928). The problem of melancholia. *International Journal of Psycho-Analysis*, 9, 420–438.

Rahman, A. & Creed, F. (2007). Outcome of prenatal depression and risk factors associated with persistence in the first postnatal year: Prospective study from Rawalpindi, Pakistan. *Journal of Affective Disorders*, 100, 1–3, 115–121.

Raja, M., Onofri, A., Azzoni, A., Borzellino, B., & Melchiorre, M. (2008). Posttraumatic Stress Disorder among people exposed to the Ventotene street disaster in Rome. *Clinical Practice and Epidemiology of Mental Health*, 4, 5.

Ramlall, S., Chipps, J. & Mars, M. (2010). Impact of the South African Mental Health Care Act No. 17 of 2002 on regional and district hospitals designated for mental health care in KwaZulu-Natal. *South African Medical Journal*, 100(10), 667–670.

Reid, G., & Dirsuweit, T. (2002). Understanding systemic violence. *Urban Forum*, 31(3), 99–126.

Reid, H. K., & Sheeby, N. (1990). The grand unification theory of alcohol abuse: It's time to stop fighting each other and start working together. In R. C. Engs (Ed.), *Controversies in the addiction field*. Dubuque, Iowa: Kendall-Hunt.

Reid, K. A., Smiley, E., & Cooper, S. A. (2011). Prevalence and associations of anxiety disorders in adults with intellectual disabilities. *Journal of Intellectual Disability Research*, 55(2), 172–181.

Reineke, M. A. (2006). Problem-solving: A conceptual approach to suicidality and psychotherapy. In F. M. Dattilio & A. Freeman (Eds.). *Cognitive behavioural strategies in crisis intervention* (3rd ed.). New York: Guilford Press, 25–67.

Reinhardt, V., & Rogers, R. (1998). Differences in anxiety between first-time and multiple incarcerates. *Journal of the American Academy of Psychiatry and Law*, 26, 375–382.

Reynolds, G. P. (1989). Beyond the dopamine hypothesis. The neurochemical pathology of schizophrenia. *British Journal of Psychiatry*, 155, 305–16.

Ribi, K., Vollrath, M. E., Sennhauser, F. H., Gnehm, H. E., & Landolt, M. A. (2007). Prediction of posttraumatic stress in fathers of children with chronic diseases or unintentional injuries: A six-month follow-up study. *Child and Adolescent Psychiatry and Mental Health*, 1(1), 16.

Rich, P. (2006). From theory to practice: The application of attachment theory to assessment and treatment in forensic mental health services. *Criminal Behaviour and Mental Health*, 16, 211–216.

Rickels, K., & Rynn, M. (2001). What is Generalised Anxiety Disorder? *Journal of Clinical Psychiatry*, 62(suppl 11), 4–12.

Ritchie, K., & Fuhrer R. (1992). A comparative study of the performance of screening: Tests for senile dementia using receiver operating characteristics analysis. *Journal of Clinical Epidemiology*, 45(6), 627–637.

Ritchie, K., & Fuhrer, R. (1994). The development and validation in France of a screening test for senile dementia. *Revue Geriatric*, 19, 223–242.

Rittenbaugh, C., Shisslak, C., & Prince, R. (1992). A cross cultural review in regard to the DSM-IV. In J. E. Mezzich, H. Fabrega, A. Kleinman, & D. Perron (Eds). *Culture and psychiatric diagnosis: A DSM-IV Perspective*. Washington, DC: APA Press, 171–186.

Robinson, M., & Wilson, G. (2011). *Toss your textbooks: Docs redefine sexual behaviour addictions*. Retrieved January 15, 2012, from http://www.psychologytoday.com

Rockwood, K., Stolee, P., & Brahim, A. (1991). Outcomes of admission to a psychogeriatric service. *Canadian Journal of Psychiatry*, 36(4), 275–279.

Rodgers, J. E. (2011). Addiction: A whole new view. Retrieved 2012, from *Psychology Today*.

Rodriguez, H., Brathwaite, D., Dorsey S. (2002). Depression and social support in the elderly population: A study of rural South African elders. *Association for Black Nursing Faculty in Higher Education*, 13(2), 45–48.

Roff, J. D., & Knight, R. (1981). Family characteristics, childhood symptoms, and adult outcome in Schizophrenia. *Journal of Abnormal Psychology*, 90, 510–20.

Rogers, R. (1988). *Clinical Assessment of Deception and Malingering*. New York: Guilford Press.

Rogers, S. C. & Clay, S. M. (1975). A statistical review of controlled trials of imipramine and placebo in the treatment of depressive illness. *British Journal of Psychiatry*, 127, 599–603.

Rogerson, (1986).

Rome, H. P. (2000). Limbically augmented pain syndrome (LAPS): Kindling, corticolimbic sensitization, and the convergence of affective and sensory symptoms in chronic pain disorders. *Pain Medicine*, 1(1), 7–23.

Root, M. P. (1990). Disordered eating in women of color. *Sex Roles*, 22, 525–536.

Ropper, A. H. (2001). Deafness, dizziness and disorders of equilibrium. In A. H. Ropper. *Adams and Victor's principles of neurology* (7th Ed.). New York: McGraw-Hill, 301–328.

Rosen, J. C. & Leitenberg, H. (1985). Exposure plus response prevention treatment of bulimia. In D. M. Gamer & P. E. Garfinkel (Eds.). *Handbook of psychotherapy for anorexia nervosa and bulimia*. New York: Guilford Press, 193–209.

Rosenhan, D. L. (1973). On being sane in insane places. *Science*, 179(70), 250–258.

Ross, C. E., & Mirowsky, J. (1989). Explaining the social patterns of depression: Control and problem solving – or support and talking? *Journal of Health and Social Behavior*, 30(2), 206–219.

Rotter, J. (1966). Generalized expectancies for internal versus external control of reinforcements. *Psychological Monographs*, 80, Whole No. 609.

Rouleau, I., Salmon, D. P., Butters, N. (1996). Longitudinal analysis of clock drawing in Alzheimer's disease patients. *Brain Cognition*, 31, 17–34.

Roy, A. (1981). Depression in the course of chronic undifferentiated schizophrenia. *Archives of General Psychiatry*, 38, 296–297.

Roy, A. (2001). Consumers of mental health services. *Suicide and Life-Threatening Behaviour*, 31, 60–83.

Ruini, C., & Fava, G. A. (2004). Clinical applications of well-being therapy. In P. A. Linley & S. Joseph (Eds.), *Positive psychology in practice*. Hoboken NJ: John Wiley, 371–389.

Rumble, S., Swartz, L., Parry, C., & Zwarenstein, M. (1996). Prevalence of psychiatric morbidity in the adult population of a rural South African village. *Psychological Medicine*, 26, 997–1007.

Ruscio, A. M., Lane, M., Roy-Byrne, P., Stang, P. E., Stein, D. J., Wittchen, H. U., & Kessler, R. C. (2005). Should excessive worry be required for a diagnosis of generalized anxiety disorder? Results from the US National Comorbidity Survey Replication. *Psychological Medicine*, 35, 1761–1772.

Rush, A. J., Stewart, R. S., Garver, D. L., & Waller, D. A. (1998). Neurobiological bases for psychiatric disorders. In R. N. Rosenberb & D. E. Pleasure (Eds.). *Comprehensive neurology* (2nd Ed.). New York: John Wiley & Sons, 555–603.

Rutherford, J., McGuffin, P., Katz, R. J. & Murray, R. M. (1993). Genetic influences on eating attitudes in a normal female twin population. *Psychological Medicine*, 23, 425–436.

Rutter, M. (2000). Genetic studies of Autism: From the 1970s into the millennium. *Journal of Abnormal Child Psychology*, 28(1), 3–14.

Rutter, M., MacDonald, H., LeCouteur, A., Harrington, R., Bolton, P., & Bailey, A. (1990). Genetic factors in child psychiatric disorders: Empirical findings. *Journal of Child Psychology and Psychiatry*, 31, 39–83.

Ryan, C., Nielssen, O., Paton, M. & Large, M. (2010). Clinical decisions in psychiatry should not be based on risk assessment. *Australasian Psychiatry* 18(5), 398–403.

Ryan, R. M., & Deci, E. L. (2000). Self-determination theory and the facilitation of intrinsic motivation, social development, and well-being. *American Psychologist*, 55(1), 68–78.

Ryff, C. D., & Keyes, C. L. (1995). The structure of psychological well-being revisited. *Journal of Personality and Social Psychology*, 69, 719–727.

Ryff, C. D., & Singer, B. (1998). The contours of positive human health. *Psychological Inquiry*, 9, 1–8.

Ryff, C. D., & Singer, B. (2003). Flourishing under fire: Resilience as a prototype of challenged thriving. In C. L. M. Keyes & J. Haidt (Eds.), *Flourishing: Positive psychology and the life well-lived* Washington, DC: American Psychological Association, 15–36.

SA History Online. 2008. SAHO Classroom: Grades 4–12.

Saavedra, L. M., & Silverman, W. K. (2004). Phobias in Childhood. *Encyclopedia of applied developmental science*. http://www.sage-ereference.com/applieddevscience/Article_n319.html. retrieved on 20 March 2009.

SADAG Conference. (April 2011). South African Depression and Anxiety Group (SADAG). 34 Key SA journalists attend SADAG conference on mental health reporting. *African Journal of Psychiatry*, 164–166.

Sadock, B. J. & Sadock, V. A. (Eds). (2000). *Kaplan & Sadock's comprehensive textbook of psychiatry* (7th Ed.). Philadelphia: Lippincott Williams & Wilkins.

Sadock, B. J. & Sadock, V. A. (2007). *Kaplan and Sadock's synopsis of psychiatry. Behavioral sciences/clinical psychiatry* (10th Ed.). Philadelphia: Lippincott, Williams & Wilkins.

Saha, S., Chant, D., Welham, J., & McGrath, J. (2005). A systemic review of the prevalence of Schizophrenia. *U.S. National Library of Medicine National Institutes of Health*, 2(5), e141.

Salovey, P., & Mayer, J. D. (1990). Emotional intelligence. *Imagination, Cognition and Personality*, 9, 185–211.

Salovey, P., Bedell, B. T., Detweiler, J. B., & Mayer, J. D. (1999). Coping intelligently: emotional intelligence and the coping process. In C.R. Snyder (Ed.), *Coping: the psychology of what works*. New York: Oxford University Press, 141–164.

Salovey, P., Mayer, J. D., & Caruso, D. (2002). The positive psychology of emotional intelligence. In C. R. Snyder & S. J. Lopez (Eds.), *Handbook of positive psychology*. New York: Oxford University Press, 159–171.

Salovey, P., Stroud, L. R., Woolery, A., & Epel, E. S. (2002). Perceived emotional intelligence, stress reactivity, and symptom reports: further explorations using the trait meta-mood scale. *Psychology & Health*, 17, 611–627.

Samelius, L., & Wägberg, E. (2005). *Sexual orientation and gender identity issues in development*. Stockholm: Swedish International Development Co-operation Agency Health Division.

Sander, J. B., & McCarty, C. A. (2005). Youth depression in the family context: Familial risk factors and models of treatment. *Clinical Child and Family Psychology Review*, 8(3), 203–219.

Sandfort, G. M, & De Keizer, M. (2001). Sexual problems in gay men: An overview of empirical research. *Annual Review of Sex Research*, 12, 93–120.

Sapolsky, R. M. (1996). Stress, glucocorticoids, and damage to the nervous system: The current state of confusion. *Stress*, 1, 1–19.

Sarason, I. G. & Sarason, B. R. (1993). *Abnormal psychology: The problem of maladaptive behavior* (7th Ed.). Englewood Cliffs: Prentice Hall.

Sartorius, N., Shapiro, R., & Jablonsky, A. (1974). The international pilot study of Schizophrenia. *Schizophrenia Bulletin*, 2, 21–35.

Sarwer, D. B., Wadden, T. A., & Foster, G. D. (1998). Assessment of body image dissatisfaction in obese women: Specificity, severity, and clinical significance. *Journal of Consulting Clinical Psychology*, 66, 651–654.

Saunders, E. (2008). *Assessment in South Africa: Finding method in madness*. Workinfo.com - human resources for today's workplace. http://www.workinfo.com/free/Downloads/36.htm. Retrieved 31 May 2008.

Schafer, W. (2000). *Stress management for wellness* (4th ed.). Belmont, CA: Thomson.

Schelling, G. (2002). Effects of stress hormone on traumatic memory formation and the development of Posttraumatic Stress Disorder in critically ill patients. *Neurobiology of Memory and Learning*, 78(3), 596–609.

Scherrer, R., Louw, D.A. & Möller, A.T. (2002). Ethical complaints and disciplinary action against South African psychologists. *South African Journal of Psychology*, 32(1), 54–64.

Schlachter, A. & Duckitt, J. (2002). Psychopathology, authoritarian attitudes and prejudice. *South African Journal of Psychology*, 32(2), 1–8.

Schmidt, U., Evans, K., Tiller, J., & Treasure, J. (1995). Puberty, sexual milestones and abuse: How are they related in eating disorder patients? *Psychological Medicine*, 25, 413–417.

Schneider, K. (1959). *Clinical psychopathology*. New York: Grune & Stratton.

Schoeman, J. B. (1989). Psigopatologie by tradisionele swart Suid-Afrikaners. In D. A. P. Louw (Ed.). *Suid-Afrikaanse handbook van abnormale gedrag*. Johannesburg: Southern Publishers.

Scholtz, G. D. (1974). *Dr Hendrik Frensch Verwoerd: 1901–1966*. Johannesburg: Perskor.

Schultz, R., Drayer, R. A., & Rollman, B. L. (2002). Depression as a risk factor for non-suicide mortality in the elderly. *Biological Psychiatry*, 52, 205–225.

Schwartz, C. C., & Myers, J. K. (1977). Life events and Schizophrenia: I. Comparison of schizophrenics with a community sample. *Archives of General Psychiatry*, 34, 1238–41.

Schwartz, M. B. & Brownell, K. D. (2007). Actions necessary to prevent childhood obesity: Creating the climate for change. *Journal of Law, Medicine, & Ethics*, 35, 1, 78–89.

Seedat, M., Duncan, N., & Lazarus, S. (2001). *Community Psychology: Theory, Method and Practice - South African and other perspectives*. Cape Town: Oxford University Press.

Segal, J. & Douki, S. (2005). CANMAT guidelines for bipolar disorder: Commentary from the African perspective. *Bipolar Disorders*, 7(3), 77–82.

Seifert, T. (2005). Anthropomorphic characteristics of centerfold models: Trends towards slender figures over time. *International Journal of Eating Disorders*, 37, 271–274.

Seligman, M. E. P. (2006). Afterword. In M. Csikszentmihalyi & I. S. Csikszentmihalyi (Eds.), *A life worth living. Contributions to positive psychology*. Oxford: Oxford University Press, 230–236.

Seligman, M. E. P. (1975). *Helplessness: On depression, development, and death*. San Francisco: W.H. Freeman.

Seligman, M. E. P. (2005). Positive psychology, positive prevention, and positive therapy. In C. R. Snyder & S. J. Lopez (Eds.), *Handbook of positive psychology*. Oxford: Oxford University Press, 3–12.

Seligman, M. E. P. and Rosenhan, D. L. (1998). *Abnormality*. New York: W.W. Norton. Publishers.

Seligman, M.E.P. (2008). Positive Health. *Applied Psychology: An International Review*, 57, 3–18 doi: 10.1111/j.1464-0597.2008.00351.x

Selye, H. (1956). *The stress of life*. New York: McGraw-Hill.

Serdula, M. K., Mokdad, A. H., Williamson, D. F., Galuska, D. A., et al. (1999). Prevalence of attempting weight loss and strategies for controlling weight. *Journal of the American Medical Association*, 282, 1353–1358.

Sheldon, K. M., & King, L. (2001). Why positive psychology is necessary. *American Psychologist*, 56, 216–217.

Sheline, Y. I., Gado, M. H., & Kraemer, H. C. (2003). Untreated depression and hippocampal volume loss. *American Journal of Psychiatry*, 160(8), 1516–1518.

Shiang, R. R. (1993). Mutations in the 1 subunit of the inhibitory glycine receptor cause the dominant neurologic disorder, hyperekplexia. *Nature Genetics*, 5, 351–358.

Shidlo, A. & Schroeder, M. (2002). Changing sexual orientation: A consumers' report. *Professional Psychology: Research and Practice*, 33(3), 249–259.
Shipton, E. (2008). The chronic pain experience. *NZ Medical Journal*, 121(1270), 9–11.
Shriver, M. (2005). Autism spectrum disorders. *Encyclopedia of School Psychology*. http://www.sage–ereference.com/schoolpsychology/Article_n20.html. Retrieved on 20 March 2009.
Sierra, M. B. (1998). Depersonalization: Neurobiological perspectives. *Biological Psychiatry*, 44, 898–908.
Silverstein, B. & Perdue, L. (1988). The relationship between role concern, preference of slimness, and symptoms of eating problems among college women. *Sex Roles*, 18, 101–160.
Simpson, R. L. & LaCava, P. G. (2007). Autism spectrum disorders. *Encyclopedia of Educational Psychology*. http://www.sage-ereference.com/educationalpsychology/Article_n23.html. Retrieved on 20 March 2009.
Sinnott, A., Jones, B., & Fordham, A. S. (1981). Agoraphobia: A situational analysis. *Journal of Clinical Psychology*, 37(1), 123–127.
Skinner, B. F. (1953). *Science and Human Behavior*. New York: Macmillan.
Slater, E. (1965). Diagnosis of hysteria. *British Medical Journal*, 1, 1395–1399.
Slavich, G. M. (2004). *Deconstructing depression: A diathesis stress-perspective*. Retrieved October 15, 2011 from http://www.psychologicalscience.org/observer/getArticle.cfm?id=1640.
Small, G. P. (1991). Mass hysteria among student performers: Social relationship as a symptom predictor. *American Journal of Psychiatry*, 148, 1200–1205.
Small, G. W. (1991). Recognition and treatment of depression in the elderly. The clinician's challenge: Strategies for treatment of depression in the 1990's. *Journal of Clinical Psychiatry*, 52, 11–22.
Smit, F., Bolier, L., & Cuijpers, P. (2004). Cannabis use and the risk of later Schizophrenia: A Review. *Addiction*, 99(4), 425–430.
Smith, D. E. (1969). Use of LSD in the Haight-Ashbury: Observations at a neighbourhood clinic. *California Medicine* (June), 472–476.
Smith, J. D. (2010). Panic stations: Brief dynamic therapy for Panic Disorder and Generalised Anxiety Disorder. *Psychodynamic Practice*, 16(1), 25–43.
Smith, K. A., Fairburn, C. G., & Cowen, P. J. (1999). Symptomatic relapse in bulimia nervosa following tryptophan depletion. *Archives of General Psychiatry*, 56, 171–176.
Smith, R. C., Singh, A., Infante, M., Khandat, A., & Kloos, A. (2002). Effects of cigarette smoking and nicotine nasal spray on psychiatric symptoms and cognition in Schizophrenia. *Neuropsychopharmachology*, 27, 479–497.
Smuts, J.C. (1926). *Holism and evolution*. New York: Macmillan.
Sneiderman, B. & McQuoid-Mason, D. (2000). Decision-making at the end of life: The termination of life-prolonging treatment, euthanasia (mercy-killing), and assisted suicide in Canada and South Africa. *Comparative and International Law Journal of Southern Africa*, 33(2), 193–204.
Snyder, C. R., Rand, K. L., & Sigmon, D. R. (2005). Hope theory: A member of the positive psychology family. In C. R. Snyder & S. J. Lopez (Eds.), *Handbook of positive psychology*. Oxford: Oxford University Press, 257–276.
Solomon, A. (2001). *The noonday demon: An atlas of depression*. New York: Scribner.
Sommer, R. (2011).The etymology of psychosis. *American Journal of Orthopsychiatry*, 81, 162–166.
South African Community Epidemiology Network on Drug Use (SACENDU). (2010). *SACENDU Research Brief*, 13(2),
South African Human Rights Commission & UNICEF (2011). *South Africa's children – a review of equity and child rights*. Retrieved March 5, 2012 from http://www.health-e.org.za/uploaded/fe94f5f04583baf7585f6701946b5ac9.pdf
Spence, C. H. (2000). Discrete neurophysiological correlates in prefrontal cortex during hysterical and feigned disorder of movement. *Lancet*, 355(9211), 1243–4.
Spiegel, D. L. (1997). Dissociated cognition and disintegrated experience. In D. Stein, *Cognitive science and the unconscious*. Washington, DC: American Psychiatric Publishing, 177–188.
Spitzer, C. B. S. (2006). Recent developments in the theory of dissociation. *World Psychiatry*, 5(2), 82–86.
Spitzer, R. L., Endicott, J., & Robins, E. (1978). Research diagnostic criteria: Rationale and reliability. *Archives of General Psychiatry*, 35, 773–782.
Squire, C. (2000). *Culture in psychology*. New York: Routledge.

Steadman, H. J., & Ribner, S. A. (1980). Changing perceptions of the mental health needs of inmates in local jails. *American Journal of Psychiatry*, 137, 1115–1116.

Stein, D. J. & Gureje, O. (2004). Depression and anxiety in the developing world: Is it time to medicalise the suffering? *Lancet*, 364(9430), 233–234.

Stein, D. J. (2006). Advances in understanding the anxiety disorders: The cognitive – neuroscience of 'false alarms'. *Annals of Clinical Psychiatry*, 18, 173–182.

Steiner, H. & Lock, J. (1998). Anorexia nervosa and bulimia nervosa in children and adolescents: A review of the past 10 years. *Journal of the American Academy of Child and Adolescent Psychiatry*, 37, 352–359.

Stice, E. (1998). Relations of restraint and negative affect to bulimic pathology: A longitudinal test of three competing models. *International Journal of Eating Disorders*, 23, 243–260.

Stones, C. (1996). Attitudes toward psychology, psychiatry and mental illness in the central eastern Cape of South Africa. *South African Journal of Psychology*, 26, 221–225.

Striegel-Moore, R. H., Silberstein, L. R., & Rodin, J. (1993). The social self in bulimia nervosa: Public self-consciousness, social anxiety, and perceived fraudulence. *Journal of Abnormal Psychology*, 102(2), 297–303.

Strober, M. (1995). Family–genetic perspectives on anorexia nervosa and bulimia nervosa. In K. Brownell & C. G. Fairburn (Eds). *Eating disorders and obesity: A comprehensive casebook*. New York: Guilford, 212–218.

Strober, M., Lampert, C., Morrell, W., Burroughs, J., & Jacobs, C. (1990). A controlled family study of anorexia nervosa: Evidence of family aggregation and lack of shared transmission with affective disorders. *International Journal of Eating Disorders*, 9, 239–253.

Strong, A., Bancroft, J., Carnes, L., Davis, L., Kennedy, J. (2005). The impact of sexual arousal on sexual risk-taking: A qualitative study. *The Journal of Sex Research*, 42(3), 185–191.

Strümpfer, D. J. W. (1995). The origin of health and strength: From 'salutogenesis' to 'fortigenesis'. *South African Journal of Psychology*, 25, 81–89.

Struwig, W. & Pretorius, P.J. (2009). Quality of psychiatric referrals to secondary-level care. *South African Journal of Psychology*, 15(20), 33–36.

Suddath, R. L., Christison, G. W, Torrey, E. F., Casanova, M. F., & Weinberger, D. R. (1990). Anatomical abnormalities in the brains of monozygotic twins discordant for Schizophrenia. *New England Journal of Medicine*, 322, 789–794.

Sue, D., Sue, D., & Sue, S. (2006). *Understanding abnormal behaviour*. Boston: Houghton Mifflin.

Sue, S., & Morishima, J. K. (1982). *The mental health of Asian-Americans*. San Francisco: Jossey-Bass.

Sullivan, G. M., Coplan, J. D., & Gorman, J. M. (1998). Psychoneuroendocrinology of anxiety disorders. *Psychiatric Clinics of North America*, 21, 397–412.

Swanepoel, M. (2010). Ethical decision-making in forensic psychology. *Koers*, 75(4), 851–872.

Swartz, L. (1986). Carl Rogers in South Africa: The issue of silence. *Psychology in Society*, 5, 139–143.

Swartz, L. (1987). Transcultural psychiatry in South Africa. *Transcultural Psychiatric Research Review*, 24, 5–30.

Swartz, L. (1991). The reproduction of racism in South African mental health care. *South African Journal of Psychology*, 21, 240–246.

Swartz, L. (1998). *Culture and mental health: A southern African view*. Cape Town: Oxford University Press.

Sweeney, D. R., & Maas, J. W. (1978). Specificity of depressive diseases. *Annual Review of Medicine*, 29, 219–229.

Szabo, C. J. (2005). Dissociative trance disorder associated with major depression and bereavement in a South African female adolescent. *Australian & New Zealand Journal of Psychiatry*, 39(5), 423.

Szabo, C. P. & Allwood, C. W. (2004). A cross-cultural study of eating attitudes in adolescent South African females. *World Psychiatry*, 3, 41–44.

Szabo, C. P. (1998). Eating disorders and adolescence. *South African Journal of Child and Adolescent Mental Health*, 10, 117–125.

Szabo, C. P. (1999). Eating attitudes among black South Africans. *American Journal of Psychiatry*, 156, 981–982.

Szabo, C. P., Berk, M., Tlou, E., & Allwood, C.W. (1995). Eating disorders in black female South Africans: A series of cases. *South African Medical Journal*, 85, 588–590.

Szasz, T. (1974). *The myth of mental illness: Foundations of a theory of personal conduct.* New York: Harper & Row.

Szasz, T. S. (1961). *The myth of mental illness.* New York: Hoeber-Harper.

Szasz, T. S. (1970). *The manufacture of madness: A comparative study of the inquisition and the mental health movement.* London: Routledge.

Szasz, T. S. (1976). 'Anti-psychiatry': The paradigm of a plundered mind. *New Review,* 3, 3–14.

Taku, K. (2011). Commonly-defined and individually-defined posttraumatic growth in the USA and Japan. *Personality and Individual Differences,* 51(2), 188–193.

Talmadge, L. D., & Talmadge, W. C. (1986). Relational sexuality: An understanding of low sexual desire. *Journal of Sex and Marital Therapy,* 12(1), 3–21.

Tandon, R., Goldman, R. S., Goodson, J., & Greden, J. F. (1990). Mutability and relationship between positive and negative symptoms during neuroleptic treatment. *Biological Psychiatry,* 27, 1323–1326.

Tangney, J. P. (2005). Humility. In C. R. Snyder & S. J. Lopez (Eds.), *Handbook of positive psychology.* Oxford: Oxford University Press, 411–422.

Tanner, C. C. (2001). Latah in Jakarta, Indonesia. *Movement Disorders,* 16(3), 526–529.

Tantum, D. (1991). The anti-psychiatry movement. In G. E. Berrios & H. Freeman (Eds). *150 Years of British Psychiatry,* 1841–1991. London: Gaskell.

Te Water Naude, J., London, L., Pitt, B., Mohamed, C. (1998). The Dop system around Stellenbosch: Results of a farm survey. *South African Medical Journal,* 88, 1102–05.

Teichman, Y. & Teichman, M. (1990). Interactional view of depression: Review and integration. *Journal of Family Psychology,* 3, 349–367.

Telch, C. F. & Argras, W. S. (2006). Obesity, binge eating and psychopathology: Are they related? *International Journal of Eating Disorders,* 15, 53–61.

Tennen, H. & Affleck, G. (2002). Benefit-finding and benefit-reminding. In C. R. Snyder & S. J. Lopez (Eds.), *Handbook of positive psychology.* New York: Oxford University Press, 584–597.

Thase, M. E., & Howland, R. H. (1995). Biological processes in depression: An updated review and integration. In E. E. Beckham & W. R. Leber. *Handbook of Depression.* New York: Guilford Press, 213–279.

The Colorado Personal Growth and Therapy Resources (1998). http://www.telosnet.com TelosNet. Retrieved 15 January 1998.

Thombs, D. (2006). *Introduction to Addictive Behaviours.* New York: Guilford Press.

Thompson, J. K. (1986). Larger than life. *Psychology Today,* 20, 39–44.

Thompson, J., Coovert, M. D., Richards, K. J., Johnson, S., & Cattarin, J. (1995). Development of body image, eating disturbance, and general psychological functioning in female adolescents: Covariance structure modeling and longitudinal investigations. *International Journal of Eating Disorders,* 18, 221–236.

Tobacco Products Control Act 1993, Republic of South Africa (1993).

Tobacco Products Control Amendment Bill 2007, Republic of South Africa (2007).

Todder, D., & Baune, B. T. (2007). Recurrence of suicidal ideation due to treatment with antidepressants in anxiety disorder: a case report. *Journal of Medical Case Reports,* 1, 166.

Tolin, D. F., Abramowitz, S., Brigidi, B. D., & Foa, E. B. (2003). Intolerance of uncertainty in Obsessive-Compulsive Disorder. *Journal of Anxiety Disorders,* 17(2), 233–242.

Tomlinson, M., Cooper, P. J., Stein, A., Swartz, L., & Molteno, C. (2006). Post-partum depression and infant growth in a South African peri-urban settlement. *Child: Care, Health & Development,* 32(1), 81–86.

Tomlinson, M., Grimsrud, A. T., Stein, D. J., Williams, D. R., & Myer, L. (2009). The epidemiology of major depression in South Africa: Results from the South African Stress and Health study. *South African Journal of Medicine,* 99(2), 367–373.

Tomlinson, M., Swartz, L., Cooper, P. J., & Molteno, C. (2004). Social factors and postpartum depression in Khayelitsha, Cape Town. *South African Journal of Psychology,* 34(3), 409–420.

Tomm, K., & Lannamann, J. (1988). Questions as interventions. *The Family Therapy Networker,* 12(5), 38–41.

Torelli, C. J. & Shavitt, S. (2011). The impact of power on information processing depends on cultural orientation. *Journal of Experimental Social Psychology,* 47, 959–967.

Treanor, M. (2011). The potential impact of mindfulness on exposure and extinction learning in anxiety disorders. *Clinical Psychology Review,* 31(6), 17–625.

Triplett, K. N., Tedeschi, R. G., Cann, A., Calhoun, L. G., & Reeve, C. L. (2011). Posttraumatic growth, meaning in life and satisfaction in response to trauma. *Psychological Trauma: Theory, Research, Practice, and Policy*. Advance online publication. doi: 10.1037/a0024204

Tsaousis, I., & Nikolaou, I. (2005). Exploring the relationship of emotional intelligence with physical and psychological health functioning. *Stress and Health*, 21, 77–86.

Tsuang, M. T. & Faraone S. V. (2000). The frustrating search for schizophrenia genes. *American Journal of Medical Genetics*, 97(1), 1–3.

Tsuang, M. T., Stone, W. S. & Faraone, S. V. (2000). Toward reformulating the diagnosis of schizophrenia. *American Journal of Psychiatry*, 157, 1041–1050.

Tully, C. (2000). *Lesbians, gays, & the empowerment perspective*. New York: Columbia University Press.

Tulsky, D. S., Zhu, J., & Prifitera, A. (2000). Assessment of adult intelligence with the WAIS–III. In G. Goldstein & M. Hersen (Eds.). *Handbook of psychological assessment* (3rd Ed.). Oxford: Elsevier Science (Pergamon), 453–470.

Turk, C. L., Heimberg, R. G., & Magee, L. (2007). Social anxiety. In D. H. Barlow (Ed.). *Clinical handbook of psychological disorders: A step-by-step treatment manual*. New York: Guilford Press.

Turner, M. (1997). Malingering. *British Journal of Psychiatry*, 171, 409–411.

Ubell, E. (1989, December 3). They're closing in on mental illness. *Parade Magazine*, 6–7.

UNAIDS/WHO. (2006). *AIDS epidemic update*. Geneva: WHO.

Ussher, J. M. (1991). *Women's madness: Misogyny or mental illness?* New York: Harvester Wheatsheaf.

Vaiva, G. B. (2003). Fright (effroi) and other peritraumatic responses after a serious motor vehicle accident: Prospective influence on Acute PTSD Development. *Canadian Journal of Psychiatry*, 48, 395–401.

Van den Broucke, S. & Vandereyken, W. (1986). Risk factors for the development of eating disorders in adolescent exchange students: An exploratory survey. *Journal of Adolescence*, 9, 145–150.

Van der Spuy, H. I. J. & Shamley, D. A. F. (1978). *The psychology of apartheid*. Washington, DC: University Press of America.

Van der Zee, K., Thijs, M., & Schakel, S. F. (2002). The relationship of emotional intelligence with academic intelligence and the Big Five. *European Journal of Personality*, 16, 103–125.

Van Dyk, A., Klompmakers, A., & Denys, D. (2010). The serotonergic system in Obsessive-Compulsive Disorder. In C. P. Müller & B. L. Jacobs (Eds). *Handbook of the behavioral neurobiology of serotonin*, Volume 21 (Handbook of behavioral neuroscience). San Diego, CA: Academic Press, 547–563.

Van Dyk, A.J. (2008). Forgiveness and the well-being of Members of the South African National Defence Force: A process for discussion. *Journal of Psychology in Africa*, 18(4), 669–674.

Van Kammen, D. P., Docherty, J. P., & Bunney, W. E. (1982). Prediction of early relapse after pimozide discontinuation by response to d-amphetamine during pimozide treatment. *Biological Psychiatry*, 17, 223–242.

Van Onselen, C. (1982). *New Babylon, new Nineveh*. Cape Town: Jonathan Ball.

Van Schalkwyk, I., & Wissing, M. P. (2010). Psychosocial well-being in a group of South African adolescents. *Journal of Psychology in Africa*, 20(1), 53–60.

Van Snellenberg, J. X., Torres, I. J., & Thornton, A. E. (2006). Functional neuroimaging of working memory in Schizophrenia: Task performance as a moderating variable. *Neuropsychology*, 20(5), 497–510.

Van Wyk, G. & Edwards, D. (2005). From trauma debriefing to trauma support: A South African experience of responding to individuals and communities in the aftermath of traumatising events. *Journal of Psychology in Africa*, 15(2), 135–142.

Vanderlinden, J., Norre, J., & Vandereycken, W. (1992). *A practical guide to the treatment of bulimia nervosa*. New York: Brunner/Mazel.

Vaughan, K. K. & Fouts, G. T. (2003). Changes in television and magazine exposure and eating disorder symptomatology. *Sex roles*, 49, 1573–2762.

Venter, F. C., Walsh, C. M., Slabber, M., & Bester, C. J. (2009). Body size perception of African women (25–44years) in Manguang. *Journal of Family Ecology and Consumer Sciences*, 37, 12–23.

Ventura, J., Nuechterlein, K. H., Lukoff, D., & Hardesty, J. P. (1989). A prospective study of stressful life events and Schizophrenia relapse. *Journal of Abnormal Psychology*, 98, 407–411.

Verhaak, P., Kerssens, J., Dekker, J., Sorbi, M., & Bensing, J. (1998). Prevalence of chronic benign pain disorder among adults: A review of the literature. *Pain*, 77, 231–239.

Verhaege, P. (1998). *Love in a time of loneliness: Three essays on drive and desire*. New York: Other Press.

Vilhjalmsson, R. (1993). Life stress, social support and clinical depression: A reanalysis of the literature. *Social Science & Medicine*, 37(3), 331–342.

Vitousek, K. & Manke, F. (1994). Personality variables and disorders in anorexia nervosa and bulimia nervosa. *Journal of Abnormal Psychology*, 103, 137–147.

Vitousek, K. M. & Gray, J. A. (2005). Eating disorders. In G. O. Gabbard, J. S. Beck, & J. Holmes (Eds). *Oxford textbook of psychotherapy*. Oxford: Oxford University Press, 177–202.

Vohs, K. D., & Baumeister, R. F. (2004). Understanding self-regulation: An introduction. In R. F. Baumeister & K. D. Vohs (Eds.). *Handbook of self-regulation: Research, Theory, and Applications*. London: Guilford Press, 1–12.

Von Krosigk, B. C. (2004). Facilitating forgiveness: An NLP approach to forgiving. Unpublished doctoral thesis, University of South Africa, Pretoria.

Wadsworth, M. E. (2005). Developmental Psychopathology. *Encyclopedia of human development*. http://www.sage-ereference.com/humandevelopment/Article_n190.html. Retrieved on 20 March 2009.

Walker, E. E, Downey, G., & Bergman, A. (1989). The effects of parental psychopathology and maltreatment on child behavior: A test of the diathesis-stress model. *Child Development*, 60, 15–24.

Walker, J. (2001). *Control and the psychology of health*. Buckingham: Open University Press.

Walker, M. T. (2006). The social construction of mental illness and its implication for the recovery model. *International Journal of Psychosocial Rehabilitation*, 10(1), 71–87.

Walker, N. (1996). *Dangerous people*. London: Blackstone Press.

Walker, S. P. (1996). The criminal upperworld and the emergence of a disciplinary code in the early chartered accountancy profession. *Accounting History*, 1(2), 7–35.

Wallace, J. M. (1999). The social ecology of addiction: Race, risk and resilience. *Pediatrics*, 103, 1122–1127.

Walsh, B. & Devlin, M. J. (1998). Eating disorders: Progress and problems. *Science*, 280, 1387–1390.

Wassenaar, D., Le Grange, D., Winship, J., & Lachenict, L. (2000). The prevalence of eating disorder pathology in a cross-ethnic population of female students in South Africa. *European Eating Disorder Review*, 8, 225–236.

Watkins, C. E., Campbell, V. L., Nieberding, R., & Hallmark, R. (1995). Contemporary practice of psychological assessment by clinical psychologists. *Professional Psychology: Research and Practice*, 26, 54–60.

Watzlawick, P., Beavin, J. B., & Jackson, D. D. (1967). *Pragmatics of human communication: A study of interactional patterns, pathologies, and paradoxes*. New York: Norton.

Weakland, J., Fisch, R., Watzlawick, P., & Bodin, A. B. (1974). Brief therapy: Focused problem resolution. *Family Process*, 13, 141–168.

Webster, E. (1986). Excerpt from 'Servants of Apartheid'. *Psychology in Society*, 6, 6–12.

Weiner, I. B. (1994). The Rorschach Inkblot Method (RIM) is not a test: Implications for theory and practice. *Journal of Personality Assessment*, 62, 498–504.

Weisman, A. G., Nuechterlein, M. J., Goldstein, M.J., & Snyder, K. S. (1998). Expressed emotion, attributions, and Schizophrenia symptom dimensions. *Journal of Abnormal Psychology*, 107, 355–359.

Weiss, J. M. (1991). Stress-induced depression: Critical neurochemical and electrophysiological changes. In J. Madden (Ed.). *Neurobiology of learning, emotion, and affect*. New York: Raven Press, 123–154.

Welch, S. L, & Fairburn, C. G. (1994). Sexual abuse and bulimia nervosa: Three integrated case-control comparisons. *American Journal of Psychiatry*, 151, 402–407.

Wells, H. (2006). *Homophobic hate crimes: Prevalence, consequence and the impact of gender*. OUT LGBT Wellbeing.

Wenar, C. & Kerig, P. (2006). *Developmental psychopathology: From infancy to adolescence* (5th ed.). New York: McGraw-Hill.

Westergaard, T., Mortensen, P. B., Pedersen, C. B., Wohlfahrt, J., & Melbye, M. (1999). Exposure to prenatal and childhood infections and the risk of Schizophrenia. *Archives of General Psychiatry*, 56, 993–998.

Westerhof, G. J., & Keyes, C. L. M. (2010). Mental illness and mental health: The two continua model across the lifespan. *Journal of Adult Development*, 17, 110–119.

Weston, S. C., & Siever, L. J. (1993). Biologic correlates of personality disorders. NIMH Conference: Personality disorders (1990, Williamsburg, Virginia). *Journal of Personality Disorders*, Suppl. 1, 129–148.

Whitman, B. Y. (1991). The roots of organicity: genetics and genograms. In P. J. Accardo, T. A. Blondis, & B. Y. Whitman (Eds.). *Attention deficits and hyperactivity in children*. New York: Marcel Dekker.

Wicks-Nelson, R. & Israel, A. C. (2006). *Behavior disorders of childhood* (6th ed.). Englewood Cliffs, NJ: Prentice Hall.

Wicks-Nelson, R., & Israel, A.C. (2009). *Abnormal child and adolescent psychology* (7th ed.). Engelwood Cliffs, NJ: Pearson Education.

Wig, N. N. (1983). DSM III: Its strengths and weaknesses – a perspective from the Third World. In R. L. Spitser, I. B. W. Williams, and A. E. Skodol (eds.), *International Perspectives on the DSM III*. Washington DC: American Psychiatric Press, 79–89.

Wildgust, H. J. & Beary, M. (2010). Review of 'Are there modifiable risk factors which will reduce the excess mortality in Schizophrenia?'. *Journal of Psychopharmachology*, 24(4), 37–50.

Willi, J. & Grossman, S. (1983). Epidemiology of anorexia nervosa in a defined region of Switzerland. *American Journal of Psychiatry*, 140, 564–567, Chapter 8.

Wilson, G. T. (1991). The addiction model of eating disorders: A critical analysis. *Advances in Behavior Research and Therapy*, 13, 27–72.

Wilson, M. (1993). DSM-III and the transformation of American psychiatry: A history. *American Journal of Psychiatry*, 150, 399–410.

Winokur, G. (1997). All roads lead to depression: Clinically homogenous, etiologically heterogeneous. *Journal of Affective Disorders*, 45, 97–108.

Winters, K. C. & Neale, J. M. (1985). Mania and low self-esteem. *Journal of Abnormal Psychology*, 94, 282–290.

Wiseman, C. V., Gray, J. J., Mosimann, J. E., & Arhens, A. H. (1992). Cultural expectations of thinness in women: An update. *International Journal of Eating Disorders*, 11, 85–89.

Wissing, M. P., & Temane, Q. M. (2008). The structure of psychological well-being in cultural context: Towards a hierarchical model of psychological health. *Journal of Psychology in Africa*, 18(1), 45–56.

Wissing, M. P., & Van Eeden, C. (1997). *Psychological well-being: A fortigenic conceptualization and empirical clarification*. Paper presented at the Annual Congress of the Psychological Society of South Africa (PsySSA), Durban, South Africa.

Wissing, M. P., & Van Eeden, C. (2002). Empirical clarification of the nature of psychological well-being. *South African Journal of Psychology*, 32(1), 32–44

Wissing, M. P., Claassens, E., & du Toit, M. M. (1998). The dynamics of cognitive styles, coping and psychological well-being in youths. In L. Schlebusch (Ed.), *South Africa beyond transition: Psychological well-being*. Proceedings of the Third Annual Congress of the Psychological Society of South Africa. Pretoria: PsySSA, 375–379.

Wittchen, H. U., Kessler, R. C., Zhao, S., & Abelson, J. (1995). Reliability and clinical validity of UM-CIDI DSM-III-R generalized anxiety disorder. *Journal of Psychiatric Research*, 29(2), 95–110.

Wittstock, B. R. (1991). Mass phenomena at a black South African primary school. *Hospital and Community Psychiatry*, 1(42), 851–853.

Wodka, E. L. & Barakat, L. P. (2007). The relationship between family support and coping in college adjustment: Implications for students with a chronic illness. *Journal of Adolescence*, 30, 365–376.

Wolf, N. (1990). *The beauty myth*. New York: HarperCollins.

Wolff, S. (2000). Schizoid personality in childhood and Asperger syndrome. In A. Klin, F. R. Volkmar, & S. S. Sparrow (Eds.). *Asperger syndrome*. New York: Guilford Press, 278–305.

Wonderlich, S. A., Gordon, K. H., Mitchell, J. E., Crosby, R. D., & Engel, S. G. (2009). The Validity and Clinical Utility of Binge Eating Disorder. *International Journal of Eating Disorders*, 42, 687–705.

Wong, P. T. P. (2011). Positive psychology 2.0: Towards a balanced interactive model of the good life. *Canadian Psychology*, 52(2), 69–81.

Wong, P. T. P., Reker, G. T., & Peacock, E. J. (2006). A resource-congruence model of coping and the development of the coping schema inventory. In P. Wong & L. Wong (Eds.), *Handbook of multicultural perspectives on stress and coping*. New York: Springer, (223–283).

Wood, A. M., & Tarrier, N. (2010). Positive clinical psychology: A new vision and strategy for integrated research and practice. *Clinical Psychology Review*, 30, 819–829. doi:10.1016/j.cpr.2010.06.003

Wood, J. M., Nezworski, M. T., Lilienfeld, S. O., & Garb, H. N. (2003). *What's wrong with the Rorschach? Science confronts the controversial inkblot test*. New York: Wiley.

World Health Organisation. (1992). *International statistical classification of diseases and related health problems* (10th Ed). Geneva: World Health Organisation.

World Health Organisation. (1993). *The ICD-10 classification of mental and behavioural disorders*. Geneva: WHO.

World Health Organisation. (2005). *Mental health policy and service guidance package*.

World Health Organization. (2004). *Global Burden of Disease*. Retrieved on March 7, 2012 from http://www.who.int/topics/global_burden_of_disease/en/

World Professional Association for Transgender Health (WPATH). (2011). *Standards of care for the health of transsexual, transgender and gender nonconforming people* (7th ed.). Retrieved February 9, 2012 from www.wpath.org/Documents2/ socv7.pdf

Wouters, A. R. (1993). Relevant psychological help in the South African context: A personal empowerment model. Unpublished PhD thesis. Soweto: Vista University.

Wright, B. A., & Lopez, S. J. (2005). Widening the diagnostic focus: A case for including human strengths and environmental resources. In C. R. Snyder & S. J. Lopez (Eds.), *Handbook of positive psychology*. Oxford: Oxford University Press, 26–44.

Wynne, L. C., Ryckoff, I. M., Day, J., & Hirsch, S. I. (1958). Pseudomutuality in the family relations of schizophrenics. *Psychiatry*, 21, 205–20.

Yach, D., Stuckler, D., & Bronwell, U. K. D. (2006). Epidemiologic and economic consequences of the global epidemics of obesity and diabetes. *Nature Medicine*, 12, 62–66.

Yates, A. (1989). Current perspectives on the eating disorders. *Journal of the American Academy of Child and Adolescent Psychiatry*, 28, 813–828.

Zabow, L. (2008). Competence and decision-making: Ethics and clinical psychiatric practice. *South African Journal of Bioethics and Law*, 1(2), 61–63.

Zabow, T. & Kaliski, S.Z. (2006). Ethical considerations In S.Z. Kaliski (Ed.). *Psycholegal assessment in South Africa*. Cape Town: Oxford University Press, 357–375.

Zabow, T. (2007). Traditional healers and mental health in South Africa. *African Journal of Psychiatry*, 4(4), 81–82.

GLOSSARY

Abstract thinking: Thinking characterised by the ability to grasp the essentials of a whole, to break a whole into its parts and to discern common properties. To think symbolically.

Acting out: Behavioural response to an unconscious drive or impulse that brings about temporary partial relief of inner tension; relief is attained by reacting to a present situation as if it were the situation that originally gave rise to the drive or impulse. Common in borderline states.

Acute Stress Disorder: Syndrome closely related to Posttraumatic Stress Disorder characterised by anxiety and dissociative symptoms after exposure to extreme stress. The only major distinctions are in duration and point of onset. By definition, ASD has an onset within one month after the traumatic event and does not persist beyond four weeks after the event.

Addiction: Refers to a dependence on a behaviour or substance that a person is powerless to stop. The term has been partially replaced by the word dependence for substance abuse. Addiction has been extended, however, to include mood-altering behaviours or activities. Some researchers speak of two types of addictions: substance addictions (for example alcoholism, drug abuse, and smoking) and process addictions (for example gambling, spending, shopping, eating, and sexual activity). There is a growing recognition that many addicts, such as polydrug abusers, are addicted to more than one substance or process.

Adjustment Disorder: A disorder found in the DSM-5 that refers to the development of symptoms in relation to a particular stressor.

Adolescence: The period between the onset of puberty and the attainment of adulthood. Determined by cultural factors that define behaviour expected of the adolescent, and in the length of time spent in this period.

Aetiology: The causes, origins, evolution, and implications of disease and other phenomena.

Affect: The subjective and immediate experience of emotion attached to ideas or mental representations of objects. Affect has outward manifestations that may be classified as restricted, blunted, flattened, broad, labile, appropriate, or inappropriate.

Aggression: Forceful, goal-directed action that may be verbal or physical; the motor counterpart of the affect of rage, anger, or hostility. Seen in neurological deficit, temporal lobe disorder, impulse-control disorders, mania, Schizophrenia.

Agitation: Severe anxiety associated with motor restlessness.

Agnosia: Impaired ability to recognise objects or people.

Agonist: Chemical substance that effectively increases the activity of a neurotransmitter by imitating its effects.

Alogia: Inability to speak (e.g., talks very little or gives brief, empty replies to questions) because of a mental deficiency such as dementia or Schizophrenia. It involves a speech disturbance in which the individual displays a general lack of additional, unprompted content seen in normal speech.

Amnesia: Loss or lack of memory.

- **Anterograde amnesia**: Loss of memory for events subsequent to the onset of the amnesia common after trauma.
- **Retrograde amnesia**: Loss of memory for events preceding the onset of the amnesia.

Anhedonia: Loss of interest in and withdrawal from all regular and pleasurable activities. Often associated with depression.

Anorexia: Loss of or decrease in appetite. In Anorexia Nervosa appetite may be reserved but patient refuses to eat.

Anorexia Nervosa: Syndrome characterised by a refusal of the person to maintain a minimally normal body weight, an intense fear of being overweight, and a misperception of one's own body size or shape.

Antagonist: A chemical substance that decreases or blocks the effects of a neurotransmitter.

Anti-psychiatry: A socio-political movement that rejects the methodologies, medical practices and underlying assumptions of psychiatry.

Anxiety: Feeling of apprehension caused by anticipation of danger, which may be internal or external./The emotion of fear linked to the anticipation of future danger or misfortune.

Apathy: Dulled emotional tone associated with detachment or indifference; observed in certain types of Schizophrenia and depression.

Aphasia: Impairment or loss of language skills resulting from brain damage caused by a stroke, Alzheimer's disease, or other illness or trauma.

Atherosclerosis: Process by which a fatty substance or plaque builds up in the arteries to form an obstruction.

Attention: Concentration; the aspect of consciousness that relates to the amount of effort exerted in focusing on certain aspects of an experience, activity, or task. Usually impaired in anxiety and depressive disorders.

Attributional style: How people explain the events of their lives, either positively or negatively.

Avolition: A common symptom associated with Schizophrenia involving the inability to begin and sustain goal-directed activity.

Behaviour: Sum total of the psyche that includes impulses, motivations, wishes, drives, instincts, and cravings, as expressed by a person's behaviour or motor activity. Also called conation.

Bereavement: Feeling of grief or desolation, especially at the death or loss of a loved one.

Biomedical model: A perspective in psychopathology that claims that all mental illnesses have a biological cause.

Biopsychosocial approach: A perspective in psychopathology that attempts to integrate biological, psychological and social factors to gain a better understanding of why mental disorders occur.

Biopsychosocial paradigm: The view that mental disorders are reactions of the personality to a combination of biological, psychological, and social factors.

Bipolar disorders: Syndromes characterised by the presence of manic, hypomanic, or mixed episodes, including Bipolar I Disorder, Bipolar II Disorder, and Cyclothymic Disorder.

Bipolar I Disorder: A mood disorder found in the DSM-5 that refers to manic and depressive mood swings. Syndrome characterised by the presence of one or more manic or mixed episodes.

Bipolar II Disorder: Syndrome characterised by the presence of at least one major depressive episode accompanied by at least one hypomanic episode.

Blackout: Amnesia experienced by alcoholics about behaviour during drinking bouts. Usually indicates reversible brain damage.

Blocking: Abrupt interruption in train of thinking before a thought or idea is finished; after a brief pause, person indicates no recall of what was being said or was going to be said (also known as thought deprivation). Common in Schizophrenia and severe anxiety.

Blunted affect: Disturbance of affect manifested by a severe reduction in the intensity of externalised feeling tone.

Body Dysmorphic Disorder: Syndrome characterised by a persistent belief that the person's appearance is somehow seriously defective. Complaints commonly involve perceived defects in the face or head, but can involve any body part.

Brief psychotic disorder: Syndrome characterised by a psychotic disturbance that lasts more than one day, but less than one month.

Bulimia Nervosa: Syndrome characterised by binge eating and inappropriate methods of preventing weight gain including vomiting, misuse of laxatives, diuretics, or enemas.

Cataplexy: Temporary sudden loss of muscle tone, causing weakness and immobilisation. Can be precipitated by a variety of emotional states and is often followed by sleep. Commonly seen in narcolepsy.

Catatonic behaviour: A common symptom associated with Schizophrenia involving marked motor abnormalities such as bizarre postures, purposeless repetitive movements and an extreme degree of unawareness.

Choreiform: Occasional jerking or writhing movements which appear to be minor problems with coordination. These movements, which are absent during sleep, worsen over time and progress to random, uncontrollable and often violent twitchings. It is a common symptom of Huntington's disease which usually appears between the ages of 35 and 50 and worsens over time.

Cognition: Mental process of knowing and becoming aware. Function closely associated with judgment.

Cognitive schemas: Learned structures of cognition used by an individual to make sense of and construct to some extent their subjective experience of the world.

Coma: State of profound unconsciousness from which a person 'cannot' be roused, with minimal or no detectable responsiveness to stimuli. Seen in injury or disease of the brain, in such systemic conditions as diabetic ketoacidosis and uraemia, and in intoxications with alcohol and other drugs. Coma may also occur in severe catatonic states and in Conversion Disorder.

Comorbidity: Refers to the simultaneous existence of two or more disorders in the same individual/more than one disorder or disease in the same individual at the same time.

Concordance rate: A quantitative statistical expression for the agreement of a given genetic trait, especially in pairs of twins in genetic studies.

Confabulation: Unconscious filling of gaps in memory by imagining experiences or events that have no basis in fact. Commonly seen in amnestic syndromes. Should be differentiated from lying.

Control: False belief that a person's will, thoughts, or feelings are being controlled by external forces.

Conversion Disorder: Syndrome characterised by pseudoneurological (somatoform and dissociative) symptoms such as amnesia, paralysis, impaired coordination or balance, localised anaesthesia, blindness, deafness, double vision, hallucinations, tremors, or seizures without medical explanation.

Convulsion: An involuntary, violent muscular contraction or spasm.

Culture: The sum total of knowledge passed on from generation to generation within any given society. This body of knowledge includes language, forms of art and expression, religion, social and political structures, economic systems, legal systems, norms of behaviour, ideas about illness and healing, and so on.

- **Culture-fair test**: A psychological test that is designed to be free of cultural bias.
- **Culture-free test**: A psychological test that attempts to minimise the effects that culture may have on a person's performance on the test.
- **Culture-bound syndromes**: Mental illnesses structured by indigenous sets of cultural schemas. Some of the mental illnesses are in fact cultural entities; they exist primarily in particular cultural contexts or are responses to certain precipitants in the indigenous meaning systems.

Cyclothymic Disorder: Syndrome characterised by numerous hypomanic symptoms alternating with numerous depressive symptoms not severe enough to warrant a diagnosis of a Major Depressive Episode occurring over a two-year period.

Delirium tremens: Acute and sometimes fatal reaction to withdrawal from alcohol – usually occurring 72 to 96 hours after the cessation of heavy drinking. Distinctive characteristics are marked autonomic hyperactivity (tachycardia, fever, hyperhidrosis, dilated pupils), usually accompanied by tremulousness, hallucinations, illusions, and delusions.

Delirium: Acute reversible mental disorder characterised by confusion and some impairment of consciousness; generally associated with emotional lability, hallucinations or illusions, and inappropriate, impulsive, irrational, or violent behaviour.

Delusion: A common symptom associated with Schizophrenia which involves false belief, based on incorrect inference about external reality, that is firmly held despite objective and obvious contradictory proof or evidence and despite the fact that other members of the culture do not share the belief.

- **Bizarre delusion**: False belief that is patently absurd or fantastic (e.g., invaders from space have implanted electrodes in a person's brain). Common in Schizophrenia. In nonbizarre delusion content is usually within range of possibility.
- **Delusional Disorder**: Syndrome characterised by at least one month of nonbizarre delusions, without other psychotic symptoms.
- **Delusion of grandeur**: Exaggerated conception of one's importance, power, or identity.
- **Delusion of persecution**: False belief of being harassed or persecuted. Often found in litigious patients who have a pathological tendency to take legal action because of imagined mistreatment. Most common delusion.
- **Delusion of reference**: False belief that the behaviour of others refers to oneself; that events, objects, or other people have a particular and unusual significance, usually of a negative nature. Derived from idea of reference, in which persons falsely feel that others are talking about them (e.g., belief that people on television or radio are talking to or about the person).
- **Mood-congruent delusion**: Delusion with content that is mood appropriate (e.g., depressed patients who believe they are responsible for the destruction of the world).
- **Mood-incongruent delusion**: Delusion based on incorrect reference about external reality, with content that has no association to mood or is mood inappropriate (e.g., depressed patients who believe that they are the new Messiah)
- **Paranoid delusion**: Includes persecutory delusions and delusions of reference, control, and grandeur.

Dementia: Mental disorder characterised by general impairment in intellectual functioning without clouding of consciousness. Characterised by failing memory, difficulty with calculations, distractibility, alterations in mood and affect, impaired judgment and abstraction, reduced facility with language, and disturbance of orientation. Although irreversible because of underlying progressive degenerative brain disease, dementia may be reversible if the cause can be treated.

Differential diagnosis: The process of distinguishing between two or more disorders with similar or overlapping signs and symptoms.

Direct observation: A method in which a researcher observes and records behaviour while something is happening.

Denial: A psychological defence mechanism whereby individuals refuse to acknowledge what has happened, is happening, or will happen, i.e., keeping any aspects of external reality out of conscious awareness because if it was acknowledged, it would produce anxiety.

Depersonalisation: Mental condition based in divided consciousness characterised by a persistent or recurrent feeling of being detached from one's mental processes or body.

Depersonalisation Disorder: Syndrome characterised by depersonalisation accompanied by clinically significant emotional distress or impairment.

Depression: Mental state characterised by feelings of sadness, loneliness, despair, low self-esteem, and self-reproach. Accompanying signs include psychomotor retardation or at times agitation, withdrawal from interpersonal contact, and vegetative symptoms such as insomnia and anorexia. The term refers to either a mood that is so characterised or a mood disorder.

Derealisation: An alteration in the perception or experience of the external world so that it seems strange or unreal. Other symptoms include feeling as though one's environment is lacking in spontaneity, emotional colouring and depth. It is a dissociative symptom of many conditions, such as psychiatric and neurological disorders, and not a standalone disorder. It is also a transient side effect of acute drug intoxication, sleep deprivation, and stress.

Detachment: Characterised by distant interpersonal relationships and lack of emotional involvement.

Diabetes: Diabetes mellitus (sometimes called 'sugar diabetes'). A condition that occurs when the body cannot use glucose (a type of sugar) normally, resulting in high levels of blood sugar.

Diathesis-stress model: A perspective in psychopathology that proposes that some people inherit or develop predispositions (diathesis) to psychopathology, although mental disorders will not emerge until stressors become intense enough to convert predispositions into actual psychological disorders.

Disease: A medical syndrome or cluster of symptoms, or a physiological disease that manifests in parts of the body. In medical terminology this refers to the diagnosis of the doctor. It is the clinician's definition of the patient's problem, always taken from the paradigm of disease in which the clinician was trained.

Disorganised behaviour: A common symptom associated with Schizophrenia involving both an inability to persist in goal-directed activity and the performance of very inappropriate behaviours in public.

Disorganised speech: A common symptom associated with Schizophrenia where speech is incomprehensible and related only remotely to the subject under discussion.

Disorientation: Confusion; impairment of awareness of time, place, and person (the position of the self in relation to other persons). Characteristic of cognitive disorders.

Dissociation: Mental condition characterised by a loss of the integration of faculties or functions that are normally integrated in consciousness. Can affect memory, sensory modalities, motor functions, cognitive functions, and personal identity or sense of self./ Unconscious defence mechanism involving the segregation of any group of mental or behavioural processes from the rest of the person's psychic activity. May entail the separation of an idea from its accompanying emotional tone, as seen in dissociative and conversion disorders.

- **Dissociative Amnesia**: Syndrome characterised by divided consciousness in which there is an inability to recall important information that is held in a separate part of consciousness.
- **Dissociative disorders**: Syndromes characterised by divided consciousness including Dissociative Amnesia, Dissociative Fugue, Dissociative Identity Disorder (formerly multiple personality disorder), Depersonalisation Disorder, Dissociative Trance Disorder, and Dissociative Disorder Not Otherwise Specified.
- **Dissociative Fugue**: Syndrome based in divided consciousness characterised by sudden, unexpected travel away from home or one's customary place of work, accompanied by an inability to recall one's past, and also a confusion about personal identity.
- **Dissociative hallucinations and delusions**: Psychotic-type symptoms based on the mental processes of trance.

Dissociative Identity Disorder: Syndrome characterised by the presence of two or more distinct identities or personality states in consciousness that recurrently take control of the individual's behaviour, accompanied by Dissociative Amnesia.

Dissociative Trance Disorder: New diagnostic category included as a disorder which is described in the Other Specified Dissociative Disorder section to accommodate dissociative syndromes, characterised by trance or possession trance symptoms.

Diuretic: Anything that promotes the formation of urine by the kidney.

Dopaminergic: Activated or transmitted by dopamine. Pertaining to tissues or organs affected by dopamine.

Dysarthria: Speech that is characteristically slurred, slow, and difficult to produce (difficult to understand). The person with dysarthria may also have problems controlling the pitch, loudness, rhythm, and voice qualities of their speech.

Dyspareunia: Syndrome characterised by genital pain before, during, or after sexual intercourse. Closely related to Sexual Aversion Disorder, Hypoactive Sexual Desire Disorder, and Vaginismus.

Dysphoria: Feeling of unpleasantness or discomfort; a mood of general dissatisfaction and restlessness. Occurs in depression and anxiety.

Dysthymic Disorder: Syndrome characterised by a chronically depressed mood lasting for at least two years. Differs from Major Depressive Disorder in that Dysthymic Disorder is a chronic illness with generally less severe depressive symptoms.

Eating disorders: Syndromes characterised by obsessive-compulsive or addictive type behaviour involving food. Persons are obsessed with ingesting or not ingesting food.

Echolalia: Psychopathological repeating of words or phrases of one person by another. Tends to be repetitive and persistent. Seen in certain kinds of Schizophrenia, particularly the catatonic types.

Egocentric: Refers to personal identity centred in the self. Persons perceive themselves as autonomous individuals with personal choices, desires, and rights, and see dependence as undesirable. In an egocentric society the 'self' becomes the primary object of interest, and personal freedom and power become the supreme values.

Elation: Mood consisting of feelings of joy, euphoria, triumph, and intense self-satisfaction, or optimism. Occurs in mania when not grounded in reality.

Elevated mood: Air of confidence and enjoyment. A mood more cheerful than normal but not necessarily pathological.

Emotion: A mental and physiological state associated with a wide variety of feelings, thoughts, and behaviour. Emotions are subjective experiences, or experienced from an individual point of view. Emotion is often associated with mood, temperament, personality, and disposition.

Epidemiology: The study of incidence, distribution, and control of diseases.

Ethnocentrism: Refers to judging other people from within one's own cultural perspective.

Euphoria: An affective state of exaggerated well-being or elation.

Exhibitionism: Syndrome characterised by a compulsion to expose one's genitals to a stranger. The typical case is a young man exposing his erect penis to unsuspecting females.

Explanatory model: Refers to the ways a set of cultural schemas explains the cause of mental illness, why the onset occurred when it did, the effects of the illness, what course the illness will take, and what treatments are appropriate. These meanings dramatically affect the lived experiences of mental patients, in many ways structuring their subjective experiences.

Expressed emotion: Refers to criticism, hostility, and emotional over-involvement directed at a mental patient by their family members.

Factitious Disorder: A disorder found in the DSM-5 that refers to the intentional production of symptoms in order to assume the 'sick role'.

False negatives: Test results that indicate no problem when a problem does exist.
False positives: Test results that indicate a problem when no problem is present.
Female Orgasmic Disorder: Syndrome characterised by a persistent absence of orgasm after normal sexual arousal that causes marked distress or interpersonal difficulty.
Female Sexual Arousal Disorder: Syndrome characterised by an inability of a woman to maintain sexual arousal during coitus. This typically results in pleasureless lovemaking, painful intercourse, avoidance of sexual activity, and marital or relationship problems.
Fetishism: Syndrome involving the use of inanimate objects (the fetish) for sexual arousal. This is typically a male disorder. Commonly used fetishes are objects associated with females, for example women's undergarments, stockings, shoes, or other articles of clothing.
Flashbacks: Sudden, intense re-experiencing of a previous, usually traumatic, event.
Flat affect: A common symptom associated with Schizophrenia involving the lack of emotional responsiveness in gesture, facial expression and/or tone of voice.
Frotteurism: Syndrome characterised by a compulsion to rub against or touch a non-consenting person in a sexual way. It usually occurs in crowded public spaces such as buses or train carriages.
Gender:
1. The behavioural, cultural, or psychological traits typically associated with one sex.
2. Sexual identity, especially in relation to society or culture.
3. The condition of being female or male; sex.
4. Females or males considered as a group
5. Traditionally, the word gender has been used primarily to refer to the grammatical categories of 'masculine,' 'feminine', and 'neuter', but in recent years the word has become well established in its use to refer to sex-based categories, as in phrases such as 'gender gap' and 'the politics of gender'. This usage is supported by the practice of many anthropologists, who reserve the word sex for reference to biological categories, while using the word gender to refer to social or cultural categories. According to this rule, one would say, 'The effectiveness of the medication appears to depend on the sex [not gender] of the patient', but 'In peasant societies, gender [not sex] roles are likely to be more clearly defined'. This distinction is useful in principle, but it is by no means widely observed, and considerable variation in usage occurs at all levels.

Gender identity: The private subjective cognition of one's gender.
Gender Identity Disorder: Syndrome characterised by an intense and persistent sense of identity as someone of the opposite gender, causing significant emotional distress and social or occupational impairment.
Gender role behaviour: The gender-specific activities that are expected in any given society. This can include such things as wearing gender-specific clothing; having a gender-specific occupation; using gender-specific forms of speech, mannerisms, hairstyles, jewellery, accessories, and cosmetics; performing gender-specific recreational activities, sexual behaviour, and household duties; and holding gender-specific socio-politico-religious offices.

Generalised Anxiety Disorder: Syndrome characterised by excessive anxiety, restlessness, inability to concentrate, and worry occurring more days than not for period of at least six months.
Hallucination: False sensory perception occurring in the absence of any relevant external stimulation of the sensory modality involved. It is symptom that is commonly associated with Schizophrenia.

Auditory hallucination: False perception of sound, usually voices but also other noises such as music. Most common hallucination in psychiatric disorders.
Gustatory hallucination: Hallucination primarily involving taste.
Haptic (tactile) hallucination: Hallucination of touch.

Mood-congruent hallucination: Hallucination with content that is consistent with either a depressed or manic mood (e.g., depressed patients hearing voices telling them that they are bad persons; manic patients hearing voices telling them that they have inflated worth, power, or knowledge).

Mood-incongruent hallucination: Hallucination not associated with real external stimuli, with content that is not consistent with either depressed or manic mood (e.g., in depression, hallucinations not involving such themes as guilt, deserved punishment, or inadequacy; in mania, not involving such themes as inflated worth or power).

Olfactory hallucination: Hallucination primarily involving smell or odours. Most common in medical disorders, especially in the temporal lobe.

Somatic hallucination: Hallucination involving the perception of a physical experience localised within the body.

Tactile (haptic) hallucination: Hallucination primarily involving the sense of touch.

Hebephrenia: Complex of symptoms, considered a form of Schizophrenia, characterised by wild or silly behaviour or mannerisms, inappropriate affect, and delusions and hallucinations that are transient and unsystematised. Hebephrenic Schizophrenia is now called Disorganised Schizophrenia.

Hyperactivity: Increased muscular activity. The term is commonly used to describe a disturbance found in children that is manifested by constant restlessness, overactivity, distractibility, and difficulties in learning.

Hyperprolactinaemia: An elevated level of prolactin in the blood.

Hypersomnia: Excessive time spent asleep. May be associated with underlying medical or psychiatric disorder (e.g., mood disorders or narcolepsy), or be primary.

Hypertension: Abnormally high blood pressure (the force of blood pushing against the walls of arteries as it flows through them). It is a major risk for stroke and heart and kidney disease that is intimately related to psychological factors.

Hypervigilance: Excessive attention to, and focus on, all internal and external stimuli. Usually seen in delusional or paranoid states.

Hypoactive Sexual Desire Disorder: Syndrome characterised by the absence of the desire for sexual activity resulting in emotional distress or interpersonal difficulty.

Hypochondriasis: Exaggerated concern about health that is based not on real medical pathology but on unrealistic interpretations of physical signs or sensations as abnormal. Hypochondriasis is a syndrome characterised by persistent and unfounded fears of having a serious disease based on a misinterpretation of normal bodily functions or minor symptoms.

Hypoglycaemia: Low blood sugar.

Hypogonadism: A condition in which decreased production of gonadal hormones leads to below-normal function of the gonads and to retardation of sexual growth and development. (The gonads are the ovaries and testes and the hormones they normally produce include estrogen, progesterone, and testosterone.)

Hypomania: Mood abnormality with the qualitative characteristics of mania but somewhat less intense. Seen in cyclothymic disorder. A hypomanic episode is a period of at least four days in which the person experiences an abnormal and persistently elevated, expansive, or irritable mood, with at least three additional symptoms such as: nondelusional grandiosity, decreased need for sleep, pressure of speech, flight of ideas, distractibility, increased involvement in goal-directed activities. Differs from a manic episode in that a hypomanic episode does not cause social or occupational impairment, and there are no hallucinations or delusions.

Hypotheses: The lowest level, most specific testable explanations for unanswered scientific problems.

Hypotonia: Diminished tone of the skeletal muscles.
Hysteria: Obsolete diagnostic category used commonly in the latter half of the nineteenth century characterised by extreme anxiety, somatoform, depressive, and dissociative symptoms such as paralyses, anaesthesias, blindness, seizures, and head and body aches, with no medical explanation, as well as dysphoria, hallucinations and multiple personalities.
Iatrogenic: Referring to a physical or mental condition caused by a physician or health-care provider which may be due to exposure to pathogens, toxins or injurious treatment or procedures.
Illness: In medical anthropology, this refers to the subjective experience of being sick, including the experience of symptoms, suffering, help seeking, side effects of treatment, social stigma, explanations of causes, diagnosis, prognosis, and personal consequences in family life and occupation.
Illusion: Perceptual misinterpretation of a real external stimulus.
Impulse control: Ability to resist an impulse, drive, or temptation to perform some action.
Inappropriate affect: Emotional tone out of harmony with the idea, thought, or speech accompanying it.
Incoherence: Communication that is disconnected, disorganised, or incomprehensive. See also 'word salad'.
Infection: Invasion and multiplication of microorganisms in body tissues.
Insomnia: Difficulty in falling asleep or difficulty in staying asleep. It can be related to a mental disorder, can be related to a physical disorder or an adverse effect of medication, or can be primary (not related to a known medical factor or another mental disorder).
Hypersomnia: An inability to stay awake; excessive sleeping.
Terminal insomnia: Early morning awakening or waking up at least two hours before planning to.
Intellectualisation: A psychological defence mechanism whereby individuals remove all emotion from their emotional experiences.
Intelligence: Capacity for learning and ability to recall, integrate constructively, and apply what one has learned. The capacity to understand and think rationally.
Intoxication: Mental disorder caused by recent ingestion or presence in the body of an exogenous substance producing maladaptive behaviour by virtue of its effects on the central nervous system. The most common psychiatric changes involve disturbances of perception, wakefulness, attention, thinking, judgment, emotional control, and psychomotor behaviour. The specific clinical picture depends on the substance ingested.
Irritability: Abnormal or excessive excitability, with easily triggered anger, annoyance, or impatience.
Irritable mood: State in which one is easily annoyed and provoked to anger. See also 'Irritability'.
Labile affect: Affective expression characterised by rapid and abrupt changes, unrelated to external stimuli.
Labile mood: Oscillations in mood between euphoria and depression or anxiety.
Magical thinking: Thinking similar to that of the preoperational phase in children (Jean Piaget), in which thoughts, words, or actions assume power (e.g., to cause or prevent events).
Major Depressive Disorder: Syndrome characterised by one or more major depressive episodes without a history of manic, mixed, or hypomanic episodes.
Major Depressive Episode: At least two weeks of depressed mood with at least four additional symptoms of depression which can include changes in appetite, weight, sleep, or psychomotor activity, fatigue, feelings of worthlessness or guilt, difficulty thinking, and recurrent thoughts of suicide or suicide attempts.

Maladaptiveness: One way of defining psychopathology that, in order to determine what is abnormal, uses the extent to which certain behaviours or experiences are maladaptive to the self or others.

Male Erectile Disorder: Syndrome characterised by a persistent inability to attain or maintain an erection sufficient for the completion of coitus.

Male Orgasmic Disorder: Syndrome characterised by a failure or delay to achieve orgasm during coitus.

Malingering: Feigning disease to achieve a specific goal, for example to avoid an unpleasant responsibility. Compare Factitious Disorder.

Mania: Mood state characterised by an abnormally elevated, euphoric, or irritable mood lasting at least one week, or less if hospitalisation is required, with at least three additional manic symptoms, which can include grandiosity, decreased need for sleep, pressure of speech, flight of ideas, distractibility, increased goal-directed activity, and excessive involvement in pleasurable activity with a high potential for painful consequences. There may be grandiose delusions and hallucinations. Seen in Bipolar I Disorder.

Mannerism: Ingrained, habitual involuntary movement.

Melancholia: Severe depressive state.

Memory: Process whereby what is experienced or learned is established as a record in the central nervous system (registration), where it persists with a variable degree of permanence (retention) and can be recollected or retrieved from storage at will (recall).

Mental disorder: Psychiatric illness or disease whose manifestations are primarily characterised by behavioural or psychological impairment of function, measured in terms of deviation from some normative concept. Associated with distress or disease, not just an expected response to a particular event or limited to relations between a person and society.

Mental retardation: Sub-average general intellectual functioning that originates in the developmental period and is associated with impaired maturation and learning, and social maladjustment. Retardation is commonly defined in terms of intelligence quotient: mild (50–55 to 70), moderate (35–40 to 50–55), severe (20–25 to 35–40) and profound (below 20–25).

Mixed episode: Episode characterised by a period of at least one week in which diagnostic criteria are met for both a Manic Episode and a Major Depressive Episode.

Models: General theories which explain a large part of the field of inquiry within a scientific discipline.

Mood: Pervasive and sustained feeling tone that is experienced internally and that, in the extreme, can markedly influence virtually all aspects of a person's behaviour and perception of the world. Distinguished from affect, the external expression of the internal feeling tone. For types of mood, see the specific term.

Mood disorders: Syndromes that have depressive or manic symptoms as their primary feature.

Mood episodes: Episodes of emotional illness and distress characterised by depression, mania, or hypomania, or some combination of these, including Major Depressive Episode, Manic Episode, Mixed Episode, or Hypomanic Episode.

Negativism: Verbal or nonverbal opposition or resistance to outside suggestions and advice. Commonly seen in catatonic Schizophrenia in which the patient resists any effort to be moved or does the opposite of what is asked.

Neologism: New word or phrase whose derivation cannot be understood. Often seen in Schizophrenia. It has also been used to mean a word that has been incorrectly constructed but whose origins are nonetheless understandable (e.g., 'headshoe' to mean 'hat'), but such constructions are more properly referred to as 'word approximations'.

Neurasthenia: A disorder referring to 'tired nerves' and including symptoms of fatigue, anxiety, and various somatic complaints. Originated in the United States, but is no longer a part of the DSM classification system. A very common diagnosis in China.

Neurogenic: Starting with or having to do with the nerves or the nervous system.

Neuroses: Mental disorders presumed to have psychodynamic origins existing toward the mild to moderate end of a spectrum of mental illnesses in the biopsychosocial paradigm.

Neurotransmitters: Chemical substances in the brain that are responsible for the communication of nerve impulses among the brain cells.

Nociception: A typical sensory experience that may be described as the unpleasant awareness of a noxious (harmful to life or health, especially by being poisonous) stimulus or bodily harm.

Nosology: Branch of medicine that deals with classification of diseases.

Obsession: Persistent and recurrent idea, thought, or impulse that cannot be eliminated from consciousness by logic or reasoning; obsessions are involuntary and ego-dystonic.

Obsessive-Compulsive Disorder: Syndrome characterised by persistent thoughts or impulses that are experienced as intrusive and inappropriate (obsessions), and repetitive behaviours (compulsions) that are performed to reduce the emotional distress associated with obsessions.

Orientation: State of awareness of oneself and one's surroundings in terms of time, place, and person.

Paedophilia: Syndrome characterised by a person sixteen years or older having recurrent sexual activity with a prepubescent child (legally this is generally thirteen years or younger).

Panic: Acute, intense attack of anxiety associated with personality disorganisation; the anxiety is overwhelming and accompanied by feelings of impending doom.

Panic Attacks: Experiences characterised by a discrete period of intense fear with at least four additional somatic or cognitive symptoms including: palpitations, sweating, trembling, shortness of breath, feelings of choking, chest pain, nausea or abdominal distress, dizziness, depersonalisation, derealisation, fear of going crazy, fear of dying, tactile sensations (paresthesias), and chills or hot flushes.

Panic disorder: Syndrome characterised by recurrent and unexpected panic attacks.

Paradigm: The highest, most general level in a hierarchy of scientific intellectual structures. A paradigm is a generally accepted view of the nature of a scientific discipline.

Paranoia: Rare psychiatric syndrome marked by the gradual development of a highly elaborate and complex delusional system, generally involving persecutory or grandiose delusions, with few other signs of personality disorganisation or thought disorder.

Paraphilias: Syndromes characterised by recurrent sexual fantasies and behaviours involving objects, persons, or situations that are considered deviant in the prevailing cultural meaning system, causing significant emotional distress and/or social impairment.

Pathoplastic: Of or pertaining to factors (i.e., culture) which exert an influence on the final presentation of a disorder.

Perception: Conscious awareness of elements in the environment by the mental processing of sensory stimuli. Sometimes used in a broader sense to refer to the mental process by which all kinds of data, intellectual, emotional, and sensory, are meaningfully organised.

Perseveration: Pathological repetition of the same response to different stimuli, as in a repetition of the same verbal response to different questions. Persistent repetition of specific words or concepts in the process of speaking. Seen in cognitive disorders, Schizophrenia, and other mental illness.

Personal distress: Distress and suffering experienced by a person.

Personality: The set of psychological traits and mechanisms within the individual that are organised and relatively enduring and that influence the individual's interactions with, and adaptation to, the environment (including the intrapsychic, physical, and social environment).

Personality disorders: Enduring patterns of pathological subjective experience and behaviour based in personality development, rather than in some specific disease entity.

- **Antisocial Personality Disorder**: Personality characterised by a persistent pattern of victimising others through theft or destruction of property, physical assault (including spouse or child abuse), or deceit to gain personal profit or pleasure.
- **Avoidant Personality Disorder**: Personality characterised by extreme social anxiety, low self-esteem, and hypersensitivity to criticism to the point that the person purposely avoids interpersonal contact.
- **Borderline Personality Disorder**: Personality characterised by a persistent instability in social relationships, self-image, and emotions. Central to this instability is fear of abandonment and rejection.
- **Dependent Personality Disorder**: Personality characterised by an excessive need to be taken care of, associated with submissive, clinging behaviour, and fear of independence.
- **Histrionic Personality Disorder**: Personality characterised by excessive emotionality and attention-seeking behaviour.
- **Narcissistic Personality Disorder**: Personality characterised by an obsession with grandiosity, an intense need for admiration, and a lack of empathy for others.
- **Obsessive-Compulsive Personality Disorder**: Personality characterised by a persistent preoccupation with order, perfection, attention to detail, rules, and control.
- **Paranoid Personality Disorder**: Personality characterised by a pervasive distrust of other people such that others are virtually always perceived as threatening or hostile.
- **Schizoid Personality Disorder**: Personality characterised by a pervasive detachment from social relationships and a restricted range of emotions.
- **Schizotypal Personality Disorder**: Personality characterised by anxiety in social relationships accompanied by eccentricities of behaviour such as superstitiousness, preoccupation with paranormal phenomena, magical thinking, or use of rituals in everyday situations.

Phenomenology: The study of phenomena, i.e., the mental construction of cognition out of raw sensory data. A phenomenon is an experience of an object by a subject. In phenomenology, it is the experience of the object that is the focus of study, not the object itself.

Phobia: Persistent, pathological, unrealistic, intense fear of an object or situation. The phobic person may realise that the fear is irrational but, nonetheless, cannot dispel it. For types of phobias, see the specific term.

- **Agoraphobia**: Syndrome characterised by anxiety about being in places in which a panic attack or other anxiety reaction might occur, resulting in a pervasive avoidance of a variety of situations./Morbid fear of open places or leaving the familiar setting of the home. May be present with or without panic attacks.
- **Social Phobia**: Syndrome characterised by a persistent fear of social situations in which extreme embarrassment may occur. Exposure to these situations provokes an anxiety response.
- **Specific Phobia**: Syndrome characterised by a persistent fear of specific objects or situations, exposure to which almost invariably evokes an anxiety response.

Polyneuropathy: A neurological disorder that occurs when many peripheral nerves throughout the body malfunction simultaneously.

Posttraumatic Stress Disorder: Syndrome characterised by prominent anxiety and dissociative symptoms following exposure to an extreme traumatic stressor.
Posturing: Strange, fixed, and bizarre bodily positions held by a patient for an extended time.
Poverty of speech: Restriction in the amount of speech used; replies may be monosyllabic.
Praxis: The ability to have interpersonal relationships and perform actions.
Premature ejaculation: Syndrome characterised by persistent ejaculation after minimal sexual stimulation and before the person or the person's sexual partner wishes it.
Proband: A term used most often in medical genetics and other medical fields to denote a particular subject (person or animal) being studied or reported on.
Prodromal: Symptomatic of the onset of an attack or a disease. Of or pertaining to the early symptoms of a disease; as, the prodromal stage of a disease.
Projection: A psychological defence mechanism whereby individuals take something of themselves and place it outside themselves, onto others.
Psychoanalysis: A means of treating patients who suffer from hysterical and neurotic conditions based on Freud's theory that psychopathology is largely caused by the repression of forbidden wishes or instinctual drives.
Psychodynamic approaches: Approaches to psychopathology that believe that the way we relate to others and ourselves is largely influenced by internal forces that exist outside consciousness.
Psychological disorder: A mental abnormality that manifests on the level of thinking, feeling or behaving.
Psychomotor agitation: Physical and mental overactivity that is usually non-productive and is associated with a feeling of inner turmoil, as seen in agitated depression.
Psychomotor retardation: Physical and mental underactivity that is typically characterised by stooped posture, very little spontaneous movement, poor eye contact, impaired coordination, slow speech, and difficulties with articulation.
Psychosis: Mental disorder in which the thoughts, affective response, ability to recognise reality, and ability to communicate and relate to others are sufficiently impaired to interfere grossly with the capacity to deal with reality. The classical characteristics of psychosis are impaired reality testing, hallucinations, delusions, and illusions.
Psychotic: The presence of delusions, prominent hallucinations, disorganised speech, and disorganised or catatonic behaviour.
Psychotic disorders: Syndromes characterised by a loss of reality testing, including Schizophrenia, Schizophreniform Disorder, Schizoaffective Disorder, Delusional Disorder, Brief Psychotic Disorder, and Shared Psychotic Disorder.
Reaction-formation: A psychological defence mechanism whereby individuals turn painful or threatening reactions into their opposite.
Reality testing: Fundamental ego function that consists of tentative actions that test and objectively evaluate the nature and limits of the environment. Includes the ability to differentiate between the external world and the internal world and to accurately judge the relation between the self and the environment. The loss of reality testing leads to a disturbance in the experience of self and one's relationship with the external physical and social environments. The presence of hallucinations and/or delusions is usually viewed as a loss of reality testing.
Reliability: The ability of separate clinicians or researchers to diagnose the same disorder consistently after observing the same pattern of symptoms in patients.
Repression: A psychological defence mechanism whereby individuals unconsciously put painful thoughts and memories out of their minds.

Ritual: In a 'normal' sense, this refers to a ceremonial activity of cultural origin. In an abnormal context it refers to a formalised activity practised by a person to reduce anxiety, as in Obsessive-Compulsive Disorder.

Rumination: Constant preoccupation with thinking about a single idea or theme, as in Obsessive-Compulsive Disorder.

Schizoaffective Disorder: Syndrome characterised by a combination of psychotic and mood symptoms in which psychotic symptoms occur in conjunction with either a manic or depressive episode, followed by at least two weeks of psychotic symptoms without prominent mood symptoms.

Schizophrenia: Syndrome characterised by the presence of psychotic symptoms for a significant portion of the time during a one-month period, and some signs of the disorder for at least a six-month period.

Schizophreniform Disorder: Syndrome characterised by a psychotic disturbance that lasts at least one month, but less than six months.

Scoliosis: A medical condition in which a person's spine is curved from side to side, shaped like an 's', and may also be rotated.

Secondary gain: Any benefit a person receives as an indirect result of having a disorder.

Seizure: Also referred to as a fit, is a transient symptom of abnormalneuronal activity in the brain. There are different types of seizures, including grand mal, absence, myoclonic, clonic, tonic, and atonic seizures.

Sensorium: Hypothetical sensory centre in the brain that is involved with clarity of awareness about oneself and one's surroundings, including the ability to perceive and process ongoing events in the light of past experiences, future options, and current circumstances. Sometimes used interchangeably with 'consciousness'.

Serological: Of or pertaining to the science that deals with the properties and reactions of serums, especially blood serum. It is the characteristics of a disease or organism shown by study of blood serums.

Sexual aversion disorder: Syndrome characterised by an aversion to and active avoidance of genital contact with a sexual partner. The typical case is a female who experiences anxiety, fear, or disgust from genital or other explicitly sexual contact.

Sexual dysfunctions: Syndromes characterised by psychophysiological problems impacting on one's ability to have satisfying sexual relations, causing marked emotional distress and interpersonal difficulties.

Sexual masochism: Syndrome characterised by sexual arousal resulting from being humiliated, beaten, or bound, or from other forms of corporal punishment.

Sexual preference: The gender(s) which an individual finds sexually arousing.

Sexual sadism: Syndrome characterised by sexual arousal resulting from inflicting physical or psychological punishment on another person.

Shared Psychotic Disorder: Syndrome characterised by a delusional belief in an individual who is influenced by someone else who has an established delusion.

Statistical deviance: One way of defining psychopathology that uses statistical norms of behaviour and experience to determine what is 'normal', and therefore what is abnormal.

Stroke: Blood flow to the brain stops, resulting in death of brain cells.

Sublimation: A psychological defence mechanism whereby individuals redirect emotions into more positive activities.

Substance: As a scientific term, an element, compound or mixture. In psychology this would refer to any chemical that is ingested, inhaled or injected that leads to a change in affect, perception, cognition or behaviour.

Substance abuse: Syndrome associated with repeated negative consequences resulting from a maladaptive pattern of substance use, such as multiple legal, social, and occupational problems.

Substance intoxication: Condition characterised by clinically significant maladaptive behavioural or psychological changes resulting from ingestion of a specific substance, such as social or occupational impairment, mood instability, cognitive impairment, or belligerence.

Substance withdrawal: Condition characterised by negative cognitive, physiological, and behavioural changes that occur when bodily concentrations of a substance decline after cessation of prolonged use.

Substance-related disorders: Syndromes associated with substance intoxication, substance abuse, substance dependence, or substance withdrawal.

Suicidal ideation: Thoughts or the act of taking one's own life.

Suppression: A psychological defence mechanism whereby individuals consciously try to put painful thoughts and memories out of their minds.

Symbol: A sign that has no logical connection to the thing it represents – an arbitrary sign. It is used simply out of convention, and its use results primarily out of historical accident.

Tangentiality: Oblique, digressive or even irrelevant manner of speech in which the central idea is not communicated.

Tension: Physiological or psychic arousal, uneasiness, or pressure toward action. An unpleasurable alteration in mental or physical state that seeks relief through action.

Theories: Specific explanations for large unanswered scientific problems.

Thought disorder: Any disturbance of thinking that affects language, communication, or thought content. The hallmark feature of Schizophrenia. Manifestations range from simple blocking and mild circumstantiality to profound loosening of associations, incoherence, and delusions. Characterised by a failure to follow semantic and syntactic rules which is inconsistent with the person's education, intelligence, or cultural background.

Thought broadcasting: Feeling that one's thoughts are being broadcast or projected into the environment.

Thought insertion: Delusion that thoughts are being implanted in one's mind by other people or forces.

Thought withdrawal: Delusion that one's thoughts are being removed from one's mind by other people or forces.

Trance: Mental condition based on a narrowed focus of attention such that what is outside attention is lost to consciousness.

Transvestic fetishism: Syndrome characterised by males deriving sexual pleasure by intermittently wearing female clothing.

Tumescence: A swelling or enlarging.

Tumour: A mass of abnormal tissue.

Unipolar mood disorder: A mood disorder characterised by episodes of depression only.

Vaginismus: Syndrome characterised by recurrent involuntary contraction of the muscles surrounding the vagina whenever vaginal penetration is attempted.

Validity: Refers to the reality of diagnostic categories. A diagnostic category (e.g., Schizophrenia) is valid when it refers to a real clinical entity independent of diagnosis, and is an appropriate means of naming that entity.

Vegetative states: In depression, denoting characteristic symptoms such as sleep disturbance (especially early morning awakening), decreased appetite, constipation, weight loss, and loss of sexual response.

Voyeurism: Syndrome characterised by a compulsion to achieve sexual arousal by observing unsuspecting persons who are getting undressed, naked, or engaged in sexual activities.

Waxy flexibility: Condition in which person maintains the body position in which they are placed. Also called catalepsy.

Word salad: Incoherent, essentially incomprehensible mixture of words and phrases commonly seen in far advanced cases of Schizophrenia.

INDEX

Please note: Page numbers in italics refer to Figures, Tables and Examples; those in bold refer to Boxes and Case studies

A

D

F

G

H

I

N

R

S

T